OCCUPATIONAL INJURIES
Evaluation, Management, and Prevention

OCCUPATIONAL INJURIES
Evaluation, Management, and Prevention

Editors

THOMAS N. HERINGTON, MD

Assistant Clinical Professor, Department of Medicine,
University of California — San Francisco,
San Francisco, California
Former Director, Occupational Injury Clinic,
California Pacific Medical Center

LINDA H. MORSE, MD, FACOEM

Chief, Occupational Medicine and Employee Health Services,
Santa Clara Valley Medical Center;
Assistant Clinical Professor, Department of Medicine,
University of California — San Francisco,
San Francisco, California

with 153 *illustrations*

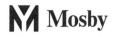 Mosby

A Harcourt Health Sciences Company

St. Louis   London   Philadelphia   Sydney   Toronto

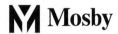

A Harcourt Health Sciences Company

Dedicated to Publishing Excellence

Editor: Laura DeYoung
Editorial Assistant: Alicia E. Moten
Project Manager: Dana Peick
Production Editor: Catherine Albright
Senior Book Designer: Gail Morey Hudson
Manufacturing Supervisor: Karen Lewis

Printed in the United States of America

Mosby, Inc.
11830 Westline Industrial Drive
St. Louis, Missouri 63146

Library of Congress Cataloging-in-Publication Data

Occupational injuries: evaluation, management, and prevention/
    [edited by] Thomas N. Herington, Linda H. Morse.
        p.   cm.
    Includes index.
    ISBN 0-8016-6805-0
    1. Wounds and injuries—Treatment.   2. Industrial safety.
3. Industrial accidents.   I. Herington, Thomas N. II. Morse, Linda
H.
    [DNLM: 1. Accidents, Occupational.   2. Wounds and Injuries.
3. Occupational Diseases.   4. Occupational Health.   WA 485 0146
1995]
RD97.5.023   1995
616.9'803—dc20
DNLM/DLC   94-36402

00 01 02 03 04 / 9 8 7 6 5 4

To
James P. Hughes, MD

mentor, guide, inspiration, and friend

Contributors

LESLEY J. ANDERSON, MD

Orthopaedic Surgeon,
Department of Orthopaedic Surgery,
California Pacific Medical Center,
San Francisco, California

JOHN BALMES, MD

Associate Professor, Department of Medicine,
University of California—San Francisco;
Chief, Division of Occupational and
Environmental Health,
San Francisco General Hospital,
San Francisco, California

WILLIAM BAUMGARTL, MD

Medical Director, Chronic Pain Program,
San Francisco Surgery Center,
San Francisco, California

GEORGE BECKER, MD

Staff, Department of Psychiatry,
California Pacific Medical Center,
San Francisco, California

LYNN BLOOMBERG, MPH

Staff, Department of Community Health Education,
University of California—Berkeley School of
Public Health,
Berkeley, California

RENATO CALABRIA, MD

Department of Plastic Surgery,
Saint Francis Memorial Hospital,
San Francisco, California

LINDA CLEVER, MD

Staff, Department of Occupational Health,
California Pacific Medical Center,
San Francisco, California

DEBORAH DOHERTY, MD

Executive Medical Director,
Kentfield Rehabilitation Hospital,

Kentfield, California;
Clinical Instructor, Department of Neurology,
University of California—San Francisco,
San Francisco, California

JOSEPH C. FARMER, MD

Professor, Department of Surgery,
Division of Otolaryngology—Head and Neck,
Duke University Medical Center,
Durham, North Carolina

JOHN FORSYTH, LCDR, MD, USNR

Staff, Puget Sound Naval Shipyard,
Bremerton, Washington

GARY FUJIMOTO, MD

Assistant Clinical Professor, Department of Medicine,
Stanford University School of Medicine,
University of California—San Francisco,
San Francisco, California;
Chairman, Occupational Medicine,
Palo Alto Medical Foundation,
Palo Alto, California

LEONARD GORDON, MD

Director, Attending Surgeon,
Hand and Microsurgery Research Laboratory,
California Pacific Medical Center,
San Francisco, California

JEFF HALBRECHT, MD

Attending Physician, Department of Occupational
Medicine,
California Pacific Medical Center;
Medical Director, Women's Pro Ski Tour;
Assistant Clinical Professor,
Department of Graduate Physical Therapy,
University of California—San Francisco,
San Francisco, California

ROBERT HARRISON, MD

Associate Professor, Department of Medicine,
Director, Occupational and Environmental Medicine,
University of California—San Francisco,
San Francisco, California

THOMAS N. HERINGTON, MD

Assistant Clinical Professor, Department of Medicine,
University of California—San Francisco,
San Francisco, California
Former Director, Occupational Injury Clinic,
California Pacific Medical Center

GERALD P. KEANE, MD

Staff, The Physiatrist Medical Group,
Menlo Park, California

JOSEPH LaDOU, MD

Professor and Director,
International Center for Occupational Medicine,
Division of Occupational and Environmental Medicine,
University of California—San Francisco,
San Francisco, California

FRANK LEONE, MD

Executive Director,
National Association of Occupational Health
Professionals;
President, Ryan & Associates,
Santa Barbara, California

GIDEON LETZ, MD

Medical Director, State Compensation Insurance Fund,
San Francisco, California

PETER LICHTY, MD

President, Western Occupational Medical Group,
San Francisco, California

BRUCE MEDOFF, MD

Assistant Clinical Professor, Department of Medicine,
University of California—San Francisco,
San Francisco, California

RICHARD MOON, MD

Associate Professor, Department of Anesthesiology,
Assistant Professor, Department of Pulmonary
Medicine,
Duke University Medical Center;
Medical Director, Duke Hyperbaric Center,
Medical Director, Divers Alert Network,
Durham, North Carolina;
President, Undersea Hyperbaric Medical Society,
Kensington, Maryland

LINDA H. MORSE, MD, FACOEM

Chief, Occupational Medicine and Employee Health
Services,
Santa Clara Valley Medical Center;
Assistant Clinical Professor, Department of Medicine,
University of California—San Francisco,
San Francisco, California

GARY PASTERNAK, MD

Internist, Valley Health Center,
San Jose, California

T. OTIS PAUL, MD

Chief, Pediatric Ophthalmology,
Department of Ophthalmology,
California Pacific Medical Center,
San Francisco, California

PETER PELMEAR, MD

Associate Professor, Department of Medicine,
University of Toronto;
Member, Active Attending Staff,
Department of Occupational and Environmental Health,
St. Michael's Hospital,
Toronto, Quebec, Canada

BARBARA POHLMAN, MD

Medical Review Officer,
Southern California Edison Company,
Santa Ana, California

MICHAEL ROKEACH, MD, FACEP

Medical Director, Emergency Department,
California Pacific Medical Center;
Assistant Clinical Professor, Department of Medicine,
University of California—San Francisco,
San Francisco, California

CORNELIUS SCANNELL, MD

Assistant Professor, Department of Medicine,
Division of Occupational and Environmental Medicine,
University of California—San Francisco,
San Francisco, California

STEVEN C. SCHUMANN, MD

Director, Occupational Health Consultants;
Director, The Stolar Group, Inc.,
Fresno, California

ELIZABETH SHERERTZ, MD

Professor and Vice Chair, Department of Dermatology,
Director, Occupational Contact Dermatitis,
Bowman Gray School of Medicine,
Winston-Salem, North Carolina

RANDALL SMITH, PhD

Staff, Department of Psychiatry,
California Pacific Medical Center,
San Francisco, California

MARK J. SONTAG, MD

Medical Director,
Sequoia Hospital Occupational Health Services,
Redwood, California

EUGENE SPECTOR, DPM

Clinical Professor, Department of Surgery,
California Podiatric School;
Chief, Department of Podiatry,
California Pacific Medical Center,
San Francisco, California

ROBERT SPENCE

President, Robert Spence & Associates, Inc.,
Portola Valley, California

EMILY SPIELER, JD

Associate Professor, West Virginia University
College of Law,
Morgantown, West Virginia

ROBERT STAMPER, MD

Chairman, Department of Ophthalmology,
California Pacific Medical Center,
San Francisco, California

SUSAN TIERMAN, MD

Staff, Department of Occupational Medicine,
Palo Alto Medical Foundation,

Palo Alto, California;
Assistant Professor, Department of Occupational
Medicine
Stanford University School of Medicine,
Stanford, California

BRYANT A. TOTH, MD

Attending Surgeon, California Pacific Medical Center;
Assistant Professor, Division of Plastic Surgery,
University of California — San Francisco,
San Francisco, California

GEORGE L. VOELZ, MD

Occupational Health Specialist,
Los Alamos National Laboratory,
Los Alamos, New Mexico

ANNETTE CAMPBELL WHITE, RN

Workers' Compensation Analyst,
California Pacific Medical Center,
San Francisco, California

JAMES C. WILSON, PhD

Chairman, Department of Psychology,
Kentfield Rehabilitation Hospital,
Kentfield, California

KAREN WOLFE

President, Health Management Technologies, Inc.,
Moraga, California

Preface

Many clinicians come to the practice of occupational medicine through a side door. With increasing frequency, general practitioners, emergency physicians, primary care specialists, and those board certified in fields such as surgery, orthopedics, and ophthalmology face injured workers who need treatment. Adding to this influx are patients from various forms of managed care contracts. These contracts for private health care coverage often include Workers' Compensation insurance in the package. Insurance providers, group practices, hospitals, and clinics are paying more attention to occupational injuries—and for good reason. Occupational injuries cost individuals, employers, and taxpayers millions of dollars in lost workdays, decreased productivity, and higher insurance premiums. As a result, most practitioners routinely see an increase of patients with work-related injuries and disabilities. These physicians, who are experienced in their respective medical specialties, seldom have received formal training in occupational medicine. Indeed, even practitioners who have been trained in occupational medicine often struggle, hampered by both the weight of administrative paperwork and a lack of clinically-relevant occupational reference materials.

It may seem that the delivery of appropriate medical care should not be affected by a patient's occupation. After all, a physician doesn't suture a wound differently because the laceration occurs from a kitchen knife at home as opposed to a box cutter at work. However, on closer examination, practitioners often find that the workplace and the patient's occupation are important variables in the formation of a thorough patient history, differential diagnosis, and management of follow-up care.

This book is intended to provide front-line practitioners with a practical, clinically-oriented approach for treating injured workers. We, as primary caregivers, do not need to know how to do complicated tendon repairs or manage serious eye injuries. We do, however, need to know how to perform a thoughtful examination, what variables to consider, what we should treat, when we should refer, and how to manage each case in the context of the patient's workplace.

Each chapter has been written with this purpose in mind. We hope that this book will be useful to hands-on practitioners and, ultimately, beneficial to our patients.

Thomas N. Herington
Linda H. Morse

Overview

Contents

Occupational Injuries
Evaluation, Management, and Prevention

SECTION I
INTRODUCTION

1 Epidemiology of Work Injury

On January 28, 1986, seven crew members were killed when the space shuttle *Challenger* exploded shortly after takeoff from Cape Canaveral. On that same day at least 16 other workers in the United States were killed at work and thousands more suffered disabling injuries.[7] Injury is the leading cause of death for persons under 45 years of age, accounting for more years of potential life lost than heart disease and cancer combined.[8] Occupational injuries constitute a significant subset of the overall injury problem and are estimated to account for one sixth of all fatal injuries to persons between the ages of 17 and 64.[22] The National Safety Council estimates that in 1988 there were 10,600 work-related deaths and 1.8 million disabling injuries,* of which 60,000 resulted in some permanent disability.[21] The Department of Labor's Bureau of Labor Statistics (BLS) reports that in 1990, the U.S. workforce experienced approximately 6.8 million job-related injuries and illnesses, which occurred at a rate of 8.8 per 100 full-time workers. Nearly half of the reported cases were serious enough to require restricted work duties or lost workdays. Approximately 60 million workdays were lost because of job-related accidents and illnesses in 1990.[4] During 1991, 368,000 new cases of occupational illness and 1.8 million job-related injuries were reported to the BLS.[4] It is estimated that on every workday 240 people in the United States die because of on-the-job accidents or protracted job-related illnesses.[20]

A recent study by the Rand Corporation estimates that the direct costs of work accidents were $83 billion for 1989 and that workers' compensation premiums cost American industry more than $60 billion annually.[13] The average cost to employers in 1978 for an injury resulting in lost workdays was $14,000.[26] The societal burden of occupational injuries is difficult to estimate, but disabled workers, instead of being wage earners, must be supported financially through the Social Security system and workers' compensation benefits. If a worker with young dependents has a serious or fatal injury, the federal government may have to provide the family with long-term income maintenance. The costs of occupational injuries in human pain, suffering, and decreased quality of life are inestimable.

CURRENT SURVEILLANCE METHODS

Information on the incidence, distribution, and causes of occupational injury is available from a variety of sources. Since data are collected for different purposes, and since capture methods, definitions, and covered populations vary, results may not be comparable. Overall estimates are undoubtedly flawed because there is no comprehensive source of information.[14]

Even the definition of work injury is variable. "Occupational injury" is generally defined as an injury arising out of or in the course of employment resulting from the action of a physically or chemically traumatizing agent. The record-keeping regulations of the Occupational Safety and Health Administration (OSHA) are more specific and define "occupational injury" as any injury, such as a cut, fracture, sprain, or amputation, that resulted from a work accident or from an exposure involving a single incident in the work environment. "Recordable injuries" under OSHA regulations involve one of the following: loss of consciousness, restriction of work or motion, transfer to another job, or medical treatment other than first aid. "Disabling injuries" involve days away from work or days of restricted work. In some countries, such as Australia, injuries of bystanders resulting from the actions of people at work are considered work related. Injuries occurring during a worker's commute to or from work are not consistently considered work related. In the United States the classification of work-related injury varies among states; currently there is no nationally accepted standard definition. This lack of consistency creates problems in the interpretation of surveillance data and hinders the development of effective prevention programs.

Despite the staggering statistics summarized in the preceding paragraphs, the number of work-related injuries and fatalities probably is seriously

---

* Defined as one that causes death, permanent disability, or any temporary total functional disability beyond the day of injury.[31]

3

underreported. The BLS has the largest dataset on occupational injury and illness. The bureau's annual survey of occupational injury and illness provides estimates of incidence rates based on logs kept by private industry employers during the year. These records reflect not only the year's injury and illness experience but also the employer's understanding of and compliance with the current record-keeping regulations. For many reasons the number of occupational injuries reported by the BLS is likely to be well below the actual number. The BLS Annual Survey is based on a random sample of the OSHA logs from approximately 280,000 employers with 11 or more employees. The data are limited because they are taken from a random sample, they exclude the smallest employers and many states (states participating range from 14 to 30 depending on the year), and the information entered on the OSHA forms is often vague.[17] Probably the most significant shortcoming of the BLS survey is that employers have a strong incentive not to report occupational injuries or illnesses because OSHA targets employers with high injury or illness rates for on-site inspections.[24]

A recent (1987) study by the Panel on Occupational Safety and Health Statistics of the National Academy of Sciences Committee on National Statistics concluded that the BLS data systems are inadequate for providing OSHA with the data it needs to implement prevention programs.[23] The panel's first recommendation was that the "BLS Annual Survey should be modified to permit the collection of detailed data on severe occupational injuries categorized as injuries resulting in death, hospitalization, or outpatient surgery."

Although many potential sources of information exist, no comprehensive, integrated nationwide system has been established to collect data on occupational illnesses, injuries, and fatalities or to provide reliable industry-specific data on incidence and prevalence of work-related disability. Occupational illnesses are clearly underreported because patients or their physicians often fail to recognize the work-related etiology of many occupational diseases. Not much has changed since 1984, when the House Committee on Government Operations issued a report emphatically stating that "since the passage of the Occupational Safety and Health Act nearly 15 years ago, a bipartisan failure of four administrations has thwarted the mandated development of an information and data collection system on occupational disease. No reliable national estimates exist . . . on the level of occupational disease, cancer, disability or deaths."[34]

FATAL INJURIES

A number of surveillance systems have been designed specifically to capture information on occupational fatalities:

1. The BLS derives estimates of workplace fatalities from its random survey of OSHA-mandated employer reports (described previously).
2. The National Safety Council (NSC) compiles statistics from multiple sources, including the National Center for Health Statistics, state health departments, and state industrial commissions.[20]
3. The National Institute of Occupational Safety and Health (NIOSH) has implemented the National Traumatic Occupational Fatality (NTOF) surveillance system, which uses death certificate data.[2] NIOSH also has the Fatal Accident Circumstances and Epidemiology (FACE) project, which focuses on electrocutions and fatal falls.[9]
4. The Department of Transportation Fatal Accident Reporting System (FARS) collects data on motor vehicle fatalities, which are the main cause of occupational death. FARS operates in all states but excludes off road accidents and deaths that occur more than 30 days after the accident.[19]
5. Employers under OSHA jurisdiction are required to report to OSHA all work-related fatalities of employees. Although these records are useful, they exclude many categories of workers (e.g., transportation workers, miners, and public employees). Events such as motor vehicle crashes, airplane crashes, and homicides are investigated by other agencies and are not routinely investigated by OSHA. Recent studies also suggest significant underreporting of fatalities that do fall under OSHA jurisdiction.[29]

Comparative studies have shown that no single source of data contains all occupational fatalities or all of the data elements necessary to describe them. The average capture rates of sources have been calculated as follows: death certificates, 81%; medical examiner records, 61%; workers' compensation reports, 57%; and OSHA reports, 32%.[30]

The variable sources of information and denominator data have produced substantial variations in the calculated death rates. For example, NTOF, using death certificate data, estimates that from 1980 to 1985 approximately 7000 work-related fatalities occurred in the United States each year. Because death certificate reporting is not accurate and consistent, NTOF data underestimate the number of occupational deaths.[7]

By comparison the NSC estimated that there were 13,000 work-related deaths in 1980 among 96.8 million workers, a rate of 13:100,000, compared with the NTOF estimate of 9.1:100,000 in the same year. The NSC data indicate a long-term decline in occupational fatality rates, from 37:100,000 in 1933 to 9:100,000 in 1988.[21] The NSC estimates do not include worker deaths resulting from intentional injuries, either homicides or suicides. Yet since 1980 at least 750 people a year have been murdered at work, and the latest statistics from the BLS indicate that approximately 17% of work-related deaths were homicides, second only to highway accidents as the cause of death. Ninety-three percent of those killed in 1992 were men, but for women murder at work was the most frequent cause of death.[32]

Despite variations in overall fatality rates, the three major sources (BLS, NSC, NTOF) show similar rankings of rates by industry. The top four industrial groups are consistently mining, construction, transportation, and agriculture (Table 1-1). These four industries account for less than 20% of the workforce but contribute more than 50% of the occupational fatalities, with average annual rates of 20 to 28 per 100,000 workers.[2]

The ratio of male to female workers killed on the job is greater than 12:1, which reflects the sex ratio in high-risk industries. Age-specific fatality rates are greatest among workers over age 60, but the largest number of fatalities occurs among workers in their twenties and thirties. Age differences vary among industries.[2]

Table 1-1 Occupational fatality rates by major industrial group, United States, 1980-1986

Industry	Number of deaths	Average annual rate*
Mining	1974	28.08
Construction	7482	25.13
Transportation	7686	23.44
Agriculture, forestry, fish	5264	20.30
Public administration	2255	6.41
Manufacturing	4917	3.58
Retail trade	3090	2.78
Service	3518	2.56
Wholesale trade	738	1.96
Finance, insurance, real estate	474	1.19
TOTAL	45089	7.54

Data from National Traumatic Occupational Fatality surveillance system, 1980-1986.
* Deaths per 100,000 workers per year.

According to the BLS data the most frequent cause of occupational fatality is motor vehicle accidents, with other causes varying by industry (Table 1-2). One study of the construction industry found that the five leading causes of death, accounting for 77% of all fatalities, were vehicle accidents, falls from elevations, workers being struck by objects, excavation cave-ins, and electrocutions.[6]

Intoxication by alcohol or other drugs certainly pays a role in occupational fatalities, although the relative significance is not clear. Various studies have reported blood alcohol levels above 0.1% in 4% to 13% of occupational fatalities.[28] Among drivers of heavy trucks involved in fatal crashes, 2% have blood levels above 0.1%, compared with 25% of drivers of cars involved in fatal crashes.

Because of the significant undercounting of occupational fatalities in the BLS survey, the BLS has recently developed the Census of Fatal Occupational Injuries (CFOI) system to improve the accuracy of data on work-related deaths. CFOI is a cooperative federal and state program. Its sources of information include death certificates, state and federal workers' compensation reports, OSHA fatality reports, and other federally mandated reports received by the BLS.[32]

NONFATAL INJURIES

Estimates of the rates and information on the distribution and causes of disabling, nonfatal occupational injury vary depending on the data source. The primary sources are the BLS and the National Center for Health Statistics. Others include the NSC, workers' compensation awards, and hospital and emergency room records. None of these sources provides a complete count of all occupational injuries.

The BLS estimates that slightly more than 6.4 million job-related injuries were reported in the private sector during 1990, which translated to a rate of 8.3 per 100 full-time workers. Of this number, nearly one half (almost 3 million cases) were serious enough for the injured worker to lose work time, to experience restricted work activity, or both. The average incidence rate for injury resulting in lost time was 3.9 per 100 full-time workers. These cases resulted in approximately 60 million lost workdays in 1990, corresponding to a rate of 78.3 lost workdays per 100 full-time workers.[5] All these measures of incidence of work-related injuries have shown increases over the last decade.

Figure 1-1 shows estimated rates of disabling injuries by major industrial group in the private sector for 1990. The highest rates typically occur in construction, agriculture, and manufacturing.

Table 1-2 Percentage distribution of occupational fatality by cause for high-risk industrial sectors, 1987-1988 average[1]

Cause[2]	Total private sector[3]	Agriculture, forestry, fishing	Mining— oil and gas extraction only	Construction	Manufacturing	Transportation and public utilities[4]
Highway vehicles	28	31	23	18	19	42
Falls	12	5	3	21	9	2
Electrocutions	9	5	4	15	5	14
Industrial vehicles or equipment	9	21	18	11	10	6
Heart attacks[5]	8	5	8	9	10	8
Struck by objects other than vehicles or equipment	8	9	32	6	13	3
Assaults	5	6	0	<1	1	1
All other[6]	—	—	—	—	—	—
TOTAL[7]	100	100	100	100	100	100

Modified from Weeks JL, Levy GS, Wagner GK, editors: *Preventing occupational disease and injury,* 1991, American Public Health Association.

[1] Results are the average of the 2 years because sampling errors for data by cause of fatality are too large to provide reliable annual estimates at the industry division level.

[2] Cause is defined as the object or event associated with the fatality.

[3] Excludes coal, metal, and nonmetal mining and railroads, for which data are not available.

[4] Excludes railroads.

[5] Heart attacks that occur at work are often considered "work related" for compensation purposes.

[6] The "All other" category includes, for example, contact with carcinogenic or toxic substances, drowning, train accidents, and various occupational diseases.

[7] Because of rounding, components may not add to totals.

Industries with the highest reported incidence rates are almost always in the manufacturing sector, with rates as high as 13.7 for the sawmill industry and 18.1 for ship building and repair (Table 1-3). The overall and industry-specific incidence rates estimated by NCHS are generally higher than the BLS estimates. These discrepancies can be related to differences in sampling methodologies and definition of injury. The NCHS estimates are derived from results of the National Health Interview Survey, which used a random sample of households in the United States. Both public and private sector workers were included regardless of size of the workplace, and an occupational injury was counted if it resulted in restriction of activity for more than one-half day.[35]

Table 1-4 shows the industry-specific annual incidence rates reported by NCHS. The highest rates were for construction (26.9 per 100 workers); agriculture, forestry, and fishing (19.1); manufacturing (14.5); and mining (13.8).

Injury rates are known to vary within each industry by a number of additional factors, including work experience, age, and size of the workforce. For example, a 10-year analysis of OSHA investigations showed that establishments with fewer than 20 employees have the highest injury rate (10:10,000) compared with less than five per 100,000 for firms with 20 to 29 employees and three or less per 100,000 employees for firms with 100 or more employees.[18] Younger, less experienced workers usually have higher injury rates. Rates are higher among nonwhites and men, but most of the variation is explained by age, occupation, or experience.[35]

The proportion of nonfatal occupational injuries associated with alcohol or other drug intoxication is not well documented. Based on available data, acutely intoxicated workers apparently have twice the risk of injury as other workers. However, the percentage of workers intoxicated while on the job is unknown, so the proportion of all injuries causally related to intoxication is not known.[28]

Data on the frequency of specific types of injury are limited. The BLS, in addition to its annual survey, also publishes information from a supplementary data system (SDS), which collects descriptive information on workers' compensation claims in OSHA-regulated states. Classification is done by industry, occupation, nature of injury, body part affected, source of injury, and type of accident.[20] Although these data include only 23 states with differing regulations concerning classification and reporting to the BLS, it is the only dataset that is nearly national in scope and classifies injury by nature of injury and body part. The box on page 9 summarizes the SDS findings for 1986. Of note

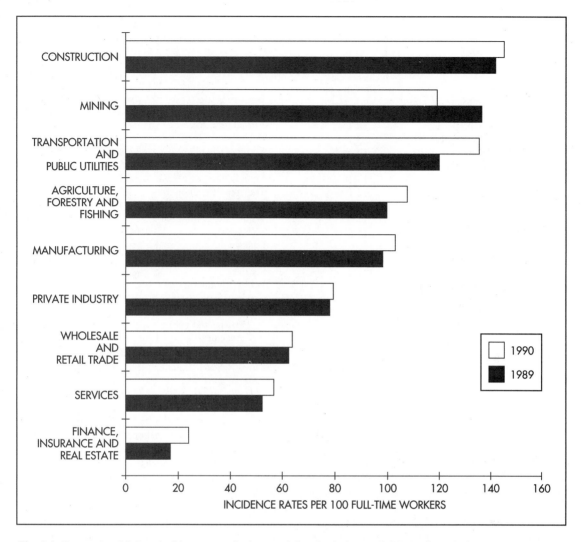

Fig. 1-1 Occupational injury incidence rates for lost workdays by industry division, private industry, 1989-90. Adapted from: Bureau of Labor Statistics, News Bulletin, 92-371, Washington, D.C. BLS, 1992.

are the high incidence of strain, sprain, back, and overexertion injuries.

FUTURE DIRECTIONS

The current systems for occupational injury and illness reporting are seriously flawed despite recent advances. We know that occupational injury is still a major cause of disability and premature death in the United States and that specific industries, particularly mining, construction, agriculture, transportation, and manufacturing, continue to experience high incidences of fatalities and disabling injuries. In certain high-risk industries such as structural metal fabrication and meat packing, every year one fourth to one third of the workforce experiences an occupational injury.

A recent review of injury surveillance discusses a number of areas that need attention to improve occupational injury surveillance in the United States:[12]

1. Detailed denominator data (including age, gender, race, industry, and occupation) are needed to better identify populations at risk for occupational injury.
2. Clarification of the distribution of physical hazards in industry is needed with collection of data on equipment, processes, and workplace physical features.
3. The coding system for recording injuries should be improved to capture facts regarding etiology and injury causation.

Table 1-3 Industries with the highest lost workday case incidence rates for injuries only, private industry, 1990

Industry	Incidence rate per 100 full-time workers
Ship building and repairing	18.1
Special product sawmills	13.7
Meat packing plants	13.4
Structural wood members	12.2
Prefabricated wood buildings	12.1
Bottled and canned soft drinks	12.1
Malleable iron foundries	11.8
Secondary nonferrous metals	11.8
Fabricated plate work (boiler shops)	11.6
Steel springs, except wire	11.6
Vitreous plumbing fixtures	11.4
Animal and marine fats and oils	11.4
Prepared flour mixes and doughs	11.3
Gray and ductile iron foundries	11.0
Steel foundries	10.9
Logging	10.7

Modified from *Occupational injuries and illnesses in the U.S. by industry, 1990,* Washington, DC, 1992, US Dept of Labor, Bureau of Labor Statistics.

Table 1-4 Number of injuries, annual average incidence rates, and number of injuries 1983-1985

Industry group	Incidence rate (per 100 workers)	Number of injuries ($\times 1000$)
Agriculture, forestry, fishing (01-09)	19.1	616
Mining (10-14)	13.8	140
Construction (15-17)	26.9	1,803
Manufacturing (20-39)	14.5	3,023
Transportation, communication, public utilities	10.1	765
Wholesale, retail trade (50-59)	7.6	1,517
Finance, insurance, real estate (60-67)	4.3	287
Services	6.5	2,038
Public administration	6.8	332
AVERAGE OR TOTAL		
Private sector	10.5	10,189
Private and public sector	10.2	10,521

Data from National Center for Health Statistics. In Weeks JL, Levy GS, Wagner GK, editors: *Preventing occupational disease and injury,* 1991, American Public Health Association.

4. Better reporting of health outcomes by health care providers is needed to more clearly delineate the pathologic effects of the injury and to ensure that all injuries at work are captured irrespective of variation among states in what constitutes a "reportable event."
5. Programs such as FACE should be expanded to attain 100% reporting of traumatic occupational fatalities and to further develop causal epidemiologic models.
6. Additional resources should be allocated to improve the analysis of causal factors through on-site investigation and modeling.

Since the mid-1980s, NIOSH has focused attention on the prevention of occupational injuries.[1] A result has been an increase in research on risk factors and in funding for surveillance systems designed to improve the understanding of the causes of occupational injuries. The ultimate goal of these programs is to identify the presence of workplace hazards so that health professionals can target specific industries for preventive interventions. To develop effective preventive programs, we need more precise information concerning exposure and the circumstances surrounding injuries and fatalities in the workplace. Only when such information is collected, analyzed, and made available in a nationally standardized database will we be able to achieve a continued decline in the disability and death rates among the American workforce. Since occupational injuries represent a substantial subset of injuries from all causes, techniques developed within the workplace will undoubtedly reduce injuries outside work.

The primary care provider has a crucial role in the surveillance and prevention of occupational injury and illness. One objective of the "Healthy People 2000" project, sponsored by the Department of Health and Human Services, is to increase to 75% the proportion of primary care providers who routinely elicit information about occupational safety and health problems as part of the patient history and who provide relevant counseling. Physicians and occupational health nurses should be actively engaged in injury prevention at various levels, including identifying previously unrecognized or unusual workplace hazards, educating injured workers and management about recognition of hazards, and advocating the implementation of prevention programs.[27]

WORKERS' COMPENSATION DATA

Workers' compensation databases are commonly used as a source of statistical information on occupational injuries, but the limitations must be appreciated. For cases to be captured by the workers' compensation system, all of the following must occur:

**PERCENTAGE OF COMPENSATION
AWARDS BY NATURE OF INJURY,
BODY PART AFFECTED, AND
TYPE OF ACCIDENT
(BASED ON AWARDS
IN 23 STATES, 1986)**

Nature of injury

Sprains, strains	41%
Cuts, lacerations, punctures	13%
Contusions, crushes	10%
Fractures	9%
Occupational illnesses	6%
Burns	3%
Amputation, enucleation	1%
Other	17%

Body part affected

Back	24%
Lower extremities	20%
Upper extremities (excluding fingers)	14%
Fingers	12%
Trunk (excluding back)	11%
Multiple parts	8%
Head, neck (excluding eyes)	5%
Eyes	3%
Body system	2%
Other	1%

Type of accident

Overexertion	30%
Struck by or against	25%
Fall	17%
Bodily reaction	7%
Caught in, under, or between	6%
Contact with radiation or caustics	3%
Motor vehicle accidents	3%
Rubbed, abraded	2%
Temperature extremes	2%
Other	4%

Modified from Weeks JL, Levy GS, Wagner GK, editors: *Preventing occupational disease and injury,* Washington, D.C., 1991, American Public Health Association.

1. A worker or the worker's physician must recognize an injury or illness as work related.
2. The worker must notify the employer that a claim is being filed.
3. The claim must be judged compensable by the employer or carrier or the workers' compensation board.*

---

* The definition of "compensable injury," unfortunately, varies from state to state, especially for cumulative trauma, occupational disease, and psychiatric claims.

Workers' compensation databases often classify claims as *specific injuries* that follow a sudden traumatic event or as *cumulative trauma* or *occupational disease* that becomes clinically evident only after months or years of work exposure. The coverage for specific traumatic injuries is consistent throughout all jurisdictions. However, the coverage for cumulative trauma and occupational disease is more variable and controversial. Some states are fairly restrictive, using scheduled diagnoses or other statutory language to limit the scope of coverage,[33] whereas others, such as California, are very permissive and may consider virtually any medical condition compensable if caused or aggravated by workplace mental stress—the so-called mental-physical claims.

In general, workers' compensation data tend to underestimate the occurrence of occupational disorders. However, the degree of underreporting varies among conditions. For specific injuries (e.g., fractures and lacerations), the correlation between reported workers' compensation claims and the true incidence of the injuries may be relatively good. However, with cumulative trauma and occupational disease the reported frequencies may bear little relationship to true incidence and prevalence. There are many reasons for this, including the following:

1. Long latency from exposure to clinical manifestations
2. Underdiagnosis by physicians
3. Difficulty in separating occupational factors from life-style stresses and aging
4. Compensability defined by statutes that may have little or no scientific basis

A number of studies have documented that a majority of workers with impairment from occupational disease (e.g., pneumoconioses) never receive workers' compensation benefits. They are more likely to receive Social Security Disability Insurance, and a recent trend has been to seek redress from toxic tort lawsuits, bypassing the workers' compensation system.[15]

On the other hand, current laws in many states have provided coverage for conditions that have a questionable relationship to work. The spectrum of what is defined as compensable injury has broadened dramatically in the last few decades to include many cases of chronic disease such as atherosclerotic coronary vascular disease (ASCVD). Many cases of chronic disease are now considered work related from a legal standpoint when in fact the scientific evidence for work relatedness is weak or nonexistent. For example, *any* disease process that is alleged to be aggravated by work-related stress can become a compensable injury under the California workers' compensation laws. This includes everything from breast cancer to rheumatoid arthritis! This trend not only distorts the occupational injury statistics but also undermines one of the original goals of the workers' compensation laws: to provide incentive for the employer to minimize hazards.[3,16]

Thus the true incidence of work-related injury and illness is unknown, and a comparison of the universe of true cases with the universe of workers' compensation claims would probably show a significant lack of congruence (Fig. 1-1).

Statistics on the frequency of workplace injuries are potentially useful for planning preventive intervention at the worksite. Inferring risk of injury from workers' compensation data is problematic, however. Studies demonstrating increased risk in certain occupational groups may actually be a reflection of *underreporting* of common conditions that are nondisabling in those occupations. For example, acute back pain in a warehouse worker will necessarily be reported because the condition is incompatible with the essential lifting functions of the job, whereas a claims adjuster with acute back pain could continue working if he or she were motivated to stay on the job.

In some jurisdictions certain conditions may actually be overreported depending on the following:

1. Economic conditions (e.g., plant closings, layoffs, and labor disputes)
2. Fraudulent practices by applicant attorneys and physicians
3. Inaccurate diagnoses (e.g., carpal tunnel syndrome) on doctor's first report
4. Permissive regulations regarding the establishment of causation (e.g., coronary artery disease and other stress-related disorders)

Although we are operating in an imperfect world with respect to data on work injuries, existing workers' compensation data have potential value in selected diagnostic categories, particularly when the diagnosis implies work relatedness and is relatively easy to confirm.[25] Examples include certain occupational diseases, such as lead poisoning and silicosis. Workers' compensation data can also be useful in a surveillance mode for some of the more common soft tissue injuries, although many pitfalls exist. For example, tendonitis may be coded as carpal tunnel syndrome, so verification of the diagnosis is critical. For other conditions such as acute low back pain, work-related injury may be difficult or impossible to separate from degenerative disease of the spine unrelated to work activity. Although the diagnosis in any one case may not be accurate, statistical clustering of claims in a given industry may indicate the need

for preventive intervention. Such analyses have been used successfully by the State of Washington, Department of Labor and Industry.[10]

ASVCD is an example of a commonly compensable condition that illustrates why workers' compensation data are of limited value in associating occupations with increased risk of a specific disease: A 56-year-old police officer has an acute myocardial infarction while escorting a combative suspect. He has no history of cardiac disease but has a strong family history, has smoked two packs of cigarettes per day for 35 years, has a blood cholesterol level of 247 mg/dl, and has borderline untreated blood pressure. This man's heart disease would be counted as an occupational illness under many state jurisdictions. The compensability is not based on scientific causation analysis. For example, in California the labor code includes a *presumption* that heart disease in peace officers is work related. This presumption is not derived from epidemiologic data. The studies on morbidity and mortality from ASCVD in police officers are mixed at best. The presumption exists because of the political influence of special interest groups representing police officers. Although lip service is paid to the stress of police work and the relation of stress to ASCVD, the available literature simply does not support such a claim. Even in jurisdictions where no formal presumption exists, this man's heart disease would likely be judged compensable simply because the acute event occurred on the job (i.e., arose out of employment). Workers' compensation judges are asked to adjudicate disputes between employer and injured worker regarding entitlement to workers' compensation benefits. When the judges are presented with the facts in the case, they are likely to infer *causation* from any temporal *association* of work and acute presentation of clinical symptoms.[11]

Even though in the preceding case the myocardial infarction undoubtedly would have occurred if the man had not been a police officer, his coronary artery disease is considered a compensable work injury. Unfortunately, such decisions undermine the safety incentive for employers. Interpreting statistics on workers' compensation claims is further complicated by the fact that *aggravation* of an underlying disease or preexisting condition is considered compensable when it occurs as the result of work activities. Of particular concern are the so-called mental-physical claims, that is, job stress that reportedly causes or aggravates a preexisting condition such as systemic lupus erythematosus. If this trend continues, virtually *any* medical condition could be considered compensable.

The reporting of true cases of workplace aggravation of preexisting disease is useful from the standpoint of preemployment screening, job placement, and reasonable accommodation. For example, an asthmatic person exposed to nonspecific dust at levels considered safe for the general population may be at risk in certain occupations. However, the reporting of most of the "mental-physical" claims has no value from a preventive health perspective.

Even risk of acute traumatic injury may not be accurately reflected in workers' compensation claims data. The example of low back pain is illustrative. An estimated 95% of the adult working population has at least one episode of disabling back pain (pain that interferes with normal work or recreational routine), but only a fraction of these episodes actually result in workers' compensation claims. Many factors may influence a worker to file a workers' compensation claim when experiencing a sudden onset of low back pain, including the following:

1. Severity of symptoms
2. Activity at the time of onset
3. Essential functions of the job
4. Psychosocial variables such as job satisfaction, relationship with supervisor, and family or financial stressors

The severity of the symptoms may be only a minor determinant in the worker's decision to file a claim. The worker's functional status in relation to the essential functions of the job may be more important than the perceived severity. Often, however, it is the psychosocial variables influencing *motivation* that tip the balance. A worker who has a low-paying job that he or she perceives as monotonous and demanding, who has little control over work flow and the general work environment, who has poor relationships with a supervisor or other co-workers, or who has significant financial or family problems may have little or no motivation to continue working during an episode of acute low back pain or to return to work after symptoms have improved. In this situation the "entitlement" aspects of the workers' compensation system predominate and the temporary disability check becomes a desirable alternative to working. Thus occupational health professionals must recognize that rising trends in workers' compensation claims may reflect socioeconomic distress, as well as the presence of physical hazards.

REFERENCES

1. Baker et al: Surveillance of occupational illness and injury in the U.S.: current perspectives and future directions, *J Pub Health Policy* 9:198-221, 1988.
2. Bell CA et al: Fatal occupational injuries in the United States, 1980 through 1985, *JAMA* 263(22):3047-3050, 1990.
3. Brandt-Rauf SI, Brandt-Rauf PW: Compensation for occupational disease: hidden agendas, *Health Affairs* 7(4):73-82, 1988.
4. Bureau of Labor Statistics: Occupational injuries and illnesses in the United States by industry, 1990, Bulletin 2399, Washington, DC, 1992, The Bureau.
5. Bureau of Labor Statistics: *News bulletin, 92-371,* Washington, DC, 1992, The Bureau.
6. Buskin SE, Paulozzi LJ: Fatal injuries in the construction industry in Washington State, *Am J Ind Med* 11:253-260, 1987.
7. Centers for Disease Control: *Occupational injury prevention,* Position Paper from The Third National Injury Control Conference, "Setting the National Agenda for Injury Control in the 1990's," Washington, DC, 1991, Dept of Health and Human Services.
8. Committee on Trauma Research: *Injury in America: a continuing public health problem,* Washington, DC, 1985, National Academy Press.
9. Conroy CS et al: *Fatal accident circumstances and epidemiology,* Report FACE-87-94, Morgantown, WV, 1988, National Institute of Occupational Safety and Health.
10. Franklin GM et al: Occupational carpal tunnel syndrome in Washington State, *Am J Pub Health* 81:741-746, 1991.
11. Hadler NM: Occupational illness: the issue of causality, *J Occup Med* 26:587-593, 1984.
12. Hanrahan LP and Moll MB: Injury surveillance, *Amer J Pub Health* 79(suppl):38-45, 1989.
13. Hensler DR et al: Compensation for accidental injuries in the U.S., Santa Monica, Calif, 1991, Rand Institute for Civil Justice.
14. Kraus JF: Fatal and non-fatal injuries in occupational settings: a review, *Annu Rev Pub Health* 6:403-418, 1985.
15. LaDou J: Cumulative injury in workers' compensation, *Occup Med: State of Art Rev* 3(4):611-619, 1988.
16. Letz G: Current problems in occupational disease compensation: is equitable distribution of benefits feasible under the current system? Presentation at 32nd Annual Western Occupational Health Conference Irvine, Calif, October 1988.
17. McNeely EM: Who's counting anyway? The problem with occupational safety and health statistics, *J Occup Med* 33(10):1071-1074, 1991.
18. Mendeloff JM, Kagey BT: Using Occupational Safety and Health Administration accident investigations to study patterns in work fatalities, *J Occup Med* 32:1117-1123, 1990.
19. National Highway Transportation Safety Administration: Fatal accident reporting system 1989: a decade of progress, Washington, DC, 1991, Dept of Transportation.
20. National Safety Council: *Accident Facts, 1992 Edition,* Chicago, 1992, The Council.
21. National Safety Council: Work injury and illness rates 1989, Chicago, 1990, The Council.
22. Office of Technology Assessment: Preventing illness and injury in the workplace (OTA-H-256), Washington, DC, 1985, US Government Printing Office.
23. Panel on Occupational Safety and Health Statistics and Committee on National Statistics, National Research Council, Pollack ES, Keimig DG, editors: *Counting injuries and illnesses in the workplace: proposals for better systems,* Washington, DC, 1987, National Academy Press.
24. Rice DP et al: *Cost of injury in the U.S.: a report to Congress,* San Francisco, 1989, Institute for Health and Aging, University of California and Injury Prevention Center, The Johns Hopkins University.
25. Rutstein DD et al: Sentinel health events (occupational): a basis for physician recognition and public health surveillance, *Am J Pub Health* 73(9):1054-1062, 1983.

26. Sheridan PJ: What are accidents really costing you? *Occup Hazards* 41(3):41-43, 1979.

27. Smith GS: The physician's role in injury prevention, *J Gen Intern Med* 5:567-570, 1990.

28. Smith GS, Kraus JF: Alcohol and residential, recreational, and occupational injuries: a review of the epidemiologic evidence, *Annu Rev Public Health,* 9:99-121, 1988.

29. Stanbury M, Goldoft M: Use of OSHA inspection data for fatal occupational injury surveillance in New Jersey, *Am J Public Health* 80:200-202, 1990.

30. Stout N, Bell C: Effectiveness of source documents for identifying fatal occupational injuries: a synthesis of studies, *Am J Pub Health* 81(6):725-728, 1991.

31. Stout-Wiegand N: Fatal occupational injuries in U.S industries, 1984: comparison of two national surveillance systems, *Am J Public Health* 78(9):1215-1217, 1984.

32. US Department of Labor: First national census of fatal occupational injuries reported by BLS, USDL 93-406, Washington, DC, 1993, The Department.

33. US Department of Labor: *State workers' compensation statutory definitions of injury and occupational disease,* Employment Standards Administration, Office of State Liaison and Legislative Analysis, Division of State Workers' Compensation Programs, Washington, DC, 1988, The Department.

34. US Congress, House of Representatives: *Report on occupational illness data collection: fragmented, unreliable, and seventy years behind communicable disease surveillance,* Subcommittee of the Committee on Government Operations, 98th Congress, 2nd Session, Washington, DC, 1984, US Government Printing Office.

35. Weeks JL: Injuries, non fatal. In Weeks JL, Levy GS, Wagner GR, editors: *Preventing occupational disease and injury,* Washington, D.C., 1991, American Public Health Association.

2 Occupational Health Care and the Workers' Compensation System: The Context in Which We Operate

Workers' compensation is a form of social insurance widely accepted in the industrially developed countries. In the United States the workers' compensation insurance system has become controversial in recent years because of the rising rate of work disability and because costs are increasingly difficult to control. The rise in work disability rates is concentrated among workers in industries undergoing contraction because of the transformation from heavy industries, such as mining and manufacturing, to service industry. More than 10% of the labor force suffered displacement during the past decade. Most of the displaced workers are older men, predominantly blue collar employees without the skills or the desire to find work in the service economy. The disability compensation system, including workers' compensation, accommodates many of these workers when it legitimizes unemployment under the mantel of illness and disability.[15]

In this time of intense international business competition, U.S. employers incurred more than $60 billion in direct workers' compensation costs in 1992, triple the amount spent a decade earlier. Counting other costs, such as production delays, damage to equipment, and recruitment and training of replacement workers, the total cost for a year is approximately $350 billion.[11]

There are large disparities between the benefits accorded federal government employees under the Federal Employees' Compensation Act (FECA) and those provided to state employees by the separate laws of the 50 states and the District of Columbia. Moreover, compensation for lost wages and medical expenses varies greatly among states, which led to a legislative attempt in 1973 to place the workers' compensation system under federal control. If the federal program for government employees (under FECA) were not so costly, federalization might appear to be the answer to the many problems affecting state workers' compensation insurance systems. Proposed federal standards for the state workers' compensation programs have been largely ignored in recent years. However, for two reasons the federal government has shown new interest in dealing with occupational diseases: (1) tort suits arising from occupational diseases have generated concern among employers, and (2) occupational diseases are an emotional topic, and public opinion is pressing politicians to support reform.[7]

Physicians who treat work-related injuries and illnesses must understand the requirements of their state's workers' compensation system and provide the necessary services to both treat the condition appropriately and efficiently and ensure the flow of benefits to the worker. Workers' compensation laws worldwide share many characteristics, but there are many important differences among the several federal and state systems in the United States. Workers' compensations systems are designed to ensure the injured worker prompt but limited benefits and assign to the employer sure and predictable liability.[13]

WORKERS' COMPENSATION LAW

The employer's financial responsibility for an employee's injury or death in the workplace was first established under Bismarck in Germany in 1884. Great Britain followed in 1897 with legislation requiring employers to compensate employees or their survivors for an injury or death regardless of who was at fault. Thus workers' compensation laws are the result of a compromise in which the employee gave up the right to sue the employer for negligence in exchange for the employer's agreement to pay the cost of medical care and to compensate the worker for time lost from work. By the turn of the century all European countries had workers' compensation laws. The workers' compensation movement did not begin in the United States until 1908, when a forerunner of the Federal Employees Compensation Act was passed. The first state laws were enacted in 1911. These initial workers' compensation systems were far simpler than today's array of programs dealing with disability, income loss, medical care, accident prevention, and vocational rehabilitation.

A major deficiency in workers' compensation laws is that they began in an era when occupational disease was not recognized. The system is relatively successful at recognizing and compensating work-related injuries. But far less than half of all occupational disease is compensated under workers' compensation systems, and its reporting by government agencies is woefully inadequate. Consequently, measures to prevent occupational diseases receive less attention than those directed at the causes of occupational injury.

Worker benefits

The objectives of workers' compensation systems are to provide employees with an income during recovery from an injury, ensure that injured workers have a competitive position in the employment market, and avoid lengthy and costly legal action. In the event of death, survivors are compensated for the loss of their provider. An injured employee is automatically entitled to medical treatment and compensation, whether the incident is the fault of the employee or the employer.*

The cost of workers' compensation benefits is considered a cost of doing business and is passed on to purchasers of the product or service. In the case of government workers' compensation systems, the costs are included in the taxes collected by federal and state governments.

To be compensable, an injury usually must "arise out of and in the course of employment." A work injury that activates or aggravates a preexisting condition also is compensable, as is recurrence of an earlier compensable injury. Depending on the jurisdiction, judicial action may be necessary to resolve questions of liability for self-inflicted injuries and suicidal acts. Similar determinations may be necessary for injuries occurring under the influence of alcohol or drugs or during entirely personal activity and fights at work.

Occupational diseases are the direct result of

work or exposure to toxic substances in the workplace. Occupational disease claims have proliferated in recent decades. In some states this situation occurs because of judicial interpretation. In other jurisdictions "presumptions" lead to the automatic acceptance of workers' compensation liability for certain diseases in designated worker groups. An example is the presumption in California law that heart disease in police and fire personnel and some other uniformed services is work related and will receive workers' compensation benefits. Throughout the United States occupational disease claims are increasing as physicians become more familiar with the discipline of occupational medicine and more confident of their diagnoses of occupational disease.

Many states recognize cumulative injury claims as occupational illnesses when the worker has sustained repeated slight physical or psychic injuries that eventually result in a disability. These broadened interpretations of illness and disability open workers' compensation systems to numerous claims of occupational stress. They also result in many new cases of repetitive motion disorder, cardiovascular diseases, hearing loss, and emotional disturbance entering the system.[5] In many states occupational physicians play a key role in resolving disputes over compensability for myocardial infarction and cerebrovascular accident, occupational and environmental exposure to toxic materials, and the occurrence of birth defects and other reproductive and developmental problems. Many physicians devote their practices to such forensic activities.[6]

Benefits to workers or their families are of several types: permanent total disability, temporary total disability, permanent partial disability, temporary partial disability, survivors' benefits, and vocational rehabilitation benefits.

Permanent total disability. Permanent total disability covers workers who are so disabled that they will never be able to work again in an open labor market and for whom no further treatment offers hope of recovery. Most states compensate such individuals with two thirds of average wages (when not taxed, this amounts to about 85% to 90% of take home wages), and some also provide additional funds for dependents. Although some states limit the duration of payments, others provide compensation for the remainder of the injured worker's life. These payments are governed by guidelines that stipulate minimum and maximum payments.

Temporary total disability. The majority of work-related injuries fall under the classification of temporary total disability; that is, the worker is expected to recover with treatment but is unable to work for a time. Benefits are paid during the re-

---

* The exception to this view of fault in workers' compensation law is a relic of the era before workers' compensation. The Federal Employers' Liability Act (FELA), passed in 1908, applies to railroad workers. It is substantially different from other workers' compensation systems in that it is a negligence-based system with no cap on damages. FELA allows railroad employees to recover damages for injuries resulting wholly or partly from a railroad's negligence. In practice, the threshold for a finding of liability against the railroad is low. Thus the railroad may have to pay damages regardless of whether it is at fault (as with workers' compensation), yet does not receive any cap on damages. Consequently the system is expensive and frustrating to administer.

covery period on the basis of average earnings, again with a minimum and a maximum of two thirds of gross or 80% of take home wages, until the individual is able to return to work (Table 2-1). There is a waiting period for this type of compensation, but it is paid retroactively if the worker cannot work for a certain number of days or if hospitalization is necessary. The waiting period serves as an incentive to return to work after less serious injuries. Thus it is like a deductible provision in other forms of health insurance.

Permanent partial disability. Permanent partial disability occurs when a worker's injury reduces her ability to compete in the labor market. In some jurisdictions benefits compensate the injured worker for losses in future earnings and are divided into two categories: scheduled injuries (e.g., loss of a limb, an eye, or hearing) and nonscheduled injuries (e.g., back injury, tenosynovitis). The first is paid according to a schedule fixed by statute (Table 2-2). Under this category, benefits are paid whether or not the individual is working. Payment is usually provided for a specified number of weeks, the length of which depends on the part of the body damaged. Benefits are based on a percentage of earnings at the time of injury and again are subject to a minimum and a maximum amount. Nonscheduled injuries receive weekly benefit payments based on a percentage of wages lost. The percentage is derived from the difference between wages earned before and after injury. In some states, however, nonscheduled permanent partial disabilities are compensated as a percentage of the total disability cases.

Temporary partial disability. Temporary partial disability occurs when a worker is injured to the degree that she cannot perform her usual work but is still capable of working at some job during convalescence. A worker in this category is compensated for the difference between wages earned before the injury and wages earned during the period of temporary partial disability, usually at two thirds of the difference.

Survivors' benefits. Dependent survivors of the employee are paid death benefits under workers' compensation. The method and size of payments vary widely among states, but all systems provide for a death benefit and some reimbursement for burial expense.

Vocational rehabilitation. Rehabilitation is provided in all states even if unspecified by statute. Vocational and psychologic counseling or retraining and job placement assistance are typical benefits, with the goal of returning the injured worker to suitable, gainful employment.

Benefits from other sources

A number of benefits are available to workers from other sources.

Social Security Disability Insurance. Social Security Disability Insurance (SSDI) supplements workers' compensation with monthly benefits.

Table 2-1 Income benefits for total disability, 1993 (selected states and the federal government)

Jurisdiction	Percent of wages	Waiting period (days)	Retroactive period (days)	Maximum weekly payment (dollars)	Minimum weekly payment (dollars)	Time limit
Alabama	$66\frac{2}{3}$	3	21	400	110	Disability
California	$66\frac{2}{3}$	3	14	336	126	TT-Disability PT-Life
Colorado	$66\frac{2}{3}$	3	14	414		TT-Disability PT-Life
Hawaii	$66\frac{2}{3}$	3	10	460	115	Disability
Illinois	$66\frac{2}{3}$	3	14	670	TT-101 PT-251	TT-Disability PT-Life
New York	$66\frac{2}{3}$	7	14	400	40	Disability
North Carolina	$66\frac{2}{3}$	7	21	442	30	TT-Disability PT-Life
Pennsylvania	$66\frac{2}{3}$	7	14	475	158	Disability
Washington	60-75, depending on conjugal status	3	14	435	46	Disability
FECA	$66\frac{2}{3}$ or 75	0	0	1248	193	TT-Disability PT-Life

Table 2-2 Income benefits for scheduled injuries, 1993 (selected states and the federal government)

Jurisdiction	Arm at shoulder	Hand	Thumb	One eye	Hearing in one ear	Hearing in both ears
Alabama	$ 48,480	$ 37,400	$13,400	$ 27,280	$11,660	$ 35,860
California	62,345	46,028	7,595	22,311	6,335	46,028
Colorado	31,200	15,600	7,500	20,850	5,250	20,850
Hawaii	143,520	112,240	34,500	73,600	23,920	92,000
Illinois	157,800	127,325	46,909	100,520	33,507	134,026
New York	124,800	97,600	30,000	64,000	24,000	60,000
North Carolina	106,080	88,400	33,150	53,040	30,940	66,300
Pennsylvania	194,750	159,125	47,500	130,625	28,500	123,500
Washington	54,000	48,600	19,440	21,600	7,200	43,200
FECA	$389,651	$304,727	$93,666	$199,821	$64,942	$249,776

Such benefits are available only after a 5-month waiting period and are calculated as if the disabled individual had reached Social Security retirement age. To be considered disabled, the injured person must be unable to work in substantial gainful employment. Furthermore, the disability must be expected to last more than a year or to result in premature death. SSDI combined with workers' compensation cannot exceed 80% of the worker's average earnings or the total family benefit under Social Security before the injury. If this is the case, Social Security benefits are reduced accordingly, although some states reduce workers' compensation benefits by all or part of the Social Security payments.

Second injury funds. Second injury funds compensate workers for injuries that are exacerbated by a subsequent injury. Other states' second injury funds compensate workers for flare ups that do not necessarily lead to total disability. These funds are established and maintained by most states in the hope that the outcome will encourage employers to hire the handicapped. Payments are made for the second injury by the employer's compensation carrier, and the fund reimburses the carrier for the additional costs.

Employers' responsibilities

Employers are responsible for providing medical treatment and compensation benefits for employees injured at work or made ill from exposure to the workplace environment. The system is based on a premise of liability without fault; that is, regardless of whether the worker, the employer, or neither is at fault, the employer is responsible for providing medical treatment and compensation benefits to the injured employee.

Workers' compensation insurance coverage is compulsory for most private employment except in New Jersey, South Carolina, and Texas. In those states employers may decline coverage, but if so

they lose the customary common law defenses against suits filed by employees (the "exclusive remedy" is the quid pro quo under which the employer enjoys tort immunity in exchange for accepting absolute liability for all work-connected injuries). Employees most likely to be exempted from coverage include domestic workers, agricultural workers, and casual laborers. Coverage is also incomplete among workers in companies having fewer than six (varies by state) employees, nonprofit institutions, and state and local governments. About 87% of wage and salary workers are covered in accordance with prevailing law.[9]

Unless exempted by the law, employers must demonstrate their ability to pay workers' compensation benefits. There are three ways of accomplishing this: insurance with a state fund, insurance through a private carrier, or self-insurance.

State insurance funds. The states have adopted two methods of meeting the problem of workers' compensation coverage. Some states require that employers insure through a state fund which operates as the exclusive provider of insurance. Other states operate their funds in competition with private carriers. A few states do not permit an employer to be self-insured.

Private insurance carriers. Private workers' compensation insurance contracts have two purposes: satisfying the employer's obligation to pay compensation and ensuring that the injured employee receives all the benefits provided by law. Once the contract is signed, the insurer is responsible for compensating the injured worker. The carrier's liability is not relieved by the insolvency or death of the employer or by any argument the carrier may have against the employer. Most state funds are similarly restricted.

Self-insurance. Large employers may decide to serve as their own insurers. This approach includes the responsibility for adjusting claims and paying benefits, although it is possible to contract these tasks out to companies that provide such services. To qualify as a self-insurer, a company must demonstrate that it has the financial ability to pay all claims that may reasonably be expected. The state agency requires that a bond or other security be posted. Since this form of insurance is time consuming to administer and requires financial reserves, smaller companies can seldom self-insure.

Companies choose to self-fund their insurance to reduce costs and maximize cash flows. Since costs of benefits, claim reserves, litigation, and administration have spiraled in recent years, many companies have concluded that they could do as well as independent carriers while saving the cost of commissions, and as a result they would enjoy greater cash flow and increased income from investments. Self-insured employers are more likely to contest injury and illness claims than are privately insured employers and state insurance funds. This tendency to litigate may erase some of the cost savings made possible by self-insurance.

Penalties for not having insurance. Employers often fail to provide workers' compensation insurance coverage for their employees. The cost of even one serious injury can erase a company's entire annual profit or even bankrupt it. Consequently, all but three states have made workers' compensation insurance mandatory. Otherwise, a company could be out of business before a seriously injured employee is fully recovered.

There are heavy penalties for uninsured employers. They can be subject to fines, loss of common-law defenses, increases in the benefits awarded, and payment of attorneys' fees. The biggest deterrent is suit at common law. A number of states will force closure of an uninsured business. All states have established uninsured employer's funds to which the injured employee can apply for benefits. Applying to such a fund does not preclude the individual from bringing action against the employer for penalties and legal fees. The uninsured employer may also be required to reimburse the fund for benefits paid to the injured worker.

The cost of workers' compensation insurance is rate adjusted for all but the smallest employers—a process known as experience rating. When fewer injuries and illnesses occur, the employer profits from lowered workers' compensation insurance costs. Experience modification provides an automatic financial incentive for employers to provide their employees a work environment free from hazards that may result in compensation claims. There are conflicting economic studies on the value of experience rating and numerous problems in the interpretation of available data.[3] Nonetheless, it is a hallowed provision of workers' compensation systems. Most large employers are experience rated, whereas small employers are typically insured in groups of similar companies.

COST OF WORKERS' COMPENSATION

Approximately 93.7 million wage and salary workers were covered under the state and federal workers' compensation programs in 1989 (the last year to undergo fiscal review by the federal government). Cash payments totaled $34.3 billion in 1989, and total cost to employers reached $48.0 billion.[9] Of the $34.3 billion in benefits paid in 1989, approximately $20.9 billion was paid as compensation for lost wages and $13.4 was paid for medical expenses (Table 2-3). In the past decade, total workers' compensation benefits increased by an average of 11.1% annually. The 1989 cost to employers through state workers' compensation programs was $336.85 per insured employee. The comparable cost to taxpayers for workers' compensation for federal employees under FECA was $417.62. The expanded benefits under the Black Lung program are even more inflationary.

About three fourths of compensable claims for workers' compensation benefits and one fourth of cash payment benefits involve temporary total disability. Permanent total disability occurs in less than 1% of compensable workers' compensation claims. Medical care costs were 7.7% above the

Table 2-3 Estimated workers' compensation benefit payment amounts (in millions), by type of benefit, 1987-1989

Type of benefit	1987	1988	1989
Medical and hospitalization	$ 9,912	$11,518	$13,424
Compensation	17,406	19,215	20,892
Disability	15,775	17,613	19,171
Survivor	1,631	1,602	1,721
Regular programs, total	25,773	29,234	32,837
Medical and hospitalization	9,794	11,401	13,299
Compensation	15,979	17,833	19,538
Disability	15,046	16,956	18,553
Survivor	933	877	985
Black Lung program, total	1,545	1,499	1,479
Medical and hospitalization	118	117	125
Compensation	1,426	1,381	1,354
Disability	698	657	618
Survivor	729	725	736
TOTAL	$27,318	$30,733	$34,316

From *Social Security Bulletin,* vol. 55, no. 1, Spring 1992.

1988 figure. In 1989, about three fifths of all benefits paid were in cash compensation and about two fifths were in medical and hospitalization benefits.

The frequency and extent of work-related disability also exert a major influence on benefit levels. Expressed as a rate per 100 full-time equivalent workers (working 40 hours a week, 50 weeks a year), the rate for 1989 remained at the 1988 rate of 8.6. In 1989, the number of workdays lost per lost-workday case was 19.6, compared with 19.1 in 1988 and 16.5 in 1980.[2]

In 1989, $19.9 billion of the $34.3 billion in benefits was paid through private insurance carriers, $8 billion through public funds (including $1.5 billion in benefits under the federal Black Lung benefits program), and $6.4 billion through self-insurance.[9] During the 1980s, benefit levels roughly tripled, with the greatest percentage gains occurring in self-insurance and private carrier payments (Table 2-4).

State and federal funds and self-insured employers each pay about one fifth of all regular benefits, whereas private insurance companies pay the remaining three fifths. The percentage paid by private insurance companies has remained about the same over the past 25 years, that paid by publicly operated funds decreased from 26% to 20% in the same time period, and the proportion paid by self-insurance increased from 12% to 20%.

The total costs to employers include the expenses of policy writing, claims investigation and adjustment, allocation to reserves to match increases in accrued liabilities, payroll auditing, and

other administrative expenses and profit. The 1989 costs to employers covered $31.9 billion in premiums paid to private carriers, $9.2 billion in premiums paid to state funds and for federal programs, and $6.9 billion in self-insurance costs—benefits paid by self-insurers plus an estimate of administrative costs.

Although covered payrolls increased less than 6% from 1988 to 1989, employer costs increased at nearly twice that rate. This difference resulted in an increase in the ratio of costs per $100 of covered payroll from $2.16 in 1988 to $2.27 in 1989. This was the fifth consecutive increase in the cost ratio following four consecutive declines. In 1984 the ratio stood at $1.66.[9]

The relationship of benefits to employer costs is one measure of the effectiveness of workers' compensation programs in providing income maintenance protection to disabled workers. When benefits financed through general revenues are excluded, the benefits/costs relationship was at a low of 54% in 1980; since 1982 it has moved in a narrow range of 67% to 71% as benefits and employer costs have increased at similar rates. In 1989 the figure was at 69.6%, indicating that nearly 70 cents of every premium dollar was returned to the worker or his or her survivors as benefit payments or medical care reimbursements.

ROLE OF THE OCCUPATIONAL HEALTH PROFESSIONAL

Employers are required to provide medical treatment as well as compensation benefits. The in-

Table 2-4 Percentage change in workers' compensation benefit payment amounts by type of insurer, 1979-1989

| Period | Total workers' compensation program | | Type of insurer (in current dollars) | | | |
| | Constant dollars | Current dollars | Private insurers | State and federal funds* | | Self-insurers |
				Total	Regular	
1979-80	2.2	13.2	14.2	7.7	12.2	22.2
1980-81	1.2	10.5	12.1	6.1	10.4	14.3
1981-82	3.1	9.0	9.8	3.8	8.4	15.8
1982-83	2.9	7.1	7.2	6.1	8.7	8.6
1983-84	7.9	12.0	14.5	6.8	11.7	13.0
1984-85	9.3	12.9	16.3	6.3	10.0	12.0
1985-86	8.2	10.9	12.0	8.8	12.7	10.4
1986-87	6.1	11.1	11.8	8.6	12.3	12.7
1987-88	8.3	12.4	13.3	10.2	14.1	13.2
1988-89	6.8	11.7	13.7	6.5	8.5	12.0
Average annual increase	5.6	11.1	12.5	7.4	10.8	13.3

From *Social Security Bulletin,* vol. 55, no. 1, Spring 1992.
* Excludes Black Lung benefits.

jured or ill employee is required to report the injury or illness as soon as possible. Typically a statute of limitations limits the employer's liability when an injury or illness is not promptly reported. The reporting requirement is met if the employer is informed by someone other than the injured individual. The employer must then provide all medical care reasonably required to alleviate the problem. In fact, the law allows for treatment even when recovery is not possible, that is, for palliative care that does not cure but only relieves.

Most states have no statutory limitations on the length of time or the cost of treatment, although a number of cost containment strategies are now being implemented by states and private insurers. These include (1) utilization review of inpatient and outpatient care, (2) hospital bill auditing of inpatient services, (3) medical bill auditing of practitioner and other services, and (4) preferred provider networks for inpatient and outpatient care.[8,10] In some jurisdictions authorities are considering the disallowance of services provided by physicians who own facilities where patients are referred for testing or treatment. A recent study of self-referral practices demonstrated that physical therapy was initiated 2.3 times more often than when the physician did not have a similar financial incentive. Psychiatric referral costs were 26.3% higher among self-referral physicians, and MRI scans were much more likely to be medically inappropriate under the same circumstances.[12,14]

Health professionals are involved in many of the required activities of workers' compensation systems, because medical treatment requires the services of physicians and nurses and frequently that of physical therapists. Hospitalization, medicines, prosthetic appliances, and surgical supplies are all paid for by workers' compensation. Many states also allow treatment by licensed psychologists, dentists, optometrists, podiatrists, osteopaths, and chiropractors. Some states even permit treatment by acupuncturists, naturopaths, and Christian Science practitioners.

Workers' compensation regulations in many states allow workers to choose their own physicians. They may be able to choose any licensed physician or may be limited to a list maintained by the employer or the state workers' compensation agency. Regardless of how the physician is chosen, the worker must submit to periodic examinations by a physician of the employer's choice. If either the employer or the worker is dissatisfied with the progress of treatment, she can ask for a new physician. Typically an employee is permitted one such change for subjective reasons alone. In contrast, the employer can be required to prove to the state agency that a change is needed. Reasons for discharging a physician include lack of reasonable progress toward recovery, inadequate or insufficient reporting by the physician, or inconvenience of the physician's practice location. If the employer selects the physician, an employee who is not satisfied with the treatment and progress may be permitted consultation with another physician at the employer's expense.

Although the employer must provide medical treatment for the injured employee, if the employee refuses reasonable treatment or surgery without justifiable cause, the employer is relieved of responsibility for any benefits related to injuries caused by the delay in or refusal of treatment. When the suggested treatment or surgery entails a significant risk, the worker's refusal is usually considered justified.

When a compensation case results in litigation, occupational health professionals become important witnesses in settling disputes.

Claims disputes

Differences of opinion often arise over workers' compensation claims. Such disputes often result from issues of insurance coverage, work relatedness of the injury or illness, provision of medical treatment, the worker's earning capacity, and the extent of the disability. The last is the most common cause of disputes necessitating a physician's expert opinion. Although the system was designed to be self-administering, many claims are subject to disputes among the employer, the insurance carrier, and the worker. Because adjudication is cumbersome, costly, and time consuming, tribunals have been established to hear claims disputes as quickly and inexpensively as possible.

In most states the worker initiates a claim and the insurer conducts the initial review. When the two parties disagree on the result, either can apply for a hearing before the workers' compensation agency. If dissatisfaction with the hearing officer's decision remains, an appeal can be made.

The states vary widely in their methods of hearing disputes, but the most commonly used methods are (1) a court-administered system, (2) a wholly administrative system, and (3) a combination of the two. The last is rapidly becoming almost as unwieldy as the common-law approach it was designed to replace.

Court-administered system

The court-administered system is closest to common-law procedure and is based on the hypothesis that the parties in a dispute are more likely to receive justice from a court than from a referee or commission.

In a court-administered system the employer may be covered either by a carrier or by self-insurance. A report of any injury or illness resulting in more than 6 days of disability must be filed within 14 days, usually accompanied by a physician's report. (Time periods, exact procedures, fee percentages, and so on are drawn from one state for the purposes of example.) The state's department of labor, through its workers' compensation division, decides whether the worker should receive compensation other than medical treatment. A form letter is then sent to the worker informing him or her of rights in case additional benefits are decided upon. Unless there is a complaint, the compensation agency takes no further action to ensure prompt payment, but the carrier must file notice when the claim is first paid. Under the system a settlement agreement must be filed even if the worker refuses to sign it. A trial court reviews that agreement to determine whether the worker is receiving his or her just benefits. If so, the agreement is approved and payments are made accordingly.

The employer has 10 days thereafter to file with the division certified copies of all relevant documents from the worker's file. If the division decides that the agreement does not provide sufficient benefits to the worker, the insurance carrier is required to adjust the agreement and have the court order modified. If the carrier refuses, the division advises the worker to take court action. Once a settlement has been approved by the court, it is binding on all parties if not contested within 30 days. However, the worker may go to trial court to contest the settlement at any time within 1 year of the injury. Compensation cases receive priority and are usually completed within 10 weeks. The case is heard by a trial judge and may be appealed to a circuit court and even to the state supreme court if the judge's finding is unacceptable to the worker. The attorney may receive 20% of the award for his or her services.

Wholly administrative system. Under a wholly administrative system the workers' compensation board pays benefits from assessments made against covered employers on the basis of payroll. Injuries must be reported as soon as possible, and benefits or the denial of benefits is determined by a claims adjudicator of a board located closest to the worker's home (again, using one state's system as an example). If the claim is denied, the worker is informed of the reason for denial and how to appeal. Either the government, without charge, or the worker's union assists in the appeal. Judgments can be appealed, in turn, to a board of review in all cases except those related to a rehabilitation decision.

The review boards are part of the state's department of labor but are totally dissociated from the workers' compensation division. They consist of a chairman and two members, one chosen by an employers' group and the other by an organization of workers (in this state's example).

The claimant must make an appeal within 90 days after the claims adjudicator's report has been received. The appeal may be in the form of a letter stating the claimant's objections, or it may be submitted on a two-page form used for that purpose. The review board studies the workers' compensation board file and any new information the board obtains in the course of its decision making. No hearing on the matter is conducted unless the claimant requests it, and such a request will be denied if the board decides that an appeal is not justified. If the board agrees to a hearing, it is held at a location most convenient for the worker. The worker may have an attorney, but the appeals process does not include payment of the attorney's fees, which is the responsibility of the worker.

Although the review board's decision is usually binding, it can be appealed to the commissioners of the workers' compensation board within 60 days by a labor union on behalf of the injured worker or by an organization of employers on behalf of the injured worker or employer. If the chairman of the review board believes that an important principle underlies the appeal, he or she may allow the worker to make an appeal within 30 days. Furthermore, if the decision of the review board is not unanimous, the worker is permitted to appeal to the commissioners on his or her own behalf within 60 days. The decision of the commissioners is binding and may not be appealed to the courts.

A medical review panel exists for purely medical issues. This panel consist of a chairman appointed by the government and two physicians, one selected by the worker and one by the employer. Decisions by this panel are final. Many states sponsor less formal panels of physicians who interview and examine the claimant, then render an opinion on disability, work restrictions, treatment, and prognosis.

Combination system. The worker's compensation agency under the combination system consists of a seven-member appeals board that is responsible only for reviewing appeals and an administrative director who is responsible for the agency's administrative functions. In California, for example, eight individuals are appointed by the governor and confirmed by the state senate.

First reports of worker injury or illness must be filed with the state's division of labor statistics and research by both the employer and the attending physician. They are usually submitted through the employer's compensation carrier or adjusting agent and constitute the initiation of a claim. Furthermore, within 5 days of the injury the employer must inform the injured worker in simple terms not only about the benefits to which she is entitled but also about the services available from the state's division of workers' compensation. The employer is further required to inform the compensation system administrator, as well as the worker, about commencement and termination dates of benefits, nonpayment of benefits, or rejection of claims. The worker must also be informed that he or she can obtain an attorney if desired. The worker must further be advised that any action must be taken promptly to avoid loss of compensation.

Thus the worker is informed of his or her rights, and, because penalties exist for the unwarranted rejection of compensation, most claims are paid automatically. The division of workers' compensation becomes involved only if either the employer or the employee seeks adjudication from the workers' compensation appeals board. Such adjudication is initiated by the filing of a simple one-page form. The application must be filed within a year of the injury or by the date of the termination of benefits, whichever is longer. If the adjudication claim is related to further trauma resulting from the original injury, the application requirement is 5 years from the date of the original injury.

Although under the system a hearing should be held within 30 days after the application, which is seldom possible because of backlog. The hearings are conducted at several locations throughout the state and are assigned to a workers' compensation judge who makes the decision. Usually, each judge reviews about 90 cases a month.

The hearings are designed to be informal, but often they cannot be distinguished from a nonjury court trial. The judges are knowledgeable in the workers' compensation process and are required to seek additional information if the evidence provided by the parties is inadequate. Medical information is usually presented in written reports. Once all the evidence is presented, the judge must present a written decision within 30 days.

If the employer or the employee is unhappy with the decision, he or she may file an appeal. This appeal, called a petition for reconsideration, must be filed within 20 days of the posting of the original decision. It is heard by a panel of three members of the appeals board. The panel is authorized to approve or deny reconsideration, issue a different decision on the original evidence, or seek additional information, including consultation with an independent medical specialist.

The decision of the panel is final unless the dissatisfied party seeks a review by an appellate court within 45 days by submitting a petition for a writ of review to the appeals court. The court is empowered to deny the review without explanation. If a review is permitted, the appeals court studies the evidence, hears oral arguments, and presents a written decision. If the party bringing the appeal is still dissatisfied, he or she may petition the state supreme court for a further hearing. However, the supreme court rarely accepts more than a few workers' compensation cases each year.

In the great majority of contested cases both parties are represented either by attorneys or by expert lay representatives. On average, those representing the worker receive 9% to 15% of the award.

Reopening of claims

Workers' compensation proceedings differ from civil lawsuits in one important aspect—the body that originally decided the award may alter its decision if the worker's condition changes or other reasonable cause exists. This process may be limited under certain conditions by state compensation laws, and most states establish a time limit beyond which a modification cannot be made. If the requirements of the law cannot be met, final decisions in compensating cases are as binding as those in any judicial proceeding.

Benefit amounts, compensable conditions, processing of claims, settlement of disputes, and general economics of each system vary widely among states. Consequently, physicians who expect to be treating occupational injuries and illnesses are well advised to learn how the workers' compensation system operates in the state in which they are practicing. A list of the workers' compensation agencies that provide information on reporting guidelines, required forms, and many other services to health care professionals is found on pages 22 through 24 and again in Appendix B. Much of the following discussion of report writing is taken from Guidelines for Medical Examination and Report issued by the California Division of Workers' Compensation. Other states have similar helpful publications.

Medical judgment is necessary to the proper settlement of many workers' compensation cases. The physician evaluates the degree of "impairment" (measured by anatomic or functional loss) and supplies an opinion to workers' compensation judges, commissioners, or hearing officers. These nonmedical people make the decision as to "disability." It is important to discuss impairment and disability separately. Disability, unlike impairment, depends on the job. For example, the loss of

DIRECTORY OF WORKERS' COMPENSATION ADMINISTRATORS

Alabama

Workmen's Compensation Division, Department of Industrial Relations, Industrial Relations Building, Montgomery, AL 36131. (205) 242-2868.

Alaska

Workers' Compensation Division, Dept. of Labor, P.O. Box 25512, Juneau, AK 99802. (907) 465-2790.

Arizona

Industrial Commission, 800 West Washington, P.O. Box 19070, Phoenix, AZ 85007. (602) 542-4661.

Arkansas

Workers' Compensation Commission, 625 Marshal St., Justice Building, State Capitol Grounds, Little Rock, AR 72201. (501) 682-3930.

California

Division of Workers' Compensation, P.O. Box 420603, San Francisco, CA 94102. (415) 703-3731.

Colorado

Workers' Compensation Section, Division of Labor, 1120 Lincoln, #1401, Denver, CO 80203. (303) 764-2929.

Connecticut

Workers' Compensation Commission, 1890 Dixwell Ave., Hamden, CT 06514. (203) 789-7783.

Delaware

Industrial Accident Board, State Office Building, 6th Floor, 820 North French St., Wilmington, DE 19801. (302) 577-2884.

District of Columbia

Dept. of Employment Services, Office of Workers' Compensation, P.O. Box 56098, Washington, DC 20011. (202) 576-6265.

Florida

Division of Workers' Compensation, Dept. of Labor and Employment Security, 2728 Centerview Dr., Ste. 301, Forest Bldg., Tallahassee, FL 32399-0680. (904) 488-2514.

Georgia

Board of Workers' Compensation, South Tower, Ste. 1000, One CNN Ctr., Atlanta, GA 30303-2788. (404) 656-3875.

Guam

Workers' Compensation Commission, Dept. of Labor, Govt. of Guam, P.O. Box 9970, Tamuning, GU 96911. 8-011-671-647-4222.

Hawaii

Disability Compensation Commission, Dept. of Labor & Industrial Relations, 830 Punchbowl St., Rm. 209, Honolulu, HI 96813. (808) 586-9200.

Idaho

Industrial Commission, 317 Main St., Boise, ID 83720. (208) 334-6000.

Illinois

Industrial Commission, 100 W. Randolph St., Ste. 8-200, Chicago, IL 60601. (312) 814-6500.

Indiana

Workers' Compensation Board, 402 W. Washington St., Rm. W196, Indianapolis, IN 46204. (317) 232-3808.

Iowa

Div. of Industrial Services, Dept. of Employment Services, 1000 E. Grand Ave., Des Moines, IA 50319. (515) 281-5934.

Kansas

Division of Workers' Compensation, 800 SW Jackson, Ste. 600, Topeka, KS 66612-1227. (913) 296-3441.

Kentucky

Dept. of Workers' Compensation, Perimeter Park Width, 1270 Louisville, Bldg. C, Frankfort, KY 40601. (502) 564-5550.

Louisiana

Dept. of Labor, Office of Workers' Compensation Administration, P.O. Box 94040, Baton Rouge, LA 70804-9040. (504) 342-7555.

Maine

Workers' Compensation Board, State House Station 27, Deering Bldg., Augusta, ME 04333. (207) 289-3751.

Maryland

Workers' Compensation Commission, 6 N. Liberty, Baltimore, MD 21201. (410) 333-4700.

Massachusetts

Dept. of Industrial Accidents, 600 Washington St., 7th Flr., Boston, MA 02111. (617) 727-4300.

Michigan

Bureau of Workers' Disability Comp., Dept. of Labor, P.O. Box 30016, Lansing, MI 48909. (517) 373-3480.

Minnesota

Workers' Compensation Division, Dept. of Labor & Industry, 443 Lafayette Rd., St. Paul, MN 55155. (612) 296-6107.

Mississippi

Workers' Compensation Commission, 1428 Lakeland Drive, P.O. Box 5300, Jackson, MS 39296-5300. (601) 987-4200.

DIRECTORY OF WORKERS' COMPENSATION ADMINISTRATORS   *(Continued)*

Missouri

Division of Workers' Compensation, Dept. of Labor & Industrial Relations, P.O. Box 58, Jefferson City, MO 65102. (314) 751-4231.

Montana

State Compensation Mutual Insurance Fund, P.O. Box 4759, Helena, MT 59604. (406) 444-6518.

Nebraska

Workers' Compensation Court, State House, 13th Flr., Lincoln, NE 68509. (402) 471-2568.

Nevada

State Industrial Insurance System, 515 East Musser St., Carson City, NV 89714. (702) 687-5220.

New Hampshire

Dept. of Labor, 95 Pleasant St., Concord, NH 03301. (603) 271-3171.

New Jersey

Division of Workers' Compensation, Dept. of Labor, Call Number 381, Trenton, NJ 08625. (609) 292-2414.

New Mexico

Workers' Compensation Division, Dept. of Labor, 481 Broadway NE, Albuquerque, NM 87103. (505) 841-8600.

New York

Workers' Compensation Board, 180 Livingston St., Brooklyn, NY 11248. (718) 802-6600.

North Carolina

Industrial Commission, Dobbs Bldg., 430 North Salisbury St., Raleigh, NC 27611. (919) 733-4820.

North Dakota

Workers' Compensation Bureau, Russell Bldg., Highway 83 North, 4007 North State St., Bismarck, ND 58501. (701) 224-3800.

Ohio

Bureau of Workers' Compensation, 30 West Spring St., Columbus, OH 43266-0581. (614) 466-2950.

Oklahoma

Oklahoma Workers' Compensation Court, 1915 North Stiles, Oklahoma City, OK 73105. (405) 557-7600.

Oregon

Dept. of Insurance and Finance, 21 Labor and Industries Bldg., Salem, OR 97310. (503) 378-4100.

Pennsylvania

Bureau of Workers' Compensation, Dept. of Labor and Industry, 1171 South Cameron St., Rm. #103, Harrisburg, PA 17104. (717) 783-5421.

Puerto Rico

Industrial Commissioner's Office, G.P.O. Box 4466, San Juan, PR 00936. (809) 783-2028.

Rhode Island

Dept. of Workers' Compensation, 610 Manton Ave., P.O. Box 3500, Providence, RI 02909. (401) 272-0700.

South Carolina

Workers' Compensation Commission, 1612 Marion Street, P.O. Box 1715, Columbia, SC 29202. (803) 737-5700.

South Dakota

Division of Labor and Mgmt., Dept. of Labor, Kneip Bldg., Third Flr., 700 Governors Dr., Pierre, SD 57501-2277. (605) 773-3681.

Tennessee

Workers' Compensation Division, Dept. of Labor, 501 Union Bldg., Second Flr., Nashville, TN 37243-0661. (615) 741-2395.

Texas

Texas Workers' Compensation Commission, 4000 South IH35, Austin, TX 78704. (512) 448-7900.

Utah

Industrial Commission, 160 East 300 South, Salt Lake City, UT 84111. (801) 530-6800.

Vermont

Dept. of Labor and Industry, National Life Bldg., Drawer 20, Montpelier, VT 05620-3401. (802) 828-2286.

Virgin Islands

Dept. of Labor, 2131 Hospital St., Christiansted, St. Croix, VI 0084-666. (809) 773-1994.

Virginia

Workers' Comp. Comm., 1000 DMV Bldg., Richmond, VA 23220. (804) 367-8600.

Washington

Dept. of Labor and Industries, P.O. Box 44001, Olympia, WA 98504. (206) 956-4213.

West Virginia

Workers' Compensation Commissioner's Office, P.O. Box 3151, Charleston, WV 25332. (304) 558-2580.

Wisconsin

Workers' Compensation Div., Dept. of Industry, Labor, and Human Relations, P.O. Box 7901, Rm. 162, 201 East Washington Ave., Madison, WI 53707. (608) 266-1340.

DIRECTORY OF WORKERS' COMPENSATION ADMINISTRATORS *(Continued)*

Wyoming

Workers' Compensation Div., 122 West 25th St., 2nd Flr., East Wing, Herschier Bldg., Cheyenne, WY 82002. (307) 777-7441.

United States

Dept. of Labor, Employment Standards Administration, Washington, DC 20210. (202) 219-6191.

Office of Workers' Compensation Programs. (202) 219-7503.

Division of Coal Mine Workers' Compensation. (202) 219-6692.

Division of Federal Employees' Compensation. (202) 219-7552.

Div. of Longshore & Harbor Workers' Compensation. (202) 219-8721.

Office of State Liaison and Legislative Analysis. (202) 219-4560.

Div. of State Workers' Comp. Programs. (202) 219-4560.

Benefits Review Board, Tech World Plaza, 5th Flr., 800 K. St., NW, Washington, DC 2001-8002. (202) 633-7500.

Alberta

Workers' Compensation Board, P.O. Box 2415, 9912 107th St., Edmonton, AB T5J 2S5. (403) 427-1131.

British Columbia

Workers' Compensation Board, 6951 Westminster Highway, Richmond, BC V7C 1C6. (604) 273-2266.

Manitoba

Workers' Comp. Board, 333 Maryland St., Winnipeg, MB R3C 1M2. (204) 786-5471.

New Brunswick

Workers' Compensation Board, 1 Portland, Saint John, NB E26 3X9. (506) 632-2200.

New Foundland

Workers' Compensation Commission, P.O. Box 9000, Station B, St. John's NF A1A 3B8. (709) 778-1000.

Northwest Territories

Workers' Comp. Board, P.O. Box 1390, Northwest Territories, Postal Code X1A 2L9. (403) 873-7745.

Nova Scotia

Workers' Compensation Board, 5668 South Street, P.O. Box 1150, Halifax, NS B3J 2Y2. (902) 424-8440.

Ontario

Workers' Compensation Board, 2 Bloor St. East, Toronto, ON M4W 3C3. (416) 927-9555.

Prince Edward Island

Workers' Compensation Board, 60 Belvedere Ave., P.O. Box 757, Charlottetown, PE C1A 7L7. (902) 368-5680.

Quebec

Commission de la Sante et de la Secuite du Travail, 524 Boudages St., Quebec, PQ G1K 7E2. (418) 643-5850.

Saskatchewan

Workers' Compensation Board, Suite 200, 1881 Scarth, SK S4P 4L1. (306) 787-4370.

Yukon Territory

Workers' Compensation Board, 401 Strickland St., Whitehorse, Yukon, Postal Code Y1A 5N8. (403) 667-5645.

Canada

Labour Canada, Federal Workers' Compensation Service, Ottawa, ON K1A OJ2. (613) 953-8001.

Merchant Seamen Compensaton Board, Labour Canada, Ottawa, ON K1A OJ2. (613) 997-2281.

---

the distal phalanx of the second digit on the left hand results in the same impairment rating in a concert violinist and a roofer, but the disability would be much greater for the musician. An individual with carpal tunnel syndrome may be disabled when considered for a job with repetitive hand movements, but not for a job that does not require extensive use of the hands.

Insurers frequently ask the physician to determine work restrictions (e.g., no overhead lifting for someone with shoulder problems, no working around moving machinery or at unprotected heights for someone with a balance problem) so that they can match abilities and disabilities to specific jobs. In some instances the exact physical restrictions are best determined by a functional capacity evaluation. A growing number of specialized centers can assist physicians with both detailed job requirement analyses and functional capacity evaluations. The insurer may authorize referral to such centers before the physician's evaluation of the employee.

Handicap, as defined in the Americans with Disabilities Act (ADA), is "an impairment that substantially limits one or more of life's activities" but also includes the individual who "has a record of such an impairment or is regarded as having such an impairment." Therefore an individual who has an abnormality on a preplacement "low back x-ray" and has been excluded from heavy lifting jobs because of the radiographic finding could be considered handicapped even though he or she has no symptoms or prior back problems and would have neither an impairment rating nor a disability.

Addressing the issue of employability is complex. Does the medical condition preclude traveling to and from work, being at work, or performing required essential functions of the job? Is the medical condition work related or not? Motivation is a factor in determining return to work status, but not for the purpose of determining employability.

When an impairment rating is requested, the examining physician should use the most current *AMA Guides to the Evaluation of Permanent Impairment.* This vital book defines impairment as "alteration of an individual's health status that is assessed by medical means."[1] Disability is "assessed by nonmedical means, and is an alteration of an individual's capacity to meet personal, social or occupational demands or statutory or regulatory requirements."[1]

Standards for disability evaluation can be found in the *AMA Guides to Evaluation of Permanent Impairment* and in schedules provided by the Social Security Administration and the Veterans Administration. Physicians who perform disability evaluations should make sure that they know which schedule is applicable in each case.

Written report

Physicians experienced in submitting current status and progress reports to employers and insurance companies should expand their experience to the reporting of definitive medical evaluations. All physicians should develop the experience and confidence to be workers' compensation medical examiners. The physician should understand exactly what the requesting party wants to know. Copies of all relevant medical records, reports, and test results should be obtained and reviewed completely. In a workers' compensation case the patient will probably see reports written by the physician. All details should be presented in unambiguous terms and in appropriate detail. Use of abbreviations and other timesavers is not appropriate in this form of medical record. Technical terms should be explained for the benefit of nonmedical readers. The history of the injury or exposure to toxic materials at work should be detailed, and the activities of the job should be completely and carefully described. All historical information should be obtained by

the physician and not by office personnel. The history should also include information about all previous employment and all nonwork activities, with particular attention to factors that might be related to the present complaints. An example often occurs in claims of toxic exposure where the claimant has a cognitive deficit corroborated by neuropsychologic testing. In such a case the individual may have had preexisting problems resulting from head injury, hypoxia at birth, or another cause, and a review of school records and previous medical history may be necessary.

In obtaining the occupational history, physicians may need information not contained in the medical file. This may be requested from the workers' compensation judge or the appropriate governmental agency, such as the state's division of industrial accidents. Additional medical reports and other evidence can often be obtained by nonmedical officials for the physician's use. The physician may need to talk with the claimant's family and with coworkers and friends. The history should be comprehensive but succinct. It is important to mention any preexisting condition that limited the ability to work or to compete in the job market, including work limitations or preclusions imposed by a physician. In the case of an injured employee reporting a back injury, for example, the physician should determine exactly what the person has done throughout his or her career that might affect the back. The job title is less useful information than a detailed description of the work activity and its duration. In a case of hearing loss, a description of noise levels in the work environment might be needed to support an opinion that the disability was probably the result of the claimed injury. Some toxic agents have long latent periods, and it may be necessary to go back 25 or 30 years in taking the history. Formal job descriptions are often available and can be useful in documenting the occupational history.

Differences among the histories obtained by various physicians should be noted and explained. The reports reviewed should be listed and summarized so the reader acknowledges having read them. The injured employee's complaints and symptoms should also be listed. Many examiners find it convenient simply to quote these verbatim, without comment.

History of the illness or injury should mention all preexisting conditions. Be precise about temporal relationships between work and the injury or between exposures and the illness. Describe other coworkers involved in both injuries and illnesses. The medical history should include relevant previous as well as concurrent conditions. List medications required by these conditions. The Social and

Family History should always include information on use of alcohol, cigarettes, and family history of problems when relevant. In the occupational history, do not ramble on with long paragraphs but rather attempt to summarize all jobs chronologically and the illnesses and injuries incurred with each. Workers' compensation claims and settlements data can be obtained by the requesting party. In some instances, historical data on major medical insurance utilization may be needed as well. Discuss required activities in the last job, including hours worked, shift work or other assignments that might have caused excessive fatigue or a circadian desynchronosis, changes in work routine that might interfere with safety and hygiene practices, and chemical and other toxic exposures in great detail. If industrial hygiene measurements are available to determine dose of exposure, these are vital to the evaluation of the employee. In the review of systems, list pertinent positives and negatives without resorting to long lists.

The physical examination requires precise, objective measurements of joint motion and any other objective signs of impairment. The ultimate rating of disability will reflect the findings more exactly if nonmedical raters are presented with readily understandable terms. If the uninjured limb to which the injured limb is being compared is itself not normal, an estimated range of normal value should be used.

In some cases the injured worker may not be making a maximal effort with, for example, a grip strength measurement. Explain the reasons for the lack of maximal effort and note the estimate of the actual grip strength. Report the loss of grip strength (for example, pain, limited joint motion, nerve injury, lack of maximal effort, etc.). Then, record an estimate of the disability percentage for each different factor.

Differential diagnosis should not be included in the report. References, unless they are critical to your conclusions, should not be cited. The total time spent with the patient should be stated.

When stating the diagnosis, the opinions should be logically and adequately conveyed by the following:

1. Summarize the case without engaging in extensive discussion of details. What is the relation between the condition(s) found and the claimed injury or occupational exposure? In this and in other answers give reasons for the opinion and be as definite as possible. "Possibly" and "maybe" are not helpful terms. "Probably," meaning a 51% or better chance that something is so, is a good word to use if it applies. If the condition found would not exist *except for* the occupational injury or exposure, (even though nonoccupational factors may have played a part) the occupational injury or exposure will be considered the cause of the condition. Nonetheless, the physician should not attempt to make legal determinations, as by saying, "Disability is due to an industrial injury"; "Disability is the result of the injury described occurring on January 10, 1993," is a more appropriate statement.

2. During what periods of time was the injured employee unable to work as a result of the medical conditions you have found? Temporary disability requires careful attention to questions of when and how long.

3. Is the condition(s) "permanent and stationary" and on what date did it become so? A practical working definition of permanent and stationary is "the condition is not going to get significantly better or worse with further medical treatment." In some states, a person has reached "permanent and stationary" or "maximum medical improvement" if symptoms have been stable for 6 months, and additional therapy will not significantly change the impairment rating. If not permanent and stationary, when will the condition become so? What medical treatment(s) and anticipated benefits are recommended?

4. Is there permanent disability now? "Disability" means anything that reduces earning capacity, such as impairment of normal use of a limb or eye, or that may be a competitive handicap in the open labor market. "Disability" may include subjective factors, such as pain that impairs ability to work, or objective factors, such as limitation of joint motion, or both. "Disability" may include work preclusion as well. Psychiatric factors must also be considered. Many states will provide physicians with their guidelines for general medical and psychiatric assessments.

5. Summarize the factors of disability, listing subjective symptoms and objective losses and limitations. In California, disabling symptoms such as pain should be referred to as "minimal," "slight" "moderate," or "severe," which are defined as follows:

"Minimal pain" constitutes an annoyance but causes no handicap in the performance of the particular employment activity.

"Slight pain" can be tolerated but would cause some handicap in the performance of the employment activity precipitating the pain.

"Moderate pain" can be tolerated but would cause marked handicap in the performance of the employment activity precipitating the pain.

"Severe pain" would preclude the employment activity precipitating the pain.

Some other words often have special meaning. In California, "occasional" means 25 percent of the time, "intermittent" means 50 percent of the time, "frequent" means 75 percent of the time, and "constant" means 100 percent of the time. In giving an opinion, do not use the words "guess" or "speculate". Instead, say "Based on my experience, my opinion is. . . ." Remember, the physician is the expert.

6. State preclusion from certain jobs or work in certain areas in exact terms. If the injured employee *should not* do certain things at work, this should be reported in the same way as if the worker *cannot*.

7. Some jurisdictions request the physician to determine apportionment. Apportionment applies only to permanent disability. The examining physician does not apportion causation, disease, or pathology. The person being examined may have disability other than that resulting from the work injury. There may be disability resulting from congenital defects, previous work or nonwork injuries, aging, or the natural progression of preexisting nondisabling conditions. When physicians attempt to apportion responsibility for disability between employers or between work-related and non–work-related causes, there is a relatively simple way to do it that avoids legal complications.

The physician should write two paragraphs, the first describing the existing disability factors (objective and subjective) and work restrictions, and the second describing the disability factors and work restrictions that would exist in the absence of the occupational injury. The hearing officer can then decide the extent of the disability represented by each of the paragraphs and, by subtraction, can decide the disability for which the employer is responsible. The physician should not attempt to figure out the percentage of disability represented by either of the paragraphs. The judge and trained raters will do this.

8. Medical treatment is an important consideration. Many workers' compensation cases are settled with "continuing medical treatment" provided as a lifelong benefit. The opinion as to the value of continued medical treatment and for what purpose it is rendered should be stated, along with recommendations for treatment if different from treatment already provided by other physicians.

9. Vocational rehabilitation may be recommended for employees who cannot return to their former job. Unless experienced in vocational rehabilitation, the physician should limit comments on this subject to identifying the worker's possible need for rehabilitation services. It should be left to vocational rehabilitation specialists to determine whether the worker will benefit from such services. If conclusions about the extent of disability have been stated clearly, experts on the physical requirements of various occupations will be able to make an appropriate decision regarding rehabilitation.

LEGISLATIVE REFORM

Many health policy experts consider the workers' compensation insurance system to be one of the most dysfunctional elements of the U.S. health care system. In the current climate of health care reform the goal of almost all legislative proposals is to extend health care coverage to all citizens. Thus an increasing number of "single-payer" legislative approaches include medical coverage for occupational injuries and illnesses in their national health insurance schemes. The "24-hour medical coverage" proposal defines an insurance system that combines the health care benefits under workers' compensation and group health insurance through coordinated claims management or through the development of a comprehensive insurance package. Legislation in this direction has been introduced in Florida, California, Alaska, and Oregon.[4]

When public and private health insurance plans are integrated to cover medical expenses for occupational injuries and illnesses, workers' access to care will be enhanced, administrative costs will be decreased, and the problem of cost shifting will be corrected. Cost shifting occurs when health care providers bill a nonworkers' compensation payer for the care of an occupational injury or illness because they want to receive a payment rate higher than workers' compensation payers provide. Regardless of what reform proposal is ultimately enacted, the workers' compensation insurance system will be needed to provide nonmedical benefits. Medical costs reflected in rate modification will no longer give the employer an incentive to provide health and safety in the workplace. This loss would require some new form of cost incentive for employers. Expanded payments of scheduled injury benefits that reflect the employer's injury and illness experience has been advanced as an alternative. Employer disability insurance is another concept being discussed.

Because the number of uninsured workers in the United States is increasing, the legislative proposals discussed here are likely to increase the costs of health insurance. Cost increases may be mitigated by savings resulting from increased efficiency and decreased administrative costs. However, the same powerful forces that seek to continue the current U.S. health care system will be at work to maintain the workers' compensation insurance system with as few fundamental changes as politically possible.

REFERENCES

1. American Medical Association: *AMA guides to the evaluation of permanent impairment,* ed 3 rev, Chicago, 1990, The Association.
2. Bureau of Labor Statistics, *Occupational injuries and illnesses in the United States by industry, 1989,* U.S. Department of Labor, 1991.
3. Ehrenberg RG: Workers' compensation wages, and the risk of injury. In Burton JF, editor: *New perspectives in workers' compensation,* Ithaca, NY, 1988, ILR Press.
4. Himmelstein J: *Workers' compensation insurance: integration with HealthAmerica,* background document prepared for Senator Edward M. Kennedy, 1993.
5. LaDou J: Cumulative injury in workers' compensation, *Occup Med: State of the Art Rev* 3(4):611-619, 1988.
6. LaDou J: The occupational medicine consultant, *Am J Ind Med* 19:257-266, 1991.
7. Larson A: Tensions on the next decade. In Burton JF, editor: *New perspectives in workers' compensation,* Ithaca, NY, 1988, ILR Press.
8. Managed care comes to workers' compensation, *Business and Health* 10:320-339, 1992.
9. Nelson WJ: Workers' compensation: coverage, benefits, and costs, 1989, *Social Security Bulletin* 55(1):51, 1992.
10. Nethercut GE: Controlling workers' compensation medical costs, *The Risk Report* XIII(3):1, 1990.
11. Olsen DA: CEOs can reform workers' comp, *The New York Times,* January 3, 1993.
12. Relman AS: "Self-referral"-what's at stake? *N Engl J Med* 327(21):1522-1524, 1992.
13. US Chamber of Commerce: *Analysis of workers' compensation laws-1993 edition,* Washington, DC, 1993, The Chamber.
14. Swedlow A, Johnson G, Smithline N, Milstein A: Increased costs and rates of use in the California workers' compensation system as a result of self-referral by physicians, *N Engl J Med* 327(21):1503-1506, 1992.
15. Yelin EH: *Disability and the displaced worker,* New Brunswick, NJ, 1992, Rutgers University Press.

3 Occupational Health Clinic

The practice of occupational medicine is rapidly changing. It is no longer satisfactory to simply provide high-quality medical care with long hours in a clinical setting. A strong, competitive, clinic-based practice now requires management skills and sophisticated planning.

Clinic-based physicians are confronted with numerous issues that complicate their practices, including the following:

1. Containing costs while providing more services and producing health care outcome data
2. Increased competition among health care providers
3. Federal and state regulations that influence patient care and referral patterns
4. Consumers (that is, employers, patients, and workers' compensation carriers) who require participation in the delivery process
5. A tendency toward increased control and participation in the delivery of care by workers' compensation carriers and insurance adjusters and companies

Occupational medicine is an evolving practice that requires a skillful approach to marketing, planning, organization, implementation, and review. However, although the responsibilities associated with the practice of occupational medicine are considerable, so are the potential personal and financial rewards. This chapter reviews the basic elements of planning and managing a successful occupational health clinic, including product line development, staffing, equipment and supplies, marketing and sales, and quality assurance.

DEVELOPING A PRODUCT LINE

The "bread and butter" of most occupational health clinics is the treatment of job-related injuries.

A clinic should be able to treat a range of injuries and illnesses that occur on the job, such as orthopedic injuries, lacerations and contusions, toxic exposure, burns, and repetitive strain injuries. The clinic also may have the ability to treat more complex problems, such as tendon injuries and fractures. Whenever possible, follow-up evaluations should be provided in the clinic; a clinic should not refer patients unless it cannot provide appropriate medical care.

Radiographic services should be available in the clinic or at a nearby location. Patient convenience often is compromised when a patient is sent to another location. Although state regulations may limit the dispensing of pharmaceuticals in clinics, providing this service enhances patient care and contributes to revenue.

A variety of examinations should be included in the clinic's product line. For example, the Americans with Disabilities Act requires a particular functional approach to the preplacement evaluation. The evaluation must assess the employee's functional ability to meet the essential job requirements. The clinic can be a valuable resource for employers in complying with this regulation and provide the employee with an accurate judgment of his ability to do the job safely.

The product line should also include periodic examinations that are appropriate to employers with workers who have potential health risks at the worksite. For example, special evaluations for asbestos exposure and pesticide and other chemical contacts may be beneficial. Finally, there may be a need for exit examinations for employees leaving the worksite through retirement, transfer, or termination. Such examinations may determine if there has been a deterioration of the employee's health as a result of his job.

A variety of surveillance services may be required by employers. These services include laboratory tests for exposure to organophosphate pesticides in agricultural environments, lead levels in some ceramic plants and foundries, and drug screens when employers are concerned about substance abuse. Periodic hearing tests are indicated for employees who are exposed to loud noise, and pulmonary function testing may be indicated in circumstances requiring the employee to wear a respirator.

Physical therapy is another important service to provide. Whenever possible, physical therapy services should be offered in the clinic or at a nearby location. On-site services are convenient for patients and facilitate physician-therapist interaction.

For acute and chronic injuries, as well as for post-surgical patients, a physical therapy program should include a variety of modalities and procedures, such as traction, massage, sonography, and gait training. Finally, a comprehensive program should offer an exercise program as the patient's disability diminishes.

Another physical therapy service is a functional capacity assessment, which tests the patient's ability to perform specific tasks, often simulating those done in the workplace. Conducting these assessments in the controlled environment of a clinic-affiliated work fitness program enables the physician to determine when the patient can safely return to the workplace with minimal risk of injury. In addition, comparative assessments of the patient's progress can be made as he recovers.

The clinic may assist in evaluating the patient's disability status by testing his ability to perform normal and customary job-related tasks. This evaluation is particularly applicable in determining the level of permanent disability or the patient's ability to perform alternative jobs for which he might be trained.

Physical and occupational therapists may also be used at the worksite to provide such services as ergonomic assessment and instruction in proper use of the back when lifting.

Vertical integration of occupational health services refers to the addition of services beyond those normally available in the clinic. For example, an orthopedic surgeon, physiatrist, or neurologist may perform consultations in the clinic on a regular basis. These services are convenient to both the patient and employer when provided in a single facility. Furthermore, the consultant has access to the patient's medical records and can often speak with the treating physician. Such collaboration may improve the patient's medical care.

Caution should be taken when using vertical services located at a site other than the occupational clinic. In some states, regulations covering "self-referral" limit the selection of some service sites, particularly if the referring source has a financial interest in the service site. This is particularly true of physical therapy and laboratory and imaging services. The problem may be obviated if the occupational clinic provides the services under the umbrella of a widely-held corporate entity, particularly if publicly owned. An attorney should be consulted for advice.

A clinic may also assist in determining the solutions to special problems. For example, employers and insurance carriers often need help to determine the direction of care for problem patients and to reach a judgment about whether a patient's health problem is related to his work.

Other services may complete the product line and may be used to develop an employer-provider partnership, with additional services available for a fixed fee. These services may include a library of books and video cassettes on topics of interest; regular staff visits to the workplace for evaluation of potential hazards; assistance with long-term health and safety planning; reduced fees for services, seminars and periodic "brown bag" lunches at the clinic to discuss subjects of interest; and vaccinations, blood pressure measurement, and other routine services at little or no charge.

It may also be possible to provide an employee assistance program (EAP). An EAP is an essential service for employees with physical or mental health conditions associated with problems such as drug abuse, divorce, and adolescent issues. The occupational health program should develop a group of appropriate providers to whom such patients can be referred.

Finally, there may be an opportunity for providing worksite–based medical services. Circumstances may exist for such care to be provided by a physician or other ancillary health care worker. The time commitment to a given employer may range from only a few hours a month to 8 hours a day. The purpose of such a program is to render a service to the employer that assists him in some way while reinforcing the clinician's relationship with the employer.

THE PROCESS OF PROVIDING SERVICES

Running an occupational health clinic successfully is a process that begins with an initial concept and ends with a successful result. There should be a vision and a purpose for the clinic that includes market analysis, careful planning, patient care, and collection for services.

Each of these phases involves several components that require attention. If any portion of the process is neglected, the result can be detrimental to the successful development of the clinic. Care should be taken not to focus on activities of interest at the expense of services that are less appealing.

The steps toward achieving a successful occupational medicine practice include the following:

- Developing the concept
- Analyzing the marketplace
- Developing a comprehensive business plan
- Constructing a sales plan
- Initiating the sales process
- Providing patient care

- Communicating with consumers
- Data processing
- Managing finances through billing and collection

Developing the concept is the first step. The practitioner must ask herself these questions: What is the clinic's philosophy? What market position do I expect my clinic to assume, given the nature of the competition? What is my real mission in establishing a clinic? A clinic philosophy should address community and public health goals, as well as profitability and positioning.

Analyzing the market is essential for constructing a business plan: What other providers are in the market, what services do they offer, what services does the marketplace want, what regulatory and contracting concerns exist? Ultimately, the product line should be molded to meet the needs of the marketplace. Although some type of formal market research is ideal, even anecdotal information can be useful in recognizing market needs (see the section, Developing a Comprehensive Business and Marketing Plan later in this chapter).

Developing a comprehensive business plan requires extensive thought. This critical document should not be neglected (a discussion of business plan development follows later in this chapter). If no business plan is drawn up, the practice may drift and lack focus. Problems would tend to be addressed by crisis management rather than planning, a situation that often is apparent to the staff and the consumer.

Constructing a sales plan is a process that flows from the business plan. It is the tactical focus for the entire staff. It looks to the target industries and the specific companies that might become clients, as well as the medical services to be offered.

Initiating the sales process is implementation of the sales plan. It is important to track the efforts of the sales staff. If inadequate or ineffective telephone and/or visit contacts are made, patient flow may be insufficient. The efforts of the sales staff must reflect both quality and quantity.

Providing patient care is the most important element in the entire process. This includes reception of the patient in the clinic, management of the visit by both physicians and nonphysicians, and provision of any ancillary services. The waiting room must be clean and pleasant; the patient's first experience with the facility is here. If the room is untidy, the receptionist impolite or hurried, and the wait prolonged or lacking in amenities, the patient will be unhappy by the time he reaches the patient care area.

A clinic might consider offering coffee and soft drinks; there should be a television and perhaps a VCR with movies or educational programs. The waiting room must be attractively, although not necessarily expensively, appointed. A "hostess" might be responsible for interacting with the patients. Occupational health is a *service industry;* the patient's experience is critical.

Once the patient is in the treatment area, care should be delivered promptly. If that is not possible, the nursing staff should explain the delay. The physician should provide the usual excellent care and display her best "bedside manner." The patient often equates quality with how well the physician listens. The physician should make eye contact and answer the patient's questions.

Communicating with consumers (that is, patients, employers, and insurance carriers) is essential. The patient must leave the office with a sense of having been heard by the physician and of having had his medical problems explained. The employer must have an explanation of the patient's condition that is sufficient for making decisions about work assignments and anticipated recovery. Finally, the insurance carrier must be able both to estimate costs related to medical care and temporary disability and to consider the possibility of job retraining or permanent disability. Each of the three have their own needs, and the occupational medicine clinic is as stable as the confidence of its consumers.

Data processing associated with the visit begins after medical care has been provided. Charges must be assembled and posted in a timely fashion, preferably within 5 working days. Billings should be appropriate, and care should be taken that no charges are missed.

Managing finances through billing and collection comes next. The clinic may use invoices, statements, or both. The billing cycle may be monthly, biweekly, weekly, or more often; the frequency depends on the clinic's office schedule and the number of patients seen. Whatever the frequency, delayed billing results in a prolonged collection period and increases the likelihood of nonpayment.

The collection effort comprises noting receipt of payment and the process of recovering difficult-to-collect charges. The clinic should assign at least one full-time staff person to this effort if receivable time exceeds 60 days.

STAFFING AND COMPENSATION

Successful management of an occupational health clinic requires appropriate staffing. Selection of the right staff members influences clinic management as well as the patient's experience.

Effective clinic management generally revolves around three key staff members: the medical director, administrator, and sales representative. The medical director should work full time in the clinic and be fully committed to the success of the practice. A physician who is board certified in occupational medicine may provide the greatest depth of experience; however, many physicians who have worked in busy hospital emergency departments or who have been general practitioners in active clinics often are strong candidates. The clinic should attempt to determine the likely needs of the employers, patients, and insurance carriers to whom it will provide service, as well as the composition of the pool of available physicians.

Compensation for the medical director, as well as other physicians, should include some type of incentive. The formula depends on the billing format for the office (fee for service, capitation, or a combination). The incentive might be based on production or profit, depending on which is more appropriate to the facility. Incentives tend to reward the physicians who are more productive and encourage seeing more patients. Consider the following guidelines:

- Total compensation to physicians for patient care should not exceed 20% of the core (excluding vertical services) gross revenue.
- Incentives should be based on charges rather than receipts, because the physicians generally do not influence collection activity directly unless overcharging and excessive write-offs are occurring.
- The incentive should not generate excessive care to increase charges.

The clinic (or program) administrator assumes as much importance as the medical director. Clinic owners may choose to refer to this person as the director or office manager. Regardless of the title, this individual is the nonphysician manager of the practice. He must be full time and have the same commitment as the medical director.

The administrator supervises all other staff members in the clinic. He must have a strong background in marketing and sales, financial management, personnel, and industrial relations. The administrator should be responsible for all the problems that the medical director does not manage. In some cases, the medical director is responsible to this person. In other cases, the reverse is more appropriate. The clinic should determine which is better for the practice.

The administrator might be compensated with a base salary and an incentive related to achieving the budget for both census and profit. Although the administrator normally is an individual with a strong sense of quality and productive effort, an incentive often is useful in maximizing that effort. The incentive might reasonably allow for approximately 10% to 20% above a monthly salary and be based on net income, because this individual should be responsible for clinic profitability.

The third key person is the sales representative. This individual is essential for generating business. She may or may not have experience in a medical clinic, but she should be an experienced salesperson. The sales representative should know how to work from a marketing plan, construct and implement a sales plan, and conduct an organized sales effort. She must be able to "close a sale." If the sales representative has medical experience, the training time will be shorter; if not, the necessary information can be learned.

Clinic owners should consider paying the sales representative a smaller base salary and larger commission. A good rule of thumb is 80% base salary and 20% leveraged or expected compensation from commission or bonus. If productive, the sales representative can be one of the clinic's most valuable assets. The incentive should be based on measurable activity: new injuries, examinations, and perhaps laboratory testing programs. Patient follow-up visits and physical therapy should not be included because these are determined by the physician and other staff members.

Additional employees fall into the categories of patient care staff, financial personnel, and administrative staff.

The **patient care staff** includes registered nurses, licensed vocational nurses, medical assistants, receptionists, clerks, x-ray technicians, and others. The selected combination depends on the clinic's particular needs for the services that will be provided. Care should be taken to select the level of staffing needed; clinics often staff at a higher skill level than necessary.

A person might be assigned to provide information to employers and insurance carriers. This person may be referred to as the patient status clerk or case manager. He is responsible for providing information about work status and for organizing the results of preplacement examinations and scheduling consultations. Having such a person obviates the need for others involved in patient care to be distracted by responding to requests for information.

Physical therapy personnel often are important contributors to the success of the practice. In general, the greatest problem is recruiting the therapists, including registered physical therapists and physical therapy assistants. These individuals are in short supply and must be offered an attractive compensation package. An incentive based on production is an excellent idea and one to which therapists often respond. There should be a base salary with the opportunity to earn an additional 25% to 40%, depending on production.

Additional support staff in the physical therapy section include exercise physiologists, massage therapists, and aides. Exercise physiologists and massage therapists serve as valuable extenders to the registered physical therapists, allowing many more patients to be seen than could be managed by the therapists alone. In particular, the exercise physiologists oversee treatment that follows the modalities and other procedures performed by the therapists.

Financial personnel include the data processing and collections clerks. Having a manager for this section may be helpful if the clinic's reporting and budgeting needs exceed the skills of data processors. Such a manager often is valuable, particularly if the clinic follows the advice offered later in this chapter about budgeting and financial tracking.

The financial staff should be organized and thorough. They should tolerate, if not enjoy, attention to detail. Accurate data processing is critical to the success of an occupational health practice. The collections clerk should develop a methodical approach to gathering the hard-to-collect billings. This person must be full time and committed to the tasks of the job.

The **administrative staff** comprises the personnel manager, transcribists, mail clerks, and other support personnel. Depending on the size of the clinic, the administrator may function as the personnel manager. This role should be filled by someone familiar with medical insurance, job descriptions, grievances, and personnel issues.

Compensation for financial and administrative personnel depends on the salary characteristics of the area in which the facility is located. In general, the medical director, administrator, and sales representative have the highest salaries, descending in that order. Each section and the individuals therein should have a salary schedule based on (1) the training and certification required, (2) contributions to billings in the clinic, (3) the availability of comparable staff in the community, and (4) the particular skills and experience of the individual.

Staff members must be selected carefully. They represent the clinic and create the impression formed by patients, employers, and insurance carriers. The clinic's success is significantly influenced by its personnel.

EQUIPMENT AND SUPPLIES

We find it useful to plan equipment by location in the clinic. The patient's first contact with the occu-

pational health facility is the waiting room. The patient experience is crucial, and a pleasant waiting area is essential. This room must be furnished attractively and comfortably with (1) chairs, (2) a bench, (3) end or coffee tables, (4) a television, (5) a videocassette recorder/player, (6) a coffee pot, (7) plants, and (8) wall decorations.

Obese patients may not fit in a standard chair, and often patients do not like to sit together. This calls for a few benches. In a busy occupational clinic, patients with less serious problems sometimes must wait when a large number of unexpected injuries or examinations arrive and need immediate attention. A video player and interesting movies or educational programs often improve this unfortunate situation. Soft drinks may be dispensed, and the coffee pot should be kept full with fresh coffee. Periodically patients should be apprised of the reason for the delay and told that, hopefully, their care would follow shortly.

The front office must be attractively and functionally outfitted with (1) secretarial chairs, (2) computer work stations, (3) a typewriter, (4) a copier, and (5) miscellaneous equipment.

The appearance of this area is important because it gives patients their first impression of the office. It should be outfitted so that the receptionists can complete the initial paperwork with the patient quickly and efficiently. The length of time the patient spends with the receptionist should be kept to a minimum. Patient information should be entered directly into the computer, if possible, limiting the requirement for manual information gathering.

Each treatment room should be planned according to its need. In general, the room's equipment will include (1) an examination table, (2) an otoscope and ophthalmoscope, (3) a gooseneck lamp or surgical light, (4) a blood pressure cuff, and (5) miscellaneous supplies.

One or more rooms should be designated for testing. These should be in a quiet part of the clinic to avoid noise that might impede audiometric testing. Testing rooms should have (1) a spirometer, (2) an audiometer, (3) an audiometric booth, (4) an electrocardiograph, and (5) a tonometer.

There is a range of spirometers from which to choose. We generally find fewer technical problems in volume measurement rather than flow measurement equipment. The clinic should choose audiometric equipment that requires patient or technician control. We prefer testing administered by the technician. The audiometric booth must meet attenuation requirements.

A trauma room should be planned that can manage moderate or more severe injuries. Equipment here should include (1) a gurney on wheels, (2) a Mayo stand, (3) a gooseneck lamp or surgical light, (4) an oxygen tank, (5) a blood pressure cuff, (6) an otoscope and an ophthalmoscope, (7) one or more arm stands, and (8) laceration trays.

Additional equipment for resuscitation may also be considered, although most occupational clinics do not require it.

The physical therapy section needs adequate equipment and is relatively equipment intensive compared with other areas in the clinic. It should have (1) treatment tables, (2) mats for the gym, (3) a whirlpool, (4) ultrasound equipment, (5) an electrogalvanic stimulation (EGS) machine, and (6) exercise equipment, including machines and free weights.

Depending on the program planned for the physical therapy department, the equipment list may be much more extensive.

If at all possible, the clinic should have its own in-house x-ray facilities. Used equipment often is satisfactory. This section should have (1) a table, overhead tube, cassette wall holder, and control panel generator; (2) a film processor; (3) a silver recovery system; (4) a view box (four bank); and (5) miscellaneous equipment, including cassettes, a cassette storage rack, a film storage bin, dark room equipment, film, and miscellaneous supplies.

The nursing station and business office will have miscellaneous equipment and supplies, including a computer system for medical records and billing. A variety of software and hardware products are available, depending on the clinics needs. A copier, fax machine, and telephone system are also necessary.

Supplies for the medical area will include (1) dressing materials, including gauze pads and wraps; (2) medications (oral, topical, and injectable); (3) splinting and casting materials; and (4) crutches, lumbar corsets, knee and elbow sleeves, ankle and wrist splints, and other orthopedic devices.

Adequate equipment and supplies are a must, and once the clinic is open, reordering should proceed in a timely fashion.

DEVELOPING A COMPREHENSIVE BUSINESS AND MARKETING PLAN

Occupational health clinics frequently are long on clinical savvy and comparatively short on business planning. In the competitive world of occupational health services, a little foresight can go a long way.

An effective business plan should begin with a fundamental understanding of the clinic's market-place. The classic market assessment involves scrutiny of three key areas: the clinic (or program) itself, the competition, and the consumer.

The clinic

The clinic (or occupational health program) inevitably has various competitive strengths and weaknesses that in turn create opportunities and limitations in the occupational health marketplace. A professional assessment should systematically list potential strengths and weaknesses.

Potential strengths include highly trained care providers, location (or locations), responsive communication policies, a full continuum of occupational health care, or an established employer client base. Rather than assessing strengths unilaterally, it often is useful to solicit the opinions of fellow staff members.

Potential limitations should be outlined in a similar way. Common barriers to a successful occupational health clinic include opposition from the physician community, limited space or a nonoptimal location, an antiquated billing system, inadequate parking, or formidable competition. When limitations are identified, it is crucial to immediately develop potential solutions and an action plan to overcome each limitation.

The competition

An occupational health clinic seldom operates in a vacuum; often a multitude of other options are available to both employers and employees for occupational health services.

The best way to assess the competitive environment is through targeted market research. Professional market research should identify the existence, breadth of services, and market penetration of potential competitors in a discrete and ongoing fashion. Using market research, a new or evolving occupational health clinic can position itself to fill service voids.

Competitive intelligence research may be completed through formal employer surveys, informal feedback from clinic sales representatives and other information sources, or a combination of the two. Intelligence should include the reputed strengths and weaknesses, array of services, and long-range forecast for each competitor.

The consumer

An occupational health clinic has numerous consumers, including the employer, the worker, and the payer. In general, however, the clinic market is primarily driven by the employer, and employers should be the primary subject of consumer research.

Although ongoing consumer research can and should be done by sending out periodic mail questionnaires, using patient satisfaction surveys at the clinic, and relying on systematic feedback from marketing and sales staff, formal professional market research is advisable. A combination of qualitative research (such as focus groups) and quantitative research (employer telephone surveys) provides a clinic with the most reliable information for making strategic decisions on location, product line, staffing, and positioning.

Employer (or payer) focus group research has several requisites:

1. *A manageable size.* A group of five to seven participants normally allows sufficient depth of discussion and seems to be optimal. Two sessions on different days should be scheduled to minimize potential bias.

2. *An experienced moderator.* Focus group moderation is an art that involves probing, follow-up, and a working knowledge of the issues. The occupational health clinic and the moderator should meet before the sessions to jointly develop a focus group agenda.

3. *Adequate notice and incentives.* Prospective focus group participants should be advised of the session 7 to 10 days in advance and should receive compensation for their involvement. We normally hold sessions at a local hotel and provide participants with a complimentary breakfast or dinner and an honorarium of $75.

4. *Targeted recruitment.* Companies should be carefully recruited to ensure that a representative group of potentially high-volume clients are present at the sessions. We have found that purchased mailing lists can be woefully out of date and misleading, so we advise clinics to call each employer to determine who is responsible for the health and safety of the workforce before a focus group is recruited.

5. *Anonymity.* We believe that focus groups are most effective when participants are guaranteed anonymity. Clinic representatives should not be present at the session; audiotapes or transcripts, or both, should be obtained from each session.

Formal employer telephone surveys can be used as a supplement tool in place of focus group sessions. An initial sample of 150 to 200 targeted employers (that is, likely high-volume users of clinic services because of industry type or location, or both), which typically generates a response rate of 60% to 70%, is adequate for obtaining meaningful information about the market.

An employer survey should address (1) current services, (2) desired services, (3) current provider preferences, (4) provider selection factors, (5) institutional (clinic) strengths, (6) business profile and associated demographics, (7) utilization volumes, and (8) preferred clinic setting.

Survey research can be used to support strategic decisions on product line offerings, staffing needs, marketing and positioning techniques, and targeted sales efforts.

Once the internal and external assessments have been completed, a business and marketing plan can be developed. We recommend the following format for an occupational health clinic marketing plan:

- *Mission statement.* A brief consensus statement on the purpose and goals of the clinic. Meaningful mission statements generally are quantitative in nature (for example, a break-even financial performance within 12 months). Care should be taken to extend beyond obvious profit motives in a clinic's mission statement. A well-rounded occupational health clinic should address the community's public health needs through surveillance, hazard abatement, and health education interventions.
- *Internal analysis.* The clinic's strengths and limitations in delivering broad-based and quality services to employers.
- *Competitive analysis.* A profile of key institutional and individual competitors, including their services, fees, and relative strengths and weaknesses.
- *Consumer analysis.* An outline of employer and employee wants, needs, and practices, including a list of the most highly targeted employers.
- *Product line strategy.* A discussion of current, short-term, and long-term service offerings and the product differentiation that would render each superior to the market norm.
- *Operational strategies.* Referral protocols and internal and external communication policies.
- *Marketing strategy.* Proposed marketing and sales activities.
- *Long-term strategy.* The clinic's concept of the future marketplace; long-term positioning strategies, including potential collaborative efforts and the services that ultimately will be offered in response to these perceptions.
- *Financial pro forma.* Volume, revenue, and expense projections for at least 3 years.
- *Results-oriented action plan.* A detailed calendar showing specific monthly activities and the individuals responsible for them.

Principles of effective sales and marketing

In the increasingly competitive occupational health environment of the 1990s, a successful clinic must market its services astutely and aggressively. Employer ignorance about the value of a strong relationship with an occupational health clinic and the complex, multidisciplinary nature of the field makes one-on-one sales the heart of successful clinic marketing. Unfortunately, few clinic administrators recognize the potential of an optimal sales effort. The following principles apply to an effective sales approach for an occupational health clinic:

- *Recruit wisely.* Occupational health clinics seem to place inadequate emphasis on the recruiting process for sales personnel. The clinic should insist on previous sales experience, ideally within health care or occupational health services.
- *Compensate well and provide incentives.* Clinics should not underestimate the value of a strong salesperson who is well paid. Incentives (either in the form of a bonus or a commission) are important and should be quota based, easy to compute, based on total revenue (rather than total calls or encounters, or new companies "acquired"), and provided frequently (quarterly).
- *Let salespeople sell.* A salesperson should be in the field at least 20 hours a week, with the remaining time devoted to preparation and follow-up. Frequently a single individual serves as both internal program coordinator and salesperson, to the invariable detriment of both functions.
- *Stratify target employers.* The sales strategy should reach out to three different-sized employers: high-profile larger employers, mid-sized employers (50 to 500 employees), and the broad remaining universe of employers. The first group may require highly customized services, lengthy negotiation periods, and team selling; the latter group involves ongoing direct mail efforts.
- *Target high-volume employers.* The market should be scrutinized to determine which employers can be expected to generate high volumes, and these should be targeted for priority contact. The more systematic the clinic, the more likely clinic volume will grow.
- *Ask the right questions and listen.* The art of selling usually boils down to an ability to ask the right questions, listen carefully, and develop solutions that match employer and employee needs with clinic capabilities.
- *Consider written proposals.* Sales calls conducted by an occupational health clinic representative should be followed up with written, benefit-oriented proposals. Proposals tend to be more effective when they portray the provider's track record and are specific in terms of fees and other commitments.
- *Effect a commitment.* Obtaining employer commitment, either formally through the development of services such as a retainer agreement, or informally through follow-up visits by the employer to the clinic, is central to occupational health sales.

Beyond the actual sales effort, there are numerous marketing techniques that should be used by an aggressive occupational health clinic:

- *Effective collateral materials.* Occupational health clinics should take care to develop first-rate collateral materials on quality stock, featuring photographs, staff biographies, and third-party testimonials from satisfied employer clients or previous clinic patients, or both.
- *Videotapes.* An occupational health clinic video can be made at a relatively low cost and can be exceptionally effective in portraying the clinic when an employer is visiting a work site.
- *Employee outreach.* Occupational health clinics should market to the employee. Providing employees with program membership and identification cards can help streamline paperwork and frequently gives the individual a sense of affiliation with the clinic. Educational programs such as emergency preparedness or first aid for employees at the work site are also useful.
- *Educational seminars.* Periodic breakfast, luncheon, half-day, or full-day seminars on a variety of key issues ("Getting the Injured Worker Back to Work," "Legal and Ethical Issues Associated with Worker Screening") are a useful way to publicize a program and generate revenue at the same time.
- *Employer advisory groups.* A council of representatives from key area employers who meet three or four times a year to discuss key health and safety issues in the workplace tends to keep a program visible and serves as an ongoing focus group.

Occupational health clinics have to come to terms with the importance of sales and marketing functions. Refusal to make marketing a high priority limits a clinic's ability to become genuinely responsive to employers' and workers' needs.

High-quality clinics should be able to describe their merits to prospective users as effectively as possible. Failure to do so is likely to limit the clinic's capacity to grow in an increasingly competitive marketplace.

FINANCIAL MANAGEMENT

Successful financial management begins with the budget process. This is consistent with the theme of general planning for the clinic in all phases. The budget is where much of the planning comes together, with estimates of the patient census from the marketing and sales staff, projection on revenue, and plans for expenses. The budget should be in place before the clinic opens to track the financial aspects of the clinic's performance. A critical goal is to identify potential financial problems as far in advance as possible.

The clinic's first step is to calculate the anticipated census. This is often done after obtaining a careful market study that evaluates the existing clients in the market and the services they anticipate (injuries, examinations, surveillance procedures, physical therapy). Anticipated census considers the use of existing services in the marketplace, the clinic's estimate of the percentage of services it will provide, and total visits generated by each visit type. This often is difficult to determine with certainty, but a relatively reasonable estimate can be based on market surveys, employer contacts, and other sources.

An alternative approach is to concentrate on the first injuries that will be seen. Thereafter, totals for other visit types can be estimated because causal relationships often occur. For example, the average first injury historically generates 1.8 to 2.6 follow-up visits. The first injury also generates approximately two physical therapy visits.

Once the census is projected, a meaningful revenue estimate is possible. On the basis of the expected visit ratio, gross revenue per visit of approximately $58 can be projected. Total projected visits are then multiplied by $58 to determine projected gross billings for the period. This allows the calculation of revenue on an accrual basis. Our experience suggests that an occupational health clinic can anticipate the following cash flow for each $100 billed, when billed at one- or two-cycle monthly billings:

Current period	10%
30-60 days	40%
60-90 days	20%
90-120 days	20%
>120 days	5%

More frequent billings will increase the collections in the current period.

We recommended that a clinic project a 3-year budget on an annual basis; thereafter, it should construct a monthly budget at the start of each year and track income and expenses through the year.

Frequently growth in census shows an initial phase of slow increase, followed by a phase of accelerated increase responding to successful sales efforts. As the marketplace becomes saturated with available providers and services, the rate of growth tends to slow. Such a pattern assumes a constant group of services. If, however, the clinic broadens its product line, the accelerated-growth phase may well continue.

Once a clinic is operating, the progress of the facility should be monitored by a regular review of the census to determine whether the clinic is meeting projections. Census data should be obtained from the preceding week on a weekly basis, and monthly patient flow should be extrapolated. In addition, determining actual gross revenue per visit allows the financial staff to project gross billings for the month.

If the clinic's projections show fewer patient visits or less revenue than planned, it should be determined which visit categories are not meeting expectations. There should be a plan for identifying problems as early as possible for timely correction.

The clinic's financial liquidity should be reviewed weekly. One method is to determine cash and cash equivalents and deduct draws on a line of credit. Should the clinic's cash position degenerate, it would be an area to review. If the clinic does not have adequate cash reserves, there could be a danger of cash shortage and its attendant problems.

At the end of the month, the patient census should be determined by visit type and by charges generated for each visit type and revenue center. Simple mathematic calculations will allow the clinic to ascertain average charges for all visits and for each visit type and revenue center. A deviation from anticipated averages may suggest an area to review. For example, the calculations may identify decreased average revenue per visit with decreased revenue for the average first injury. This could be explained by a change in the patient mix, with injuries generating lower charges.

The clinic's end-of-the-month review should also include assessment of aged accounts receivable. The aging pattern should be reviewed to determine whether the balance over 90 days is increasing, in percentage and/or absolute amount. If so, collection efforts may need to be increased. Further, if the days in accounts receivable is increasing, the collection effort might need enhancing.

The clinic should have procedures for managing cash, as well as data processing to ensure security. Daily cash accounts must be reconciled by totaling the previous day's cash collection and accompanying charge sheets. Posting of charges should use manual totals from log and charge sheets and comparison with computer-generated batch totals.

Receipt management should involve manual totals by the mail clerk with comparison to a manual total by at least one other individual. The computer-generated batch total must balance to the manual total and reconcile to the bank statement or other similar report.

QUALITY ASSURANCE

Maintaining quality medical care is the core of the clinic's service to patients, employers, and insurance carriers. The clinic should develop a series of steps to ensure excellent medical service.

Medical protocols should be established to foster a consistent level of care. Protocols constitute an outline of management for the most common diagnostic problems. By encouraging physicians and other care providers to use these protocols, the clinic would ensure that conditions are managed with the most appropriate diagnostic maneuvers and therapeutic steps, minimizing the likelihood of insufficient or excessive care. In addition, although not diminishing the physician or other provider's role, it increases the likelihood that patients will be treated consistently in the clinic.

The clinic should complete a periodic scan of medical records for satisfactory use of protocols. An appropriate number of medical records for a particular diagnosis should be selected, and charts should be critiqued to ensure that the care regimen followed the protocol.

Deviations should be discussed with the physician. If variations from the protocol are appropriate, no further action is indicated. Otherwise, it may be useful to review care with the provider. Further, it is useful to peruse medical records for legibility, completeness, and organization. Deviations from reasonableness should be followed up as needed.

There should be a program of "outcomes analysis" in the clinic. It is valuable to track groups of patients by diagnosis to ensure that the pattern of care in the clinic is appropriate. For example, it is useful to know how much is being spent on various diagnostic conditions or groups of conditions.

The clinic should determine how often laboratory and x-ray procedures are being ordered, as well as their cost. The average number of days of disability and the total time in treatment before discharge should be calculated. By constructing such a pattern, a clinic can compare patterns of care, both within the clinic among providers and to other facilities. Of course, retrieving such data nearly always requires a computer.

One staff member, preferably a nurse, might be designated to review charts of patients with prolonged or complicated care or situations where permanent disability is anticipated. Periodically, chronic patients are forgotten, and "case management" ensures timely and appropriate care.

We recommend the establishment of a quality assurance committee. The committee should be composed of both medical and nonmedical staff. They may be charged with reviewing care by protocol, or they may explore quality of service in less organized ways. For example, the committee might address the quality of the patient experience by looking at such factors as the length of time patients spend waiting, conditions in the clinic, employee working conditions, and employee group activities.

Questionnaires are a valuable source of feedback on consumer satisfaction. Regular inquiries of patients, employers, and insurance carriers should be considered. Their opinion can be sought in brief personal interviews or written forms. This approach to evaluating care is perhaps the most valuable information the clinic can obtain and should be the basis for improving or enhancing the program.

ALTERNATIVE CLINIC MODELS

As the employer-provider interface becomes more common and sophisticated, the number of alternate models become larger. There are five primary types of clinic models, each with unique advantages and disadvantages.

- *Private clinic.* Numerous occupational medicine clinics are owned by a small group or even an individual practitioner. These clinics have the advantage of greater control over the consistency of care, often easy access for injured workers, and ease of operation. However, as the trend in provider-employer relationships moves toward one-stop shopping and continuity of care, the solo or small practitioner assumes an ominous disadvantage. In general, clinics of this type are advised to consider relationships with other entities that might allow the clinic to increase its scope of services.
- *Group practice.* In many respects a group practice model mimics a private clinic model, with the added advantage of greater potential for more highly coordinated patient care be-

yond the initial encounter. However, even group practice settings seem to lack the ability to intervene across the entire occupational medicine continuum of care: injury and illness prevention, acute care, and rehabilitation.

- *Hospital emergency department–based facility.* Any hospital emergency department that sees injured workers, either episodically or routinely, has an occupational medicine component by default. The 24-hour availability of services and immediate access to ancillaries and other associated services are positive attributes in such settings. However, a classic emergency department setting frequently tends to offer inconsistent care, follow-up, and levels of provider expertise.
- *Hospital-based clinic.* Hospital-based clinics centered outside of the emergency department are a rapidly growing segment of the occupational medicine market. When organized ef-

fectively, they can offer consumers a broad-based, highly integrated series of services. Frequently, however, chronic hospital inertia and the inability to genuinely measure a true return on investment hamper the development of such programs.

- *Chain clinic.* Groups of related occupational medicine clinics, either within a geographic region or spread among multiple regions, are also becoming more common. Chain clinics have the potential to attain economies of scale in operations, patient tracking, administration, and marketing, thus holding down costs.

Any type of model is workable provided it combines the principles of sound clinic management, a commitment to the practice of sound occupational medicine, and a willingness to listen and respond to the genuine needs of occupational medicine clients.

4 Administrative Aspects

Good patient care requires meticulous attention to processing paperwork and effective communication with all parties involved in occupational injuries. In addition to the traditional issue of communication between physician and patient, appropriate information must be transmitted to the employer and compensation carrier adjustor, and often to a nurse case manager, vocational rehabilitation coordinator, or union representative as well. Many excellent care providers fail to recognize the importance of this communication flow. As a consequence of indifferent or poor reporting, treatment authorization may be delayed or denied, disability payments may be withheld, or the patient may be sent to another physician. In addition, workplace hazards may not be promptly corrected, and reimbursement of clinic fees may be delayed or denied.

Patient referral sources. Patients may be referred to the physician from any of several sources. Although the current trend is away from in-house company medical departments, some companies do maintain a staff physician or nurse to administer first aid, formulate internal medical policy, perform job placement examinations, establish and monitor medical surveillance programs, evaluate and select medical care providers, coordinate case management and early return to work for sick or injured workers, and triage injured workers to preferred occupational medicine clinics, urgent care clinics, emergency rooms, or private practitioners for treatment. In companies that do not have internal medical departments, employers may refer injured employees directly to the preferred medical facility.

Self-referral is another source of patients. An employee may seek treatment for a complaint that she feels is the result of a work injury or exposure. However, a self-referred employee may not have reported the injury to her employer. In such cases obtaining prior treatment authorization is critical, particularly in states where the employer has some degree of control over early medical intervention.

Finally, personal physicians may refer patients directly for further evaluation and treatment of a medical condition that has been deemed work related.

Regardless of the referral source, good communication starts with good information. Each clinic should have an indexed list of local companies who use the clinic's services, with all compensation carrier information, including the name and telephone/fax number of the specific adjustor for that company, whenever possible. Some carriers assign adjustors to specific companies, and others assign adjustors to patients alphabetically by the claimant's last name. Adjustor attrition and reassignment of cases from one adjustor to another may make communication challenging for a busy clinician who is trying to track down the appropriate claim worker. Whenever possible, the adjustor's name and the insurance company's claim and case numbers should be noted in the chart because the switchboard operator at the insurance company will ask first for the claim number. If the company has a nurse or physician who does worker's compensation case management, that person's name and phone number should be included in the chart. Any special instructions, such as limited duty, outside referrals, and physical therapy, should also be available. This may be stored on a Rolodex, in the computer, on a wall poster, or in a policy and procedure manual, but it must be readily accessible to the front desk, nursing, clinical, and billing staff.

Even if the clinic accepts walk-in traffic, employers and workers should be encouraged to call ahead for appointments so that a degree of control over patient flow and waiting time is maintained. Long waits in crowded, sterile waiting rooms offend patients and their employers who wish to keep time away from work at a minimum.

Treatment authorization. When a patient calls or comes to the clinic for treatment of an industrial injury, the clerk should ensure that the visit is authorized and note on the schedule or in the chart who authorized it (for example, Jane Doe, supervisor; John Jones, adjustor, Great Comp Company).

When the patient registers at the clinic, the clerk should ensure that all information regarding the date of injury, the employer's name and phone number, and the workers' compensation carrier is entered into the chart correctly. Formats vary, depending on the clinic's resources. Some clinics have a large rubber stamp outlining the informa-

41

tion, which the clerk stamps on the inside jacket of the chart and then fills in. Others use a computer-generated coversheet or a separate registration sheet. The important point is that the information should be part of the patient's chart and immediately accessible for the nurse and clinician.

Obtaining treatment authorization can be frustrating and time consuming. Many clinics insist on written authorization in advance. Companies with which the clinic has contracts can be given treatment authorization forms for the supervisors to complete and send with the patient (Figs. 4-1 and 4-2). For medical-legal evaluations, it is wise to require an advance letter from the carrier formally referring the patient and outlining the specific questions to be answered. Of course, all related medical records from other hospitals, clinics, and practitioners should be sent to the evaluator before the patient's appointment.

The most difficult cases to deal with are also the most common: an injured worker shows up from a small company about which the physician has no information. We advise such patients who call first for an appointment to obtain their supervisor's permission and workers' compensation information before they come; however, an acutely injured patient from a small, chain-affiliated fast-food restaurant often shows up with no idea what the physician is talking about. In these cases the restaurant manager may be young, inexperienced, and even hostile to the notion of workers' compensation, and he may be resistant or unable to provide the necessary information. Our policy is to treat the emergency and to track down the information later. Some clinics require the patient who may not be covered by workers' compensation insurance (for example, a self-employed contractor) to sign a form accepting financial responsibility if treatment coverage is denied by the insurance company.

Sleuthing correct carrier information may require a phone call to the company's corporate or district office or, in states with state compensation plans, which frequently cover small businesses, a call to the carrier's regional office. Most states have some form of uninsured worker coverage that the physician can use if the employer is not covered. This information should also be available at the front desk.

Doctor's report of injury. All states have some version of a form for the physician to fill out documenting the injury (Fig. 4-3). It is important to have a stack of these available or in the computer. They must be processed in a timely, legible man-

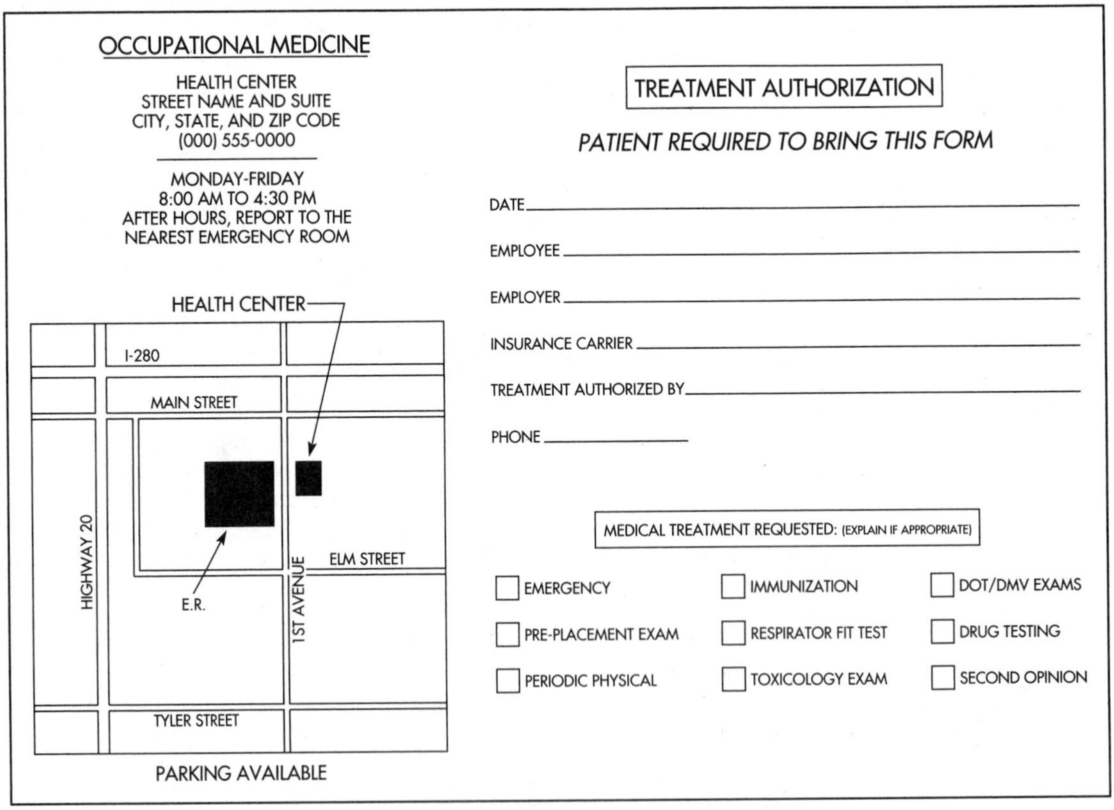
OCCUPATIONAL MEDICINE

HEALTH CENTER
STREET NAME AND SUITE
CITY, STATE, AND ZIP CODE
(000) 555-0000

MONDAY-FRIDAY
8:00 AM TO 4:30 PM
AFTER HOURS, REPORT TO THE
NEAREST EMERGENCY ROOM

PARKING AVAILABLE

TREATMENT AUTHORIZATION

PATIENT REQUIRED TO BRING THIS FORM

DATE ______

EMPLOYEE ______

EMPLOYER ______

INSURANCE CARRIER ______

TREATMENT AUTHORIZED BY ______

PHONE ______

MEDICAL TREATMENT REQUESTED: (EXPLAIN IF APPROPRIATE)

☐ EMERGENCY ☐ IMMUNIZATION ☐ DOT/DMV EXAMS
☐ PRE-PLACEMENT EXAM ☐ RESPIRATOR FIT TEST ☐ DRUG TESTING
☐ PERIODIC PHYSICAL ☐ TOXICOLOGY EXAM ☐ SECOND OPINION

Fig. 4-1 Sample treatment authorization.

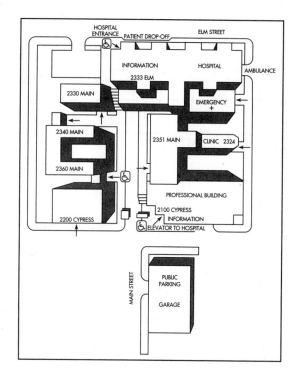

Fig. 4-2 Sample treatment authorization.

ner. All the information on the form must be filled out carefully. This documentation initiates several critical processes. First, it notifies the employer (usually through the insurance carrier) of a new injury and describes the injury. The Occupational Safety and Health Administration (OSHA) requires employers to keep a record of injuries for regulatory purposes and to identify areas for intervention. Writing "slip and fall" is ambiguous and does not allow the employer to identify and correct possible hazards as readily as would writing "slip and fall on broken stair riser." Second, the document notifies the payer of an impending claim so that funds can be allocated to pay medical bills, make indemnity payments, set aside reserves for future medical costs, and investigate questions about liability.

Causality is also a key part of the form. The patient or clinician, or both, must provide the link between the injury and the job, must determine that the injury arose out of and in the course of employment. The clinician who fails to make this relationship clear risks denial of the claim and payment for his services. Readable typed forms or carefully written ones are crucial so that the adjustor can reach you if she has a question. Physicians who scrawl signatures and do not legibly type or stamp their name and phone number on paperwork frustrate the adjustor's attempts to reach them.

Copies of this form (titled, perhaps, "Physi-

cian's First Report of Injury") are to be kept in the chart and sent to the compensation carrier and any other agency as required. We have found it helpful to give the patient one for her files and to keep one in an alphabetical "First Report" file for use when the chart cannot be located or when the physician wants to pull all charts from a particular company or all charts with a particular diagnosis but does not yet have a computerized database.

Occasionally an employer may wish to reimburse medical costs directly and may ask the physician not to file a first report or a claim with the workers' compensation carrier. Such requests come from employers whose insurance premiums are "experience rated," so that fewer claims mean lower premiums. This practice is condemned, not only because it is illegal in some states, but also because seemingly minor medical problems can become complicated and entangle the patient, physician, employer, and insurance carrier in a dispute over reimbursement and liability.

Similarly, employees may ask the physician not to file a claim because they fear losing a job as the result of reporting a work injury. Although it is illegal for an employer to lay off an employee because of a work injury, such practices do occur. Nonetheless, the practitioner must explain the reporting requirements to the patient at the initial visit to avoid subsequent misunderstanding about legal and reimbursement issues.

DOCTOR'S FIRST REPORT OF OCCUPATIONAL INJURY OR ILLNESS

Within 5 days of your initial examination, for every occupational injury or illness, send this report to **insurer or employer (only if self-insured).** Failure to file a timely doctor's report may result in assessment of a civil penalty. **In the case of diagnosed or suspected pesticide poisoning,** send one copy of this report directly to the Division of Labor Statistics and Research; and notify your local health officer by telephone within 24 hours and by sending a copy of this report within seven days.

	PLEASE DO NOT USE THIS COLUMN
1. **INSURER NAME AND ADDRESS**	
2. **EMPLOYER NAME**	Case No.
3. Address: No. and Street City Zip	Industry
4. Nature of business (e.g., food manufacturing, building construction, retailer of women's clothes)	County
5. **PATIENT NAME** (First name, middle initial, last name) 6. Sex ☐ Male ☐ Female 7. Date of Mo. Day Yr. Birth	Age
8. Address: No. and Street City Zip 9. Telephone number ( )	Hazard
10. Occupation (Specific job title) 11. Social Security Number	Disease
12. Injured at: No. and Street City County	Hospitalization
13. Date and hour of injury or onset of illness Mo. Day Yr. Hour ____ a.m. ____ p.m. 14. Date last worked Mo. Day Yr.	Occupation
15. Date and hour of first examination or treatment Mo. Day Yr. Hour ____ a.m. ____ p.m. 16. Have you (or your office) previously treated patient? ☐ Yes ☐ No	Return Date/Code

Patient please complete this portion, if able to do so. Otherwise, doctor please complete immediately. Inability or failure of a patient to complete this portion shall not affect his/her rights to workers' compensation under the Labor Code.
17. **DESCRIBE HOW THE ACCIDENT OR EXPOSURE HAPPENED** (Give specific object, machinery or chemical. Use reverse side if more space is required.)

18. **SUBJECTIVE COMPLAINTS** (Describe fully. Use reverse side if more space is required.)

19. **OBJECTIVE FINDINGS** (Use reverse side if more space is required.)
    A. Physical examination

    B. X-ray and laboratory results (State if none or pending.)

20. **DIAGNOSIS** (If occupational illness, specify etiologic agent and duration of exposure.) Chemical or toxic compounds involved? ☐ Yes ☐ No

21. Are your findings and diagnosis consistent with patient's account of injury or onset of illness? ☐ Yes ☐ No
    If "no," please explain.

22. Is there any other current condition that will impede or delay patient's recovery? ☐ Yes ☐ No
    If "yes," please explain.

23. **TREATMENT RENDERED** (Use reverse side if more space is required.)

    If further treatment required, specify treatment. Estimated duration

24. If hospitalized as inpatient, give hospital name and location. Date Mo. Day Yr. admitted | Estimated stay

25. **WORK STATUS** Is patient able to perform usual work? ☐ Yes ☐ No
    If "no," patient can return to: Mo. Day Yr.
        Regular work _____
        Modified work _____ Specify restrictions _____

Doctor's Signature _____ Date _____ License Number _____
Doctor Name and Degree (Please Type) _____ IRS Number _____
Address _____ Telephone Number ( )

Fig. 4-3 Sample doctor's first report of injury.

Federal and state medical reports. From time to time the clinician may be requested to complete other kinds of forms. Federal employees are covered by a separate insurance system with its own distinct—and lengthy—forms. For example, the U.S. Postal Service uses special forms to outline work restrictions or modified duty and to report work injuries or disability. These forms may be brought to the clinic by the employee or may be obtained by the clinic from the government employer. Patients also may ask the practitioner to complete private disability insurance forms because, for example, union insurance policies may supplement the limited income from workers' compensation temporary disability payments (see the discussion on Disability Paperwork).

Finally, the practitioner may need to complete State Disability Insurance (SDI) forms for a patient whose workers' compensation case has been delayed pending investigation. Such individuals face a complete loss of income, because they are not receiving temporary disability payments. The State Disability office may put a lien on the workers' compensation carrier and often is reimbursed if the claim is ultimately accepted as work related. Completing this form allows the injured worker on temporary disability to receive some income during the weeks or months of administrative processing and investigation.

Work status report. In addition to the first report, a work status slip is provided at the first visit and at each one thereafter (Figs. 4-4 and 4-5). This form can be computer generated, preprinted on NCR paper, or photocopied. The purpose is to inform the employer and compensation carrier about the patient's work status and future care plan. It also gives the patient written documentation of future appointments. Many clinics use a time clock to stamp patient arrival and departure times on the slip so that both the physician and the employer know how long the employee spent at the clinic. This slip is distributed to the patient, employer, insurance carrier, and is included in the chart.

Although requirements vary by state, it is prudent to provide the compensation carrier with written reports periodically. For complicated or lost-time injuries (chemical exposures, cumulative

Health Center
Occupational Medicine Clinic
Employee Health Service
Street Name and Suite
City, State, and Zip Code

WORK STATUS REPORT

IMPRINT CARD

(PATIENT) (COMPANY)

(DATE OF INJURY) (INDUSTRIAL CARRIER)

Patient was seen on ____________ .

PATIENT'S STATUS IS:

☐ Discharged to full work on ____________ , no further care indicated.
☐ Returned to work on ____________ , follow-up clinic visit on ____________
☐ Returned to limited duty on ____________ (describe limitations) ____________ for an estimated ____________ days, follow-up clinic visit on ____________ .
☐ Excused from work today and the next ______ calendar days, follow-up clinic visit on ____________ .
☐ Consultation has been requested with ____________ M.D. On ____________ .
☐ Referred to ____________ M.D. for further care. On ____________ .
☐ **PHYSICAL THERAPY:** Frequency ____________ Duration: ____________ .

COMMENTS: ____________

____________ STAFF PHYSICIAN

(STAFF CLINICIAN)

White copy: RETURN TO EMPLOYER Canary copy: MEDICAL CHART Pink copy: To Patient Goldenrod: Worker's Compensation

Fig. 4-4 Sample work status report.

```
┌─────────────────────────────────────────────────────────────────────────┐
│ MEDICAL CENTER                              PATIENT STATUS REPORT          │
│                                                                           │
│                    OCCUPATIONAL INJURY CLINIC                             │
│                 Street Name, Suite, City, State, and Zip Code             │
│ ─────────────────────────────────────────────────────────────────────── │
│                                                                           │
│                                                                           │
│ ─────────────────────────────────────────────────────────────────────── │
│ DATE:  IN _____  OUT _____ │
│ NAME _____│
│ EMPLOYER _____│
│ DATE OF INJURY _____│
│ WORK STATUS                                                               │
│     ☐ Return to full work _____│
│     ☐ Unable to return to work _____│
│     ☐ Return to modified duty with restrictions _____│
│         _____ Seated/standing work only                              │
│         _____ Alternate position (sit, stand, walk)                  │
│         _____ No/Limited climbing, bending, stooping                 │
│         _____ No/Limited overhead reaching                           │
│         _____ No/Limited        use of       right/left    hand/arm  │
│         _____ No lifting, pushing, pulling over                      │
│                 _____ 0-15 lb.                                           │
│                 _____ 15-30 lb.                                          │
│                 _____ 30-40 lb.                                          │
│         _____ Other _____│
│                   Other _____│
│ PHYSICAL THERAPY_____│
│ OCCUPATIONAL THERAPY_____│
│ DISPOSITION                                                               │
│     ☐ Return to clinic_____│
│     ☐ Discharge_____│
│     ☐ Consultation_____│
│ DIAGNOSIS _____│
│ COMMENTS _____│
│                              _____, M.D.       │
└─────────────────────────────────────────────────────────────────────────┘
```

Fig. 4-5 Sample work status report.

trauma, reaggravation of previously closed injury claims), a dictated report, in addition to the First Report form, is prepared after the first visit and updated periodically by dictated or handwritten progress reports. These supplemental reports should be sent to the insurer for any of the following:

1. Any notable change in diagnosis, prognosis, or treatment

2. Any change in work status

3. Hospitalization, surgery, or a medical emergency

4. The patient is referred to another physician for consultation or further treatment

5. To report progress every 2 to 3 weeks, even if the case appears uncomplicated

6. The patient's condition becomes permanent and stationary

In an era of tight resources, a legible, handwritten progress report form can serve simultaneously as the chart progress note and report to the carrier (Fig. 4-6). If the practitioner chooses to communicate by photocopying handwritten chart progress notes or supplemental report forms, he should still dictate a brief note summarizing the patient's progress and anticipated course every few visits. These progress reports are read and used mainly by adjusters and occasionally by nurse case managers or company nurses. Therefore, when dictating, it is important to use appropriate technical medical terminology, but also to explain in lay language simultaneously. "Phalen's test negative" may mean nothing to the adjustor, but "Phalen's test for carpal tunnel syndrome negative" communicates something meaningful. As always, effective communication demands the sensitivity to address the audience rather than oneself.

These reports should go to the patient, the chart, and the compensation adjuster, but not to the employer unless there is a company medical unit (nurse or other medical person) that can ensure confidentiality and can deal with supervisors or personnel staff as needed. Thought must be given to the appropriateness of reports transmitted to the employer (or any other third party) that disclose medical information about the employee. In many states, diagnoses and other medical details regarding work-related injuries are considered to be in the domain of "public record," but there are legal and ethical questions about whether the employer needs to know specific diagnoses. (Please refer to Chapter 6 for further discussion about the issue of confidentiality and release of medical records.)

DISABILITY PAPERWORK

Patients who are off work often have other short- or long-term disability plans, including a short-term loan, life insurance, or mortgage disability insurance that covers their payments when totally disabled, and union or other supplemental disability plans, for additional income. Because compensation temporary disability payments rarely approach a person's salary, it is critical to the patient that the clinician fill out these forms. It is also aggravating for the clinic staff because the forms are all different, come at different times, require different ways of providing the information, and all come with a plea of urgency from the patient. Some clinics refuse to fill them out or charge a small fee for each one. Both of these policies are inappropriate, as far as we are concerned. Excellent, rather than adequate, patient care embraces all facets of the work injury: physical, psychologic, and administrative.

We have found the following procedure to work reasonably well:

The patient is given or sent a copy of all paperwork concerning her case, including the first report, work status slips, dictations, and supplemental reports. Patients on disability are counseled to identify any other types of insurance they may have (frequently they forget what policies they have been paying for over the years) and are told that they must bring all copies of their clinic paperwork when they bring the forms in for completion. We prefer to do this during a scheduled visit; however, if the patient must have it done sooner, she is instructed to call the clinic and arrange to bring the form with all compensation paperwork to the clinic at a time when the treating physician is present. An appointment is not required, but the patient is informed that she may have to wait. The patient's packet is presented to the receptionist, who brings it to the attention of the physician's nurse. The nurse fills out what she can and gives it to the clinician between patients. After the physician completes and signs the form, it goes back to the front desk, where copies are made for the patient and the chart. The original, the copy, and the packet are returned to the patient. For updates, the patient is required to bring in the copy of the first version of that form, making it much easier for the nurse or physician to copy and update. It is the patient's responsibility to mail all of these forms. We take responsibility only for compensation-related paperwork. Having a firm policy of requiring the patient to bring in her paperwork and doing it on the spot, with the patient mailing it, reduces the stress and work load for the physician and the clinic staff. It also eliminates the risk of losing the papers or delaying completion until the chart is found and the patient's physician is at the clinic.

Many companies have superb disability plans to supplement both occupational and nonoccupational disability. These plans are regulated by the federal Employment Retirement and Income Supplementation Act (ERISA). Because this law requires more documentation about the disability than other types of plans, automatically sending the agency appropriate to the patient's particular plan a copy of all dictations and updated progress reports to the insurance carrier responsible for the long-term disability plan will greatly help the patient preserve her income protection. It is also a key point of information for the physician, because these plans cover 80% to 100% of the pa-

Medical Center
Street Name and Suite
City, State, and Zip Code
(000) 555-0000

MEDICAL CENTER

DOCTOR'S SUPPLEMENTAL REPORT

PATIENT: _____   SCVMC #: _____

D/INJURY:_____   D/EXAM: _____

EMPLOYER: _____

INSURER: _____   CL. #: _____

CURRENT COMPLAINTS: _____

_____

_____

_____

FINDINGS/DIAGNOSIS: _____

_____

_____

_____

TREATMENT (type, frequency and duration): _____

_____

_____

_____

_____

DISABILITY STATUS: _____

_____

_____

_____

_____

REMARKS: _____

_____

_____

_____

_____

_____

CLINICIAN'S SIGNATURE: _____   DATE: _____

Fig. 4-6 Sample report to insurance carrier.

tient's income, much more than most supplemental disability insurance plans, and can be a real barrier to return to work.

Finally, depending on the clinic's resources, all the above chart and paperwork that is now done by hand could be done by dictation, computer transcription, and subsequent fax or E-mail distribution to companies and carriers. (Please see the discussion of computer application in Chapter 5.)

PERSONAL CONTACT WITH THE EMPLOYER

Telephone contact with the employer and claims adjustors is important. Ideally the employer or compensation carrier, or both, should be called by the nurse or clinician when any patient is not returned to full work after an occupational injury or illness. This allows timely processing of the carrier's paperwork to get the temporary disability payments and the physician's fees paid. It also allows the employer to plan for the employee's absence and to arrange necessary coverage or redistribution of work tasks.

Employers should be carefully questioned about the availability of modified work or alternate assignments. Frequently the patient may not know that alternative work exists. Company policies regarding modified duty may change rapidly, and what was true last month may be completely different this month. A discussion with the supervisor about restrictions or options frequently identifies productive work that the patient can do during recovery.

Many clinics have a policy of trying to visit each contract company at least once a year. The best combination is to send both the clinic manager and a physician or nurse practitioner. Key parts of the facility should be toured and a meeting held with personnel, employee or union representatives, and any medical staff on site. Attention should be paid to work processes, including exposures and hazards. The meeting should explore how the company feels about the clinic's services and what they would like done differently. The clinic may not be able to meet their requests, but at least it can be explained why not. Information gained from this visit should be written up and added to the database on that company in the clinic's computer or contract files. The practitioner's interest and effort are excellent marketing tools also.

PERSONAL CONTACT WITH THE COMPENSATION CARRIER'S ADJUSTER

Direct communication with the adjuster is important not only for temporary disability cases but also for complicated ones, such as chemical exposures or cumulative injuries. The adjuster can then discuss causality, ask questions about disease or injury processes, and get to know the practitioner and how he thinks. It also allows the physician to explain atypical cases or to request help from the adjuster to gather information not available to the clinician. The adjuster can also guide the physician through the administrative options available to the doctor and the patient when cases do not progress as anticipated. We find most adjusters an invaluable help in case direction and resolution, and we have found that most simply want the physician's honest, objective medical opinion.

Should the physician have a concern about personal life-style issues or stressors interfering with the patient's recovery or suspect that malingering or actual fraud may be involved, additional information or assistance might be requested from the claims examiner. The adjusters can subpoena and send the physician copies of the patient's records from all other providers or can arrange a sub rosa investigation with a private investigator. Fortunately, this is rarely needed, but in frustrating cases such resources are available to the clinician.

However, the practitioner's role is that of medical care provider for the patient. (See Chapter 20, The Challenge of Patient Management). The clinician should not cast himself as a private detective. In short, administrative and legal questions are best investigated and handled by administrative and legal personnel.

If the physician has difficulty with a particular adjuster, he can call later and ask to talk to the senior claims manager, requesting intervention. This action should not be routine and should be done only if the clinician has already provided all appropriate documentation required. Many compensation carriers have a physician consultant or medical director who can be contacted in difficult cases, but again, this approach should be used with caution. For example, if the clinician has a classic case of hand-arm vibration syndrome and the adjuster, disagreeing, denies the claim, the clinician might then wish to contact the senior manager or consultant for assistance.

All compensation carriers have regularly scheduled educational sessions for their adjusters, who have to handle medical decisions without medical background. If someone in the clinic has the skill to present technical medical material in clear, practical lay language and knows the compensation system rules, he can offer to give free educational sessions to groups of adjusters and to provide free brief telephone consultation. This again makes the clinician known and accessible for direct referral, because adjusters often channel patients to specific clinics. Moreover, insurance administrators are less likely to delay or deny a patient's claim if they know the clinician and feel comfortable with his judgment.

For the most part, medical training does not emphasize the business or administrative aspects of a practice. Physicians rely on the expertise of an office manager or on their own instinct to establish and maintain office systems. Practitioners thrive on sleuthing a diagnosis and guiding appropriate treatment but too often view paperwork as a waste of precious physician time. They may not attend to the flow of charts, forms, and reports until the stacks on the desk approach the maximum weight-bearing load or the office manager threatens.

Clinicians therefore must recognize that when they agree to provide medical care in the workers' compensation setting, they also embrace a set of administrative responsibilities that must be fulfilled with the same alacrity and concern accorded to practicing medicine. In fact, in the context of occupational injuries, administrative issues and paperwork should be viewed as an integral part of practicing medicine, as opposed to an annoying obligation. Prompt attention to these administrative duties facilitates the delivery of medical care and helps ensure prompt distribution of benefits to the injured worker.

No discussion about administrative policies and procedures would be complete without a look at the future. As we write this, health care reform is foremost in the news, with the Administration's latest proposal under scrutiny. Some form of managed care clearly is part of our future, and workers' compensation certainly will be included. Reform may dramatically reduce paperwork, with consolidation of claim forms into a single version; however, stricter requirements for prior authorization could make our work more onerous. We need to think about the directions our field is taking and prepare for the future.

WORKERS' COMPENSATION AND MANAGED CARE

This section provides background information on how payers have applied medical cost containment methods that were originally developed for group health plans to workers' compensation medical benefits. Understanding the theory and practice of managed care hopefully will allow the treating physician to deal more smoothly with the payers in a cooperative effort to manage costs without compromising quality of care.

Inflation in the cost of health care has reached crisis proportions. During the past decade, group health medical benefits have nearly doubled every 5 years, and many large corporations have seen erosion and even elimination of profits because of rising health care costs. By 1986 the medical component of the Consumer Price Index (CPI) surpassed the overall CPI by a margin of 7 to 1—the largest differential between the two indices ever recorded. In response, both government and private health insurers have introduced a variety of measures designed to control costs. In fact, virtually all group health insurance payers now have extensive medical cost containment programs. This has given rise to an entire new industry of "managed care" vendors, who are constantly searching for innovative ways to control health care costs.

The common features of managed care are familiar to any practitioner who participates in preferred provider organizations (PPOs) or health maintenance organizations (HMOs). Bill audits and preauthorization requirements for hospitalization, specialist referral, surgery, or other high-cost procedures are now common features of fee-for-service medicine.

The application of managed care techniques to workers' compensation has been relatively recent, however. In the past, increased medical expenses were simply passed on from the insurance carrier to the employer in the form of higher premiums, but now employers are complaining that escalating workers' compensation costs are eroding their ability to compete with foreign companies. It is true that the medical costs in workers' compensation have shown a *differential* rate of rise even above that seen in health care generally. By 1990 medical costs had exceeded indemnity benefits in most states, and the annual inflation rate has been estimated at 13% to 15%, almost double that seen for health care generally.

Many factors contribute to the differential increase in workers' compensation medical costs, including the following:

1. The lack of cost sharing in workers' compensation compared with group health creates incentives for patients (employees) and physicians to shift costs to workers' compensation.

2. Supply and demand are *not* independent in health care: an increase in the supply of physicians *creates* an increased demand for services. This is exaggerated in fee-for-service reimbursement systems and in the absence of cost sharing. Both of these conditions exist in workers' compensation.

3. Because reimbursement levels for the newer high-tech diagnostic treatment procedures are relatively high, they tend to be overused. This results in higher costs without better outcome (such as use of MRI in the management of patients with back pain). This problem is exaggerated in workers' compensation, which traditionally has not had utilization controls.

4. The presence of litigation in workers' compensation results in prolonged treatment and increased use of medical services to maximize the permanent disability rating. The system thus rewards illness behavior, and care continues despite failure to improve.

5. In the workers' compensation system the amount and nature of care are not specified or limited by contract, as in group health. For example, the Labor Code in California allows reimbursement for any care that is "reasonable and necessary." Because insurance personnel have been reluctant to second guess providers, *all* services rendered traditionally have been presumed reasonable and necessary. This has resulted in wasteful and outright abusive medical practice.

6. A common misconception exists among injured workers (as well as most patients) that more care is necessarily better. This combined with a psychologic sense of entitlement (the employer owes benefits to the injured worker) causes increased use of medical services in workers' compensation.

7. Workers' compensation benefits include wage replacement and vocational rehabilitation, which creates an incentive for shifting to industrial coverage. This is exaggerated when negotiated labor contracts provide for full pay while the employee is off work for an industrial injury (for example, the state of California "Industrial Disability Leave").

8. There is some degree of free choice of physician in workers' compensation, whereas group health has increased the use of PPOs and HMOs, which limit selection of the provider.

9. The significant increases in the cost of health care generally have resulted in decreased group health benefits provided by employers. Consequently, there has been a shifting of costs by employees and providers to the workers' compensation system to cover expenses no longer paid by group health plans.

Various strategies have been used in group health to control medical costs. The federal government initiated controls of inpatient costs (through Medicare and Medicaid) in the early 1980s by creating a prospective reimbursement system based on diagnosis-related groups (DRGs). This provided an incentive for hospitals to reduce costs. However, there has been a resulting increase in the costs of physician services and outpatient and home health services so that the overall impact of DRGs on medical costs is not known.

Most third-party payers currently are using the various other mechanisms to control inpatient costs. They can be lumped under the generic title of "utilization review" and include four elements:

(1) retrospective review, in which monitoring is done to identify billing errors, inappropriate levels of treatment, and excessive fees; (2) concurrent review, in which the length of hospital stay is monitored; (3) preadmission certification, which is designed to reduce the use of hospitals for procedures that can be done on an outpatient basis; and (4) discharge planning (done in conjunction with concurrent review) to maximize the use of home therapy, extended-care facilities, and hospice care.

Utilization review has also been applied to outpatient services, both retrospectively (audits of fees and levels of service) and prospectively (by reviewing treatment plans and applying practice guidelines).

Alternative delivery systems have been widely used in group health as a strategy to improve provider efficiency and control medical costs. HMOs merge the insurance and provider functions to create an incentive to provide more efficient care. Independent physician associations (IPAs) operate in the context of an HMO, whereby physicians' fees are determined by the profitability of the HMO.

PPOs are also popular. They usually are based on fee discounts in exchange for guaranteed volume of patients, but they can also incorporate utilization review and monitoring of practice patterns. To the extent that there is employer control of provider, these alternative systems are now being applied to the workers' compensation system.

Wellness programs have also been considered as a mechanism to reduce health care costs by emphasizing prevention programs. They may be relevant to workers' compensation in areas of stress, substance abuse, heart disease, and "repetitive trauma" musculoskeletal injuries.

A primary goal of any medical cost containment program should be to move the injured worker out of the health care system and back to the workplace as efficiently as possible. The emphasis should be on *quality of care* because it is best for the injured worker, maximizes the chances for return to work, and ultimately is the most cost effective. There is a need to use all necessary, but not more than necessary, medical resources. Improved communication with the injured worker is essential to the success of any program designed to control medical costs.

Regulations do not preclude workers' compensation carriers from implementing programs that prospectively and concurrently monitor providers to ensure that injured workers are receiving reasonable, appropriate, and necessary care. Cost control methods first developed in group health settings have been used in workers' compensation with apparent success, including inpatient utilization review and hospital bill audits. Utilization review of outpatient services has also been gaining in popularity, although the impact on cost has not been adequately evaluated. Utilization review must be grounded in "technology assessment" and ideally supported by scientifically sound studies of outcome.

It has been clearly demonstrated that controlling fees by whatever method offers little long-term benefit unless it is combined with utilization review. The analogy is that of a ball of rubber: if squeezed at one end, it will balloon out somewhere else. If fees are controlled, utilization rates will increase to compensate for the reduced fees. Fee schedule audits and PPOs based solely on fee discounts are therefore not rational as isolated mechanisms to control costs.

The term "managed care" has been used to describe a concept that combines utilization review with strategies to make the treating physician a partner in the goal of efficient return to work.[1] Managed care should be a cooperative effort among the medical provider, the patient, and the payer to optimize outcomes in a cost-efficient manner. The starting point can be a select physician network based on provider understanding of return-to-work issues and willingness to follow established practice guidelines. In most states current regulations do not preclude workers' compensation carriers from implementing preferred arrangements for delivery of medical benefits. However, the degree of legislatively mandated employer control over medical providers may be a limiting factor in achieving high penetration into the network.

An important impediment to the development of more long-term solutions is the lack of outcomes data.[2] For many common industrial conditions, such as low back pain, more information is needed to refine diagnostic and treatment protocols. Data collected by workers' compensation insurance carriers may offer a unique opportunity to accumulate information on medical outcomes. The advantages of the workers' compensation data is that it includes the readily definable outcome of return to work. A disadvantage, however, is that variables other than quality of medical care may profoundly affect the patient's return to work (especially motivational factors). Outcome data are also useful for provider monitoring. Ideally, participation in a preferred provider network should be based solely on outcomes rather than intensive prospective monitoring, which is time consuming and costly for both physician and payor. If case-rate reimbursement mechanisms based on diagnosis or even capitated payment schemes can be applied to workers' compensation (both of which put the physician at some financial risk), prospective utilization review and bill audits can be minimized.

REFERENCES

1. Medical Committee, International Association of Industrial Accidents Boards and Commissions: The role of managed care in workers' compensation: Medical Committee annual report, Baltimore, Md, September 1989, The Association.
2. Gots RE: Managing the quality and cost of health care in workers' compensation, *National Council on Compensation Insurance (NCCI) Digest* 5(1):35-40, 1990.

SUGGESTED READINGS

Gapen P: Whittling down workers' compensation costs, Business and Health: 35-40, Oct, 1989.

Herzlinger RE et al: How companies tackle health care costs, Harvard Business Review 63:69-81, 1985.

Iskowe DS: Workers' compensation medical benefits: a practical framework for implementing new cost containment strategies, Brentwood, Tenn, 1992, Focus Healthcare Management.

Iskowe DS et al: The workers' compensation insurance crisis: a call for new initiatives in medical management, Brentwood, Tenn, 1992, Focus Healthcare Management.

Milstein A et al: Controlling medical costs in workers' compensation, Business and Health pp 34-36, March, 1988.

National Council on Compensation Insurance: Cost containment: report of the Cost Containment Committee of the Workers' Compensation Congress, NCCI Digest 4(4):25-49, 1989.

Taulbee P: Coralling runaway workers' compensation costs, Business and Health pp 46-55, April, 1991.

Workers' Compensation Research Institute (WCRI): Medical cost containment in workers' compensation: trends and interstate comparisons, WCRI Pub No WC90-4, Cambridge, Mass, 1989, The Institute.

5 Information Management and Computer Application in the Occupational Health Clinic

Computerizing American business and industry has brought about dramatic changes in the way people work, the way decisions are made, and how resources are allocated. While computerizing the occupational health aspect of American industry is late in joining the information movement, it is now poised to bring about exponential change in occupational health as a professional specialty. Computerizing occupational health programs will positively affect medical costs and quality of worklife and will result in a significant shift toward injury prevention and increased worker productivity.

These advances will come about not because occupational health professionals use computers. They will occur when occupational health professionals experience a paradigm shift in understanding how to use computers effectively through reorganizing work, allocating adequate management support, and expanding expectations about what computerization can achieve.

COMPUTERIZING OCCUPATIONAL HEALTH

Until recently, computerizing occupational health programs seemed to mean task automation. Many computer hopefuls expected an immediate eradication of the paper maze and reduced labor costs. Many used the time-savings rationale to justify the cost of computerization—a position that has proved wrong. Saving time through task automation is too narrow a view to justify the significant expenditures of dollars and human energy involved in computerization.

Although computerizing eliminated repetitive manual tasks, it did not eliminate the need to address other operational issues. The time-savings rationale overlooked the fact that dedicated personnel time is required to input data and failed to take into account a fundamental change in the way work is accomplished. Assuming that workers at all levels should be able to incorporate computeri-

zation into the daily routine, management neglected to weigh the effects on work style. A computerized approach, which is multitiered and nonlinear, differs significantly from the manual, repetitious methods to which people were accustomed.

Naive or misguided approaches to computerizing any application can lead to monumental problems and failures. More important, a shortsighted view can result in poor implementation and unmeasured costs. Inevitably, the whole notion of computerizing is either dropped or confined to a minor portion of the work. Effective leadership is as important to the automation process as are the computer hardware and software.

The advent of microcomputers in the early 1980s gave ordinary people access to the power of computerization. Computers became affordable and accessible at the application level where the actual work is accomplished. Programming (program design and structuring) could be accomplished by professionals in the application domain rather than by remote computer programming experts.

To remain competitive, the occupational health clinic must be run as an efficient business, effectively communicating with its business constituency. How computerized information is presented can influence employers' perceptions of medical competence and quality of occupational health services. The way to impact employers' perception of quality is through the new paradigm of information management, using a computerized process to gain the information advantage. The shift in nomenclature reflects a broader scope, but also highlights the possibilities. Computerized information provides a common language between people of divergent concerns and goals, as between employers and occupational health professionals.

Ironically, although much of the work of occupational health management is information management, the concept itself has not been widely embraced by occupational health professionals. This reluctance is partially the result of the problems and surprises that people encounter when computerizing. Awareness of these problems and misconceptions can help one avoid them and can point to more effective approaches.

Operational problems

We might assume that current operational problems will be eradicated with the use of computers to streamline work. One must separate management, operational, and personnel issues from the computerization process itself. Difficult issues cannot be solved by hoping that users will be distracted or uplifted by the excitement of computerizing. In fact, computerizing almost always surfaces new operational issues or those that have been overlooked or avoided.

For example, simple management decisions such as where to place a workstation can seriously and significantly affect its use. A manager might decide to limit computer access, either to prevent damage or to control its use. This management style reflects inappropriate use of a new technology, because one of the most powerful aspects of computing is accessibility. Artificially limiting access highlights an underlying issue of resource mismanagement.

Computerizing the work process can also identify conflicts in operational procedures. In fact, management should be alerted to look for and expect operational issues to surface during the implementation process. For instance, people might have completely different understandings of a regulatory imperative, such as correct documentation of the Occupational Safety and Health Act (OSHA) log or frequency of laboratory testing in medical surveillance. Under a manual process, these discrepancies in understanding procedures may never be uncovered. Computerizing also uncovers redundant or inconsistent criteria for manual list keeping.

Conflicts also emerge around decisions to import or export electronically specific data elements. Which department has the information first? Which should share the information with other departments? Answers may reveal internal factionalism or basic confusion about where given information belongs. Resolving these problems can be challenging; the answer does not always lie in the realm of expediency or logic.

Medical-legal issues

Medical-legal and confidentiality issues are potentially significant. Specific steps can be taken to solve questions of security against text alteration, to protect confidentiality during transfer, and to ensure medical-legal integrity.

An effective way to approach the problem is to identify the ways manual records are protected and to apply similar protections to the electronic record. The issues are accessibility and text alteration. Electronic access can be protected by means of password security systems. If the system is a part of a network, then network access protection is available through the network software system. Further security is available on most commercially available application software at varying levels of detail: system level, menu level, record level, and field level. Determining the need to access and granting access are not technology functions but management's responsibility.

Once users are cleared to enter the system, text and record alteration protection should be available. Some set a grace period following data entry after which the document is automatically transformed into a view-only format: users can read it but not change it, and the record cannot be deleted. Others are more strict: the record is saved and rendered view-only immediately. Another common way to deal with the problem of text protection is to print, sign, date and place the record in the medical chart. Although the method is effective, it dilutes the benefit of paperless computerization.

User identification or electronic signatures can also be applied. Unfortunately, these safeguards limit accessibility and ease of use. Putting obstructive mechanisms in place should be weighed against the need for productivity. Potential medical-legal problems can be overengineered, leading to dissatisfaction and reluctance to use the system.

Decisions about accessibility should be considered with legal counsel. Acceptable standards are needed for the entire health care industry. Just as standards have been set for manual systems, where, for example, a line is drawn through altered chart text and initialed or signed, a similar but technically feasible method must be established for electronic records. Chapter 6 further discusses medical record confidentiality.

Only now, after little more than 10 years of microcomputing, is awareness heightened regarding what computers can achieve in occupational health. Separating management and operational issues from the computerization process of information management remains challenging, but understanding this distinction is critical to success.

GUARANTEEING SUCCESSFUL COMPUTERIZATION

What guarantees success in computerizing occupational health programs? How can the benefits be maximized? What knowledge and planning are required? The essential prerequisite is to recognize that the effective computerization of any business is not a single-level operation. Four distinct management functions demand attention.

First, clearly identify the specific purposes and goals for computerizing, clarifying the rationale to eliminate vague notions or questions regarding purpose. Only by articulating purpose and goals will staff become engaged in the process. No one can follow a path that has not been clearly defined.

Second, select appropriate hardware/software on the basis of current uses and future goals. These decisions involve choosing particular equipment and mapping appropriate placement and use. Again, employees must be involved, and leadership must be aware of organizational and operational issues that are likely to surface in the selection process.

Third, thoughtfully plan implementation. Detail the steps involving how the system will be made operational, and set realistic expectations for management and staff. Decide how training will occur and who will be trained. Defining accountability is essential; when responsibilities are vague, no one accepts them. Premanage the anticipated implementation problems by communicating expectations and procedures.

Fourth, craft outcome measures to monitor the system's success on every level. How do people know when they are successful? Employees must understand their jobs and what is expected of them. Outcome measures can quantify success in implementation and identify problems that must be addressed to maximize benefit.

When even one function is overlooked in planning, the investment opportunity is jeopardized. On the other hand, addressing computerization with a comprehensive management approach can result in profound success. We will therefore examine the four areas in detail.

Setting goals for computerizing

Successful computerization demands that one establish clear purposes and goals. Avoid the tendency to be simplistic or esoteric rather than pragmatic. Be honest about true purpose and aware of future possibilities. The following are examples of purposes and goals.

Goals one through seven describe common views of automation advantages in occupational health—certainly acceptable reasons for pursuit. Goals eight through twenty-two show a much broader scope of deliverable outcomes from computerization.

Task automation. To computerize strictly to automate tasks or save time is a mistake. Important task automation advantages are possible, but when that is the only goal users are misled into thinking the ultimate goal is reached, and the full possibilities of computerization are lost.

Computers remember things with reassuring accuracy and consistency. The database is a reservoir of information available for manipulation. Data entered into the system once can yield a variety of outputs. Examples include reports of injury for Workers' Compensation, the OSHA-200 Log, or a frequency analysis.

The time saved depends on the software design and hardware architecture and the accuracy and completeness of data entry. Success in task automation requires dedicated, trained personnel for data entry. This issue is discussed later in this chapter in the section on implementation.

Electronic medical records. Medical record documentation imperatives are regulatory and professional. Complete computerization of medical records should include all physical exams, medical and occupational health histories, workers' compensation and medical disability data, and all medical surveillance information such as audiometric exams, immunizations, chemical or biological exposures, potential exposure screening, and health maintenance. Adequate disk space must be planned to incorporate the data.

Like other health care personnel, most physicians have learned to document with a pen or through dictation. Relying on manual input in an electronic environment requires a second step and another person to interpret the data for entry. This redundancy may adversely affect productivity and accuracy. Less desirably, physicians may directly enter notes themselves. If time saving and efficiency are the only computerization goals, they may not be realized.

Alternate methods of data entry, such as voice entry or light pens, are becoming available. Voice entry is on the threshold of practical implementation.

Retaining historical and medical data requires great amounts of computer hard disk space. Nevertheless, electronic medical records detailing clinical visits, medical history, occupational history and medical surveillance are feasible even on microcomputers. What should be computerized and what should remain on the hard copy chart is an operational decision driven by hard disk size, projected number and size of records to be kept, and whether purging or archiving tactics can be implemented. Computer performance will be diminished with large amounts of data, regardless of the hardware and software.

Selective documentation. One way to avoid overwhelming disk consumption is to selectively or incrementally incorporate elements of medical record documentation. Satisfy regulatory demands first. Additional documentation, particularly of medical surveillance, can be added as the software format and discretionary disk space allow. Analyze priorities and select those that will bring the most immediate benefit to the organization or those that will not cause undue hardship later in terms of compliance or data retrieval in a high-risk situation. If unlimited disk space is available, document everything electronically.

Hardware disk capacity is available, is inexpensive, and can be enhanced. However, execute good planning from the beginning by calculating exactly the amount of disk space needed. Most software developers and vendors will supply information regarding required disk space for each portion of the software program. Table 5-1 displays a sample method for sizing the system.

The record size and the header account for the screen lay-out, labels, and format. These capacity elements are built in by the programmer. When multiplied by the estimated number of records, the hard disk consumption can be very accurately determined.

Documentation for retrieval. Electronically documenting medical records carries some attractive benefits. Data elements, such as years of audiometric scores or months of blood pressure readings can be instantly retrieved if the appropriate database software format has been used. Word processing alone will not do. Information in a word processing format, which is a flat file similar to hard copy, only serves to simplify the clerical function. Selected data cannot be retrieved from word processing, which contributes nothing to leveraging information for decision support, analysis, or review. The only way to position documented health information for future use is to structure a database to capture key data elements in the same format over time.

Such a database places each important factor in a cell, known as a field, to be recalled later and compared with other similar cells. Long notes, even if electronic and eloquent, are useless in the context of data retrieval. They can be retrieved, of course, if they are printed and read individually. The use of word processing to support or clarify data elements is entirely acceptable, but it should not be relied on in the powerful information management context.

To economize when planning and using electronic medical records, users must organize their thinking and present material in a concise manner. Medical histories are suited to electronic data management, but only if they are properly interpreted in a database format. Dictation notes are adequate for their traditional purpose, but they cannot produce information such as trending or analysis. Input format can be engineered for ease, speed, and standardization, so that the resulting gain is using the data elements to compare events and cases, to interpret and forecast trends. Searching for trends or predicting outcomes can be easily, often instantly, accomplished. Data fields populated by predetermined lists, such as injury type or International Classification of Diseases (ICD) 9 code, allow the retrieval of specific, standardized information from which new information can be derived.

Medical surveillance is particularly well suited to electronic documentation. In fact, the federal government long ago acknowledged this when it first mandated that audiometric program data be computer stored. Electronically stored readings can be automatically compared with shifts and aggregate trends.

An obvious benefit to electronically managed medical surveillance is instant retrieval of data to manage regulatory audits and avoid fines. The time saved in data retrieval argues in favor of task automation. More important, data credibility, along with the speed and accuracy of presentation, is persuasive.

Table 5-1 Hard disk usage planner for occupational health medical records

Required data	Record size*		Number of records		Header space size*		Hard disk space required*
Employee records	(559	×	_____)	+	1570	=	_____
Clinic visit record	(631	×	_____)	+	1250	=	_____
Visit notes record	(3500	×	_____)	+	738	=	_____
Medical surveillance record	(3550	×	_____)	+	1560	=	_____
Job analysis record	(2275	×	_____)	+	9289	=	_____
Functional capability	(2117	×	_____)	+	9845	=	_____
Employer file	(758	×	_____)	+	2146	=	_____
Insurer file	(391	×	_____)	+	482	=	_____

* Numbers are bytes.

Employer reports. Employers often prefer the distilled executive summary or one-page letter. The fact that information is medical, mandated, or even interesting has no bearing on the basic fact that if it is long, it is less likely to be read. Presenting usable information to business management is essential to the ultimate gains, financial and otherwise, of any occupational health entity. Computerization allows presentation of concise, readable, understandable information to business management in a common language format.

More important to most physicians is the fact that information derived from a database can be crafted to protect confidentiality. Data elements can be trended, identifying contributing factors such as department, supervisor, location, or time of day when the injury occurred. In this way, medical information is transformed into a useful information tool.

Standardized data. Using electronic medical data elements rather than narrative descriptions is not new. It demonstrates a way to organize all medical information so that objective data elements can be statistically analyzed to project outcomes and appropriate standards of care defined. It requires disciplined and organized thinking to design medical observations into standardized essential data elements. However, it is the basis for developing normative data leading to standardized guidelines for treatment and duration of disability.

To date, few in occupational medicine have organized data in a standard format that can be compared broadly. The use of ICD 9 or other simple, standardized coding methods is imperative to initiate this process and establish a common platform. Once a standard format is accepted, adding data elements (such as length of disability following an injury, type of work, specific industry, and geographic location) to the diagnostic code rounds out a clear picture of events, procedures, and outcomes.

Normative disability data have been previously unavailable because only workers' compensation insurers or third party administrators collected injury data electronically, using accepted risk management or loss control terminology. Standards do not exist. Injuries are generally coded in terms of type (abrasion, sprain, strain); body part (leg, arm, back); and cause (contact with, struck by or against, and fall against). Even those identifiers would be helpful if they had been standardized. Medical professionals have the advantage of well-established and widely accepted coding standards, such as ICD and CPT, already in place.

Tracking and monitoring. Computers are useful in case management because they remember (document) where the employee has been referred, the diagnostic tests and treatments ordered, and the results. Proactive, comprehensive case monitoring that addresses all providers, resources, and other case participants fits into the more aggressive framework of today's managed care environment. The computer is used to map the case, identifying all services, resources, and persons involved in the process. It offers a view of the entire case, not simply the activity within the clinic walls.

Demonstrating cost savings. Because workers' compensation is a legal system rather than a simple medical benefit, cases are more difficult to control and cost control strategies are more difficult to apply than for similar cases paid for by medical benefits. This presents an opportunity for occupational health professionals to demonstrate how they affect cost on the employer's behalf. Using information systems designed to manage and report to employers the savings from their efforts offers significant advantage to physicians.

A computerized system performs best as a vehicle to report cost savings because of consistent documentation and common language. Business professionals do not think like medical professionals. The disciplines, jargon, and the values and stakes are different. Detailed medical summary reports do not offer employers options. Medical condition reporting needs to be reframed around what the recipient wants to know. Employers appreciate loss-control information, accounts of specific cost-savings measures, accounts of what the physician is doing on their behalf rather than diagnosis and number of visits. Case-specific, encounter-specific measurable medical decisions that directly affect costs will avoid later conflict with others involved in the case and will appropriately allocate responsibility. Treating physicians have overwhelming influence over case severity (a risk management term referring to duration and cost) and outcome. From a competitive viewpoint, physicians will do well to find a credible and respectable way to report what they have done on the employer's behalf.

Stated another way, employers prefer information that they can use, that they can do something about, or that assists in their planning. Loss control information in the form of incident frequency, severity, and trend analysis is amazingly useful to employers.

Cost savings can be measured and reported. In the course of providing treatment, cost-controlling decisions are made regularly by physicians and their staffs. Documenting and quantifying those decisions on a transaction by transaction basis is not only possible but necessary. Using a computer system can make it an honorable, straightforward process, understood and appreciated by employers.

Begin by creating a set of cost-savings assumptions and share them with employers to ensure agreement about how the savings are being measured. Once the process is clarified, it can be monitored and reported. Creating a database to document dollar savings or the number of days saved simplifies the process of accumulating, comparing, allocating, and distributing the information regarding cost savings for client employers.

Marketing advantage. Occupational medicine is widely acknowledged as a rapidly growing industry. In a competitive market, physicians are frequently asked to become involved in the marketing effort to gain and retain employer clients. Many practitioners find marketing distasteful or a poor use of their time; moreover, most physicians have not been trained for marketing activities. Having an effective information system can help.

Good marketing techniques involve understanding what is desired or needed by clients and supplying it. In that context, employers want information for loss control and decision support. Using computers as a marketing tool creates unprecedented gains with little, if any, additional effort or cost. All it requires is advanced planning and thoughtful data collection.

Loss control. Employers want data that suggest the next action. Reports that tick the number of clinic visits do not supply a basis for decisions. Reports should help them make decisions, identify problems, and point to solutions. Good information reports can even underscore supervisor and manager accountability. Reports should reflect recent incidence, rather than that of several months ago, to instill urgency so that corrective action can be taken.

For example, one employer received a loss control report from the occupational medical clinic that pointed to a specific supervisor associated with an unusual number of cases. The employer had not made the connection because the supervisor's assignment had been rotated frequently during the period. The trend was elusive until the computer system identified the connection and presented the information impartially.

Another example of a loss control report is to trend injuries by job class. In one case, this type of analytical reporting was able to document reduced injury frequency after an ergonomic change was made on the assembly line.

Other loss control reports might trend key variables associated with injuries and illness, such as age of the employee, length of service, and specific job or cost center. Loss control consultation based on hard data offers the opportunity to identify additional cost-savings interventions.

Insurers or insurance administrators may provide loss control reports directly to employers. These reports can be challenged on the basis of their timeliness alone. Although the report might be dated the most recent month, the data contained are often 3 months old. Insurers are often the last to know about an injury or illness, whereas medical providers are the first to know.

Management reports. The objectivity that computerized data afford is particularly valuable to employers for fair and unbiased interventions and employee evaluations. With the advent of the Americans with Disabilities Act and other equal opportunity legislation, employers must rely on objective information about injury trends and hazards of specific jobs. Computer data are relatively unbiased and can support fair and unprejudicial management decisions.

Behavior change tool. Information can empower the employer's efforts at injury prevention. Computerized information becomes a tool for behavior change and a platform for safety, loss control, and continuous quality improvement.

Workplace accidents are not caused by dark hallways, slippery floors, or malfunctioning equipment; they result from attitudes and relationships in the workplace. The California State Highway Patrol makes it a practice to survey persons with moving traffic violations or accidents regarding their mood at the time of the event. According to state highway patrol records, over 80% admit to being angry or upset just before the incident.

Similarly, when people at work are angry or frustrated, they work less safely and accidents occur. Negative attitudes generate carelessness. Lifting classes and safety training will not affect this phenomenon. Even management leadership classes alone will not reduce or eliminate injuries.

Studies conducted by Habeck and colleagues at the University of Michigan demonstrated factors within the company that affect workers' compensation and disability experience. Companies that recognize employee needs, offering caring kinds of services such as Employee Assistance Programs (EAPs) have significantly fewer workplace accidents and other disability costs. The study shows that management attitudes toward employees carry a hefty impact on workers' compensation costs.

Supervisors do need training about the strength of their influence on workers' behavior and how to use this influence as a positive force. Providing leadership tools and reinforcing leaders with feedback information for benchmarking progress is a powerful intervention.

Loss information, or information reports about injuries and illnesses that are detailed to the cost center or department level, is influential. It has a "heads up" effect, sometimes referred to as the sentinel effect, allowing supervisors to mark their progress, rather than ignore it. The information feedback to supervisors must be timely and distributed at regular intervals.

The same criteria can be applied to provider performance. Using information to report by ICD code the number of work days lost, the number of modified workdays, and costs by specific providers will clearly identify the outliers in terms of treatment performance. As with managers and supervisors, the information speaks for itself to change behavior; yet, it is nonconfrontive and noninvasive.

Information is so powerful that even if outlying providers are not personally identified, performance shifts toward the mean in subsequent reporting periods. The power of information to change behavior is much like biologic or behavior feedback. A response (change decision) is based on the incoming data. With a little imagination and creative application, information can become a broadly applied, potent behavior modification tool.

Occupational physicians who can embrace information as a tool will deliver new and effective services to their employer clients. Using a tool already in place for other purposes is an intriguing suggestion. The investment takes the form of willingness to explore a new paradigm.

Normative data. People frequently ask about disability treatment and duration guidelines that are derived from normative data. As observed earlier, normative disability data are nonexistent at the time of this writing; data have yet to be collected in significant quantities to establish standard criteria. Occupational health professionals are the most logical persons to collect that data; claims adjusters have not offered leadership in this area. Occupational health professionals are the participants who can assign diagnostic codes appropriately, create treatment patterns, and control frequency of visits and duration of the disability. When the diagnostic code is collected with a severity factor along with actual treatment, frequency, and duration, the normative data become reality. Normative guidelines that result will serve to drive down inappropriate costs. These data will support legitimate care and undermine opportunistic or inappropriate treatment.

Those most interested in normative data fall into one of two groups. The first consists primarily of occupational health entities and professionals using it as a prerequisite to quantify cost savings and as a marketing stimulus. The other group consists of third-party entities, primarily insurers, insurance administrators, health maintenance organizations (HMOs), preferred provider organizations (PPOs), utilization reviewers, and case managers who use the information to withhold treatment or payment. Normative data is best used to form guidelines that keep workers' compensation system abusers in check.

Information as gatekeeper. The term "gatekeeper" was a popular and important term during the 1980s to describe the primary physician managing the case. In that context, the term is one that can be expanded, establishing occupational medical physicians as information gatekeepers. Instead of discontinuing case management when referral is made to a specialist, the occupational health information gatekeeper (acting as case manager) continues to manage case information, monitoring and mapping it throughout its course.

In this way, the occupational physician retains administrative supervision of the case without offending the current treatment provider after the referral. Data are collected and used to make decisions, influence other providers, and bond with clients.

Electronic report transmission. Electronic transmission of mandated and requested reports is an exciting and efficient option available from computerization. Many use facsimile transmission or a combination of computer and fax. Modem transmission of summary reports or formal workers' compensation reports streamlines the process. Reports are transmitted directly and instantly, computer to computer, bypassing mailrooms and problems that may cause unnecessary delays. Indeed, a new business has emerged, electronic data transmission companies, providing services to both medical providers and employers.

Although many more important reasons exist to computerize occupational health, this may be the one to get the job done. Electronic transmission may be a prerequisite for payment in the future.

Peer review. As noted earlier, reporting provider performance can affect behavior. In this manner, peer review can be almost fully automated. When norms are established, performance profiles will be run against them, highlighting the outliers. The computerized process requires little additional cost and is useful beyond the peer review outcome.

Outliers or problem cases trigger a notation, "flag," or report that lists issues for review. Problem physicians, identified in terms of use of diagnostic, therapeutic, and other medical service utilization measured against standard protocols, will be automatically noted. Once again, the objectivity of such a report makes it much easier to confront the physician or other provider in the peer review process. Disparate variables can be discussed and evaluated on a collaborative, rather than embarrassing or punitive, basis.

Managed care, case management. The terms "managed care" and "case management" are exploited by nearly everyone in health care. Many believe that managed care and case management (or what may be referred to as utilization management) is accomplished only with an information system as backup. When HMO and PPO companies enter the workers' compensation and occupational health delivery system, their first action is to obtain an applicable computerized system. What are the implications for other occupational health practitioners?

This continuing movement toward computerized managed care by those established in information management suggests that without an information system, one cannot claim to be offering case management or managed care. Case management is essentially a third party function, not necessarily an insurance third party. The issues must be addressed comprehensively, engaging employers in the process. Case management or managed care cannot begin and end with medical visits.

Network management. Referring patients to cost-effective providers is, indeed, beneficial. The difficulty comes in identifying the cost-effective providers. Too often, those selected are the ones who are best known to the organizer or who offer the least resistance to discounting.

Notwithstanding the peer review and performance appraisal capabilities of a system, the benefits of using a computerized system for managing the network itself cannot be overrated. Credentialing; monitoring agreements; ticking contract renewals; identifying providers, including specialists in desired geographic areas; identifying clinics with special characteristics such as those with Spanish speakers or with evening office hours make the system indispensable for managing care.

Reimbursement. Hospitals and many larger, independent medical groups invested heavily in computerized reimbursement systems and now lag behind in application, end-user computing because they are busy defending past costs and excess capacity. The old systems cannot keep up with new marketing demands of network discounts, PPO network management, and consolidated billing. Energies and resources are directed to patching new capabilities to old systems.

As managed care expands into all medical arenas, methods of reimbursement are undergoing dramatic changes. Certainly with government determined to reform healthcare, the way practitioners are paid is sure to change dramatically. Those best positioned to tolerate or benefit from the changes, however, are those who are poised to premanage the future. An appropriate accommodation to the future is a good information system that will handle a variety of purposes and goals, not the least of which is reimbursement.

Cost accounting. Physicians must consider cost accounting to participate in marketing opportunities, specialty networks, and fee discounting. One must know whether a profit is to be made in any given activity. Delivering more services could mean losing more money unless services are quantified in terms of personnel time and fixed overhead. Simple income and expense calculations may not be enough in the future. Occupational health professionals must justify their own time and that of their staff members, their overhead (including space and equipment). They must compare with those of outside, contracted occupational health providers.

Changes in the way services are authorized and remunerated will necessitate major changes in delivery practices and systems. Practitioners will be required to demonstrate efficiencies of service delivery to participate in the new delivery system. Cost accounting is a computerized decision support mechanism that will select the survivors.

Other products. Possibly a curious but exciting outcome of computerizing is to generate new service products based on the technology itself. An example of using occupational health information systems as a service product is contracting with employers to manage their OSHA reporting or workers' compensation reporting. Collecting the required data electronically on behalf of client companies can produce the OSHA log, benefit summaries, and loss control reports.

With a sophisticated computerized occupational health information system, additional services might include inputting and evaluating historical OSHA data for trend analysis. Assisting employers' compliance with the ADA (Americans with Disabilities Act) by keeping job analysis databases for them is another service product. The information system is literally converted to sellable products.

Client bonding. New technology can lead to new client services. Being on line with clients through modems, transferring data between them and the occupational clinic, offering computer/fax reports such as those for work status or instant OSHA logs, and generally keeping the electronic lines and more traditional lines of communication open have intriguing marketing and functional qualities. Offering clients access to specific view-only data creates a sense of participation and control. More important, the psychological bonding that can be produced with these gestures of partnership cannot be underestimated.

CHOOSING APPROPRIATE HARDWARE AND SOFTWARE

Technology. Changes and new breakthroughs in computer technology occur daily. Hardware technology is constantly on the move, as are operating systems and application software. Information published about technology is likely outdated by the time it reaches a reader.

The best that computer trade journals can do is report user experience with specific products and manufacturers' and developers' claims about products and product releases. That being the case, great care should be taken before relying heavily on what the popular press says about existing and future products.

What can be said about purchasing hardware and software is that to wait until price and technology stabilize will perpetually postpone the purchase. Prices for hardware will continue to decline (or more technology will be available for the same price), and prices for software will increase because performance has shifted from hardware to the software. The approach for purchasers presented here is a rational, disciplined, logical process for decision making.

Consistent trends in computerization. Besides the shift of performance from hardware to software, a few other significant trends are irrefutable. Awareness of the trends helps in selecting hardware and software because the trend line points to the future. The fear of purchase can be minimized by understanding what is likely to occur.

The trend over the past 30 years is that size, and the cost of computer hardware has been and continues to be on a downward slope, while utility and accessibility has increased just as significantly (Fig. 5-1). The trends are consistent, regardless of brand or platform, whether mainframe, midrange, or microcomputer, and regardless of operating system and software.

Size trends are the most obvious. Essentially, the difference among mainframe, midrange, and personal computers is size, measured in disk capacity. Mainframe computers that once occupied whole rooms can now be housed in relatively tiny spaces. A major early breakthrough initiated the downsizing trend when vacuum tubes were replaced by microprocessor chips with integrated circuits. Computers that recently required as many as 200 integrated circuits like those using the Intel 386 chip now offer equal or better performance with 15 or fewer integrated circuits. That is why some notebook size computers are as powerful and have as much capacity and speed as early mainframe computers.

Price of hardware correlates with the downward trend in size. Particularly in the case of microcom-

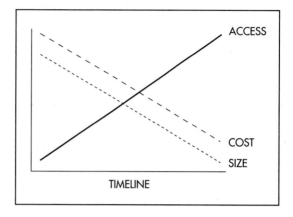

Fig. 5-1 Computer hardware trends.

puters, prices have dropped significantly. A desktop computer in the mid 1990s sells for about one fourth or less than the price of desktop computers in the early 1980s, and they are exponentially more powerful than earlier mainframe computers.

With decreasing size and increasing power, is the trend toward accessibility. When personal computing was offered in the early 1980s at a fraction of the price for standard computers, computing was suddenly available to nearly everyone. Until that time, only the scientific elite had access. Understanding computers and how to get them to perform was complex in the mainframe world, requiring specialized training. This exclusivity created an elite, monastic order of computer programmers and analysts.

Business managers, chief executive officers (CEOs), and chief financial officers (CFOs) were forced to subscribe to the expertise of the elite who owned access to necessary information. A major shift took place when control over assets meant control over information and the distribution of information and when the personal computer, whose name implies access, was introduced in 1979. The power of information management no longer evolved out of withholding access. It now came from gathering and sharing information.

The fundamental concept behind how computers function has never changed. All computers have only three elemental functions: data input, data manipulation, and information output. These three processes occur regardless of the housing and engine, regardless of the use or application, and regardless of how complex the software is.

Data input is the process whereby data is entered into the system. Data usually are entered by means of the keyboard. As the typing occurs, it can be viewed on the monitor. The process is the same, regardless of the program or platform. As technology advances, however, options other than keying data are more available and serve to increase information accessibility and sharing. The new advances include scanning with light pens or bar codes, voice entry, digital photography, and video and interactive video. Regardless of how the data are entered, it must find its way into the system so that it can be read and understood by the machine.

Once the data are in the system, the software running the application program takes over for the second of the three standard computer functions. The data are "crunched," manipulated, stored, moved, combined with other data, transmitted to other systems, or operated on in numerous other ways.

Output, the third function, occurs in the form of reports, digital readouts, or graphic displays. Output might be visible on the screen, sent to the printer for hard copy, or put into a standard (ASCII) coded format which can be transmitted through a modem, fax cable, or by means of wireless cellular transfer. The software program determines the output's structure and format.

An approach for decision making

The decision process is a business planning process whereby business and operational decisions are made in advance. As with any business endeavor, the business plan determines objectives, budget, implementation of resources, and payback period. Only by setting explicit goals can payback (return on investment) be determined. Shortchanging the planning process will almost guarantee dissatisfaction. Expectations must be clear so that all can contribute their enthusiasm and support to the project.

Purchasers are usually advised to first choose the required software and then pick the hardware to fit. This simplistic approach implies that the system will be autonomous with no need to consider existing hardware or software systems. Because general access to complex schemes is available, the task is to determine what needs to be accomplished, what outputs are desired, and what functional or geographic participation is needed. State desired outcomes explicitly. Once the plan is in place, then look for software and hardware.

Intervening factors such as systems that are already in place, the degree of commitment that has been made by the organization, management preference, and availability of system support will all come into play in the planning process. Computing has been around long enough that many organizations have investments, loyalties, and sometimes egos tied to former decisions. If a new

system is being purchased without any of these encumbrances, then look not only at the specific anticipated application but at more general use in the market. In other words, keep future applications in mind, such as being on-line with the customer base. Consider general business preferences so that communication will be feasible.

Hardware. Three general hardware platforms are mainframe, midrange, and microcomputers (PCs, or personal computers). The differences are in size and in operating system. The laptop or notebook computers might make up a fourth platform except they use the same operating system as PCs. Unique operating system languages differentiate hardware platforms which is why communicating between and among them has been difficult to date. Also, each has special advantages unique to that platform. The differences, however, are continually blurring, while the similarities increase.

The chief distinguishing factor and advantage of mainframe computers is their size, reflected by the large amount of data they can capture, manage, and store. Their central value is to store data, using microcomputing as the user interface. PC capacity expands almost daily. Growth occurs by adding disk capacity, by connecting to a server, and eventually by using client server technology whereby larger systems (mainframe or midrange computers) act as the server, providing data storage. PC workstations then generate data calls to the client server to retrieve specific data, perform operations on them, and return the altered data to the client driver, all in real time.

Speed, cost, and utility are the remaining differences between hardware platforms, and speed is the incremental gain. That leaves cost and utility as the main distinguishing factors among hardware.

Cost is the most important consideration when evaluating mainframe technology. Whereas most occupational health departments will not entertain the notion of purchasing a mainframe, they must decide whether to use the supplier's or client's excess mainframe capacity for occupational health. In this case, cost is not in the purchase but in using the mainframe. Most companies charge access time to users of the mainframe to help support the MIS (management information systems) or DP (data processing) department. Mainframes are complex and difficult to manage, requiring substantial technical staff. Maintenance is also expensive, lending credence to the notion that anyone using the mainframe must support its cost.

The cost of participation may be bearable in itself, but what is the trade-off? Most mainframe computers are difficult to access and are not flexible in use. Developing software programming for occupational health tends to be unsatisfactory, or, at the very least, incomplete. If the choice is using the mainframe or having no computing capability at all, use the mainframe. Very little else would support the decision to select the mainframe platform. Computing literature, in fact, notes the trend toward downsizing, moving away from larger computers to smaller ones, primarily the microcomputer, without losing capacity or speed while gaining affordability, access, flexibility, and ease of use.

Midrange computers are best known as the IBM System 34, 36, or 38 series and now the IBM AS/400 group, DEC, SUN and others. These computers, generally fast and functional, are midrange in capacity, smaller than mainframes, larger than personal computers. Most are reliable workhorses. On the downside, compared with microcomputers, they are more difficult to program, program changes are more expensive and time consuming, and programming must be completed by someone skilled in the specialized language. Support and general maintenance is generally more expensive. Midrange computers, however, are an excellent choice for client server architecture if larger capacity and speed are required.

The microcomputer hardware category has expanded rapidly and continues to evolve. With the microcomputer, computing has been put into the hands of end users, the application specialists. Even program adaptation and report design can be accomplished by users. The cost, by comparison, is minimal. One study describes relative cost in terms of less than one dollar for 600,000 kilobytes (about the size of a floppy disk) of storage on a microcomputer compared with seven dollars for the same amount of storage on a mainframe. This equates to reducing initial costs from hundreds of thousands, even millions of dollars, to only a few thousand dollars. Maintenance and support costs are also comparably less.

Network and client server technology. Networking technology allows microcomputers to support larger applications than ever before. Networks provide for intercommunication between workstations and allow each workstation to access an integrated database on a larger computer, the server. In other words, multiple computers can be linked together, all using the same software systems which reside on the central server. Productivity is dramatically enhanced with the use of networking because everyone shares one database, rather than multiple, discrete manual, or electronic systems. It far surpasses the clumsy "sneaker-net" technology whereby data is passed from one computer to another by saving to diskette on one com-

puter and transferring it by copying the diskette into the next computer.

Servers can be added to servers to enlarge the computing capability by means of technology known as bridging or "mirroring." Networks can be local area networks (LAN), where the workstations are literally cabled to each other, or wide area networks (WAN), meaning the workstations exist long distances from one another and are connected in real time by means of special twisted fiber in telephone wiring.

Microcomputer servers are similar to other workstations except they are usually larger, in excess of 1 gigabyte, and dedicated to managing the distribution of data to the participating network users. Disk capacity represents only small marginal cost; therefore, purchasing the most capacity possible makes good sense.

Of course, not everyone requires powerful network capability. For small networks, two to five workstations, a server with around 320 MB (megabytes) might be adequate. A network of that size would comfortably serve an average one- or two-physician occupational health clinic for 2 to 3 years, depending on the number of functions for which the system is used.

Some people double the function of the server by using it as an operating workstation, as well. Doing so, however, degrades speed performance. The beauty of networking is that capacity and function can be added incrementally, permitting users to begin computerization on a limited level, then expanding the hardware along with implementing accelerated function and utility.

The issue of connectivity, of allowing computers to communicate, is on the threshold of major advances. Utility will be gained by combining the best features of the larger computers, mainframes, and minicomputers with the functionality and flexibility of microcomputers. Specifically, the use of client server technology will become commonplace, with the larger hardware being used for storage and speed, and with PCs or microcomputers used for daily transactions—all sharing the same database for different but related operations.

Cost performance. Defining cost performance in combination with the preferred software application is the way to decide between hardware platforms and operating systems if other issues (personality and politics) can be isolated or remain constant. A method that will aid in decision-making is to list all the costs associated with each of the platforms and then list performance qualities and capabilities, positive and negative. Remember cost includes more than the price tag. In the case of hardware or software, consider soft costs: training, support, maintenance, warranties, and guarantees.

Product research, of course is good only for the short term because new products will be on the market as soon as a choice or purchase is made. The pace of technology development and competition among hardware manufacturers make decisions difficult but not impossible. Murphy's Law of computer hardware guarantees that the price will fall shortly after purchase. Waiting for the market to stabilize is futile and a means to avoid decision making altogether. Take the plunge. The chosen system may be considered outdated by some as soon as purchased, but outdated does not mean unusable. Do not prolong the research agony. A guaranteed right decision is an elusive goal. Aim for the best equipment and most capacity possible, keeping an eye on current and future goals.

Cost versus price. The one directive about hardware is to purchase the most capacity and speed that can be afforded to prolong usability. Taking advantage of a sale sometimes grants the best opportunity to the retailer removing old inventory. Some exceptions to this caveat do exist. The buy-the-best approach is particularly important when purchasing a server or client server, but sometimes purchasing less expensive but fully compatible equipment for network workstations is a way to economize without jeopardizing the system. Do not, however, cut costs by purchasing "dumb" workstations, with no disk capability of their own. Newer, more powerful software, particularly operating system software such as Windows, requires intelligence (disk capacity) at the workstation level.

Be sure to consider total costs, not only the purchase price. Total costs include installation, training, maintenance, and support. The soft costs are important and should not be ignored or avoided. Were they not separated in line items, they would be buried in the price. People who trim costs by cutting down on training or support shortchange themselves in value. Users who do not understand how to fully use a system cannot maximize the power that was purchased. Budget for retraining, as well, to adjust for staff turnover.

Effective computing is not cheap; value has a cost. If the goal is important, then the resources should be allocated accordingly.

Software. Users need to understand three different and necessary kinds of software: disk operating system software (like DOS), network operating software (like Novel), and application software (like word processing, spreadsheet, or occupational health application software). They are identified as three separate kinds of software be-

cause people sometimes confuse them or think they can do without one of them. Each is supplied by different vendors and each is purchased and managed separately. The industry is consolidating by broadening the effect of each of the types of software. Ultimately, the operating system software will perform the functions of network and even application.

Discussion of software will concentrate on microcomputer software, acknowledging the identified trend in hardware downsizing and accessibility. Concentrating on microcomputer software also recognizes PC cost and function, which makes it more appealing and accessible from an economic standpoint to most occupational medical practitioners.

Operating systems. A major driver in software expansion is operating system software, a rapidly growing technology. DOS (disk operating system), for instance, was developed in the late 1970s for the first personal computers, many of which had 64 kilobytes of memory and no hard disk capacity. That means they had 64 kilobytes to support DOS plus the application software. Since that time, DOS has been enhanced to 640 kilobytes and more by borrowing additional memory through memory extender software utilities. Much more RAM (random access memory) is needed to meet new demands for expanded functionality. (Note: Memory [RAM] is required to run the computer, to initiate and manage application software. Capacity, on the other hand, is disk storage.)

New operating systems such as OS/2 from IBM and Windows from Microsoft offer far greater capability, but they require from 2 to 10 megabytes of memory. With the new operating systems, windowing, multitasking, direct navigation by means of "hot keys," graphics, and much larger application programs all require large amounts of RAM. For instance, large Lotus spreadsheets cannot be managed by DOS alone but require expanded memory.

Graphical user interface (GUI, pronounced gooey) such as that provided by Windows and OS/2 operating systems is increasingly popular. The GUI emulates the preeminent Macintosh interface. The screen flexibility provides for pixel level (tiny dots on the screen) use rather than the 80 character limitation of DOS programs. GUI also makes substantial use of the mouse (which many users prefer) to click on selections or icons, minimizing keystroking.

Network management software. Users are recognizing that productivity is enhanced by networking using LAN (local area network) and WAN (wide area network). In fact, asking workers to share equipment has been shown to significantly and negatively affect productivity and employee attitude. Attempting to computerize an operation by asking several people to use the same computer is self-defeating. Some try to solve the problem by adding another computer without spending the money to establish a network so that information can be shared. Multiple workstation computing, however, demands intercommunication through a network if benefits are to be realized.

Network management software is required for networking and is usually offered as a separate product. Now, however, Microsoft Windows NT is promising built-in network capability and OS/2 LAN Manager offers the same. Integrating the network management software with the operating system makes a great deal of sense and, in fact, is much cheaper and appears to be easier to manage. Network management is complex and should not be discounted in the human resource allocation process.

Whenever a network is in place, a network administrator should be designated. Usually, technology requirements are not as demanding as are operational and leadership requirements. In other words, the network administrator must be available to assign passwords, to ensure that network server backups are done on a timely basis, and to serve as liaison between the users and the technical support, most often provided by the network vendor.

Application software. Application software allows users to do the job at hand and specifically meet the business goals and falls into four categories: word processing, spreadsheets, desktop publishing, and databases. Application programs may differ widely and the uses may overlap somewhat, but the important thing is to know the difference. Word processing and spreadsheet programs were the first available for general use on PCs followed by databases. Word processing provides powerful typing and editing capabilities. Most word processing programs now have some limited graphics capability as well.

Spreadsheets, on the other hand, are primarily numeric and financial. They allow instant, updated calculations. Both word processing and spreadsheet software have powerful macro capabilities, allowing users to set their own template, merely changing a few characters or numbers to update the entire format.

The type of word processing or spreadsheet format chosen will have to match the operating system in place. Windows, OS/2, or Macintosh operating systems, for instance, can run Microsoft Excel, whereas DOS cannot. On the other hand, only Windows, OS/2, and Macintosh run desktop publishing and other substantial graphics programs. Another fact to remember is that only Mac-

intosh will run Macintosh programs, and only those designed for PCs will run on PCs. In other words, software developers are developing as much for operating systems as they are for the hardware platform. Industry consolidation, however, will soon blur the lines further. IBM and Apple have established a corporate partnership to facilitate some software integration.

Database software, on the other hand, offers another distinct and powerful form of computing. Databases are required for storing data, reorganizing it, and reporting it in another fashion. As opposed to word processing and spreadsheet formats in which output exactly reproduces input (without modification), database formats use the power of the database to retrieve information in a myriad of configurations.

Differentiating between word processing and database computing is important because uninitiated users prefer word processing, which is more akin to their familiar manual, unidimensional format. Word processing contributes little to information management because data elements cannot be accumulated, trended, and measured against a standard. The only way to reuse word processing is to read it again. Word processing is a fabulous editing tool (few would return to the typewriter), but it is not an information management tool. Learning to use database systems as opposed to word processing systems takes some understanding.

Database management makes mainframes and minicomputers powerful. In fact, one of the major reasons for selecting a more powerful operating system such as OS/2 is that the database manager is the same as the DB2 used by mainframe technology. Powerful database management programming includes SQL, an integrated language that allows users direct access to the database to create their own data calls for report formats.

Apple Macintosh has not performed as well as the IBM and compatible PCs in the business world partly because it has not, until recently, offered powerful database management. This limitation must be balanced against the allure of its ease of use. Moreover, because PC-based systems are moving closer to emulating DB2 mainframe database format, the promise of connectivity and communication with mainframes and minicomputers is closer to reality. A smart solution might be to offer both Macintosh and PCs on a network, with the use of some of the new integrating capability, while being specific about why each is there. Macintosh supports graphics and word processing far better than it manages databases.

The make-or-buy software decision. After considering all possible variables, select application software. Now is the time to write the request for proposal (RFP) to software vendors. List only the functions and features required by the computing business plan. Accept responses only from vendors who support the designated operating system (DOS or Windows). If the plan is specific and if appropriate business decisions are made in advance, confusion resulting from too many choices can be eliminated. Do not ask for responses to everything possible because the responses will produce confusion preventing precise decision-making. Make the essential operating system and hardware decisions to establish the first cut and narrow the field.

Tossing out a list of complex requirements and selecting on the basis of price are inadequate approaches, bound for dissatisfaction. When it comes to software, one of the most critical business decisions is to make or buy. While the trend is away from developing new software it might make sense as an interim step. The cost, however, is usually greater than expected, support is insufficient, and outcome is questionable.

Too often the make-or-buy decision is based on price. To avoid purchasing software, someone in the organization is asked to build it. The someone is usually a representative of the data processing or information systems department, a person with little or no knowledge of occupational health application. A feature of microcomputers is that they do not require systems engineers to program the software; they can be programmed by someone with limited expertise. Be aware of the problems that can arise with this decision.

If the programmer is to be someone with no knowledge of occupational medicine, then an occupational health professional will need to interpret systems' needs and work with the programmer to reach the desired outcome. Unfortunately, the professionals do not usually possess the specialized communication skills required to translate the current and future information management needs into systems. Therefore, a great deal of time will be required from the translator and must be calculated into the cost.

Another problem is timeliness. Too often the occupational health department has no priority over other company or hospital departments, leaving them with little or no support and last-in-line status. Ongoing maintenance and support lags.

On the other hand, if occupational health professionals attempt to write the program, they often do not know the standards of programming such as systems application architecture, which allows the system to grow and remain functional over future hardware and technological migration. Moreover, some assurance (possibly an indenture sys-

tem) is important to allow for future support. Rarely can another person adequately supplant the original programmer, especially if programming standards and source code technical documentation are not in place.

Occupational medicine is complex, and designing suitable programming is not for part-timers or for those whose real job is something other than programming and support. Program changes will be required to meet changing state and federal regulations. Provisions for changes must be made in the process of deciding to make the software.

The decision to make software. The foregoing are some of the reasons for avoiding the make decision. Because some will choose to build their software, a few suggestions about how to write specifications for program design might be helpful. Essentially, nonsystems persons attempting to design software programs should follow six steps.

1. *Decide on the desired outputs.*

   The best method for describing to technical programmers what you want is to provide a picture of your desired output. The picture should represent the reports you want and the detail of each. Show column headings, column subtotals, and totals.
2. *List data elements.*

   List all the data elements in all the outputs desired and all data that is likely to be needed, but not yet formulated, in a report or output format.
3. *Create tables, combining appropriate data elements; determine and describe their relationship to one another.*

   This process is key to how the system will function and flow. It establishes databases within the system, the data hierarchy, and the relationships between and among them. Design the flow of the program, which is how the data fits into hierarchical relationships. If this step is not completely analyzed and adequately communicated to the programmer, the system is in jeopardy.
4. *Design menu or user interface screens.*

   Design the menu or other user interface that seems the most straightforward; however, it must match the data flow already established, and its use must be almost intuitive to the user. A program considered user friendly hinges on the simplicity of user access.

   When alternative input devices are to be incorporated, design them into the system. If the data will be scanned from another database, detailed programming specifications must be written. Each data element must be defined in terms of field length and other attributes such as alpha, numeric, date, or currency.

5. *Normalize the system.*

Review the system to ensure that no data element appears in more than one place. Be sure standard conventions are used for dates and time, names, addresses, and other demographic variables. Consider needs for retaining historical data, addressing issues like the next century and distinguishing date information, and capturing multiple encounter or claim data. These common problems are often overlooked by amateur program designers. Also, be sure database relationships are workable and appropriate.

6. *Detail system outputs.*

Return to step one and detail the outputs or reports. If specific formats are required, such as a regulatory agency mandated report, include it as an example. For each output, clearly identify where in the system the data element can be found.

Determine the selection criteria for each report, describe how the data elements should be arranged, and show examples of the arithmetic. If work days lost are to be automatically calculated, for instance, define the assumptions for beginning and ending date selection. Include all samples possible.

The complex process of designing and building a system is the same whether the platform is mainframe or PC. As a result, systems that appear to users to be the simplest, even simplistic, are probably the ones that are best designed. User friendly systems are that way because the design and interface has the user in mind, not the programmer. Moreover, those systems considered user friendly are user forgiving. The user is allowed to make mistakes without catastrophic results or without being thrown out of the system, another function of design.

The same deliberate process for writing design specifications is effectively applied to making requests for system enhancements or customization. Attempts to redesign the relationships of the databases are not recommended because costs are likely to be outrageous and have poor results. However, do begin with the specific outcome or outputs required. Be specific about data elements and how they are to be used in the output, including all the calculations. Be sure the data requests are not duplicated somewhere in the system. Work with the programmer to reach a conclusion or understanding of where new data fields should be placed in the system. Again, do not attempt to explain rationale to programmers, but be detailed about desired output.

Potential software designers and developers who are not systems professionals eventually have difficulty with the specificity required for software programming. Health professionals tend to think in whole concepts; computer programmers think in bytes. Stating *why* a particular process is requested will not usually produce results. The request must state *what* in painful detail. Expect delays and frustration if you determine to build the software system.

The decision to buy software. Designing a system requires disciplined planning and thinking; so does selecting software. As stated earlier, it is important to first determine the business goals, the systems already in place, and future business plans. List the functions required to achieve the business goals and predetermined factors such as existing platform. If no predetermined factors exist, the choice will be wider and probably more difficult.

If you find software that meets your stated needs, do not forget to ask the vendor about training, support, maintenance, migration, and other factors such as availability of the source code. Source code is the line-by-line written instruction that produces operating software. Source code is not normally available to users because when it is altered, the developer has no way of knowing what has changed and, consequently, cannot support it thereafter. Do not ask about source code without a specific plan or protocol for its use because it will be expensive and probably unusable. A better question is whether the source code is documented and available through an escrow arrangement.

The purpose of an escrow arrangement or statement in the contract is to protect against the software vendor no longer being able to meet obligations of supporting the software. Producing and supporting software is a business. Businesses can be sold or owners could simply decide to no longer offer services. An escrow agreement defines what happens to the system thereafter.

COMUG (Computers in Occupational Medicine Users Group) prepares an annual directory of occupational safety and health software which is useful in beginning the selection process. The directory is usually available at the AOHC (American Occupational Health Conference) or by contacting the group directly (804/977-3784). Particularly helpful is a decision grid format used as a worksheet to identify needs criteria and to assist in the selection process.

Occupational health entities associated with larger organizations such as hospitals sometimes make the mistake of allowing their information services department to independently and arbitrarily prepare their RFP. This is a mistake because questions are often asked that have nothing to do with the application or with anything but mainframe computing. In some cases, the inappropriateness of the RFP has prevented appropriate software vendors from responding.

Quantifying the decision. The most important and simplest thing to be said about cost or price is that to base decisions on price alone may sabotage the goal. Computing is not cheap. Information has value and value has a price. If the business goal is important, then allocate appropriate resources.

It helps to prepare a decision grid to clarify needs and quantify the decision. First prepare a list of requirements, features, and functions for the designated platform. Second, score each feature or function in terms of its importance or priority in meeting business goals. Third, expand the grid by scoring each software package available on each individual element to compare like items to like items. Fourth, establish a scoring scheme: 5 fully satisfies the need; 4 mostly satisfies the need; 3 slightly satisfies the need; 2 indicates software is available through vendor by means of customization at an additional charge; and 1 indicates that software is not available.

Highlight the scores that match feature desirability with feature availability. Flag items considered high priority, but not available from a vendor. This step alone will reduce the participant field. Multiply the priority by the availability and sum the scores for each vendor. The totals suggest the decision, but they are not absolute. Remember to consider the soft features and costs. Table 5-2 displays an example and suggested format. Implementing a grading tool is also useful in justifying decisions for upper management. Also, in the future, rationale for why a decision was made can be quickly articulated.

Table 5-2 Purchase decision matrix for occupational health software

Feature/Function	Vendor 1		Vendor 2		Vendor 3	
	Priority	Availability	Priority	Availability	Priority	Availability
Visit worksheet	5	5	5	5		
Doctors' notes	5	5	4	5		
History	4	4	3	5		
Audiometric	3	5	5	4		
Drug screen	2	5	5	1		
Random selection	2	5	5	1		
Other surveillance	5	3	4	2		
Accounts receivable	1	5	5	1		
Case management	1	5	4	1		
Job analysis	1	5	5	5		
Mandated reports	5	5	5	5		
Activity reports	5	5	3	5		
Accounting reports	5	5	5	5		
Employer reports	3	5	5	5		
Accountability	1	5	5	5		
Ad hoc reports	5	1	4	1		
Network capability	5	5	4	2		
Data import/export	3	3	4	1		
Archive capability	2	1	5	1		
Remote transmission	3	1	5	1		
Security system	5	5	5	1		
Vendor support	5	5	5	5		
Customization	3	4	5	1		
Documentation	3	3	5	5		
Back-up support	3	3	5	1		
Vendor client list	5	5	4	5		
Vendor history	5	5	4	3		
Training	5	5	5	2		
Cost	5	5	5	1		
Column total	105	123	133	85	0	0
TOTAL POINTS*	12915		11305			

* Total points are relative units used only to compare systems.

Implementing the system

A case has been made for differentiating cost and price for both hardware and software. The price might not include sufficient soft costs, installation, training, support, and maintenance. These are important considerations in determining overall, long-term costs, but they are also indirect costs over which managers and directors have full control.

Management planning for implementing a system is as important as system selection in the overall scheme of costs. The finest system might be selected, but poor implementation will ruin it. The degree of management planning is allocated to the implementation process is 100% positively correlated to the success of fully implementing the utility of the system and meeting business goals.

Note that the emphasis is on management planning and implementation. Indeed, vendors of hardware, software, and network systems have a responsibility to provide adequate documentation and to appropriately train personnel who use their systems. Without strong management backup, without clearly stated management expectations, and without full management support, the system will be a failure because staff will not be totally engaged in the process.

After the decisions are made regarding the system design, the network configuration, and the software, several other management decisions are necessary. Every system has multiple levels of implementation. The first, of course, is planning and scheduling the computer, network, and software installation. At another level is a series of operational decisions: How will the tasks be allocated? Who will do what and when? What is the sequence of activity for data entry? Where will the computers be placed in the office? Where will printers be? Who should have access to what information? How will confidentially be maintained? Where will the necessary information be obtained? These questions have little to do with the specific system, but they have everything to do with how satisfactorily the system will be implemented.

Those who actually use the system will do a better job if the business goals are shared with them. This is not a suggestion that system implementation should be democratic. Instead, leadership should be decisive and clear.

Management must communicate that working with the computer for documentation *is* the job. Otherwise health care personnel tend to believe it is an as-time-permits task, meaning it is avoided until the end of the day, preferably until the day is over. To communicate effectively, managers must own the same notion, that this *is* the job. When the managers' attitudes are confronted, they are often found to retain bias or fear about the systems. Probably, the best approach is to offer specialized training for managers in advance, so they are better prepared to lead.

Inadequate dedicated personnel time will result in poor outcomes. Individual accountability and responsibility for keying specific information should be established and communicated. Keyboard skill levels will affect the time-saving goal, but normally only in the short term. By defining each individual range of responsibility for entering data, goals other than saving time are communicated to users.

In a busy clinic, carving out time to computerize data is the best, sometimes only way to communicate importance, priority, and permission. Health care professionals find it difficult to let a patient stand in front of them while entering data. They feel they are not doing what is needed for the patient. Moreover, anxiety mounts when someone is looking over the keyboard. The staff must recognize that information management (in this case, data entry) is a key part of patient care, particularly in workers' compensation. People are accustomed to waiting for the computer at the bank, the gas station, the department store, and nearly everywhere else. Patients will quickly accustom themselves to the process.

Health professionals are taught from day one to pick up a pen and note whatever is happening. Changing that behavior to move directly to the computer requires changing a long-standing, well drilled habit. Fully learning the computer habit can take as little as 2 weeks if coupled with a positive attitude, the intention to master the change, and applied energy.

Assign responsibility. Make assignments for staff members regarding the specific information which they are responsible for entering into the system. Approaching implementation with a plan and communicating the scope of responsibility for each person allows people to understand that they are not personally responsible for everything and will not be blamed for omissions outside their scope of responsibility. On paper, draw a diagram of who is responsible for completing which screens in the system; the sequence of data entry; and who is responsible for editing, correcting, and printing reports. Clarify the purposes. Good management allows for clear and reasonable accountability with feedback tools for self-evaluation and adjustment.

Similarly, establish procedures for seeking help. Not everyone should pick up the phone to call vendor support, particularly if charges will be made for such services. The bill could be rather sizable, and management would not have a mechanism for determining where the problems are. Interdependence and communication is healthy and important among staff, but management has to know where the weak points are. Otherwise, working within the group can provide camouflage for the weak link. The goal is information management so that if one is not contributing, the results are obvious.

A hands-off management model does not work when implementing computerization, especially if computing is new for the group. When managers try to stay out of the process, it usually means the manager also has fears and users sense it. Beware of managers or key people who refuse to touch the keyboard, thinking their status excuses them. They misunderstand the importance of information management, and the results will be disappointing.

Finally, train, train, and train. Never shortchange the training process. Ask the trainer how the sessions will be organized and who should attend and when. Provide the trainers with graphs showing individual responsibilities so that training is directed logically. Arrange for follow-up training if needed. The degree to which people feel comfortable with the system and the processes in the system reflects its usefulness.

Designing outcome measures and goals

The one irrefutable fact and predictable outcome in computerized technology is change. Change will occur because of technology migration, regulatory demands, and the dynamic process of user experience, expertise, and expectations. When selecting hardware, software, and network configuration, keep a clear eye on the future. The future is not a remote matter left to sorcerers; it is created by the goals set and pursued. The future of occupational health, as with all businesses, is information management. But short sighted goals produce short sighted results. Expertly implementing and managing the future is the key to business success.

Cost of information. When the system is fully implemented, evaluate the result compared with the goals set. Are the goals being achieved? Where are the shortcomings? Are the desired outcomes being experienced? Are the outcomes consistent with the goals? Were the original goals shortsighted? Should the goals and outcomes be rearticulated or rewritten? Rarely will all the goals be met the first time.

Sometimes conditions change so that the initial goals set are no longer appropriate or should no longer be primary goals. Goals are guides and should be revisited frequently. Too often, once the

system is in place, management walks away thinking that their job is done. However, implementation is only the mobilization phase of the long term.

Information management in occupational health is a business within a business. Where occupational health is concerned, the information itself is part of both the treatment and the marketing process. Information is a loss-control tool, a compliance tool, a marketing tool, a behavior change tool and, remarkably, a prevention tool. It will serve to bond the employer-provider relationships and help control costs while supporting provider participation. Engaging employers in partnership through the intelligent, creative use of information solidifies the relationship and achieves the greater goals.

SUGGESTED READINGS

Abramson L: Better quality through accountability, *Business and Health* 64, 8(11), Nov 1990.

Baker HE, Coltrin SA: HRM students need adeptness in HR software, *HR News* 7(6):A4, Dec 1992.

Bednarz AJ: GUI: a love story, *HR/PC* 7(7):1-5, 1992.

Betts M: Serve or else, *Computer World*, pp 29-30, Dec 1992.

Blum K: Software user training: a critical step in the success of your system, *HR/PC* 6(9), Aug-Sept 1991.

Britton D: Job evaluation: a sound and simple computerized approach, *HR/PC*, pp 4-8, July-Aug 1992.

Carroll J: The good news about interfacing human resource systems, *HR/PC* 6(2):1-5, 1991.

Cascade Technologies: Interactive voice response system, *HR/PC* 4(11), Aug 1992.

Cayne DA: PC scenario: toward the user workbench, Gartner Group, 1988.

Charbuck D: Time to upgrade, *HR/PC*, Aug-Sept 1990.

Diers CD: Make the HRIS more effective, *HR/PC* 6(2):1-5, 1991.

Discola J: Microcomputer applications in health care delivery: focus on cost containment aspects, *AAPPO Journal* 2(4):11-16, 1992.

Drury D: Disability management in small firms, *Rehabilitation Counseling Bulletin* 34(3):243-256, 1991.

Frieden J: What's ahead for managed care? *Business and Health* 9(12):43-48, 1991.

Glatzer H: A good buy, *Human Resource Executive* pp 28-31, Dec 1992.

Gleckman H et al: The technology payoff, *Business Week* pp 56-68, 1993 (special report).

Habeck RV et al: Employer factors relate to workers' compensation claims and disability management, *Rehabilitation Counseling Bulletin* 34(3):210-226, 1991.

Harris N: Managed care is right course, employers say, *Business and Health* 10(9):32-41, 1992.

Howe N: The resident report writer expert, *HR/PC*, Oct-Nov 1992.

Hungate R: From managed care to measured care, *Business and Health* 77, 9(13), Dec 1991.

Hunt HA et al: Employer control of workers' compensation costs, *The Business Outlook Discussion Paper* 5:2, 1989.

Huntly D: Key injuries hurt companies, *HR/PC*, Aug-Sept 1990.

Kapel C: Data sharing: key role in HRIS in '90s, *HR/PC*, Feb-March 1991.

Katz F: Making a case for case management, *Business and Health* 9(4):75-77, 1991.

Krebs V: Everybody wins with Windows 3.0, *HR/PC*, Jan-Feb 1991.

Lukes EN, Wachs JE: Use of computers among occupational health nurses: results of a survey, *AAOHN Journal* 40(8):365-369, 1992.

Mahal DG: Running out of disk space? *HR/PC*, Oct-Nov 1991.

Mann G: The move to integrated managed care, *Risk Management*, pp 41-45, Jan 1993.

McDonald M: You can control your disability costs, *Business and Health*, pp 21-36, May 1990.

Neibel S: Building better systems with postimplementation reviews, *HR/PC*, Feb-March 1992.

O'Leary MA: Information and its influence on decision making, *AAOHN Journal* 40(1):42-43, 1992.

O'Hara K: Case management evolves into partnerships, *NAOHP Visions* 3(2):1-17, 1992.

Perry S: A look at future PC-based human resource information systems, *HR/PC*, July-Aug 1989.

Peterson KW, David LF: Directory of occupational health and safety software, version 4.0, American College of Occupational Medicine, April 1992.

Reilly JT: Using optical disk technology for human resource and payroll information, *HR/PC*, Oct-Nov 1991.

Resnick R: Managed care comes to workers' compensation, *Business and Health* 10(10):32-39, 1992.

Riley CT, Moellring G: Economic crisis in health care changes the way companies look at benefits, *HR/PC*, Aug 1991.

Ritter S, Leclair SW: The small employer disability management consortium as a case management and consultation alternative, *NARPPS Journal and News* 5(4):15-24, 1992.

Sanders BD: Assessing system usability, *HR/PC*, Aug-Sept 1992.

Sherlund RG: Software industry trends, *Goldman Sachs Investment Research*, Feb 1988.

Simpson R: Managed care is more than cost containment, Special report: integrating managed care, *Business and Health*.

Special report: artificial stupidity, *The Economist*, Aug 1992.

Special report: the caveman's laptop, *The Economist*, Feb-March 1991.

Special report: data watch: outcomes research is growing dramatically, *Business and Health* 6-7.

Special report: employers get involved in outcomes research, *Business and Health*, pp 25-28.

Special report: How outcomes projects are changing medicine, *Business and Health*, pp 16-21.

Taulbee P: Corraling runaway workers' compensation costs, *Business and Health*, pp 46-55, 1991.

Verity JW et al: Taming the wild network, *HR/PC*, Jan-Feb 1991.

Willey BL, Winstead WW: Computer-based clinical charting and patient case management, *Caring* 9(6):44-47, 1990.

Williams FS et al: Implementing computer information systems for hospital-based case management, *Hosp Health Serv Admin* 36(4):559-570, 1991.

Wittek MC: How to get good independent data, *Business and Health* 9(4):2-4, 1991.

Wolfe K: The benefits of computerized health information systems: why computerize? *AAOHN Journal* 37(11):479-481, 1989.

Wolfe K: Asset management opportunity, *AAOHN Journal* 38(1):37-39, 1990.

Wolfe K: Computerized information management, *AAOHN Journal* 38(4):186-187.

Wolfe K: Computerized information management. II. Hardware and software: making the right choice, *AAOHN Journal* 38(5):243-245, 1990.

Wolfe K: Using information to maximize loss control, *AAOHN Journal* 39(1):40-41, 1991.

Wolfe K: Revisiting the information technology rationale, *AAOHN Journal* 39(5):253-254, 1991.

Wolfe K: Getting a grip on computerphobia, *AAOHN Journal* 39(7):352-353, 1991.

Wolfe K: Data base or word processing: knowing the difference can make the difference, *AAOHN Journal* 40(4):194-195, 1992.

Wolfe K: Software documentation: variations and users, *AAOHN Journal* 40(7), July 1992.

Wolfe K: Using information to optimize case management, *AAOHN Journal* 38(10):504-506, 1990.

Woodhull D et al: Successful loss control programs require management's time, money, *Occupational Health and Safety* 60, Sept 1987.

Yenney SL: Solving the health data management puzzle, *Business and Health* 9(9):41-50, 1990.

6 Legal Issues in Occupational Medicine

Physicians often express anxiety or confusion about treating patients with occupationally caused injuries and illnesses. This anxiety is not generally rooted in the medical issues raised by the provision of health care itself: in fact, medical treatment of work-induced health problems is essentially no different from treatment of equivalent health problems that are not work related. The American Academy of Orthopaedic Surgeons has advised, "The treating healthcare provider should be the advocate for the medical well-being of the injured worker; the physician/patient relationship should be the same whether or not the injury occurred at work."[1]

It is the legal and ethical context for the provision of occupational health services that presents particular problems for the treating physician. When treating a patient for a minor illness or injury contracted at home, the physician can deal directly with the patient; the cause of the problem and its treatment will likely be within the patient's control. Health problems caused at work, on the other hand, present greater legal, economic, and social complexities. Neither the physician nor the patient can ignore the external forces that will influence the patient's progress and prognosis. Neither the patient nor the physician has control over the workplace design and the hazards that may be causing the medical problem. The employer's attitudes and policies regarding workplace hazards and workplace-induced disabilities, the extent of job security which the employer offers during periods of disability, and the availability of monetary benefits will influence the course of the patient's recovery. Ultimately, any successful attempt to deliver health services to working people must consider the roles played by the employer and the employer's representatives (including employer-retained attorneys and physicians). The patient's job security, job mobility and economic prospects must also be considered.

Employers, attorneys, insurers, and various state and federal health, safety, and compensation agencies look over the shoulder of the treating physician when a patient's medical problem is derived from work. It is the interest of these others in the patient encounter that causes the spe-cial legal problems associated with occupational injuries.

The purpose of this chapter is threefold: to assist physicians in making legally defensible decisions in the provision of care to occupationally injured patients; to provide physicians with legal information to help them assist these patients; and to alert physicians to the general scope of public health laws that may affect occupational health services. The first part of this chapter discusses potential legal pitfalls involved in the interaction between patient and physician. In particular the legal issues involving the release of medical records and the provision of medical reports to a variety of outside people significantly complicate the physician-patient relationship when an occupational injury or illness is involved. The second part addresses the physician's potential involvement in the legal issues that may confront an occupationally injured patient. Each patient's economic and employment status will depend on whether the physician is willing to provide documentation regarding the occupational causation or the degree of impairment resulting from the health problem. The patient may need assistance from the physician to be excused from work, to return to work, or to obtain compensation or disability benefits and medical insurance coverage during the course of treatment. The patient's trust in the physician — and therefore the degree of compliance with medical instructions — will be influenced by the physician's understanding of the surrounding legal issues, as well as the physician's willingness to provide assistance to the patient. Ignorance of the patient's situation and the surrounding legal rules may lead to serious adverse consequences for the patient, including discharge from employment.

It is critical for treating physicians to remember that their ethical and legal obligations run to the patient first. The economic interests of other people and entities, including the patient's employer, are well protected by the legal system. It is therefore essential for physicians who treat individuals with occupationally-induced health problems and who are concerned about their patients' long term health to become familiar with the various legal rules that govern requests for information by others and requests for assistance that will come from their patients.

Finally, the third part of this chapter provides a brief summary of physicians' public health responsibilities when diagnosing occupationally caused health problems. Available resources under occupational safety and health laws available to assist physicians who treat occupationally injured workers are also summarized.

LEGAL ISSUES IN PROVIDING PATIENT CARE
Record keeping and confidentiality

The legal obligations regarding the maintenance of medical records and their disclosure to the patient or to others are governed by state law and vary considerably from state to state. In general, these legal rules are no different when a patient's health problem is occupationally caused. The legal and ethical problems regarding records in occupational health cases arise primarily when requests for information are made by third parties.

Maintaining records. The requirements for the maintenance of records in situations involving occupational injuries and illnesses do not differ from the general legal requirements for medical records that are exhaustively described in other sources. Records document and justify treatment provided to a patient. In many instances, they provide the foundation for defense of any legal action brought by a patient on the basis of the claim that the physician was negligent in providing care.

The history provided by the patient, including the patient's description of the cause of the medical problem, should be included in the record. The fact that the patient describes or the physician suspects occupational etiology does not change the physician's general obligation to maintain complete records of all patient encounters. The fact that the physician cannot verify the specifics of this patient-provided information does not relieve her of including it in the record; this rule is the same for occupational and nonoccupational illnesses and injuries. The physician should, as always, be specific in describing the nature, extent, causation, and prognosis of the patient's problem.

The physician must exercise some extra degree of care in the maintenance of records relating to occupational injuries and diseases. This extra diligence is generally necessary because it is likely that the medical records will end up in the hands of a variety of people during the course of treatment. First, physicians should exercise some discretion as to which of a patient's comments to include in the record. Offhand comments ("My supervisor is unfair. . . . I can't stand my work") may be irrelevant to the medical care but have ma-

jor consequences if included in the record for later release to employers or insurance carriers.

Second, a patient will provide considerable confidential medical information that may be important for treatment but irrelevant both to any later legal proceedings and to the patient's ability to perform her job. For example, a simple inquiry regarding the medications that a patient is taking yields substantial information about the patient's underlying health status. An indication in a record released to the employer that a patient is currently taking azidothymidine (AZT) for treatment of acquired immunodeficiency syndrome (AIDS) or Dilantin for seizure control may have significant impact on the patient's later employment opportunities, despite the current legal prohibitions regarding discrimination on the basis of disability. Release of this kind of sensitive, nonoccupational information may also lead to legal liability for breach of confidentiality. In view of this, physicians should, when possible, maintain separate notes regarding work-related and non–work-related aspects of the patient's history and treatment.

Development of a complete record regarding occupational safety or health problems may require the physician to obtain material safety data sheets, which provide specific information regarding the hazards of materials used in the workplace, and environmental or medical records maintained by the patient's employer. Patients are guaranteed a right of access to employers' records by the Hazard Communication Rule under the Occupational Safety and Health Act (OSHA), but only when they relate to exposure to toxic substances or harmful physical agents. The patient does not have a right to get information that involves any of the employer's trade secrets.

The OSHA rule does, however, allow treating physicians to obtain this trade secret information directly from the employer. In cases involving medical emergencies, the employer must identify the specific hazardous chemical to the health care provider immediately, without regard to the confidential nature of the trade secret information. If there is no medical emergency, the provider must make a written request to the employer, spelling out in reasonable detail an occupational health need for the information requested. Valid reasons for making this request include a need to assess the chemical hazards to which employees will be exposed; to conduct or assess sampling of the workplace atmosphere to determine exposure levels; to assess the adequacy of personal protective equipment or engineering controls instituted by the employer; to conduct studies to determine the health effects or exposure; or to perform adequate preplacement or periodic medical surveillance examinations. The provider must also execute a written confidentiality agreement guaranteeing that the trade secret information will be kept confidential.

The particular problems involving medical records in the context of occupationally caused illness and injury arise primarily because these records are likely to be sought by and seen by many third parties. As a practical matter, this means that physicians should be careful to provide clear and adequately specific findings and documentation of the findings in the record. In addition, substantial care must be exercised to avoid inappropriate release of the information related to the particular occupational health problem and the general medical chart.

Releasing information to the patient. In most states patients have a legal right of access to medical records. Conceptually, the provider owns the physical record, but the information in the chart belongs to the patient. Although state law may allow some latitude for physicians to deny unlimited access to psychiatric records, patients cannot be denied access to information regarding their health status; in most states, physicians have no right to prevent release of information in medical records to patients. This general rule is consistent with the need for the patient to be able to give informed consent to all medical treatment.

Legal liability may exist for failure to disclose medical information to a patient who continues to be occupationally exposed to a toxic substance. In one famous California case, the failure to disclose to workers that their x-ray films showed asbestos-related lung abnormalities, when the workers continued to be exposed to asbestos in the workplace, resulted in corporate liability. Lawsuits of this nature have occasionally been brought by workers against physicians retained by employers as well.

Some primary care physicians have been reluctant to provide occupational diagnoses to patients because they fear the patients lack sufficient job mobility to obtain alternative employment. It is essential that physicians recognize that the physician's duty is to disclose all the relevant information; it is the patient's decision as to whether to assume the additional risk of continued exposure.

Releasing information to third parties. The medical records involving an occupationally injured patient will be of significant interest to everyone concerned about the patient's status. This may include the patient's employer, the employer's lawyer, the physician retained by the employer, the patient's lawyer, the workers' compensation insurance carrier, the carrier's lawyer, and others involved in any claim for benefits filed by the patient. As a result, the worker's treating physician is often asked to provide medical reports and copies of the patient's medical records or to engage in telephone conversations regarding the patient with third parties. Not all of these people will have the patient's best welfare at heart.

This diversity of interest in the patient record creates a number of special legal and ethical quandaries for the treating physician. In the treatment of disease or injury that is not occupationally related, the primary transfer of patient documents is to other referral physicians whose interest is focused on providing the patient with maximally beneficial medical care (or to health insurers to obtain third-party reimbursement for services). In contrast, requests for medical records regarding occupationally impaired individuals are often unrelated to the desire to provide or pay for beneficial medical care.

Information released to third parties regarding occupational injuries and diseases is likely to show up in unanticipated places. Ethical and legal guarantees of confidentiality do not follow the records to their ultimate destination after they have been released to nonmedical third parties. Employers and their attorneys may, for example, share the information with the patient's direct supervisors and others at work who live in the same community as the patient. The release of the information can become a release to the general community, and gossip results.

These problems are magnified when the treating physician has maintained a longitudinal relationship with patient. In this case, the medical records for the patient contain information unrelated to the specific occupational injury. Release of this unrelated information to someone who is not providing health care to the patient will magnify the effects of any breach of confidentiality. Clearly, information about family problems or sexual dysfunction should not be released to the employer or allowed to wander through the community. Of equal importance, a careless release of medical information under these circumstances can also do damage to a physician-patient relationship that may have been established over a period of years.

Releasing records with patient authorization. It is generally recognized that patients have a reasonable expectation of privacy in medical treatment records. This expectation is limited to those

---

A physician should never release confidential medical information to any one other than the patient unless *either* the patient has provided specific, preferably written, authorization for the release *or* the physician is under a legal compulsion to provide the information.

records that are kept as part of the therapeutic relationship between patient and provider; it does not, for example, extend to records created at the request of employers or other third parties who are paying for the generation of medical information about the individual patient.

The ethical duty to maintain the confidentiality of medical records is well established. The specific legal rules regarding the confidentiality of medical records vary considerably from one state to another, however. Most states have statutes providing that information developed in a physician-patient relationship is entitled to a legal testimonial privilege, that is, a physician may not be forced to testify in legal proceedings regarding the medical records unless the patient consents or the physician is under a specific legal compulsion to release the information. This privilege prohibits physicians (and other health care providers) from disclosing confidential medical information in a civil court case unless the patient waives the privilege.

In addition, many states impose legal requirements that the privacy or confidentiality of patient records be maintained. This obligation is broader than the physician-patient privilege because it applies to situations that do not involve civil litigation. A breach of confidentiality can create liability for any health care professional who releases medical information without explicit authorization from the patient unless required to do so by law. This liability is often drawn from the physician's general ethical duty and from physician licensing statutes that require the maintenance of confidentiality of records. Some states have no explicit case or statutory law governing physician-patient confidentiality. The fact that a state has not yet specifically addressed the potential liability issues raised by unauthorized release of private medical information does not mean, however, that a physician will necessarily be shielded from liability if private medical records involving medical treatment are released to third parties without the consent of the patient.

It is important that physicians learn the specific legal rules governing confidentiality in the state where they practice. There are, however, several rules of thumb which will assist physicians in making defensible legal and ethical decisions regarding the release of information to third parties.

First, the provider should remember that *everyone other than the patient is a third party*. This includes the patient's own attorney, members of the patient's family, all other health care providers, the patient's employer, and any representative of the employer. Some states, reflecting a certain degree of common sense, recognize that the need for confidentiality when a physician is dealing with a patient's authorized representative is less acute than when dealing with other parties.

Second, *liability for the inappropriate release of confidential information only arises if medical records are released without the patient's consent.* Therefore, adequate proof that the patient has consented to the transfer of the information is always a defense to any charge that legal rules regarding confidentiality have been violated.

Third, *liability generally does not arise when a physician refuses to release information if the patient has not explicitly consented to the release.* In other words, obtaining and following explicit instructions from the patient maximizes the legal protection for the provider. The only clear exception to this rule arises when there is a specific legal requirement for a physician to release records. These legal requirements are discussed later in this chapter.

Fourth, *oral communications regarding the patient's status or diagnosis constitute a release of information.* Physicians should exercise particular care when called on the telephone by insurance carrier representatives or by attorneys or physicians who are working for the employer. Several courts have explicitly held that attorneys, who represent interests adverse to those of the patient, cannot informally interview the treating physician. Some of these states forbid informal conversations even when the patient has signed an authorization for release of medical records or when the workers' compensation statute includes a blanket authorization for release of medical records relating to an occupational injury or illness.

Fifth, *medical records should be reviewed by the physician or a trained staff member to ensure that the information released is within the scope of the patient's release and is relevant to the request made.*

Sixth, *copies of releases and requests for information should be carefully maintained in the medical chart.* This record should include an indication of the scope of the information released.

These general rules do not vary according to who makes the request or the manner in which it is made. For example, in most states the patient's attorney is not entitled to review the patient's medical records without providing a copy of a signed release from the patient. The physician retained by the employer is not entitled to have a friendly professional telephone discussion with a treating physician about the patient's health status or prognosis unless the patient has explicitly authorized this conversation.

There are, however, situations in which the patient may prefer that medical information be released. Medical information will often be required to substantiate that the patient is absent from work for medical reasons or that the patient may be entitled to workers' compensation or other monetary benefits. As in all aspects of medical treatment, the provider is well advised to discuss these issues with the patient in advance and obtain proof of informed consent regarding the release of information. Often, an explicit office or clinic policy that advises patients regarding their obligation and right to provide limited authorizations to release information can assist in ensuring that records are released when necessary.

SCOPE OF INFORMATION TO BE RELEASED.   There is almost no clear legal guidance regarding the precise form that a release from a patient must take to authorize disclosure of confidential medical information. It is well accepted, however, that all releases of medical information should indicate at a minimum the patient's name, the records to be released, and the name of the person to whom they are to be released and should be signed and dated. Some states require notarization.

In theory, a release from a patient should represent the patient's informed consent for the distribution of private medical information to others. Questions may therefore arise regarding the exact intended scope of the patient's authorization. The physician can best defend the decision regarding release of information by erring on the side of protecting the confidentiality of the records. For example, if a release provided to the physician specifies that only certain medical records should be released (such as those relating to treatment for a specific occupational injury) then clearly only those records should be provided to the third party. Similarly, a patient who signs a release when applying for workers' compensation benefits may not intend to release all personal medical records.

Often, however, patients will sign broad general releases indicating that all of their records should be provided to the person indicated. These releases may have been signed at some date in the past. The patient may not have been advised regarding the implications of a release of an entire medical record. For example, a patient may provide her attorney with a broad release at the time of their first meeting; this attorney then provides a copy of the release to others. Treatment, perhaps unrelated to the initial legal consultation, may occur long after the release was signed. It is up to the physician to determine the appropriate response to a broad release of this nature. A patient obviously could not knowingly release information to someone if the release had been signed before the treatment was provided. Because little legal guidance exists on this issue, the physician or her staff may want to discuss with the patient the appropriate response

to a request and have the patient execute a more specific release for inclusion in the patient chart.

This is particularly true if the signed authorization is old or was not executed within the context of current litigation; the patient may simply not recollect having signed it and may not intend to authorize the release of current information. In these situations, the development of an office or clinic policy regarding responses to releases can be of considerable assistance to the physician, the patient, and the physician's office staff in assessing each particular situation. As pointed out elsewhere, "A vigilant and sensitive physician should refuse to disclose information clearly irrelevant to the legal issues or outside the scope of the patient's authorization. Absent an order from the court, or a more specific consent from the patient, a physician should remain steadfast in a refusal to disclose information of questionable relevancy."[2]

Releasing records without patient authorization. In some specific situations, a law or legal proceeding will require the release of personal medical records without individual authorization by the patient. These situations vary from one state to another. Two particular situations may arise in the context of treatment for occupational injuries or diseases.

Special rules on releasing medical records in workers' compensation claims.   The workers' compensation laws of many states include a general statutory authorization for the release of medical information to the various parties interested in the outcome of a patient's claim for workers' compensation benefits. These laws assume that by filing for benefits a worker has essentially waived any right to the medical record's confidentiality which may otherwise have existed. Relying on these laws, the patient's employer or employer's attorney will often claim an absolute legal right to receive copies of all medical records regarding the patient. Two notes of caution are therefore in order.

First, these laws almost always authorize only the release of medical records related to the treatment of the particular occupational injury or illness that is the subject of the application for benefits. Release of an entire medical chart by a primary care physician is likely to result in the release of information that is personal and unrelated to the specific injury. Information other than the records of the specific treatment should be released on the basis of the patient's explicit signed authorization; the workers' compensation laws do not appear to require or authorize the broad release of information that the employer or insurer may request. In these situations, clear office policies governing release of information and separation of work-related and non–work-related information in the medical record will make it easier to identify relevant records.

Second, these legal requirements for release of records may not encompass telephone or other conversations with employers, other nontreating physicians, or attorneys. At least one court has explicitly held that the statutory authorization in a workers' compensation law for the release of records does not include authorization for more informal contact between the treating physician and the employer, insurer, or their representatives.

Legal proceedings and responding to subpoenas and orders. In addition to the provision of medical information in relation to workers' compensation claims, physicians may be legally required to provide copies of medical records in the following circumstances.

Court orders and subpoenas. Orders from courts may be of two types. A judge may sign an order that explicitly requires a health care provider to provide a patient's medical records. Generally, providers should exercise care to comply with the specific provisions of any court order and to document in the medical chart the receipt of the order and the release of the information.

The more common scenario is that a physician is served with a subpoena that orders the physician to appear in court or for a deposition and give testimony or a *subpoena duces tecum,* ordering the physician or the keeper of the records to appear and/or produce medical records. The legal privilege that protects the confidentiality of the physician/patient relationship in civil litigation is not automatically extinguished on the issuance of a subpoena. On receiving an unexpected subpoena, it is entirely appropriate for the physician to contact the attorney who sent it to find out more about the proceedings. It is not appropriate, however, to discuss the patient with the lawyer over the telephone.

Rules governing response to subpoenas vary from state to state. In some states, physicians who receive subpoenas or court orders are released from any liability for the release of medical information. Some states, however, require that a subpoena for medical information be accompanied by a signed authorization from the patient or that records be released without authorization only if the patient is a party to the legal proceedings. Again, physicians should take care to know the specific rules in their own states regarding release of personal medical records in response to subpoenas.

Physicians should also be aware that subpoenas are generally issued at the request of an attorney without any review regarding whether the attorney is entitled to the information sought. Although technically issued by a court, subpoenas are not signed by judges; they are generally signed by the clerk of the court at the request of an attorney. In general, the patient or the patient's legal representative will also have been notified that the court order or subpoena has been issued. It is advisable to communicate with the patient or her attorney regarding the request for medical information before releasing any records, particularly if the request or the accompanying patient authorization appear to require the release of highly personal information unrelated to the occupational injury. When faced with legal documents like subpoenas, physicians or their office staff should not relax their usual vigilance to maintain, whenever possible, the confidentiality of medical records and to ensure that patients have given informed consent when authorizing release.

Legal proceedings. Some (but not all) states regard the bringing of a lawsuit in which an individual's health status is an issue to constitute a specific waiver of any right to confidentiality regarding that individual's medical records. This constructive waiver is conceptually similar to the specific provision for waiver in workers' compensation claims. Again, the physician must guard against excessive disclosure of information that is irrelevant to the issues in the legal case.

Developing a clinic policy on confidentiality. Physicians who regularly treat occupationally injured patients know that their offices may be inundated with requests for information and subpoenas. The sheer volume of these requests often leads to blanket instructions to clerical and nursing staff and results in release of medical records that should have remained confidential. The development of a policy establishing the appropriate response to different types of requests and informing patients about their obligations to provide up-to-date releases can be of considerable assistance to staff, physicians, and patients.

Any policy will need to be adapted to the specific legal rules of the state in which the physician practices and to the particular circumstances of the office or clinic in which it is to be used. In drafting a policy, the following should be considered:

- If the majority of requests for information come because of pending litigation, particularly claims for workers' compensation benefits, it is essential that the specific rules regarding these programs be considered.
- To the extent possible, the office should develop and insist on using a medical release or authorization tailored to its own procedures and recordkeeping. For example, if work- and non–

work-related matters are separated in the records, then the release should specify which information is being released. It is acceptable to reply to requests for records by requesting that the patient be asked to sign the particular form of authorization developed for that practice setting.

- One primary concern will be the extent to which the physicians (or, where relevant, nurse practitioners and physician assistants) are willing to become involved in reviewing medical records prior to any release. If the health care professionals are not involved, any policy will need to be adequately clear to provide guidance to nonprovider staff in deciding which portions of records should be released.

- Subject to the specific rules in the state, all policies should provide that no medical information will be released without written authorization from the patient; that no personal medical information will be given over the phone to anyone unless the patient has given explicit instructions; and that copies of signed authorizations will be filed in the medical chart together with a record of what information was released.

- All policies should explicitly state the scope of release of information in response to written requests. In particular, the policy should state whether general, predated releases from patients will be honored.

The following suggested policy represents an attempt to provide maximum possible protection to the confidentiality of medical records in a primary care setting.

Although this particular policy may not be applicable to all practice settings, it was successfully adopted by at least one primary care clinic that served large numbers of working coal miners in rural West Virginia. After initial hostility, particularly from attorneys, the various individuals who made routine requests for information from the clinic adapted to the policy's requirements. The protection of the confidentiality of the patients was thereby substantially improved.

Consent for treatment and liability for errors

The legal rules regarding both consent and liability for negligence are the same for occupational medicine cases as for all other medical cases. Physicians who provide treatment for occupationally caused health problems—whether they were previously the worker's primary care physician or are chosen as the treating physician by the employer, the insurer, or the worker for the specific injury—must exercise the same standard of

SAMPLE CLINIC POLICY ON RELEASE OF INFORMATION[3]

1. No personal medical information will be released to anyone except the patient himself or herself unless the clinic receives written authorization from the patient. This includes release of medical information to family members.

2. No personal medical information will be released in response to a telephone call, except to confirm that a medical excuse has been issued for a worker who has missed work due to illness. This confirmation will consist only of the following: that an excuse was issued, what days the excuse covered, and when the patient was released to return to work.

3. When a written release is received, only those medical records predating the date of the signing of the release will be released. This clinic operates on the assumption that a patient cannot sign a valid release for something that did not exist at the time the release was signed. Therefore, records of encounters that happened after the release was signed will not be released. The person requesting the records will be informed of this, and a current release will be requested where applicable.

4. When a written release is received, it will be routed to the health care provider who sees the patient on a regular basis. The provider will evaluate the record and maintain the confidentiality of any information that is not material to the request and that would be embarrassing or humiliating to the patient if it is released. For example, if a release is received concerning a particular occupational injury or disease for which the patient has been seen at the facility, information regarding irrelevant personal psychological or sexual problems will not be released. In this situation, when a medical chart is copied, such information will be obscured.

5. All written releases will be filed in the patient's medical chart, and a notation made on them as to the action taken and the information released in response to the request. This action will be communicated to the patient at the next encounter.

6. Any persons regularly requesting information from medical charts will be encouraged to use the release form developed by the clinic.

7. This policy will be made available to anyone requesting information regarding this clinic's policy on release of information. Questions regarding this policy should be routed to the administrator; questions regarding release of particular information should be routed first to the health care provider involved and then to the medical director.

care as is required for treatment of all patients. Other sources deal extensively with issues of consent and medical malpractice and a detailed discussion of these issues is beyond the scope of this chapter.

Physicians are in general expected to impart to a patient sufficient information regarding medical treatment for the patient to make an intelligent, informed choice. Informed consent for treatment should be obtained from patients in all situations except those involving emergencies.

In situations involving minors, including those suffering from work-related injuries, consent should be obtained prior to treatment from the minor's guardian or parent. Most states provide specific exceptions to this rule. These exceptions include allowances for the provision of emergency care and delivery of care to emancipated minors, such as those who are married or who are themselves parents or who are fully self-supporting. Some states provide a specific age, below the general legal age of majority, at which minors can consent to treatment on their own. No special provision appears to be made in any state for unemancipated minors who are working and are injured at work. Notably, illegally employed minors are eligible for workers' compensation benefits if they are injured at work.

Although issues of liability for negligent treatment when a patient suffers from an occupational injury are no different from general issues of liability, the treating physician may find that the treatment decisions made for occupational injuries are subjected to a higher level of scrutiny by patients. Physicians treating occupational injuries are, in some states, designated by employers or insurers to provide care to the patient for the workers' compensation injury. Without the benefit of the patient's free choice of provider, the physician may find the patient more hostile than would be the case in a more traditional therapeutic relationship.

A more complex question arises when a physician is called on to advise a patient regarding whether to return to a work situation which poses a continued health risk. Patients sometimes press physicians to allow them to return to work environments that are not healthy; physicians sometimes believe that patients are excessively reluctant to return to work. As noted earlier, there is no question that patients are legally entitled to be warned of the risks attendant to returning to work, although these risks are outside the health care provider's control. Physicians have, of course, been held legally responsible for failing to provide adequate information to patients. Company physicians, physicians employed by the patient's employer, have been held responsible when workers were not advised regarding diagnoses of occupational diseases and the dangers of continued exposure and when they inappropriately advised an employee to return to work after an injury.

Some treating physicians have raised the concern that they may be held legally responsible if they release a patient to return to work in a setting that may adversely affect the patient's health. In many states, a claim in this situation would be barred because workers' compensation provides the exclusive remedy for any subsequent on-the-job injury. It is unlikely that liability will result if the provider has made full disclosure and has documented the disclosure regarding the risks. The ultimate decision as to whether an individual should return to work rests with the individual patient/worker and the employer, not with the physician.

Physicians may also be confronted with situations in which patients are suspected to be abusers of drugs or alcohol or for some other reason may pose a significant threat to the safety of others and to themselves in the workplace. There is no easy legal solution to the obvious dilemmas posed by this situation. As always, frank disclosure and discussion with the patient, although difficult, must be pursued before any disclosure is made to others regarding these issues. Thereafter, the physician must decide whether to include this information in any report provided to the employer or the workers' compensation program. The ultimate decision regarding whether to continue the employment of the individual rests with the employer.

Obtaining payment for treating occupational injuries

A pragmatic problem—how to get bills paid—presents some particular twists when the patient has a medical problem caused by her work. In general, when an employee is absent from work the employer is not obligated to continue to provide health insurance, unless required to do so under a contract with the patient or a labor union. Some employers continue this insurance voluntarily. In addition, occupationally injured employees may have several guarantees regarding the availability of third-party payment.

Workers' compensation medical benefits. Workers' compensation in every state provides medical coverage for treatment of the occupationally caused medical problem; in general, this medical benefit covers the health care costs associated with the particular occupational injury or disease for the worker's lifetime. The medical costs associated with workers' compensation claims have risen more quickly than the general inflationary rise in health care costs and now constitute about 40% of all workers' compensation costs. As a result, workers' compensation insurance carriers and state-administered funds have almost universally instituted a variety of cost-containment measures in an attempt to slow this inflationary spiral.

Three types of cost-restricting measures have been used. First, states put limits on the aggregate cost or the duration of the medical benefit in association with a particular claim. Although this practice has largely been abandoned, some states still allow the parties to agree to limit the duration of medical care when settling a claim. Second, states instituted fee schedules and a variety of preauthorization procedures that mirror cost containment efforts generally used by health insurers. Third, states regulated who can provide treatment to an injured worker by controlling the process for choosing the treating physician. Although a majority of states still allow the injured worker to select her own treating physician, some states require the worker to select a physician from a list compiled either by the employer or the insurer. In a small minority of states, the employer designates the treating physician; even in these states, however, workers often end up seeing their own primary care physician. The effectiveness of restricting the injured worker's right to choose the treating physician in achieving cost containment is questionable. In any event, the procedure for selection of a treating physician for work-related health problems is likely to change if Congress enacts national health care reform. It is likely that patients' own managed care programs will provide these services.

Independent of how the treating physician is chosen, a physician generally needs to be the designated or authorized treating physician on a claim to obtain workers' compensation insurer or fund payment for treatment delivered to an injured worker. This presents a particular problem for a primary care physician in those states in which treating physicians in workers' compensation claims must be selected from lists provided by the employer, the state agency, or the insurer. The procedures for getting onto these lists vary. Most states also restrict the ability of the patient to change treating physicians during the course of a claim. It is essential for health care providers to learn the particular rules in their own states regarding the mechanisms for obtaining authorization to treat when payment is expected from the workers' compensation program.

Finally, it is the employer's obligation to provide workers' compensation insurance, including medical benefits, to injured workers. This means that the injured worker is not required to pay any part of the cost of the care. Most states do not allow health care providers to bill any portion of a bill directly to the patient for treatment, including the amount in excess of the fee schedule.

Employer-provided health insurance. Workers and their families continue to need general health insurance during periods of the worker's disability.

Recognizing this, the Family and Medical Leave Act requires continuation of health insurance for the duration of any leave of absence granted under the provisions of that law. These leaves may last for a maximum of 12 weeks.

Before 1992, several state legislatures had enacted laws that required employers to provide continued health insurance coverage when a worker was absent due to a work-related injury compensable under the workers' compensation statute. Because of federal preemption of regulation of benefit plans, however, these state laws have been held to be unenforceable.

Medicare. Workers who are totally disabled for more than 12 months may also qualify for disability coverage under the Social Security Disability (SSD) program. Once found eligible for SSD, the worker will become eligible for Part A Medicare coverage (which covers primary hospitalization costs) after 24 months of qualified disability. Medicare coverage will provide general health insurance for treatment, whether or not it is related to the occupational disability.

PHYSICIAN'S INVOLVEMENT IN THE PATIENT'S LEGAL DILEMMAS

In addition to being asked to provide copies of medical records, the physician will often be called on to provide reports or certification of the patient's ability to work in order for the patient to claim eligibility for benefits or to establish some legal entitlement to her job. A remarkable number of programs require the worker's treating physician to act as a gatekeeper in ways that are different from the traditional physician-patient relationship.

A refusal to provide requested certification of the work-relatedness of the patient's medical problem or of the patient's level of impairment or functional capacity will result in a denial of benefits or eligibility for job protection for the patient. On the other hand, certification of eligibility may only provide the patient with a foot in the door; the employer or insurer will still have the opportunity to develop and submit alternative medical data indicating that the patient is ineligible. This adversarial process means, however, that the treating physician may be called on to defend her conclu-

---

A treating physician who is interested in assisting occupationally injured patients through the myriad of programs for which they may be eligible *must learn the specific rules of the program in question.*

sions; to do so, it is essential for the physician to understand the particular legal rules associated with any given program.

Rules governing workers' eligibility for different programs vary considerably. Medical notions about what constitutes proof of causation or disability are not the same as legal definitions. Perhaps more troubling is the fact that the legal definitions may be very different from one program or statute to another. As a result, well-intentioned physicians who attempt to assist a patient in obtaining legal protection often fail to provide the appropriate documentation. Physicians must therefore learn the particular rules governing specific, often state-based, programs.

Some programs require that a worker be disabled from performing any substantial gainful employment to be considered disabled. Others require only that the worker be currently unable to perform the preinjury job. In yet others, the patient must demonstrate that impairment limits the ability to perform a major life function, although not necessarily one that affects the ability to do the job at issue.

There are also critical differences between legal definitions of "disability" and "impairment." In general, impairment is a physical or mental limitation in function resulting from a disease process or injury. Disability, on the other hand, represents a judgment regarding the affected individual's loss of capacity to function as a result of the impairment and requires evaluation of an individual's level of physical, social, vocational, and psychologic functioning. According to Arthur Larson, a leading authority on workers' compensation, "Disability is not a purely medical question: It is a hybrid quasi-medical concept, in which are commingled in many complex combinations the inability to perform, and the inability to get, suitable work."[4]

Laws providing monetary benefits, like workers' compensation, as well as those providing job security guarantees, like the Americans with Disabilities Act, require physicians to be aware of these distinctions. Many of these programs recognize that the same impairment may cause different degrees of disability depending on an individual's age, education, and job requirements. Benefit programs often expect a physician to provide an assessment of disability, not just impairment.

In particular, the definitions of "disability" governing eligibility under different programs vary considerably.

The development of knowledge regarding these medico-legal issues is especially important for primary care physicians providing medical care for the occupationally injured worker within the context of a long-term relationship. These physicians have greater knowledge about their patients' general health status than one-shot evaluating physicians may have. As a result, many agencies will give greater weight to the treating physician's conclusions and recommendations than to the conclusions reached by a physician called in only to evaluate the specific injury or illness.

As noted previously, a physician may be legally and ethically obligated to provide copies of medical records developed during the course of treatment to those who request them, subject to appropriate release by the patient. Physicians are not, however, legally obligated to provide separate medical reports to substantiate a patient's legal claims. Patients may nevertheless expect that a treating physician will provide necessary documentation to the extent that the physician's conclusions do, in fact, support the patient's claims. Many treating physicians, of course, regard the provision of such reports to others, when requested by the patient, as within the reasonable scope of treatment.

Medical certification of disability to preserve job security

Most physicians are unaware that employees have remarkably little guaranteed job security once they have been injured on the job. In many circumstances, injured workers are not legally entitled to a job transfer to accommodate a partial disability. Even the Americans with Disabilities Act, which provides the most comprehensive legal protection to workers with disabilities, provides only limited rights to job reassignment. Employers are not legally required to provide light- or modified-duty programs. In general, workers' compensation laws make it illegal for an employer to discharge an injured worker in retaliation for filing for compensation benefits; in most states, however, the law does not outlaw discharge for lengthy absences, even if the absence is the result of a compensation-related injury. Although legal restrictions on the right of employers to discharge individuals with disabilities have grown, the protections offered are not consistent and almost always require that the worker have the assistance of a physician who will certify that she meets the particular requirements of the specific program.

As a practical matter, injured workers usually know the extent to which they can expect their employers to provide job security during temporary periods of disability. The answer from a patient will depend on a number of variables, including whether they have any job security under a labor contract, the general past practice of the employer, state law, and the extent to which recession generally—or economic problems of the particular enterprise—is pressuring the employer to maximize efficiency without regard to worker longevity.

Eligibility for job protection under an employer-specific program or under any of the following laws will depend on the treating physician's assessment as to whether the patient is capable of performing the work in question. Any indication from a treating physician that an individual is not capable of performing a particular job or particular job functions may result in adverse employment consequences for the patient. It is essential that the physician discuss the implications of these findings with the patient before providing a written report.

Obtaining information about job functions. The physician may be called on to provide medical certification regarding the patient's ability to work under any of the laws and programs described in the following section. Knowledge regarding the specific functional job duties (not simply a job description) may be essential in evaluating the patient's ability to perform the job. None of these laws makes specific legal provision requiring the employer to provide the necessary information to the physician regarding job duties and functions. Most employers will respond voluntarily to requests for information, however. If a physician is treating a number of patients from the same workplace, a tour of the workplace will often be of significant assistance in making these determinations. The more understanding that a physician has regarding the jobs which a patient may be called on to perform, the better he or she will be able to provide medical advice to the patient and the better she will be able to give the necessary specific information called for in each of the following programs. In general, if an employer fails to provide necessary descriptive information about a patient's job, the physician is justified in relying on the patient's descriptions.

Americans with Disabilities Act and state disability discrimination laws. The Americans with Disabilities Act (ADA) forbids discrimination by employers (with 15 or more employees) against individuals who currently have disabilities, are incorrectly perceived as being disabled, or have a record of disability. Workers who qualify for this protection must meet the general requirements for the job (education, experience, skills) and be able to perform the essential functions of the job with or without reasonable accommodation. In other words, qualified disabled workers under the ADA include only those who are able to work.

Workers who are injured at work or suffer from an occupational disease may be qualified for protection under the ADA. Not every occupationally injured worker will be considered disabled within the meaning of the ADA, however. Many injured workers who qualify for workers' compensation benefits will not be protected under the ADA.

To qualify, the worker must suffer from an injury or illness that results in a physical or mental impairment substantially limiting a major life activity such as caring for oneself, doing manual tasks, walking, seeing, hearing, speaking, breathing, learning, or working. If the life activity at issue is the individual's ability to work, he or she must be unable to perform a class of jobs or a broad range of jobs. For example, the inability to perform a specific job, as a result of a job-specific allergy, may not, therefore, qualify for protection under the ADA. Infectious diseases, including human immunodeficiency virus (HIV) positivity, AIDS, tuberculosis, and hepatitis, may constitute disabilities within the meaning of the ADA. Legal protection is not, however, extended to people who perform food handling functions and suffer from infectious diseases listed by the Centers for Disease Control and Prevention (CDC) as being communicable through food handling jobs; HIV and AIDS are not on the current CDC list.

Temporary health problems such as strains and sprains from workplace injuries will not, in general, qualify as disabilities under the ADA. The extent, duration, and impact of the impairment must be assessed to determine whether the worker suffers from a disability within the meaning of this law. The Equal Employment Opportunity Commission (EEOC), the federal agency charged with enforcement of the ADA, gives the following example:

> A broken leg that heals normally within a few months, for example, would not be a disability under the ADA. However, if a broken leg took significantly longer than the normal healing period to heal, and during this period the individual could not walk, she would be considered to have a disability. Or, if the leg did not heal properly, and resulted in a permanent impairment that significantly restricted walking or other major life activities, she would be considered to have a disability.[5]

Workers with temporary impairments that do not qualify as disabilities under the ADA may nevertheless be protected from adverse actions by their employers under the Family and Medical Leave Act discussed later.

Workers with diagnoses of disorders that do not currently cause impairment (such as nondisabling congenital abnormalities, pleural plaques seen on chest x-ray films, or benign arrhythmias demonstrated by electrocardiography) and workers who have a record of prior disability (including a record of filing workers' compensation) but who are otherwise qualified to perform the job in question are also entitled to protection under the ADA. An employer is prohibited under the ADA from refusing to hire or rehire an employee because of the worker's history of injuries or because the employer fears that the worker may manifest problems in the future, unless the future risk is more than speculative.

If the patient suffers from a qualifying disability, the patient must be able to show that he or she is able to perform the essential functions of the job, with or without reasonable accommodation. Essential job functions include only the fundamental duties of the job. Employers are expected to analyze jobs to determine which duties are in fact essential. The fact that a job has historically included certain peripheral duties does not mean that the employer can insist that it continue to include those duties.

If the patient is unable to perform the preinjury job without modification, the employer may be required to make changes in the job to meet a statutory duty to provide reasonable accommodation to the worker. Reasonable accommodation may include modifying the work environment, eliminating nonessential tasks from a job, or transfering the disabled worker to another vacant position that she can perform. For example, an employer may be required to make existing facilities physically accessible, modify work schedules, or acquire or modify equipment. This includes providing mechanical devices to assist in lifting and moving heavy objects. The determination of the need for and the scope of reasonable accommodation is intended to be made through a flexible, interactive process that involves both the employer and the disabled worker. This process requires the individual assessment of the particular job and the specific limitations of the individual.

If an individual requests accommodation and the employer does not believe the accommodation is needed, the employer may request documentation of the individual's functional limitations to support the request. It is here that the physician who is treating an occupationally injured worker enters the picture.

If the employer is unable or unwilling to provide the recommended accommodation, the employer may argue that the changes will result in undue hardship. Employers who can successfully show that the accommodation would lead to such hardship will not be required to make the changes.

Employers may also refuse to employ or reemploy an individual who poses a direct threat to safety where reasonable accommodation cannot adequately reduce the risk. The statutory language of the ADA would only allow an employer to reject a worker if that worker posed a safety threat to others; the regulatory language developed by the EEOC expanded this definition to allow exclusion of workers who pose a direct threat to their own safety or that of others.

The direct threat must be based on individualized, objective evidence and must involve a high probability of imminent and significant risk of substantial harm. In determining whether to exclude a qualified individual from a job, the employer must consider the duration of the risk, the nature and severity of the potential harm, the likelihood the harm will occur, and the imminence of the potential harm. In providing technical assistance to employers, the EEOC gives this illustrative example: A physician's evaluation of an applicant for a heavy labor job that indicates the individual had a disc condition that might worsen in 8 or 10 years would not be sufficient indication of imminent potential harm. In determining whether to employ or reemploy a worker, employers may not base decisions on a speculative future risk, the individual's history of filing workers' compensation claims, or the potential future costs of workers' compensation.

PHYSICIAN'S ROLE UNDER THE ADA. The ADA should change the way in which occupational health professionals, employees and employers work together. Physicians can now assist injured workers in returning to work, in addition to playing a role in the patient's application for monetary benefits. Under the ADA, physicians are called on to determine whether an individual has a qualifying disability, to assess an individual's functional abilities and limitations in relation to job functions, and to evaluate whether the individual poses a direct threat to health and safety. Medical certification of both the existence and extent of the disability is essential for the patient/worker to qualify for a job or to pursue a claim under the ADA.

Workers with disabilities may be required by their employers to provide medical documentation about their disability and their ability to work. In general, this documentation will consist of a written report from a health care professional regarding the individual's functional impairments. In providing this information, the health care professional will need to be specific. For example, mechanical assistance may be available to accommodate an individual's inability to lift, as opposed to carry, objects over a specified weight limit; the physician should, therefore, specify that the limitation relates to carrying but not lifting.

To reach this level of specificity, physicians should obtain from employers job descriptions that include accurate functional job analyses. The job description should include the specific mental and physical functions the job requires, the amount of time spent on each, the environmental factors in the area at the worksite (temperature, dust, ventilation, noise), the type of equipment used, and so on. Using these descriptions, a physician can then describe the aspects of any particular job that the patient can perform with or without reasonable accommodation. In the event the employer does not provide the necessary information, the physician will be forced to rely on the patient to provide information regarding the work environment.

In evaluating the safety risks in employment of the patient, the physician should remember that future speculative risk of injury (such as the possibility that a past back injury may predispose a patient to future injury) is not the intended target of the direct-threat language in the ADA. Treating physicians will nevertheless want to discuss the issues of future injury carefully with patients before supporting the patient's application to return to work.

The ADA explicitly forbids an employer from making employment decisions based on medical problems that are unrelated to the applicant's ability to perform the job in question. Preplacement physicals can be performed only after a conditional offer of employment has been made by the employer. An employer can require fitness for duty medical examinations before returning employees to work after an injury, but these examinations must be limited to job-related capabilities. The employer may not refuse to allow an injured worker to return to work because the worker is not fully recovered from the injury unless the worker is unable to perform the essential functions of the job or the worker would pose a direct threat to the safety of self or others. Medical information that is not job-related may not be the basis for any decision by the employer and should not be included in any report provided to the employer. The physician who performs these examinations must use the information about the job requirements to focus the evaluation on the ability of this patient/worker to do the particular job in question.

It is not the physician's role to make employment decisions, to decide whether it is possible to make reasonable accommodation, or to determine whether modifications in the work environment will be excessively costly for the employer. Ultimately, it is the employer who is charged under the ADA with making the final determination as to whether an individual is qualified to perform a job and whether the risk involved in employing or reemploying the individual will be too great. On the basis of a medical examination, if the patient/worker cannot perform the essential functions of the job with or without reasonable accommodation or if the patient poses a direct threat to self or others, the employer may then refuse to hire or rehire that individual.

State law in some states also forbids employment discrimination on the basis of handicap or disability. State provisions are increasingly parallel to the provisions of the ADA. Physicians may be called upon to provide medical information for the patient to support both federal and state claims if the patient is charging the employer with discrimination on the basis of disability.

Family and Medical Leave Act. The Family and Medical Leave Act (FMLA) became effective on August 5, 1993. In general, the act entitles employees who have worked for employers with 50 or more employees for more than 1 year to up to 12 weeks of unpaid leave per year for the birth or adoption of a child, to care for a spouse or an immediate family member with a serious health condition, or when unable to work because of a serious health condition. A serious health condition requires either inpatient care or continuing treatment by a health care provider and can include those that are work-related. The Department of Labor's interim regulations require, when inpatient care is not involved, that the absence from work be for a period of more than 3 days in addition to requiring the continuing treatment of a health care provider.

The FMLA can provide guaranteed job security for workers who are temporarily disabled by occupational injuries. This protection is separate from any benefits a worker may receive through a workers' compensation program and distinct from the prohibitions against discrimination under the ADA. Instead of providing cash benefits or extending protection against discrimination solely to those with substantial impairments, the FMLA simply entitles eligible employees the guaranteed right to return to work after an absence. Employers covered by the law are required, once the leave period is concluded, to reinstate the employee to the same or an equivalent job—one in which the pay, benefits, and other terms and conditions of employment are equivalent. Employers are also required to maintain any preexisting health insurance coverage during the leave period.

PHYSICIAN'S ROLE UNDER THE FMLA. To be eligible for a leave under the FMLA, injured employees must have medical certification from a health care provider (generally defined as a medical or osteopathic physician) that they are either unable to work at all or are unable to perform any of the essential functions of the position. Leave may be taken by the employee whenever medically necessary. The employee need not, however, be so incapacitated that she is unable to work at all. An employee may also request intermittent leave or a reduced work schedule to accommodate planned medical treatment; the health care provider must then certify that this type of leave is medically necessary and stipulate the expected duration and schedule of the leave. Employers who want a health care provider to review an employee's ability to perform essential job functions have the option of describing these functions in a position description provided to the health care provider for this purpose. Failure of the patient to obtain medical certification for the leave may result in denial of the leave and, in some situations, discharge.

Medical certification in support of the employee's leave request must be provided to the employer within a reasonable time. The physician may use an optional medical certification form available from the Department of Labor. When certifying that the injured employee's own health status justifies a leave under this law, the physician must provide the following information:

- The date the serious health condition commenced and the probable duration of the condition
- The diagnosis
- An indication as to whether hospitalization is required
- A brief description of the treatment prescribed
- A statement that the employee is unable to perform the essential functions of her position, on the basis of information provided by the employer or, if not provided by the employer, based upon conversations with the worker/patient.

The interim regulations specifically provide:

> If an employee submits a complete certification signed by the health care provider, the employer may not request additional information from the employee's health care provider. Rather, an employer who has reason to doubt the validity of a medical certification may require the employee to obtain a second opinion at the employer's expense.[6]

When the patient is ready to return to work, the employer may also require a fitness-for-duty medical certification, consisting only of a simple statement that an employee is able to return to work.

Legal guarantees of the right to return to work after a job injury. A minority of state workers' compensation laws and the Federal Employees' Compensation Act provide that injured workers have a legal right to return to work after an absence for a compensable injury. In most of these states, the treating physician must certify that the patient is fit to return to work. Although any serious functional limitations should be noted when a patient is seeking to return to work (for example, lifting or bending restrictions), the physician and the patient should be aware that the lack of availability of light duty positions may jeopardize the patient's ability to find work. This is true despite the expanded protection now available under the Americans with Disabilities Act. Although an employer is required to make reasonable accommodation for a disabled worker, employers are not required to create jobs to accommodate them.

Employer's absence policy requirements. Employers may also require that an employee obtain a medical note verifying that the employee is ill or unable to perform her own job for a period of days. Failure to provide these notes can result in disciplinary action against the worker. The physician should discuss with the patient the specific requirements imposed by the employer regarding this verification of temporary illness. In general, verification of the period of illness and readiness to return to work are essential. Employers vary as to whether a diagnosis is also required to verify the medical absence. If the diagnosis is not required, it should not be provided, in keeping with the general rights of the patient to maintain confidentiality over medical information.

Medical certification of disability for receipt of benefits

Most workers injured on the job have three primary concerns: to recover physically from the injury or illness, to maintain their job security and get back to work, and to obtain medical certification of disability to qualify for some form of wage replacement or other disability-based benefits. Because workers are rarely paid full wages by their employers when they are off work due to illness or injury, it often appears that a prime motivation of the worker in seeking medical care is to get a physician's help to obtain monetary compensation. In fact, such patients are in a difficult situation. The need to obtain monetary assistance may be paramount in their minds, simply because their economic livelihood has been cut off. The patient's economic support is contingent on the physician's willingness to cooperate in providing the necessary forms to workers' compensation or other insurance programs.

The medical certification of disability is, however, fraught with legal confusion. Patients may be eligible for a variety of disability programs. The definitions of qualifying disability or impairment may differ substantially among these programs. Some programs require physicians to give an opinion as to whether the health problem is work-related; others do not. Some programs require assessment only of the level of impairment; others require an assessment of disability. Some programs require a physician to predict the potential duration of disability. To determine whether a patient should be supported in a claim for benefits, physicians must become familiar with the particular requirements of each program.

Confusion also flows from the potentially contradictory roles that a physician may play. Treating or primary care physicians will be asked by their patients to support claims for benefits or eligibility for job protection. They may also be asked by employers or others to perform disability, preplacement, or reemployment medical examinations or to be a source of information regarding the patient's medical history. It is certainly true that "physicians cannot be all things to all patients."[7] It is therefore essential that physicians determine which role they are assuming and that they communicate this decision to the patient.

The following section briefly describes the role of the physician in the most common benefit programs: workers' compensation, Social Security Disability and Supplemental Security Income, employment-based disability programs, and disability insurance. Patients may also seek benefits from veterans programs, which are not discussed in this text.

Workers' compensation. Workers' compensation is a state-based program of social insurance that provides a variety of benefits to workers injured at work or who suffer from occupational-caused diseases. Rules governing these programs vary considerably from one state to another. Federal workers' compensation programs also cover federal employees, workers covered by the Longshoremen and Harbor Workers' Act, and coal miners with lung disease caused by exposure to coal mine dust.

Benefits under these programs generally fit into four categories:

- Wage replacement during period of inability to perform the preinjury job (temporary total disability benefits)
- Permanent total disability benefits in cases in which individuals cannot return to work, although the extent of these benefits and the rules for eligibility vary from one state or program to another
- Medical benefits for the specific injury or illness, generally not limited as to duration
- Some compensation for the permanent level of

disability or wage loss resulting from injury or illness (permanent partial disability benefits), intended to compensate the worker for loss of function and loss of competitiveness in the labor market (this also varies substantially among programs).

Not all occupationally disabled individuals actually receive workers' compensation benefits. Their ability to obtain benefits will depend on the particular rules governing proof of eligibility in the state or federal program that covers their employment. Often, eligibility will turn on what the treating physician says about the injury or illness. The final determination regarding eligibility is not, however, made by the physician. In every program, final adjudication of eligibility is decided by the insurer and ultimately by a designated state or federal agency.

Workers' compensation is the primary benefit program that always requires the worker to demonstrate both that she is impaired and that the impairment is work-related. Physicians are called on to make reports regarding the etiology and the extent of impairment and disability. The physician may rely upon the history provided by the patient in determining whether an injury occurred at work. The etiology of diseases that also occur in everyday life is, of course, more difficult to determine. Proof of causation to establish eligibility for benefits is not equivalent to scientific certainty, however. A statement that it is more likely than not that the injury or illness is job related is generally adequate to establish causation.

The primary care physician is in a unique position to evaluate causation in workers' compensation claims. Because of the existence of an ongoing relationship with the patient, the primary care physician can contribute information regarding the worker's health status prior to the injury or regarding the effect of workplace exposures on the progression of disease. This information will assist in establishing a relationship between the workplace and the impairment. Unfortunately, many primary care physicians have been reluctant to diagnose and treat occupationally caused injuries and illnesses. Some feel that they have not been adequately trained to provide this care or prefer not to deal with the legal and ethical issues that these patients present. With the expanded focus on managed care, however, primary care physicians are likely to be called on to play an expanded role. To the extent that these physicians have greater familiarity with the patient and her needs, they will be able to make an important contribution to the provision of occupational medical care.

Workers become eligible for medical benefits from workers' compensation when any medical treatment is needed for an injury or illness determined to be work-related. No documentation of temporary total or permanent impairment or disability is required for eligibility for medical benefits. In fact, many workers' compensation claims are for minor injuries that involve only medical benefits.

If the worker is unable to work, temporary total disability benefits are paid when the patient/worker is temporarily unable to perform his or her regular job. After the injured worker returns to work or is unable to return to work because of residual effects of the injury, the physician may be called upon to assess the level of permanent impairment or disability from the injury. Forty-two states ask physicians to use the American Medical Association (AMA) *Guides for the Evaluation of Permanent Impairment* in evaluating the residual effects of injuries. This publication, while valuable, only provides guidance for the evaluation of impairment, not disability. In fact, a lower court in Texas ruled the use of the AMA guides for the evaluation of disability to be unconstitutional, noting that "disability is a legal term which expresses the loss of earning capacity, diminished earning capacity . . . impairment does not equal disability." Physicians need to determine whether the expectation of their states' workers' compensation program requires an assessment of disability or one of impairment and whether their state uses the AMA guides.

Social Security Disability benefits. Social Security Disability Insurance is a federal insurance program. Workers contribute to it through a payroll tax and their benefit amount is based upon the amount of their contribution. Disabled workers may also apply for and receive Social Security Disability (SSD) benefits during the same period in which they receive workers' compensation benefits. There are, however, both federal and state limits on the total amount of weekly benefits a worker can receive from the different programs. To be eligible for benefits, the worker must:

- Be under 65 years of age
- Have insured status as a result of having worked in covered Social Security employment for an adequate amount of time
- Have a current qualifying disability (or, if the worker has recovered, the period of disability must have lasted at least 12 months and ended less than 12 months before she applied for benefits)

Again, medical certification of the extent of disability is required for an individual to establish eligibility for benefits. Particular weight in the Social Security program is given to the opinion of the treating physician, especially when the opinion is supported by medically acceptable diagnostic techniques and is not in conflict with other evidence. Primary care physicians knowledgeable about the process may have important impact on the outcome for the patient.

For the purposes of the SSD program, disability means that the worker is unable to engage in substantial gainful activity as a result of severe, medically determinable physical or mental impairment that has lasted or can be expected to last for at least 1 year or will result in death. The worker must be unable to do his or her previous job or any other substantial gainful activity that is available in the national economy. Individuals with severe impairments who have only marginal education and have worked exclusively in jobs involving unskilled physical labor will almost always be considered disabled for the purposes of this program. A person who is currently employed is obviously not eligible for benefits. The extent of disability required for eligibility for SSD benefits is considerably more severe than the extent required for eligibility for temporary total disability benefits from workers' compensation programs. Eligibility for SSD benefits does not require that any impairment be caused by the patient's work.

Physicians may make a determination of disability by relying on the patient's history and description of symptoms, including pain. Ultimately, a designated state agency in each state will make the determination of eligibility, including an evaluation as to whether the patient's description of symptoms is consistent with the medical signs, laboratory results, and other diagnostic findings.

SSD is considerably different from workers' compensation programs. Eligibility may be based on the patient's total disability resulting from a combination of impairments. Physicians therefore should document all health problems of the patient, not just those that are work-related. This creates a record-keeping problem for those patients who file simultaneous claims for workers' compensation and SSD, because only the records related to the occupational injury or illness should be made available in any litigation over workers' compensation eligibility.

Disabled individuals who are extremely impoverished may qualify for Supplemental Security Income (SSI) benefits. The determination of disability status is the same as for the SSD program. Eligibility is not based on payment of Social Security taxes or an employment record. Instead, SSI is a need-based program that requires demonstration of poverty and disability. Most workers suffering from disability related to occupational injury or disease, who are severely disabled, will meet the requirements of the SSD program and should not meet or need to meet the need-based requirements of the SSI program.

Sickness and accident and disability insurance; disability pensions. Disability insurance, sickness and accident programs, and disability pensions are provided by some employers as fringe benefits to employees. Some workers also purchase disability insurance, particularly to cover payments on vehicles or home mortgages in the event of disability. Most of these programs require medical certification by the treating physician of the worker's inability to work. They do not generally require that the inability to work be occupationally caused.

All of these programs are governed by their own specific plans, and eligibility determinations are made by a private plan administrator. Waiting periods and the definition of disability are set out in the plan itself. In general, short-term disability policies define disability as the inability of the employee to engage in his or her usual occupation. The physician need only certify that the worker is currently unable to do her own job. Longer term disability policies or disability pension plans may require that the worker demonstrate that she is unable to perform any remunerative work at all. Generally, patients will obtain the necessary forms from the disability insurer and provide them to the physician. The forms provide direction regarding the necessary medical certification and documentation. Again, the medical records relating to the disability will often be sought by the plan administrator.

PUBLIC HEALTH LAW AND THE PROVISION OF OCCUPATIONAL MEDICINE SERVICES

Physicians who provide occupational health services or who act as primary care physicians to groups of workers from particular workplaces are often in the best position to report individual cases that represent sentinel events in occupational health and to discern patterns or clusters of illness or injuries related to workplace hazards. Physicians are not, however, in a position to engage in primary prevention. Employers, not doctors or patient/workers, control the level of risk in the workplace. Patients may also not be able to remove themselves from workplace exposures. Most patients need their jobs.

Nevertheless, physicians in primary care and occupational medicine settings can generate valuable surveillance data. State public health agencies maintain registries for the reporting of a variety of public health statistics. Traditionally, these registries collected birth and death certificate data, information generated by autopsies and coroner inquiries into unexpected deaths, and infectious disease data. Disease registries are now maintained in many states for cancers or occupational illnesses. In addition, a number of states have been engaged in developing the Sentinel Event Notification System for Occupational Risks (SENSOR) with the National Institute for Occupational Safety and Health (NIOSH). Except in cases of infectious disease outbreaks, physicians in most states do not have a legally enforceable duty to report occupational-induced injuries or illnesses. Reporting of these cases is, however, often helpful in developing a more adequate understanding about the frequency and severity of occupational-induced health problems. Physicians should obtain a list of reportable diseases from their state public health agencies. County and state health departments often have extensive but rarely used powers to confront public health hazards.

How should a physician go about reporting information regarding occupational safety and health diagnoses to expand the public health knowledge and fuel preventive activities? First, the physician must determine whether any report will identify the patients involved. Clearly, identification of affected individuals lends support and credibility to any report. Except in cases involving mandatory reporting of diseases under public health laws, the physician must obtain from the patients who are involved full consent to the release of this confidential medical information.

Second, to whom should the report be made? Obviously, required reporting of occupational diseases and injuries should be provided to the designated state public health agencies. There are, in addition, several agencies whose mission is to address workplace health and safety hazards. The Occupational Safety and Health Administration regulates hazards in general industry, pursuant to the Occupational Safety and Health Act. Many state governments have obtained approval from OSHA for a state plan and have assumed OSHA regulatory functions within their states. In these states, federal OSHA does not enforce the law. OSHA or the state agency can conduct inspections of covered workplaces when there is a claimed violation of an employer's obligation to comply with specific health and safety standards, to provide a workplace that is free from recognized hazards likely to cause death or serious bodily harm under the general duty clause of OSHA, or when there is a risk of imminent danger to employees. Inspections can be conducted at the request of employees, their representatives, or others, including physicians. OSHA is inadequately funded and sometimes fails to respond quickly or adequately to all requests. Nevertheless, some primary care physicians do report considerable success in working with OSHA area offices. The Mine Safety and

Health Administration, pursuant to the Mine Safety and Health Act, similarly regulates occupational health and safety in the mining industry. State governments in mining states also have regulatory agencies that function in addition to MSHA. A list of addresses of state and federal regulatory agencies can be found in Appendix A. In addition, employers are required to report all incidences of occupational illness and disease to OSHA and MSHA.

OSHA and MSHA are empowered only to regulate known hazards. NIOSH, an institute within the Centers for Disease Control and Prevention, conducts research regarding occupational safety and health hazards and is charged with developing recommended occupational safety and health standards for both mining and general industry. As part of its mandate, NIOSH can conduct health hazard evaluations (HHEs) in workplaces where hazards are suspected. These evaluations may include both environmental and epidemiological studies of the worksite. NIOSH has a right to obtain access to the workplace to conduct these studies. Requests for these worksite evaluations cannot be made by physicians, however. They must come either from the employer, a designated representative of the workers (generally a labor union), or a group of at least three workers. Physicians must therefore work with their patients' labor organizations or with a group of patients in obtaining assistance from NIOSH. Individual workers who make these requests can request that NIOSH protect their anonymity. Once the formal request for an HHE has been made, NIOSH will welcome any information from the treating physician regarding the observed effects of the workplace hazard.

NIOSH also provides technical assistance to physicians who are confronted with occupational health problems. The institute has issued numerous written reports on workplace hazards. In addition, the toll-free NIOSH telephone number (1-800-35-NIOSH) provides physicians with access to scientists and physicians with technical knowledge regarding occupational safety and health.

Finally, NIOSH can provide on-site technical assistance at the request of other federal and state governmental entities. Physicians in the field can work together with their county or state health departments to generate a request for NIOSH field assistance in evaluating occupational safety and health problems. The ability of NIOSH to conduct workplace investigations when these requests are made depends on the requesting agency's legal right of access to the workplace or upon the cooperation of the employer.

Physicians should remember that individual workers are often reluctant to request assistance from outside agencies because of fear that their employers will retaliate against them. Although illegal, retaliation is unfortunately a commonplace occurrence. This fear is not overcome by assurances of anonymity, which are often ineffective, particularly in small workplaces. Physicians should therefore not be surprised if their patients are not always eager to support a public report of the existence of a suspected workplace hazard.

Because of the patients' potentially legitimate concerns about job security, physicians also should exercise caution in contacting external agencies or employers directly without the full consent of the employees who are involved. The patient/worker is likely to have the best idea about the likely consequences of direct contact with the employer.

SUMMARY

The physician who treats patients with occupational injuries and diseases is presented with a complex array of demands. In addition to the usual provision of adequate medical care, the physician should at all times be attentive to three issues: preserving the confidentiality of the patient's records; addressing the needs of the patient for medical certification of her health status; and always communicating clearly to the patient regarding what she can expect the physician to do.

REFERENCES

1. American Academy of Orthopaedic Surgeons: *Working it out: the workshop report,* p 74, Nov 1992.
2. Bisbing SB et al: Disclosures about patients. In Falk K, et al, editors: *Legal medicine: legal dynamics of medical encounters,* ed 2, St. Louis, 1991, Mosby-Year Book, p 231.
3. Spieler EA: Legal and Ethical Issues in Occupational Health (Module 5). In National Health Service Corps: *Clinical and community issues in primary care,* 1982, p 188.
4. Larson A: *The law of workmen's compensation,* New York, 1992, Mathew Binder, pp 15-426.220.
5. Equal Employment Opportunity Commission: Technical assistance manual to Title I of the Americans with disabilities act, 1992, 2.2(a) (ii).
6. Dept. of Labor Wage and Hour Division: Family and medical leave act interim regulations, 1993, 29 Code of Federal Regulations §825.307.
7. Carey TS, Hadler NM: The role of the primary physician in disability determination for social security insurance and workers' compensation, *Annals of Internal Med* 104:706-710, 1986.

SUGGESTED READINGS

Bruce JA: *Privacy and confidentiality of health care information,* ed 2, Chicago, 1984, American Hospital Publications.

Carey TS, Hadler NM: The role of the primary physician in disability determination for social security insurance and workers' compensation, *Annals of Internal Med* 104:706-710, 1986.

Falk K et al, editors: *Legal medicine: legal dynamics of medical encounters,* ed 2, St. Louis, 1991, Mosby-Year Book.

Freund E, Drachman JG: Mandatory reporting of occupational diseases by clinicians, *J Am Med Assn* 262:3041, 1989.

Greenwood J, Taricco A, editors: *Workers' compensation health care cost containment,* Horsham, Pa, 1992, LRP Publications.

Larson A: *The law of workmen's compensation,* New York, 1992, Mathew Binder.

Richards EP III, Rathbun KC: *Law and the physician: a practical guide,* New York, 1993, Little, Brown.

Roach WH Jr et al: *Medical records and the law,* Rockville, Md, 1985, Aspen Publishers.

Rozovsky FA: *Consent to treatment: a practical guide,* Boston, Toronto, 1984, Little Brown.

Tomes JP: *Health care records: a practical legal guide,* Dubuque, Ia, 1990, Kendall-Hunt.

Vevaina J et al, editors: *Legal aspects of medicine,* New York, 1989, Springer-Verlag.

Weeks J, Wagner GR: Compensation for occupational disease with multiple causes: the case of coal miners' respiratory diseases, *Am J Pub Health* 76:58, 1986.

Ziporyn T: Disability evaluation: a fledgling science? *J Am Med Assoc* 250:873-80, 1983.

LEGAL READINGS

United States Code (USC); Code of Federal Regulations (CFR).

Americans with Disabilities Act of 1990, 42 USC §§ 12101-12113, 1992.

Equal Employment Opportunity Commission: Regulations to Implement the Equal Employment Provisions of the Americans with Disabilities Act, 29 CFR § 1630, 1992.

Equal Employment Opportunity Commission: Technical Assistance Manual to Title I of the Americans with Disabilities Act, 1992.

Family and Medical Leave Act, 29 USC §§ 2601-2619, 1993.

Dept. of Labor Wage and Hour Division: Family and Medical Leave Act Interim Regulations, 29 CFR 825, 1993.

Mine Safety and Health Act, 30 USC §§ 801-878, 1988.

Occupational Safety and Health Act, 29 USC §§ 651-678, 1988.

Occupational Safety and Health Administration: Occupational Safety and Health Standards, Hazard communication, 29 CFR § 1910.1200, 1992.

Public Health Service, Department of Health and Human Services: Occupational Safety and Health Research and Related Activities, Requests for Health Hazard Evaluations, 42 CFR §85, 1992.

Social Security Act, 42 USCA §§ 301-1395, 1992.

Employees Benefits, Social Security Administration: Federal Old-Age, Survivors and Disability Insurance, Determining Disability and Blindness, 20 CFR § 416, 1993.

7 Ethical Issues in Occupational Medicine

Balancing competing interests is a challenge for health professionals who are part of the worker/employer/health care triad. Differing priorities, expectations, knowledge, goals, and values can be difficult to manage. To ensure the best care for injured workers, occupational health professionals must have outstanding clinical skills and an exceptional ability to communicate. They must also be aware of and embrace principles of ethics.

DEFINITION OF A PROFESSION

The term "trade" has linguistic roots meaning "path" or "track." It came to mean a course of action and, then, one's business, calling, livelihood, or occupation. "Craft" first referred to strength and skill and came to mean an occupation, trade, or pursuit that requires manual dexterity or artistic skill. "Profession" has origins that imply a public affirmation or avowal and suggest devotion to a life of service that is demanding and difficult and "thereby engages one's character, not merely one's mind and hands."[1]

Several elements distinguish a profession from other enterprises. Service, duty, altruism, public interest, compassion, integrity, trust, knowledge, and competence are some commonly accepted attributes. L. D. Brandeis, justice of the U.S. Supreme Court, defined a profession in 1914:

First. A profession is an occupation for which the necessary preliminary training is intellectual in character, involving knowledge and to some extent learning, as distinguished from mere skill.
Second. It is an occupation which is pursued largely for others and not merely for one's self.
Third. It is an occupation in which the amount of financial return is not the only measure of success.[2]

A more recent definition of a profession by R. P. Foa includes these principles:

1. The activity of the profession is intellectual with material drawn from science and learning, yet dependent on the performance of individuals.
2. The activity must embody virtues (honesty, courage, justice, creativity) essential to the achievement of excellence and lead to internal rewards for that achievement. . . .
3. The activity must receive the acknowledgement of society because it fulfills the above criteria and because

the activity of the profession as a whole furthers goals set for it by society.[3]

Our work is valued by society because it embodies more than the application of science and knowledge in behalf of patients. Our work is valued because of our values, values brought to life by ethical guidelines and practice.

MEDICAL ETHICS

P. G. Derr, when writing about ethics in occupational medicine noted, "A dominating concern for the life and health of the patient is . . . not only justifiable, it is required. And it is required not only (or primarily) by a legally defined fiduciary relationship . . . It is required by the physician's own commitment to medicine as a profession."[4] The American College of Physicians addresses other ethical considerations that apply to the workplace.

The patient's welfare and best interest must be the physician's main concern. The physician should treat and cure when possible and help patients cope with illness, disability, and death. In all instances, the physician must help maintain the dignity of the person and respect the uniqueness of each person. . . . The physician's obligations to the patient remain unchanged even though the physician-patient relationship may be affected by the health care delivery system or the patient's state.[5]

"Legal" versus "ethical"

Plainly, the fact that an act or policy is legal does not necessarily mean that it is ethical. The American College of Physicians further notes, "The law does not always establish positive duties (what one should do) to the extent that professional (especially medical) ethics does. . . . [Furthermore] When conflicts arise, the moral principle is clear. The welfare of the patient must at all times be paramount, and the physician must insist that the medically appropriate level of care take primacy over fiscal considerations imposed by the physician's own practice, investments, or financial arrangements."[5] For example, although laws may not restrict giving an injured worker's personal health information to an employer, the ethic of confidentiality forbids this without the patient's consent. In this age of computers, faxes, and multiple copies of forms, protecting confidentially requires nothing less than zeal.

Review of medical ethics

In their classic text on biomedical ethics, T. L. Beauchamp and J.F. Childress note that although awareness of morals is not sufficient when making an ethical decision, a review of morals is probably necessary and certainly relevant. In the struggle to make a moral decision versus one based on self-interest, one must consider three guidelines: supremacy (the overriding "ought", the thing to do that dispassionate observers would acknowledge as "right"); universalizability; and protecting and promoting human welfare. These moral guidelines, at least partly determined by society, constitute the underpinnings of medical ethics. Thus, ethical decisions depend on identifying moral problems, as well as collecting reliable facts and examining assumptions, commitments, and values.

Beauchamp and Childress list four basic ethical principles: respect for autonomy, nonmaleficence, beneficence, and justice.[6] A brief summary of their descriptions of each principle follows.

Autonomy. Patients must have the freedom to determine their own future without pressures. Assuring this freedom requires that patients know they are making a decision and that they do so intentionally. They must also know and understand the effects that their choice or decision will have and all of the risks and opportunities that are part of it. Perhaps the best way to ensure respect for autonomy is to respect each patient, to be respectful of each patient. Fully informed consent allows patients to exercise their autonomy.

Autonomy can be assured and honored by obtaining informed consent. Typical components of informed consent include: disclosure, understanding, volunteering, competence, and consent. The terms "autonomy" and "competence" do not refer only to patients; they also refer to health professionals. Physicians must have clinical autonomy. Those who give the information, choices, and possibilities involved in informed consent must also be competent.

Nonmaleficence. The best way to define nonmaleficence is to call forth perhaps the longest standing tenet of medicine, primum non nocere: above all, do no harm. Harm may come from acts of omission and comission and from action(s) unrelated to consent or medical treatment. Harm may also result from breaches to confidentiality and other mistakes that undermine workers' privacy and dignity.

Beneficence. To act with beneficence, a health professional should prevent evil or harm, remove evil or harm, and do or promote good.

Justice. The final basic ethical principle is justice. This means treating each person fairly. Although this can also be characterized as giving everybody what they deserve, prejudice and bias can enter into assumptions of what they deserve. For example, some people wrongfully think that those with acquired immunodeficiency syndrome (AIDS) are getting what they "deserve." Therefore, one should think in terms of fairness or equitability. In order to ensure fairness, efforts must be made to counteract forces that may put a person at a disadvantage, such as poverty, age, sex, and lack of education. Another useful concept is that "there is a right to a decent minimum. . . .[6]

Codes of ethics in occupational medicine

Guidelines, codes, and standards that are rooted in ethics and excellence, are action-oriented, and are shared can help assure good care of injured workers. Some commentators believe that published occupational medicine codes only recommend behavior or outline responsibilities and are not based on a deep understanding of ethics. Some have questioned the social and political viewpoints of authors as well as the breadth of their experience. The statements are, however, reasonable starting points.

Occupational health professionals must present a statement of ethics to employers with whom they are associated. The goal is to have its full discussion and mutual endorsement, adoption, and assimilation. As we know, prevention is preferable to treatment. Prevention saves pain, suffering, and money. Thorough discussion of ethics before the first patient is seen from a particular worksite prevents a great deal of misunderstanding and dispute and saves a great deal of pain, suffering, and money.

Several statements of ethics formulated by organizations in the field of occupational health are displayed in Table 7-1.[6]

Figure 7-1 is the statement by the American College of Occupational and Environmental Medicine outlining principles intended to aid physicians in maintaining ethical conduct in providing occupational medical service.[7]

Figure 7-2 presents applications of the Canadian Medical Association Code to occupational health services.[8]

Figure 7-3 is the Code of Ethics of the American Association of Occupational Health Nurses.[9]

Donald Whorton, MD, Morris Davis, JD, and Ephraim Kahn, MD, believed that the American Occupational Medical Association's statements had substantial weaknesses (personal communication). They believe that the recommendations are not active enough; physicians should not only observe but they should intervene. They were of the

Table 7-1 Recent efforts in North America to establish voluntary codes of conduct pertinent to occupational health services

Agent	Activity	Area of emphasis
American College of Epidemiology	Proposed guidelines	Occupational epidemiology
American Public Health Association	Occupational Health Section	Occupational medicine
Canadian Medical Association	Code of Ethics for Occupational Medicine	Occupational medicine
American College of Occupational Medicine	Code of Ethics	Occupational medicine
American Medical Association	Statement to U.S. OSHA	Occupational health and exposure records
National Commission on Confidentiality of Health Records	Federation of 26 organizations concerned with medical records	Occupational and exposure records
Canadian Centre for Occupational Health and Safety	Proposed guidelines	Monitoring and surveillance

opinion that the statements should insist upon objective data rather than only observations or honest opinion and should emphasize that physicians should be independent and not bound by salary, stock options, or other benefits. They also said that the statements should state strong "musts."

Although many debate I. R. Tabershaw's assertion that the physician is an agent of the employer, he presents an activist approach to ways physicians can practice ethically:

1. Know the hazards of the work environments for which he[sic] has accepted responsibilities.

2. Carry out medical examinations adequate to determine a [person's] health and fitness for the particular job and the health risks involved, if any.

3. Inform the worker of the hazards of the job, if they exist, in language the worker can understand.

4. Advise and work with management to minimize the risks at work.

5. Bear in mind [the] responsibility . . . to safeguard the health of the worker who looks upon [the] physician whose legal, social and ethical responsibility is to the individual (which can be breached only on indisputable evidence that the public welfare is endangered)."[10]

Although the advice is otherwise practical, these statements can be criticized because, unarguably, all jobs have risks and risks should be eliminated, not simply minimized.

L. Rosenstock and A. Hagopian highlight arenas in the physician/worker/employer triad in which conflicts can arise. These include loyalty, confidentiality, patient advocacy and disclosure. They note that "the health of the worker and the health of the company can no doubt come into con-

flict."[11] Indeed, daily discussions with employers and workers about return-to-work decisions may convince a health professional that a conflict exists. This is not so. Companies need healthy workers and workers need to be healthy. This is in everyone's best interest. One way to ensure that workers are healthy is to have complete information about their jobs so that job placement is appropriate.

Rosenstock and Hagopian also note that information about the job description should be available so that advice about initial employability is based on sound judgment.[11] This also applies to return-to-work recommendations. To give a good, ethical opinion, a physician must know the job analysis, not only the job description; precisely how a job is performed; opportunities for light duty (including company policies about how long a person may be on light-duty status). Nothing substitutes for visiting the workplace to establish firm ground on which to base return-to-work recommendations. It must be said that even with mounds of objective, accurate data, unknowns may determine a worker's successful return to work. Factors such as a patient's motivation, personal and family problems, relationships with supervisor, and a company's ability to adhere to advice may set the course.

Statements by professional organizations about ethics can help clarify health professionals' responsibilities. As noted previously, however, these statements are not perfect and invite revision. Furthermore, viewpoints change and, as D. Walsh says, "Occupational medicine invites ambivalence."[12] P. W. Brandt-Rauf also confirms

CODE OF ETHICAL CONDUCT FOR PHYSICIANS PROVIDING OCCUPATIONAL MEDICAL SERVICES*

These principles are intended to aid physicians in maintaining ethical conduct in providing occupational medical service. They are standards to guide physicians in their relationship with the individuals they serve, with employers and workers' representatives, with colleagues in the health professions, and with the public.

Physicians should:

1. Accord highest priority to the health and safety of the individual in the workplace.

2. Practice on a scientific basis with objectivity and integrity.

3. Make or endorse only statements which reflect their observations or honest opinion.

4. Actively oppose and strive to correct unethical conduct in relation to occupational health service.

5. Avoid allowing their medical judgment to be influenced by any conflict.

6. Strive conscientiously to become familiar with the medical fitness requirements, the environment and the hazards of the work done by those they serve, and with the health and safety aspects of the products and operations involved.

7. Treat as confidential whatever is learned about individuals served, releasing information only when required by law or by over-riding public health considerations, or to other physicians at the request of the individual according to traditional medical ethical practice; and should recognize that employers are entitled to counsel about the medical fitness of individuals in relation to work, but are not entitled to diagnoses or details of a specific nature.

8. Strive continually to improve medical knowledge, and should communicate information about health hazards in timely and effective fashion to individuals or groups potentially affected, and make appropriate reports to the scientific community.

9. Communicate understandably to those they serve any significant observations about their health, recommending further study, counsel or treatment when indicated.

10. Seek consultation concerning the individual or the workplace whenever indicated.

11. Cooperate with governmental health personnel and agencies, and foster and maintain sound ethical relationships with other members of the health professions.

12. Avoid solicitation of the use of their services by making claims, offering testimonials, or implying results which may not be achieved, but they may appropriately advise colleagues and others of services available.

---

* American College of Occupational and Environmental Medicine.

Fig. 7-1 Principles to aid physicians in maintaining ethical conduct.

the anguish that physicians practicing occupational medicine can feel. The low response rate to his questionnaire probably reflects lack of awareness of ethical issues and limits conclusions that can be drawn from his study. Nonetheless, results are disturbing. Of the 37% of members of the American Occupational Medical Association who responded to his questionnaire, 21% reported that in their practices they had ethical dilemmas frequently or always and almost half reported that these conflicts sometimes arose. The most staggering finding was that 25% of physicians reported that the primary loyalty was to themselves always; 2% said it was to management always; and only 56% reported that it was to patients always. Respondents recommended several ways to change the situation such as better role models, better role definition, changes in training and more codes of ethics.[13]

Codes of ethics or statements of behavior, responsibility, and philosophy are necessary but not sufficient. Ethics must be practiced: each step, each decision in the care of injured workers must be viewed from an ethical standpoint. Above all, primum non nocere.

Ethical issues in occupational medicine

Dilemmas in the care of injured workers are not the only ethical challenges in occupational and environmental medicine.

- Ethical issues are prominent in health promotion. For example, is there subtle coercion of workers to participate? Do classism, racism, and bias enter the picture?
- Biochemical, mental, genetic, drug and alcohol screening have ethical components.
- Privacy and confidentially present basic ethical issues as do AIDS and reproduction.
- Research is permeated with moral and ethical concerns. How and to whom are results distributed? Are data and conclusions published without interference from sponsoring agencies?
- Psychiatric history and evaluation raise important ethical points. Can a worker's history of erratic or threatening behavior accurately predict future problems in the workplace? If psychiatric injury is a possibility, can an accurate history be obtained when confidentiality is not guaranteed?

Even if workers are not injured, the possibility of personal and environmental contamination raises broad concerns about community health. The ethics of environmental medical practice need to be amplified with an eye to long-recognized principles. In 1875 Reverend Charles Brigham wrote, "What makes any occupation of man unhealthy—dangerous to health in a community?

APPLICATIONS OF THE CANADIAN MEDICAL ASSOCIATION
CODE OF ETHICS TO OCCUPATIONAL HEALTH SERVICES

Consider first the well being of the patient.

- Accord highest priority to the health and safety of the individual in the workplace.

Honor your profession and its traditions.

- Strive continually to improve medical knowledge and make appropriate reports to the scientific community.
- Avoid allowing medical judgment to be influenced by any conflict of interest.
- Actively oppose and strive to correct unethical conduct by any person or group.

Recognize your limitations and the special skills of others in the prevention and treatment of disease.

- Seek consultation whenever it is indicated.
- Avoid usurping the position of the family physician, but offer information, assistance, and cooperation in the medical management of the worker.
- Refrain from verifying the genuineness of sickness absence on behalf of the employer.
- Cooperate and consult with others outside the medical profession to prevent illness and promote health to the extent that they are competent and have similar intent and ethics with respect to the health and well-being of the workers.

Protect the patient's secrets.

- Treat as confidential whatever is learned about the worker as a patient; release information only when it is required by law or when it is clearly needed by others to preserve health and life; release information to other physicians according to traditional medical practice.
- Keep the medical records secure; be clear, through written agreement, on who is responsible for the custody of records in your absence and on what happens to them in the event of changes in the health service staff or in the status of the firm; do not permit access to medical records by persons outside the service unless required by law to do so.
- Communicate your judgment to both the employer and the worker when the worker has undergone a medical assessment for fitness to perform a specific job; however, do not give the employer specific details or diagnoses unless the worker has so requested.
- Grant a request by a worker to release medical information to employers or others only if the request has been made without duress; specifies the nature of the information, the purpose for its release, and the person to whom it may be released; and states the time for which it is valid.

Teach and be taught.

- Become familiar with the medical fitness requirements, the environment, the hazards of the work, and the health and safety aspects of the production and operations.
- Advise management and workers or their representatives of hazards to health and of opportunities to improve employee well-being, and assist in necessary actions.

Fig. 7-2

- . . . The conditions and processes of the work [not only harm the worker] but are a nuisance and a danger to the neighborhoods and to persons not working.
- "That the products and the results of the work minister to disease and undermine and destroy the soundness of those who use them." [14]

Despite their importance and fascination, these public health segments of occupational/environmental medicine do not pertain directly to the ethical care of injured workers. They should play a role in framing our medical decisions, however, and need our continued attention and understanding.

Two points of ethics outlined by the American College of Physicians and little noted in occupational health need to be considered along with basic principles. These pertain to the need for physicians to reach out for assistance and also to participate in determining the future of the profession. "Physicians should obtain consultation when they feel a need for assistance in caring for the patient or when it is requested by the patient or a legally authorized representative." [15]

An ethics-based decision about returning a patient to work may well require consultation. Physicians, accustomed to making assertions and thinking that they know a great deal while being embarrassed to admit ignorance, may not seek this consultation. This is unethical. Care of an injured worker may well require consultation with health professionals including medical subspecialists, occupational and physical therapists, hand surgeons, radiologists, psychologists, and/or pain treatment specialists.

"The physician should help develop health policy at the local, state, and national levels by expressing views as an individual and as a professional. Through professional activities and associations, as well as through the political process, physicians should participate in health policy decisions."[15]

Workers' compensation reform and safety and health programs are policy areas calling for physician action now. Whether policy is made by a company or agency, at the local or national level, the perspective and experience of physicians are essential. There is no escaping this ethical requirement.

Ethical issues in the care of injured workers

Managing patients and employers is difficult especially when expectations, hopes, and goals clash. Tension mounts when discomfort, time, and expenditures mount. In the occupational setting, health practitioners diagnose, treat, heal, and, often mediate. Most physicians who care for injured workers must interact with many employers, since almost 56% of employees work in places with fewer than 100 employees[16] and nearly 90% of employers have fewer than 20 employees.[17] Numerous mediations may be underway at once. This complex situation alone makes the physician as "double agent" untenable, even though "the private practitioner . . . may be anxious to accommodate the interest of the business client."[18] It is too demanding to be a double agent in a single situation, much less many simultaneous situations. Furthermore it is impossible for an ethical professional to provide anything less than patient-centered care.

The physician cannot always do exactly what patients want, of course. Patients' requests may not be medically appropriate. Patients may request time off from work when the injury does not warrant it.[19] Conversely, an injured worker may wish to return to work even if the physician disagrees. In addition, public health and safety concerns may conflict with patients' preferences. If a bus driver wishes to return to work despite a hand injury that prevents a strong and dependable grip on the wheel, and power steering is unavailable, how does a physician make an ethical decision that benefits all? Who comes first? A process involving therapy, patient education, and job accommodation will usually lead to a congruence of interests and a mutually agreeable return-to-work date. Should all else fail, the lesser of the evils is to delay returning the worker to full duties until it is safe to do so. This responsibility for public health and safety is the only legitimate dual relationship in occupational health. A. R. Jonsen, M. Siegler and W. J. Winslade note that while this difficult relationship exists, and although patients probably expect it, the physician must disclose the dual responsibilities and its implications to patients while being certain that "employers will allow them to abide by the ethical code."[20] Having dual responsibilities (for worker health and public health) do not suggest that the physician is a double agent. The overarching "ought" is toward health.

The elements of a good doctor/patient relationship include honesty, trust, loyalty, openness.[21] These elements should be practiced in a symmetrical fashion among patient, physician, and employer. One way to encourage honesty is for physicians to inform patients about the purpose of the evaluation and for patients to sign a release of information. This may not be required for strictly work-related matters but is definitely required if personal health matters may be part of the information flow. Workers must also know the implications of any testing and diagnosis before agreeing to the procedure or signing a release. Some practitioners believe that virtually every permission for health information to be released to an employer is coerced. Workers risk being labeled uncooperative and may fear job jeopardy by not consenting to the release of information to the employer.

A final example of the ethical care of patients with an occupational injury is prescribing drugs. Antiinflammatory agents, pain medications, and antibiotics are commonly used in treating injured workers. Prescribing drugs requires that health professionals remember basic moral principles of respect for autonomy, nonmaleficence, beneficence, and justice, as well as the profession's own responsibility for being data-based and not self-serving. With this in mind, one must decide which drug to use and analyze how that decision was made. What was the influence of advertisements, drug representatives, symposia, medical literature, grand rounds, or discussions with colleagues? Who sponsored the symposia? Lecturers, research and honoraria were funded by whom? Was there full disclosure about these fiscal matters? Professionals need to know if there are incentives for using particular medications. A gift giver may expect a certain response: there are no free lunches, dinners, or trips. Are the drugs the best and the least expensive available? Are they generic; are they over-the-counter; are they store brands? Prices vary wildly and quality may vary also.

One of the most important ways to ensure the ethical practice of occupational medicine is to ask oneself probing questions about who benefits from one's recommendations about diagnosis, treatment, and return to work. It should always be the patient.

Six guidelines are suggested for health professionals in the practice of occupational medicine:

- Know thyself. Health professionals should know their own values and beliefs. They should be interested in doing what is right for patients and society.
- Collect data from history and physical examinations. Despite advances in technology, 88% of diagnoses are made on the basis of histories and physical examinations.[22] A psychosocial history is crucial especially in the light of increasing evidence that pain syndromes in adults may be associated with violence in their childhood. Additional important data include the job analyses and company policies such as the availability and duration of light-duty assignments.
- Explore the possibility that ethics could play a part in the decision. Are there conflicts between the worker and employer and physician? Is the issue precedent-setting? Is the situation murky for some reason? Any of these criteria suggests that an ethical dimension exists.
- Determine the choices, the conflicts, and the consequences of any decision.
- Consult with others.
- Before making a decision, test it against your own values. You may be choosing between two evils. At least choose the lesser one.

Health professionals who are part of the worker/employer/health triad should consider 10 practical actions in providing occupational medical service.

1. Before entering into any agreement, describe your ethical positions to the company and gain full endorsement and adoption. Try to be sure that your ethical statements are accepted by companies as bone-marrow deep, not skin deep.
2. Respect patients. Welcome their questions and answer them fully and honestly. Honor requests.
3. Constantly learn about basic and clinical science, about new approaches and new technologies, about new ways to understand the healing of tissues, attitudes and behaviors. Admitting ignorance is a sign of strength when you pursue knowledge.
4. Insist on complete information. You need to receive it; you need to give it.
5. Good decisions require openness and daylight. Secrets, deficient data, and distortions will lead to unethical decisions and to situations that fail the practical headlines test. ("How would it look in the headlines?")
6. Ask yourself tough questions every day. What do you tell to whom about whom? Who really needs to know versus who wants to know, and why do they want to know?
7. Apply a common sense test. Would your interpretation of data differ or would your diagnosis and treatment differ if you were in practice, in a university, or working for a corporation?
8. Recognize and mitigate any financial incentives.
9. Know that reputation is paramount. Health professionals may have fluctuations in income; workers and companies may be irritated at various times. If health professionals

can be counted on for reliable, objective, ethical decisions and the highest quality care, they, their patients, and companies will flourish. Don't swerve from the medical straight and narrow.

10. Engender trust. Fostering and maintaining trust with all parties is essential in order to return workers to health in the complicated world of the workplace.

REFERENCES

1. Kass LR: Professing ethically: on the place of ethics in defining medicine, *JAMA* 249(10):1305-1310, 1983.
2. Brandeis LD: *Business: a profession,* Boston, 1914, Small, Mayard.
3. Foa RP: Are physicians professionals? *Pharos* 49:21-23, 1986.
4. Derr PG: Ethical considerations in fitness and risk evaluations, *Occupational Medicine: State of the Art Reviews* 3(2):193-208, 1988.
5. American College of Physicians: American College of Physicians Ethics Manual, ed 3, *Ann Intern Med* 117(11):947-960, 1992.
6. Beauchamp TL, Childress JF: *Principles of biomedical ethics,* ed 3, New York, 1989, Oxford University Press.
7. American College of Occupational and Environmental Medicine: Code of Ethical Conduct for Physicians Providing Occupational Medical Services. Reaffirmed by ACOEM Board of Directors, October 28, 1988.
8. Guidotti TL, Cowell JWF, Jamieson GG: *Occupational health services: a practical approach,* Chicago, 1989, American Medical Association.
9. American Association of Occupational Health Nurses: AAOHN code of ethics, *AAOHN Journal* 34(8):365, 1986.
10. Tabershaw IR: How is the acceptability of risks to the health of the workers to be determined? *J Occup Med* 18(10):674-676, 1976.
11. Rosenstock L, Hagopian A: Ethical dilemmas in providing health care to workers, *Ann Intern Med* 107(4):575-580, 1987.
12. Walsh D: Divided loyalties in medicine: the ambivalence of occupational medicine practice, *Soc Sci Med* 23(8):789-96, 1986.
13. Brandt-Rauf PW: Ethical conflict in the practice of occupational medicine, *Br J Ind Med* 46:63-66, 1989.
14. Brigham CH: The influence of occupations upon health, *J Occup Med* 18(4):235-241, 1976.
15. American College of Physicians: American College of Physicians Ethics Manual, ed 3, *Ann Intern Med* 117(11):947-960, 1992.
16. US Bureau of the Census: Statistical abstract of the United States, ed 112, Washington DC, 1992.
17. US Bureau of the Census: Statistical abstract of the United States, ed 110, Washington DC, 1990.
18. McCunney RJ, Brandt-Rauf P: Ethical conflict in the private practice of occupational medicine, *J Occup Med* 32(1):80-82, 1991.
19. Holleman WL, Holleman MC: School and work release evaluations, *JAMA* 260(24):3629-3634, 1988.
20. Jonsen AR, Siegler M, Winslade WJ: *Clinical ethics,* ed 3, New York, 1992, McGraw-Hill, Inc.
21. Holleman WL, Holleman MC: School and work release evaluations, *JAMA* 260(24):3629-3634, 1988.
22. Peterson MC et al: Contributions of the history, physical examination, and laboratory investigation in making medical diagnoses, *West J Med* 156(2):163-165, 1992.

SECTION II
OCCUPATIONAL INJURIES

Because the hand is so exposed, it is the most frequently injured part of the body. The frequency of hand injuries must not distract from their seriousness, however, because even a relatively minor hand injury if not managed properly can result in lost time, productivity, and permanent functional impairment. Proper management rests on understanding the hand's complex structure and function and on familiarity with the local anatomy. From that perspective, this chapter outlines an approach to the diagnosis and treatment of work-related injuries in the hand.

ACUTE INJURIES
Soft-tissue injuries

Lacerations. A routine and detailed history must be obtained. It is important to determine whether the patient uses anticoagulants and other medications, as these can alter the management of a hand injury. For the same reason, it is essential to document the presence of diabetes, immunosuppressive disorders, and other illnesses that may predispose to infection, poor healing caused by vascular compromise, neuropathy, and other problems. One should obtain the history of tetanus prophylaxis and determine whether there has been a previous hand injury. The patient's recovery depends on their age, occupation, and hand dominance, so this information is obtained as well. Finally, the details of the injury are carefully documented, including exactly how, when, and where it occurred.

The patient should be examined lying down with the extremity elevated. This position will stop bleeding in most cases. If bleeding continues, however, there may be a partial laceration of a major artery, and direct pressure should be placed on the wound. A tourniquet can be used if the amount and duration of tourniquet pressure can be carefully monitored. Vessels should not be clamped until the full extent of the damage can be visualized; otherwise, nerves and other structures may be damaged.

The examination begins distal to the laceration, avoiding any temptation to probe the wound. By examining the distal parts first, an accurate diagnosis can almost always be made. If the injuries require a formal operation, detailed exploration and probing of the wound in the emergency setting may be skipped; instead, the wound need only be irrigated and dressed. If a diagnosis cannot be made, the wound should be cleansed and inspected for foreign objects and damaged structures. The hand examination must include evaluating the skin, nerves and vasculature, taking x-ray films to assess the integrity of the bones and joints, and testing for compartment syndrome. After assessing sensory and motor nerve function, a local anesthetic should be administered.

Splinting. After treating most injuries, the hand is temporarily immobilized. Toward this end, it is fitted with a static resting splint that places the wrist in slight extension, the metacarpophalangeal (MCP) joints in flexion, and the interphalangeal (IP) joints in extension. In this position, the collateral ligaments of the MCP and IP joints are kept tight, which avoids further tightening and later contracture. The duration of immobilization depends on a variety of factors. For example, if the patient has an unstable fracture, a splint must be worn for approximately 3 weeks to avoid displacing the bone fragments when the hand and fingers move. In the presence of a flexor tendon or nerve injury in the palm, the fingers must not be extended for a period of about 3 weeks to avoid rupturing the repair. It is important to minimize the period of immobilization, however, because experience has shown that doing so enables the resumption of normal movement and function sooner and more easily. (This same principle underlies the management of unstable fractures; internal fixation with plates or screws provides stability of the fracture site while allowing the initiation of hand and finger movement and exercise within a few days.) In a few situations, the hand must be completely immobilized for up to 3 weeks, but in most cases, mobilization of one type or another should be initiated within 7 to 10 days of the injury to begin restoring normal function.

The first goal of the mobilization and exercise program is to establish range of motion, and only when this has been accomplished should a strengthening regimen begin. Range of motion is

103

best provided by light continuous traction to reeducate the scar tissue. Rapid repetitive movements or very forceful activities are to be avoided because they may promote swelling. When full range of motion is not possible, partial range of motion should be instituted to keep the finger joints supple and mobile. For example, hands with a flexor tendon injury are placed in a dorsal block splint, which prevents finger extension; this limitation protects the tendon repair but allows the finger joints to be passively flexed (the so-called Duran protocol). Another method is to attach a rubber band to the bandage in the palm and to a hook on the fingernail; the rubber band causes the finger to flex passively but also permits it to be actively extended by the patient within the limited range of motion allowed by the splint (the so-called Kleinert protocol).

A well-conceived hand therapy program includes dynamic splinting for contractures, active and passive range-of-motion exercises, and other specific modalities. The patient can often do much of the therapy at home, so their motivation to comply with the rehabilitation program is a vital factor in regaining good function.

Flexor tendon injuries. A damaged tendon in the hand is a serious injury and must be treated with a great deal of respect. Such an injury can occur in association with a skin laceration and so appear trivial at first, but it can require the patient to be off work for quite some time if their job involves much hand activity (Fig. 8-1). Frequently, a tendon injury can lead to permanent functional impairment and even a significant disability that can prevent the patient from returning to the original occupation. For this reason, an accurate diagnosis, early effective treatment, a carefully planned hand therapy program, and a return-to-work program are essential if a successful outcome is to be achieved.

The diagnosis can be made by examining the posture of the hand as it lies on the examination

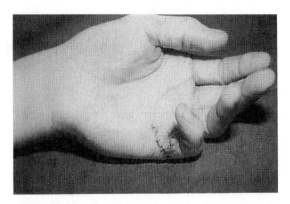

Fig. 8-2 A flexor tendon injury can be diagnosed by examining the posture of the hand as it lies on the examination table.

table (Fig. 8-2). The resting position of the fingers in an uninjured hand are partly flexed with a normal arcade of increasing flexion from the index to the small finger. A digit with a flexor tendon injury will not profile with the normal cascade but will lie in a relatively extended position. This lack of continuity is accentuated with the application of pressure to the flexor surface of the forearm; a normal finger will flex further into the palm, but the injured digit will be unaffected by this action. This test is useful in inebriated patients and in children who are uncooperative (Fig. 8-3).

Because the normal excursion of flexor tendons is 5 to 7 cm, a tendon may appear to be intact at the base of the wound yet actually be injured. If a flexor tendon was lacerated when the finger was firmly clenched into a fist, the level of the skin laceration will be considerably more proximal than that of the tendon laceration. Conversely, if the laceration occurred when the finger was in extension and the finger is examined while in a rela-

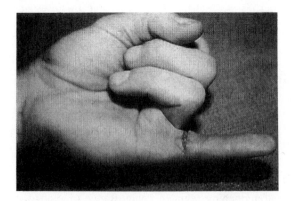

Fig. 8-1 Tendon laceration.

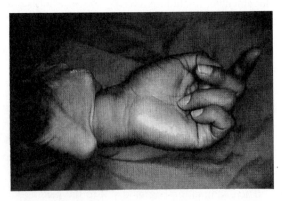

Fig. 8-3 Applying pressure to the flexor surface of the forearm causes a normal digit to flex into the palm; a digit with a flexor tendon injury is not affected by this action.

tively flexed position, the tendon laceration will be more proximal than the skin laceration. Thus, it is important to test tendon function to rule out injury.

The flexor digitorum profundus (FDP) tendon is tested by stabilizing the middle phalanx and asking the patient to flex the distal interphalangeal (DIP) joint. The flexor digitorum superficialis (FDS) is tested by holding the adjacent fingers in extension at the DIP joint (thereby inactivating the FDP to the injured finger because all of the FDP tendons are connected) and asking the patient to flex the injured finger at the proximal interphalangeal (PIP) joint. The FDP to the index finger is separate from the FDP tendon to the other fingers; this makes it difficult to exclude its function to test the FDS to the index finger. The latter is tested by asking the patient to strongly pinch the index finger against the thumb; the more strongly this finger is flexed, the less the DIP joint will be used and the more action is required of the FDS of this finger. The flexor pollicis longus is tested by stabilizing the proximal phalanx of the thumb and asking the patient to flex the IP joint. The flexor carpi ulnaris, flexor carpi radialis, and palmaris longus tendons are tested by palpating each as the patient flexes the wrist against mild resistance.

Once a tendon laceration has been diagnosed, it is important to determine its location, as the site of injury has a bearing on the treatment and the patient's prognosis. For this purpose, the hand has been divided into zones (Fig. 8-4).

Zone I. Zone I encompasses the FDP tendon from its insertion into the distal phalanx to the proximal portion of the middle phalanx. A tendon

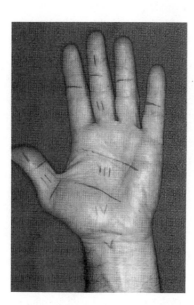

Fig. 8-4 Classification of tendon injuries of the hand.

laceration in zone I or a rupture of the FDP from its insertion in the distal phalanx is known as a "jersey finger" because it often occurs in football players when they grab an opponent's jersey. As the finger is being forcibly flexed, the jersey pulls the finger with equal force into extension; this combination of forces stresses the attachment of the tendon in the distal phalanx, and a spicule of bone may pull off as the tendon moves proximally in the finger. An x-ray film may show the fleck of bone in the proximal part of the finger and thereby aid the diagnosis.

Zone II. Zone II, which stretches from the mid-palmar flexion crease to just distal to the PIP joint region, is the area of the fibrous, flexor tendon pulleys. In this zone, the FDS divides into two tails and passes deep to the FDP to insert into the base of the middle phalanx. The FDP passes through the divided FDS, proceeds distally along the course of the middle phalanx, and inserts into the distal phalanx. Zone II has been termed "no man's land" because tendon repair in this region is difficult and is prone to problems, especially adhesions, which prevent normal gliding within the pulleys. Flexor tendon injuries in this zone should be repaired in the operating room by a hand specialist (see Fig. 8-1).

Zone III. Zone III extends from the distal margin of the flexor retinaculum to the midpalmar crease. Injury to the FDP in this region can cause an abnormal pull of the lumbrical muscles, resulting in what is known as a lumbrical-plus finger. When the patient attempts to flex the DIP joint, the lumbrical muscle attached to the contracting FDP tendon moves more proximally, but because this muscle inserts into the extensor expansion of the finger, the IP joints extend rather than flex.

Zones IV and V. Zone IV lies beneath the flexor retinaculum, and zone V is proximal to the carpal tunnel.

The flexor tendons are deeper and more difficult to repair than the extensor tendons. When lacerated, they should be repaired in the operating room to ensure a thorough exploration, a secure repair, and no damage to other structures. Repair should be performed promptly. If immediate repair is not practical and the wound is clean, the skin may be closed, the patient given antibiotics, and the repair done within a few days.

CASE STUDIES

Case 1

A 23-year-old delicatessen worker lacerated the palmar surface of the proximal phalanx of her small finger as she was cutting a sandwich. Although the 1 cm wound appeared benign, the tendon and ulnar digital nerve had been divided. This injury was serious because of its location in "no man's land," and because the ul-

nar digital nerve to the small finger provides sensation to the surface of this finger, which has fairly frequent contact with objects. The patient required urgent surgery by a hand surgeon to repair the nerve and tendon. Despite early, vigorous postoperative therapy, adhesions developed, and the patient required tenolysis 3 months later. Good sensation returned, and she ultimately regained full range of motion. She was off work for 3 months after the surgery and for 6 weeks after the tenolysis.

This case illustrates that even with appropriate and immediate treatment by a specialist, a substantial amount of time off work is required after a simple laceration that involves tendons and nerves.

Extensor tendon injuries. Extensor tendon injuries are often simple to treat, and recovery of normal function is fairly rapid. The most frequent functional problem following repair is stiffness in the affected digit—a complication that underscores the importance of minimizing the period of immobilization and implementing a carefully planned postoperative exercise program. As in the case of flexor tendon injuries, the implications of extensor tendon injuries vary with the site of laceration.

Zone I. Zone I of the extensor mechanism is that area from the insertion of the central slip in the proximal part of the middle phalanx to the end of the finger. When the tendon in this zone is either sharply lacerated, severed in a crush injury, or ruptured as a result of forcible flexion of the DIP joint, the DIP joint lies in a flexed position. This deformity is called a mallet finger because the injured digit has the appearance of the hammers that strike piano strings. An avulsion of the extensor tendon insertion into the distal phalanx can also cause a mallet finger, and this particular injury is accompanied by a fracture that can be demonstrated on an x-ray film. The vast majority of closed mallet finger injuries are treated by splinting with the DIP joint in extension. Crush injuries may require debridement, whereas avulsion fractures that involve more than 30% to 50% of the joint and are also markedly displaced may occasionally benefit from open reduction and internal fixation, especially if the DIP joint is subluxed. In most cases, though, the position of the bone fragment is such that the fracture is appropriately treated by closed methods.

Fractures in Zone I will heal in about 4 weeks, but mallet deformities caused by soft tissue injury alone generally take 8 to 12 weeks to heal, and *continuous* splinting is required for the entire period. If the splint is removed and any extension lag remains at the DIP joint, splinting should be continued for a longer period—generally until the joint has active extension.

If a mallet deformity is left untreated, the volar plate of the PIP joint will stretch out over time and cause the joint to hyperextend; the increased extensor forces across this joint combined with the incompetence of the tendon at the DIP joint create a swan-neck deformity (Fig. 8-5). This problem requires more complex reconstruction, so it is best to avoid it by early treatment of the mallet deformity.

Zone II. Zone II is the area from the distal metacarpal to the proximal part of the middle phalanx. It includes the insertion of the central slip, the lateral bands that run from the intrinsic muscles to join the extensor expansion, and the sagittal bands at the level of the MCP joints. The sagittal bands, which hold the extensor tendon central, pass around the finger, insert into the volar plate, and are responsible for extending the MCP joint. The lateral bands are held in position by their attachment to the transverse retinacular ligaments. The extensor mechanism in this zone is called the extensor hood mechanism because of its shape.

The insertion of the central slip can suffer a sharp laceration or be damaged when an extended PIP joint is forcefully flexed. When this tendon is disrupted, the lateral bands tend to migrate palmar to the axis of flexion of the PIP joint. As a result, the joint herniates between the lateral bands on either side, much like a button through a buttonhole. For this reason, the problem is known as a boutonnière deformity (Fig. 8-6). Any attempt by the patient to extend the PIP joint is futile because the central slip that enables this action is not functional. The migration of the lateral bands adds to the problem; normally they would assist extension, but their abnormal position results in further joint flexion.

What often occurs after an injury to the central slip is that the lateral bands remain in their normal

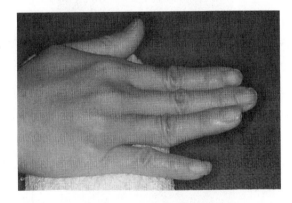

Fig. 8-5 A swan-neck deformity results when a mallet deformity is left untreated. The swan-neck configuration is caused by hyperextension of the proximal interphalangeal (PIP) joint coupled with incompetence of the tendon at the distal interphalangeal (DIP) joint.

position, leaving the PIP joint temporarily unaffected. Over the course of weeks or even months, however, the bands sublux palmarward, causing the deformity to develop gradually. It is for this reason that injuries on the dorsal side of the PIP joint must be carefully monitored even if tendon function initially appears to be intact.

The splinting of digits with a boutonnière deformity need only include the PIP joint. The lateral bands distally are pulled taught and dorsal as the DIP joint flexes; for this reason, this joint should be encouraged to flex to reduce the likelihood of stiffness and keep the lateral bands mobile and more dorsal. The late treatment of boutonnière deformities is complex, requiring release of the retinacular ligaments, lysis of the lateral bands, and sometimes further reconstruction of the central tendon slip (Fig. 8-6).

Laceration of the sagittal bands can cause subluxation of the extensor tendon either radially or ulnarly with an abnormal pull on the finger. The laceration should be surgically repaired to restore the extensor tendon to its central position.

Case 2

A 38-year-old construction worker was injured when a window fell on the proximal interphalangeal (PIP) joint of the long finger. X-ray films showed no fracture, and the patient was able to flex and extend his finger. No splint was applied, and he returned to work 3 days later despite fairly severe local swelling. He was able to continue working, but over the next 2 to 3 weeks he noticed a deformity developing at the joint, and he slowly lost the ability to extend the joint as a result of a 45-degree flexion contracture. Over the next 2 months, a reciprocal hyperextension deformity developed at the distal interphalangeal (DIP) joint. This deteriorating boutonnière deformity resulted from a laceration of the central extensor tendon, which initially was compensated for by the lateral bands that extend the PIP joint. As contraction of the transverse retinacular ligaments caused these lateral bands to migrate to a more volar position, they moved volar to the axis of flexion of the PIP joint, and flexed the joint instead of extending it.

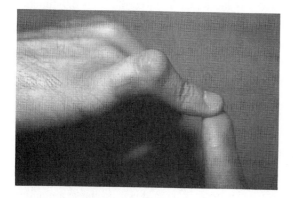

Fig. 8-6 Boutonnière deformity.

In this case, therapy helped the patient regain passive extension of the PIP joint. Good flexion and extension were regained after surgery was performed to release the transverse retinacular ligaments, bring the lateral bands into a more dorsal position, and reconstruct the central tendon.

Zones III, IV, and V. Zone III is that area from the distal aspect of the extensor retinaculum of the wrist to the metacarpal neck. Zone IV lies beneath the extensor retinaculum, and Zone V is proximal to it. Tendon injuries in these regions are similar to one another and can be diagnosed as follows:

FIRST DORSAL COMPARTMENT. The function of the abductor pollicis longus is halfway between extension and abduction of the thumb. During this action, the tendon can be observed to tent the skin, and it can also be palpated to determine its integrity. The extensor pollicis brevis is tested by asking the patient to extend the thumb and then comparing extension at the MCP joint with that in the opposite hand.

SECOND DORSAL COMPARTMENT. The extensor carpi radialis longus and brevis are tested by palpation during forceful extension of the wrist against resistance.

THIRD DORSAL COMPARTMENT. The extensor pollicis longus is examined with the palm of the hand flat on the examining table. If the patient is able to lift up the thumb from the table, the tendon can be observed to contract and be palpated. It should be remembered that when the thumb is flexed across the palm, the intrinsic muscles (i.e., the abductor pollicis brevis and flexor pollicis brevis) extend the IP joint. This movement should not be confused with that enabled by the extensor pollicis longus tendon, which extends the IP joint when the thumb is extended away from the palm.

FOURTH AND FIFTH DORSAL COMPARTMENTS. The extensor digitorum communis is tested by asking the patient to extend the MCP joint with the IP joint in extension. As in the thumb, the intrinsic tendons extend the IP joint. Incomplete extension at the MCP joint may occur if a lacerated extensor tendon communicates with an adjacent extensor tendon through the juncturae tendonae. Isolated lacerations of the juncturae tendonae are unimportant and do not require repair. The extensor digiti minimi and extensor indicis proprius are tested by asking the patient to make a fist and extend the index finger alone and then the small finger alone. Flexing the long and ring fingers into the palm incapacitates the extensor digitorum communis and allows the function of the aforementioned tendons to be demonstrated. The integrity of the extensor carpi ulnaris, which is in the fifth dorsal compartment, is tested by palpating the tendon as the patient extends and ulnar deviates the wrist.

Lacerations of these tendons should be repaired and the hand placed in a palmar protective splint with the fingers and wrist extended. Protected movement is initiated within 7 to 10 days of the injury. If one or two lacerated extensor tendons on the dorsum of the hand are visible in the wound, repair can be done in the emergency department. The involved finger should be allowed only limited flexion to prevent tendon rupture.

Nerve injuries. All nerve injuries in the hand and upper extremity are serious because they may result in decreased sensation, diminished muscle power, and considerable functional impairment even if the patient receives optimal treatment. The outcome of nerve repair depends on many factors, the most important of which are the patient's age, the nature and site of the injury, and the specific nerve lacerated. A detailed consideration of these factors and the method of nerve repair are beyond the scope of this chapter, but the principles of treatment are reviewed here.

Neuropraxis refers to a lesion in which nerve conduction is blocked for physiologic reasons and not because it has actually been severed. It occurs with a closed injury such as a stretch or crush injury in which the nerve is damaged, causing abnormal sensation or motor weakness, but there is a spontaneous return of function within 1 to 3 months. *Axonotmetsis* refers to a lesion in which there is axonal disruption, resulting in wallerian degeneration distal to the site of injury. Recovery from this type of damage may be slow because of the time required for reinnervation of the distal nerve, skin, and muscle. Axonotmesis frequently occurs in gunshot wounds and in stretch injuries with displaced fractures. *Neurotmesis* refers to a lesion in which the nerve is completely disrupted or lacerated, and a decrease in function can be expected. This type of damage requires surgical repair. Following treatment, the nerve will regenerate at a rate of approximately 1 mm per day, with a longer time to reinnervation and a poorer prognosis the more proximal the lesion.

Most nerve injuries should be repaired acutely. Priority is given to any open wounds, which are cleaned and provided with soft tissue cover. Most nerve lacerations should be repaired on the day of the injury, but if a hand or finger wound is clean, it can be closed, the patient given antibiotics, and the repair done within a few days. If other damage requires more immediate attention or if soft tissue cover must be provided immediately, a secondary repair of the nerve can be done within the next 2 to 3 weeks. A nerve gap in which the severed nerve ends cannot be brought together without considerable tension should be treated by sural nerve grafting, which is generally performed as a secondary procedure.

Distal sensation is tested by pinprick and two-point discrimination. The latter is evaluated by placing the two blunt ends of a paper clip 1 cm apart along the longitudinal axis of the finger on either the radial or ulnar side in the region of the pulp. Normal two-point discrimination is between 4 and 5 mm, but the patient in whom the nerve has been transected will have a two-point discrimination of more than 2 cm. This test is frequently used to assess the time and completeness of nerve regeneration.

The most commonly injured nerves in the body are the digital nerves in the hand. Of these, the border digits—the digital nerves of the thumb, radial aspect of the index finger, and ulnar aspect of the small finger—are most often involved. These nerves are functionally important and should be repaired under the operating microscope. In general, the other digital nerves in the hand should also be repaired, but the decision to do so depends on the patient's occupation, functional requirements, and personal preference. For example, a laceration of the ulnar digital nerve to the ring finger will not cause substantial functional impairment in most individuals, so repair of this nerve in a laborer who must return to work as soon as possible will probably be seen as unnecessary. In other locations, nerve repair may be less a matter of choice than of feasibility. Approximately 5 mm proximal to the base of the nail, the digital nerve arborizes into three small branches; nerve repair distal to this level is always difficult and sometimes impossible. Injuries to the superficial palmar arch or the tendons in the region of the palm are often associated with injuries to the common digital nerves in the palm, and these should always be repaired.

The median nerve is extremely important, as it supplies the palmar surface of the thumb, the index finger, the long finger, the radial side of the ring finger, and the thenar muscles. When this nerve is lacerated, its motor and sensory function must be evaluated. In the hand, motor function is tested by palpating the thenar muscles as the thumb abducts away from the palm. The integrity of this nerve proximal to the forearm region can be assessed by testing the function of the flexor pollicis longus and FDS tendons.

The ulnar nerve provides sensation to the small finger and the ulnar side of the ring finger, whereas its motor function consists of the intrinsic muscles of the hand; these can be tested by assessing abduction of the index finger away from the long finger and radial or ulnar abduction of the long finger when the hand is palm down on the examination table. Motor function can be tested by asking the patient to pinch firmly together the index finger and thumb. If the intrinsic musculature is incompetent, sharp flexion of the IP joint will result as the patient compensates by using the flexor pollicis longus. This phenomenon is known as Froment's sign (Fig. 8-7). The integrity of the ulnar nerve proximal to the forearm region can be assessed by testing the function of the FDP to the ring and small fingers.

The radial nerve is tested by having the patient extend the wrist while palpating the tendons in the forearm that perform this function. The same can be tested by extending the MCP joints with the IP joints in extension.

Partial nerve lacerations must be repaired as urgently as complete lacerations, and they can produce deficits that appear inconsistent. Patients with a Martin-Gruber anomaly have an anastomosis between the median and ulnar nerves in the midforearm region. When such individuals sustain a high laceration of the median nerve, they may experience damage to the ulnar-innervated muscles of the hand; conversely, a high laceration of the ulnar nerve may leave functional the ulnar-innervated intrinsic muscles of the hand. Likewise, an anastomosis between the median and ulnar nerves in the palm (a Riche-Cannieu anastomosis) can produce confusing results of sensation tests in the fingers.

In addition to paralyzed muscles and lack of sensation, several other serious complications can result from nerve injury. Painful neuromas can occur at the site of nerve damage and at the end of amputation stumps (Fig. 8-8). Certain nerves are notorious for their potential to produce neuromas of exquisite sensitivity, which can render an extremity useless. The sensory branch of the radial

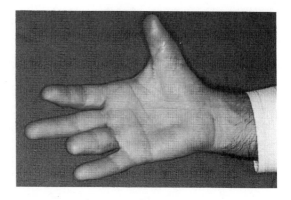

Fig. 8-8 Neuromas can form at the end of an amputation stump.

nerve in the region of the wrist, and the dorsal branch of the ulnar nerve in the distal forearm and hand are two such nerves, but other nerves are capable of this problem as well. Neuromas can sometimes be managed through reconstructive techniques such as nerve grafting or burying the nerve in a different position. Neuromas-in-continuity are especially difficult to treat if there is distal function. Resection of the neuroma may improve the pain locally, but distal function may be lost, at least temporarily. Neurolysis can improve the patient's condition in some cases.

A particularly dreaded complication of nerve injury is reflex sympathetic dystrophy with resultant vasomotor instability. This condition causes severe pain, swelling, discoloration, and stiffness caused by increased sympathetic outflow (Fig. 8-9). Early treatment and referral to an experienced occupational therapist and/or anesthesiologist is essential.

Case 3
A metal worker suffered a crush injury of the radial side of the wrist when he was struck by a falling piece of metal. At the time, a laceration of the sensory branch of

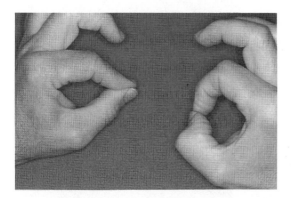

Fig. 8-7 Froment's sign, which indicates incompetence of the intrinsic musculature, is elicited by asking the patient to firmly pinch together the index finger and thumb.

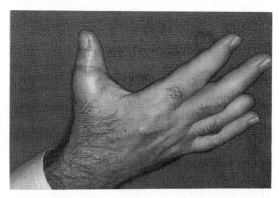

Fig. 8-9 Reflex sympathetic dystrophy following neuroma formation at amputation stump.

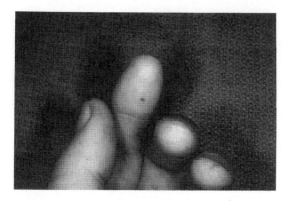

Fig. 8-10 High-pressure injection injury.

the radial nerve went unrecognized, and only the skin was repaired. Several weeks later, he began experiencing a shock-type sensation as neuroma developed. Six months later he was experiencing exquisite tenderness and was completely unable to use his hand or even wear long-sleeved shirts. A diagnosis of possible reflex sympathetic dystrophy was made. He was treated with stellate ganglion blocks and desensitization therapy for 3 months, but the condition did not improve. In an effort to reduce the sensitivity, surgery was performed to resect the neuroma and place a small nerve graft. His condition improved after this procedure, and he regained limited use of his hand. However, he also required treatment at a pain clinic for over 4 months. He ultimately was referred for vocational rehabilitation and resumed work at a lighter job 18 months after the original injury.

This case emphasizes the need for accurate diagnosis and nerve repair, and it illustrates the exquisitely painful neuromata that can be produced by the superficial sensory branch.

High-pressure injection injuries. High-pressure injection of paint, grease, or other substances can injure the fingers and hand so severely that amputation of the affected part may be necessary. This type of injury usually occurs when a worker tests a high-pressure spray gun with their fingertip over the nozzle. The pulp of the index finger of the nondominant hand is, therefore, the most frequently affected site. The wound may only be a small puncture that causes little alarm, which is why the patient may not present immediately after the injury (see Fig. 8-10). Its appearance is deceiving, however, for few injuries are as treacherous.

The extent of damage depends on several factors. One is the nature of the substance injected, which is usually highly toxic. Grease and oil produce extensive local necrosis, but even water can produce this effect. The force of injection, which can range from 100 to 1000 pounds per square inch, causes the fluid to track along the planes of

the tissue and flexor tendon sheath. In this way, it can travel from the fingertip throughout the hand and even proximally into the forearm. If the agent does travel proximally, it produces an intense inflammatory reaction that causes great pain and tenderness. Systemic effects may result if there is absorption through extensive synovial and soft tissue contact. The extent of damage to the finger should be assessed by evaluating its sensation, motor function, and vascularization. If the substance injected is radiopaque, x-ray films may show the extent of infiltration.

Other potential complications of this injury are neurovascular compromise, and, at a later stage, the formation of draining sinuses and secondary infections caused by the sloughing of soft tissue. Prompt and aggressive surgery is vital in patients with this type of injury. They should immediately be referred for emergency hand surgery to undergo radical debridement, decompression, and removal of the noxious substance (Fig. 8-11).

Case 4
A patient suffered a high-pressure injury of the tip of his nondominant index finger while testing a small grease gun. The wound appeared benign to the initial treating physician, who cleaned and bandaged it. Twenty-four hours after the accident, the patient was referred to our service by the Emergency Department and was immediately taken to surgery. A major debridement was performed because grease had infiltrated all the way proximal to the carpal tunnel. Meticulous care was used to remove as much of the grease as possible, after which carpal tunnel release was performed. The wounds

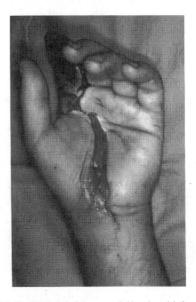

Fig. 8-11 Radical debridement following high-pressure injection injury to index finger.

were left open. Despite this extremely vigorous treatment, the index finger necrosed and ultimately required amputation.

As this case shows, high-pressure injection injuries must be recognized immediately and treated as soon as possible. It is questionable, however, whether more prompt treatment would have salvaged this patient's finger.

Fingertip injuries. The fingertip—that portion of the finger or thumb distal to the insertion of the long flexor and extensor tendons—is a sophisticated organ of touch, containing many nerve endings, a specialized nail, and a nail bed. Injuries to this region are probably the most common of all hand injuries. Although they may appear to be minor, they can be painful and result in functional impairment and prolonged disability, especially if not managed properly.

The scheme of Allen categorizes injuries of the fingertip by location:

Type 1—Injuries to the skin and subcutaneous tissue distal to the nail
Type 2—Injuries distal to the distal phalanx involving the nailbed
Type 3—Injuries distal to the lunula, through the phalanx, nail bed, and pulp
Type 4—Injuries proximal to the lunula

Treatment should provide for adequate soft tissue coverage, a maximum of finger length, the prevention of neuromas and bone prominances, adequate sensibility, good joint motion, and as normal an appearance as possible. Ninety percent of fingertip injuries can be treated by allowing healing by secondary intention and epithelialization or by skin grafting. Type 3 and 4 injuries are treated with local flap procedures, although their management does depend somewhat on the angle of the injury.

Type 1 and 2 injuries in which the defect is less than 1 centimeter are allowed to heal by secondary intention. The wound is debrided under local anesthetic, and a dressing of nonadherent petrolatum-based gauze is applied. Healing is achieved through rapid epithelialization from the periphery of the wound and dermal scar contracture. This simple method provides good skin texture, good sensibility, and allows early mobilization. It is also the method of choice for children because of their excellent regenerative potential.

When the defect is too large to comfortably allow healing by secondary intention, skin grafting is performed after the wound has been adequately debrided. In general, skin grafting is preferable to reattaching the amputated fingertip because it provides immediate coverage and expedites healing. If a thin, split-thickness skin graft is used, it will contract from the wound margins like a wound that heals by secondary intention, and good sensibility will be achieved. Skin grafting is more comfortable for the patient than healing by secondary intention because repeated dressing changes of an open wound are not needed. Skin for the graft can be taken from the medial aspect of the ipsilateral forearm, the volar wrist crease, or the hypothenar region, the latter two sites providing the best color match. The graft is anchored with sutures and a stent dressing and left undisturbed for 5 to 7 days, barring infection or other problems.

Type 3 and 4 injuries, which penetrate the phalanx, nail bed, and pulp, are treated with flaps, although primary closure of the wound can sometimes be achieved if intact skin can be brought over the distal injury. In cases of amputation within 5 mm of the lunula that involve more than 50% of the distal phalanx, the bone should be trimmed, the nailbed tissue ablated, and the wound closed primarily. Injuries in which significant pulp, skin, and subcutaneous tissue have been lost but sufficient bone and nailbed tissue remain are managed with either a local, V-Y advancement flap or, occasionally, the lateral V-Y flap from one or both sides of the finger (Fig. 8-12). A volar advancement flap (Moberg flap) can be used to cover distal defects in the thumb. A regional pedicle flap such as a thenar flap, cross finger flap, or, on rare occasion, a distant flap may also be necessary.

Nail bed injuries and their subsequent deformities are a source of significant morbidity. A hematoma that occupies less than 25% of the subungual space may simply be drained with the use of a hot paperclip to provide adequate relief. Larger subungual hematomas should be treated by removing the nail and inspecting the underlying nail bed for lacerations; those that need repair are sutured with 6-0 chromic catgut under loupe magnification, and the nail is replaced to maintain the nailfold and prevent it from healing over. If neces-

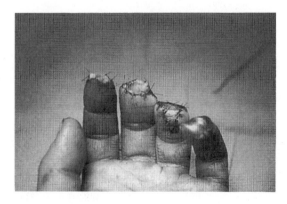

Fig. 8-12 Fingertip injury.

sary, a piece of plastic can substitute for the nail and be maintained (or held in place) for about 3 weeks. Avulsions of the proximal nailbed and the germinal matrix should be repaired with half-buried mattress sutures. Although an underlying comminuted tuft fracture may be treated as a soft tissue injury, a displaced distal phalangeal shaft fracture implies a nailbed disruption and should be treated by reduction and repair. Handled carefully, these injuries will usually heal without severe problems.

Case 5

A worker suffered a crush injury of two fingertips in a punch press. A split-thickness skin graft was placed on the finger with the smaller lesion, and a V-Y advancement flap was placed on the finger with the more substantial defect. The wounds healed well, although considerable sensitivity remained at the tips of the fingers for about 6 months. The long finger sustained a fracture of the tuft of the distal phalanx, but this eventually healed without further treatment. However, despite good healing, fingertip injuries can result in long-term morbidity; this patient was unable to return to work for 6 months.

In cases such as this one, a patient's ability to return to work depends on his desire to do so and the employer's ability to provide light work that does not require use of the fingers for heavy grasping or contact of the sensitive areas.

Vascular injuries. The vessels of the upper extremity are subject to different types of damage. A crush injury may cause thrombosis and, with it, the risk of thromboembolism. Partial lacerations may lead to excessive blood loss, which should be managed by applying pressure until the damage is repaired under the operating microscope. Damage to either the axillary or brachial artery is limb-threatening, but injury to the radial or ulnar artery usually is not because the two vessels compensate. A laceration of either of these vessels should usually be repaired, but it is essential in certain individuals who, because of a congenital or acquired anatomic variation, have all or part of the hand supplied by one vessel only.

Injury to the superficial or deep palmar arches or the common or proper digital vessels may or may not result in ischemic changes distally. The need for vascular reconstruction depends on the specific location of the damage and the clinical presentation. An embolism from a thrombosed proximal vessel can occlude distal vessels and cause ischemia. If diagnosed early, the vessel damage or thrombosis can be treated by endarterectomy or vein grafting, depending on the cause of the injury and quality of the damaged vessel. If the vascularity of the hand is at all in question, the patient must be promptly referred to a specialist.

Repetitive injury to blood vessels can produce substantial symptomatology. For example, a worker who sustains repeated trauma to the ulnar aspect of the wrist may develop an ulnar artery thrombosis with resultant ischemic pain (the so-called ulnar hammer syndrome). Early diagnosis and treatment of a thrombosis or aneurysm is advised because the results of late repair are generally unpredictable.

Compartment syndrome. Local swelling can result from an open or closed injury or from ischemia due to vascular compromise more proximally. When swelling occurs within a closed fascial compartment, the increase in pressure causes compression of the veins and lymphatics and, eventually, the arteries. As venous outflow is curtailed, the pressure within the compartment increases further, causing what is known as compartment syndrome (Fig. 8-13). If this condition is not treated immediately, permanent nerve damage and muscle fibrosis will result.

The diagnosis of compartment syndrome can be confirmed by measuring local pressure with a Wick catheter inserted under the fascia of the involved part. In general, a reading above 30 mm Hg indicates the need for immediate surgery. If the reading is equivocal, passive stretching of the flexor compartment of the forearm is done, and, in the hand, stretching of the intrinsic muscles. The latter is accomplished by hyperextending the MCP joints and flexing the PIP joints. If passive stretch causes pain and the compartment feels firm, surgery should be performed to avoid the serious complications of sustained increase in pressure within a closed compartment. It is important to realize that the arterial pulse may be present as the syndrome develops and may persist until the late stages. By the time pressure in the compartment exceeds arterial pressure, irreversible damage has already occurred.

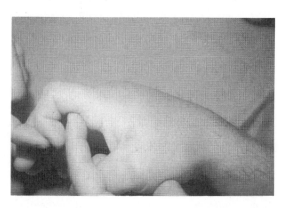

Fig. 8-13 Compartment syndrome.

Case 6

A man was changing a tire at work when the jack malfunctioned and the car wheel fell on his hand, crushing it and keeping it pinned for approximately 5 minutes. No fractures were evident, and the hand had good sensation and circulation. About 2 to 3 hours later, though, the hand was massively swollen and a severe compartment syndrome had developed, with tightness of the intrinsic muscles (tightness of these muscles is shown by extending the metacarpophalangeal [MCP] joint and passively flexing the PIP joint). The carpal tunnel and intrinsic muscle compartments were released from the dorsum of the hand, and therapy was begun immediately thereafter. Within a month the hand was fully healed, and the patient returned to work full time with no further problems.

This case illustrates the value and necessity of diagnosing and treating compartment syndrome immediately.

Bone and joint injuries

Before discussing specific bone and joint injuries and their treatment, it is necessary to understand the range of fracture types and certain principles of fracture management.

Fractures may be either closed or open, depending on whether the skin has been breached. Open fractures have a greater propensity for infection and always need thorough irrigation and antibiotic coverage. For this reason, they should be treated within 4 to 6 hours of the injury. Patients with an intraarticular fracture, a fracture that involves the articular surface, may develop an incongruous joint surface and thus be more prone to stiffness and late arthritis. Extraarticular fractures are located in the shaft, base, or neck of the bone and may be transverse, oblique, spiral, or comminuted. It is important to determine the geometry of the fracture line(s) because this will give some indication of how likely it is the fracture will displace with movement. Angulation, generally defined by the direction of the apex of the fracture, may be in the dorsal-volar direction or the ulnar-radial direction.

Range-of-motion exercises should be initiated soon after treatment to maintain joint mobility and tendon gliding. Fractures that will displace with motion are, therefore, managed by open reduction and internal fixation.

Fracture and dislocation of the thumb. A Bennett's fracture is a relatively unstable intraarticular fracture at the base of the thumb metacarpal. It results from traction at the attachment of the abductor pollicis longus tendon as the stout ligament holds the ulnar portion of the articular surface in place. This action causes proximal displacement of the radical portion of the joint and metacarpal. Reduction and cast support may occasionally be adequate, but the fracture tends to displace as the swelling subsides. For this reason, optimal treatment consists of pinning the fracture after open reduction with a direct view of the articular surface.

Orlando's fracture is a Y- or T-shaped fracture at the base of the thumb metacarpal. This fracture line implies some comminution, which, if too extensive, is not amenable to internal fixation. This fracture is more likely to result in an irregular joint surface and lead to late arthritis.

Transverse fractures at the base of the metacarpal are extraarticular, usually stable if undisplaced, and, thus, amenable to treatment in a cast. Some displacement of the fracture can be tolerated if mobility is present.

Ligamentous injuries of the MCP joint are common and usually caused in a fall with the thumb abducted. Because such injuries often occur in skiing accidents, an acute tear of the ulnar collateral ligament at this joint is known as a skier's thumb. The ligament should be repaired immediately if it is completely disrupted. If it goes unrecognized and untreated, late instability will result and reconstruction of the ligament will be required.

Approximately half of all complete tears of the ulnar collateral ligament will be found with the ligament lying external to the adductor aponeurosis. In this position, the ligament is not in contact with its counterpart or the bone, so there is no potential for healing without operative intervention. This type of injury is known as a Stener lesion. A "gamekeeper's thumb" may occur in individuals who repeatedly abduct their thumb, chronically subjecting the ulnar collateral ligament to minor trauma that eventually causes incompetence of the ligament. A much rarer injury is that to the radial collateral ligament at the MCP joint, which generally results from forceful ulnar deviation of the thumb against resistance.

Phalangeal fracture and dislocation. Fractures of the distal phalanges, which are also common, are generally managed by splinting in extension for 3 to 4 weeks. Closed treatment is adequate in most cases, but other measures are required for those caused by a severe crush injury and are accompanied by open wounds, and those with marked displacement, especially if the nailbed is involved. Irrigation is required in such cases, as is pinning of the fracture to improve the likelihood of healing and decrease the patient's pain. Any intraarticular fracture of the DIP joint involving 30% to 50% of the joint or more should be reduced as accurately as possible and pinned in this position to restore the articular surface. Should fracture fixation fail and arthritis develop at this joint, joint fusion can be performed.

If the PIP joint suffers this same fate, however, fusion would severely impair the function of the entire hand as well as the finger. For this reason, fractures at the PIP joint must be handled more aggressively to avoid such functional impairment. The treatment of other fractures must be determined by their position and configuration. Oblique fractures with good bone contact and no shortening of the bone can be treated by cast support. Transverse fractures tend to displace, though, and often require open reduction and internal fixation.

Interphalangeal joint injuries. Tears of the collateral ligaments of the IP joints require careful splinting to avoid stressing the damaged ligament. Buddy-taping the adjacent finger often provides such support while allowing mobilization of the joint.

Amputations and crush injuries

Methods of repairing major injuries—microvascular repair of small nerves and vessels, techniques of providing better soft tissue coverage, early therapy, and rehabilitation—have enhanced the possibility of functional restoration even in patients with serious crush injuries and amputations. There are circumstances, however, in which surgery is not appropriate, and amputation not only provides the best result but is also the quickest way to restore good function.

Replantation is expensive, requires considerable recovery time, and may not always be in the patient's best interest. The decision to replant an amputated part must be based on a clear understanding of the indications for this procedure, as well as a number of other factors. First, the patient may have other injuries that contraindicate digital replantation, so their general condition—mental as well as physical—is of paramount importance. Personal considerations such as the patient's occupational requirements are particularly important, and their avocational interests should also be taken into account. Every person views the loss of a body part differently, and one's attitude around this issue may be at least partly related to cultural values. Considering that replantation generally requires a longer hospital stay (1 to 2 weeks) and rehabilitation period (2 to 6 months), some patients prefer amputation/closure. Amputation/closure, however, will not end the patient's problem, as neuroma formation, skin adherence or sensitivity, poor sensation, lack of dexterity, and poor pinch and grasp can all complicate the postoperative picture.

The indications for replantation depend on the site and type of injury and the likely functional outcome. Replantation of a single amputated finger should be performed in the occasional patient who has strong cosmetic, psychologic, and cultural reasons for wanting the procedure done or when there are unusual functional considerations, such as if the patient is a performing musician. Otherwise, single-digit replantation should generally be performed only when the amputation is distal to the PIP joint. These guidelines stem from the fact that replantation proximal to this level will most likely result in a stiff PIP joint that will disable the replanted finger to the point of compromising function in the rest of the hand. Multiple finger amputations result in considerable disability, and, for that reason, should be replanted if at all possible. For the same reason, an amputated thumb should be replanted if at all feasible, even if a considerable amount of shortening is necessary (Fig. 8-14).

An avulsion injury in which the soft tissue has been partially or completely avulsed from the bony structures can sometimes be salvaged, and salvage should be attempted if this injury occurs in conjunction with a multiple-digit amputation or a thumb amputation. When such damage occurs in the ring finger, as in a ring avulsion injury, salvage may occasionally be appropriate, but ray amputation and transfer of the small finger to the long finger position are usually preferable. If a ring avulsion injury causes devascularization but not complete amputation, the digit can usually be salvaged with good results. Transmetacarpal wrist and forearm amputations should be replanted if possible and a functional amount of sensation restored to the amputated or crushed part.

Replantation is often not feasible in multiple-level injuries or when the proximal nerves have been damaged so severely that the part will have no sensation, as occurs in severe brachial plexus injuries. Amputations proximal to the wrist in which the part contains a considerable amount of muscle tissue should not be replanted if the cold ischemia time exceeds 6 hours.

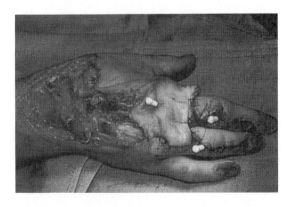

Fig. 8-14 Multiple amputation.

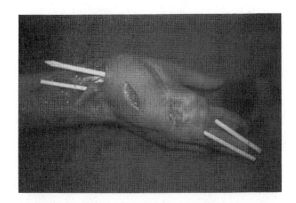

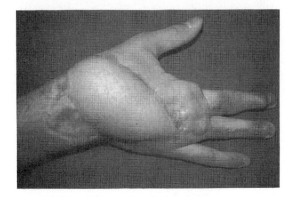

Fig. 8-15 Crush injury and reconstruction.

Each replantation center has its own protocol for managing amputated parts before arrival at the replantation center. Prior to treatment at California Pacific Medical Center in San Francisco, the part is kept in a dry container that is placed in a larger one filled with ice; this maintains the temperature of the part at 6° to 10° C. The patient is given antibiotics, and the extremity is dressed with a moist dressing, splinted, and elevated.

Surgical repair of these severe injuries is the province of specialists. So too is the postoperative rehabilitation and therapy program, which is essential for the restoration of maximal function. The interested reader is directed elsewhere for further information on these aspects of patient care.

CASE STUDIES
Case 1
A man amputated his nondominant thumb at the interphalangeal (IP) joint in a saw accident. He was referred to our replantation service, where the bone amputation site was fixed with Kirschner wires, and nerve and vascular repairs were performed under a surgical microscope. Motion at the IP joint was not anticipated because the joint had been severely damaged; thus the flexor and extensor tendons were not repaired. A fusion of the joint was performed that required shortening the thumb by approximately 1 cm.

In this type of case, shortening the thumb by 1 cm does not present a functional problem as long as motion is good at the MCP and carpometacarpal (CMC) joints. Unlike with the fingers, thumb function does not depend on motion at the IP joint.

Case 2
A patient suffered a massive crush injury of his hand when a truck rolled onto it. All of the dorsal structures from the wrist to the level of the proximal phalanx were avulsed. The hand was debrided, and the crushed index finger was amputated. Skin from the amputated finger was used to cover some of the wound, and a microvascular free flap was taken from the patient's scapular region to cover the remainder. These measures allowed tendon reconstruction to be done approximately 6 months later. The reconstructive process was lengthy, lasting approximately 14 months, but the hand regained excellent function, and the patient returned to work as a laborer (Fig. 8-15).

With crush injuries, if well-vascularized tissue is transferred to a region of severe damage, good function can be restored even in the most extreme cases.

CUMULATIVE TRAUMA DISORDERS
Cumulative trauma disorders, also known as repetitive strain disorders and overuse syndromes, have become a frequent work-related problem that accounts for a significant amount of time off work, medical expense, and permanent disability. The incidence of these problems has increased exponentially in the past 10 years because of changes in employment practices, work activities, and equipment. Today, many individuals are in occupations involving keyboard data entry, assembly line activity, or other tasks that require highly repetitive movements for hours on end.

Definition
Cumulative trauma disorders are problems of nerves, muscles, tendons, and bones that are caused, precipitated, or aggravated by repeated movements of the body. This medically varied group of musculoskeletal problems includes entrapment neuropathies, tendonitis and synovitis, and vascular injuries.

Etiology
Although repetition is an important factor in the pathogenesis of cumulative trauma disorders, it is not the only one. Stressful postures such as extremes of flexion or extension of the wrist, full pronation or supination of the forearm, flexion of the elbow, or abduction of the shoulder above the horizontal plane can all predispose the upper ex-

tremity to this type of problem. The force applied during task performance also contributes to the development of an overuse syndrome. Specific situations have known associations with particular problems, such as the use of vibrating tools and carpal tunnel syndrome. For these reasons, the physician must obtain a detailed and careful history of the patient's activity requirements on the job — specifically those that involve the hands and upper extremities.

Factors unrelated to the work situation can also have a bearing on the patient's condition, so a detailed history of the patient's home activities should be obtained as well; this includes hobbies and activities of daily living. Finally, it is important to be aware that underlying systemic diseases such as diabetes, rheumatoid arthritis, and thyroid malfunction may render the extremities more susceptible to this type of problem.

Entrapment neuropathies

Nerves can be compressed as they exit the spinal cord or at any of several specific points along their course in the upper extremity. These points are generally located within the fibroosseous canals or tunnels through which the nerves run. The patient's clinical presentation depends on the site of compression and the nerve involved.

Median nerve. The median nerve is most frequently compressed at the level of the elbow or just distal to it (pronator syndrome, anterior interosseous nerve syndrome), or at the wrist.

Carpal tunnel syndrome. Carpal tunnel syndrome, the most common of the nerve entrapment problems, refers to the group of clinical findings associated with compression of the median nerve at the level of the wrist. It occurs on average at about age 55, but occupational cases tend to occur in younger individuals because of the stress placed on the wrist and hand at work. Women are affected twice as often as men, and the problem is bilateral in about half of the cases. When the problem is bilateral, one must determine whether both hands have patterns of use consistent with the development of this problem or whether important nonindustrial factors such as an underlying systemic disorder have been involved.

ETIOLOGY. The median nerve passes through the carpal tunnel as it travels from the forearm into the hand. This nonelastic tunnel, which measures approximately 2 to 2.5 cm in diameter, contains the long flexor tendons to the fingers and thumb, the median nerve, and, occasionally, an abberant median artery. The floor of the canal is formed by the carpal bones, the ulnar side is formed by the hook of the hamate and pisiform bones, and the radial side is formed by the trapezium and scaphoid. The roof is formed by the stout transverse carpal ligament, or flexor retinaculum. When the contents of this nonelastic canal expand, the pressure within the canal rises and causes compression of the soft and pliable median nerve; this, in turn, causes functional impairment of its motor, sensory, and sympathetic fibers. Thus, the development of this problem depends on the volume of the structures within the canal in relation to the dimensions of the canal itself. Swelling from trauma, synovitis from rheumatoid arthritis, tumors, or inflammation may all cause carpal tunnel syndrome.

A change in the boundaries of the carpal tunnel may occur with a wrist fracture, which, combined with the accompanying swelling, frequently causes an acute carpal tunnel syndrome. Although the effect of cumulative trauma is not completely understood, it is thought to cause a slow but progressive swelling and synovitis within the canal. Whether it is flexion and extension or ulnar and radial deviation, abnormal patterns of wrist use repeated thousands of times a day may produce such changes, and the effect produced is exacerbated when great force is also used. Firm grasping, awkward positions of the wrist, the use of hand-held tools that vibrate or require awkward positions of the wrist, and direct pressure on the wrist may all cause work-related carpal tunnel syndrome.

Hypothyroidism, renal failure, and pregnancy are among the systemic conditions that may predispose an individual to carpal tunnel syndrome by causing fluid retention. Diseases such as diabetes and rheumatoid arthritis render the median nerve more susceptible to this problem by altering local circulation.

CLINICAL PRESENTATION. The signs and symptoms of carpal tunnel syndrome are sensory, motor, and autonomic. It is essential to carefully check the hand for atrophy of the thenar muscles, dryness of the skin supplied by the median nerve, and scarring. Usually, the patient first complains of sensory symptoms like pain and tingling in the median nerve distribution (the thumb, index, and long finger, and the radial side of the ring finger). Numbness is sometimes associated with the pain and tingling, and it frequently occurs at night, causing the patient to awaken. Motor symptoms consist of weakness and decreased grip strength to the point of being unable to open jars and dropping objects. The latter can be a function of decreased sensation in the fingers as well as weakness.

The sensory signs consist of decreased sensation in the median nerve distribution, which can be assessed by testing sharp-dull discrimination, Weber static or moving two-point discrimination, or the Von Frey pressure test with the use of

Semmes-Weinstein monofilaments. The patient's ability to feel vibration is measured with a variable amplitude vibrometer operated at a fixed frequency of 120 Hz, and the threshold of feeling is compared with that in the contralateral hand. The Semmes-Weinstein monofilament pressure test and vibration testing were conceived by Szabo, who showed that 80% of cases tested abnormally, whereas only 50% had abnormal two-point discrimination. (No test is completely reliable, however, and the diagnosis is made by considering all of the clinical findings.) Motor function is tested by assessing the strength of the thenar muscles. The patient is asked to abduct the thumb away from the plane of the palm against resistance. As the thumb is abducted, the contraction of the thenar muscles can be palpated to assess their strength.

Special tests may be used to confirm the diagnosis. *Phalen's test* is performed by asking the patient to maximally flex the wrist for 60 seconds. A tingling sensation, primarily in the median nerve distribution, occurs in the majority of patients with carpal tunnel syndrome. *Tinel's sign* is elicited by tapping over the median nerve in the region of the carpal tunnel. A tingling sensation in the distal distribution of the median nerve, especially in the fingertips, confirms the sensitivity of the median nerve and, thus, the presence of carpal tunnel syndrome. The median nerve compression test is performed by applying direct pressure over the median nerve at the level of the carpal tunnel. If symptoms develop within 2 minutes, the test is considered positive. These tests will sometimes produce confusing results. For example, while the physician conducts the Phalen's test, the patient may complain of pain in the wrist or discomfort in the forearm, and testing for Tinel's sign may cause tingling in the proximal portion of the extremity. Such test results are difficult to evaluate and may be considered equivocal.

Special studies may be used in situations where the diagnosis remains in question. An electromyogram of the thenar muscles may show some denervation of the thenar muscles, whereas a nerve conduction study can show slowing of median nerve conduction across the carpal tunnel region. The nerve conduction study may be negative after prolonged splinting and rest, even in the face of carpal tunnel syndrome. For this reason, it is best performed after some provocation, such as prolonged flexion of the wrist. It is possible, however, to obtain many false negative results and, occasionally, false positive results. Magnetic resonance (MR) imaging is still experimental with respect to carpal tunnel syndrome and, at present, does not aid the diagnosis. However, MR imaging is useful when there is suspicion of a specific tumor, some other type of space-occupying lesion, or an unusual cause of alteration in the shape or size of the carpal tunnel that cannot be assessed on x-ray film with either a routine or carpal tunnel view.

TREATMENT. The first line of treatment, especially if the patient is seen in the early stages of the problem, is to address the cause. Underlying disease processes that can cause fluid retention should be brought under control. The patient's activities can be modified by rotating assignments at work, improving the ergonomic conditions of the workstation, modifying the keyboard, limiting the amount of continuous time spent doing repetitive activities, and redesigning the tools used. There is little evidence of the efficacy of ergonomic alteration in the treatment of early carpal tunnel syndrome. Traditionally, health care providers have believed that alteration of any causative factors should accompany other medical treatment.

The treatment of carpal tunnel syndrome focuses on decreasing the inflammation, which is accomplished by resting the wrist in a splint at night and either part or full time during the day. Work duties can also be modified to incorporate less force and repetition. If these measures are not adequate, part-time work or a complete rest from work for a time may be necessary. Antiinflammatory medication can be administered systemically, but an injection of cortisone into the carpal tunnel is more effective. Depot forms of cortisone should be avoided. The injection is given with a 25-gauge needle placed 1 cm proximal to the wrist crease on the radial side of the palmaris longus tendon and angled 45° distally. This placement generally delivers the cortisone in exactly the correct location. Injection frequently succeeds in alleviating the symptoms at least somewhat. There is evidence that a cortisone injection may indeed be curative within the first 3 to 4 months after the onset of symptoms as long as the underlying cause of the problem is addressed. In addition, improvement following a cortisone injection may indicate the greater likelihood of a successful outcome if surgery is required at a later time. If symptoms have been present for more than 6 months, cortisone injections usually do not provide lasting relief, but an improvement in the symptoms confirms the diagnosis. Cortisone is therefore used not only as a therapeutic modality but also in a diagnostic and prognostic capacity.

A failure of adequate conservative measures over approximately 3 months with the patient unable to work or do daily activities and experiencing ongoing symptoms of pain, discomfort, and numbness, or muscle wasting and increasing weakness in the hand are all indications for surgical release of the transverse carpal ligament. Because a patient with an occupation that requires highly repetitive wrist and hand movements may not be able to return to full work following surgery, rest and a simple job and activity change is sometimes as effective as surgery. Job modification is frequently required and may obviate the need for surgery in some cases.

In cases requiring surgery, there is a current controversy as to whether endoscopic carpal tunnel release is better than the standard tried-and-true open procedure. Some have claimed a quicker return to work with endoscopic release, although the long-term results of this procedure are not thought to be much different from those of standard open release. The benefit of less scar tenderness and possible earlier return to work must be weighed against an increased incidence of digital nerve laceration with the endoscopic technique, the greater likelihood of an incomplete release, and the inability to visualize the carpal canal. The open technique affords the advantage of being able to take a synovial biopsy specimen to determine the possibility of unusual causes or remove an aberrant muscle or a tumor.

CASE STUDIES

Case 1

A 45-year-old office worker developed pain in her wrist region that frequently woke her up at night. This problem began near the end of her pregnancy, but substantial deterioration in her condition coincided with an increased amount of data entry at work. She was off work for 3 months after the birth of her child, and the problem improved. She was treated with splinting and a cortisone injection into the region of the carpal tunnel. After she had been back at work for approximately 3 weeks, the symptoms recurred, with numbness that awakened her at night, tingling in the fingertips, and poorly localized pain in the wrist and hand. She also complained of shooting pains that traveled up toward her elbow. A nerve conduction study was done, and the results were positive for carpal tunnel syndrome. A carpal tunnel release was performed, which required her to be off work for 2 months.

Considering that this patient was doing 8 hours of data entry a day, it was recommended that she not return to this highly repetitive activity. It had brought on the carpal tunnel syndrome, and there was concern that the problem would recur if she went back to her old job. She underwent vocational rehabilitation and found a job that required less intensive and repetitive use of her right hand.

Pronator syndrome (anterior interosseous nerve syndrome). Median nerve compression in the proximal forearm can produce clinical findings similar to those in carpal tunnel syndrome, so it is sometimes a challenge distinguishing between the two. The median nerve can be compressed in the proximal forearm at one of four sites: (1) in the distal part of the upper arm beneath the supracondylar process and the ligament of Struthers; (2) beneath the bicipital aponeurosis, or lacertus fibrosis; (3) beneath the superficial and deep heads of pronator teres (hence, the term for compression in this region); and (4) after the nerve exits from the pronator teres muscle where it passes beneath the arch of the FDS. Ganzer's muscle is an accessory head of the flexor pollicis longus and can also compress the nerve.

CLINICAL PRESENTATION. Patients with compression of the median nerve in this region generally complain of aching in the proximal and midforearm. They also have numbness, pain, and tingling in the median nerve distribution in the hand. These sensations do not awaken the patient at night as frequently as occurs in carpal tunnel syndrome. As in carpal tunnel syndrome, abduction of the thumb is weak. Tinel's sign is generally positive over the region of compression in the proximal forearm, and negative in the region of the carpal tunnel. The possibility of compression at both sites must always be kept in mind because distal entrapment is more likely the more proximal the compression. The development of symptoms with resistive pronation of the forearm may indicate the site of entrapment. Pain also is provoked with resisted flexion of the PIP joint of the middle finger, thereby tensing the FDS. If symptoms are reproduced with forearm supination, compression under the bicipital aponeurosis may be present.

Compression of the anterior interosseous nerve causes motor paralysis and aching pain in the forearm. The patient is unable to flex the IP joint of the thumb or the DIP joint of the index finger because of weakness or paralysis of the flexor pollicis longus and FDP of the index finger. When the elbow is flexed, the pronator teres muscle becomes ineffective, and pronation of the forearm occurs by contraction of the pronator quadratus. This muscle, because it is supplied by the anterior interosseous nerve, is weak or absent in patients with anterior interosseous nerve syndrome. Nerve entrapment around the elbow can be distinguished from nerve entrapment at the carpal canal by testing for Tinel's sign, performing Phalen's test, and administering the provocative tests described. Also, in pronator syndrome, the nerve is affected more proximally. There is aching in the proximal forearm, lack of sensation, and sometimes paraesthesias over the thenar eminence from the palmar cutaneous branch of the median nerve.

TREATMENT. As with carpal tunnel syndrome, treatment is initially conservative. Occupational and other daily activities should be modified, antiinflammatory medication administered, and the region splinted and rested. Surgery may be indicated if symptoms continue and prevent the patient from working and functioning reasonably. Electrodiagnostic studies can be used to confirm the diagnosis, but false negative results are not unusual.

Ulnar nerve

Ulnar nerve syndrome. The ulnar nerve can be compressed at the level of the spinal cord or at any of three sites along its course through the upper extremity. These sites are at the level of the thoracic outlet, the cubital tunnel on the medial aspect of the elbow, and the ulnar tunnel on the medial aspect of the wrist.

Thoracic outlet syndrome. The brachial plexus can be compressed as it passes between the clavicle and the first rib. This usually affects the lower part of the brachial plexus as the nerves pass out of the thorax and over the first rib, through the so-called thoracic outlet. Because the subclavian artery also travels with these nerves, vascular compression can accompany the nerve compression. The clinical presentation stemming from pressure on these nerves is known as thoracic outlet syndrome.

ETIOLOGY. The exact cause of compression in this region is unknown, but it is probably a combination of factors that is responsible for this result. These factors may be structural, such as an extra rib in the neck (cervical rib) or a tumor in the area. In most patients, no specific cause is found, and the problem is thought to be related to poor posture that places persistent stress on the neck and shoulder musculature. Occasionally, direct trauma with swelling can precipitate the problem.

CLINICAL PRESENTATION. Pain is often vague and poorly localized. It may occur only when the arms are elevated above shoulder level because this position closes the space between the clavicle and the first rib. Patients may have unusual sensations and complaints such as a feeling that "the blood is not getting to my hand." Other symptoms may be located in the ulnar nerve distribution (i.e., numbness in the ring and small fingers, weakness in the hand, and a weak grip). Occasionally, symptoms related to the median and other nerves may be experienced and cause a presentation similar to that in carpal tunnel syndrome.

A great variety of specific tests have been described, but none is universally reliable. Each physician should become familiar with several of those available.

Abduction/external rotation maneuver

The shoulder is placed in this position and the pulse is palpated at the wrist. If the pulse disappears as the shoulder is externally rotated, some compression of the nerves and vessels in the tho-

racic outlet is likely. Twenty percent of "normal" people will have a loss of pulse, but only if it is accompanied by the patient's symptoms is the test considered positive. There are a number of variations of this test, including Roos' test and Adson's test.

Special tests

First, x-ray films are obtained to determine whether a cervical rib is present. Second, EMG and nerve conduction velocity studies are done with the shoulder in the abducted/externally rotated position to get a positive result. Third, finger plethysmography is performed in the normal resting position and then with the shoulder in the abducted and externally rotated position. In thoracic outlet syndrome, the latter position will diminish the pulse and precipitate symptoms.

SPECIAL DIAGNOSTIC CONSIDERATIONS. There are two confusing aspects to the diagnosis of thoracic outlet syndrome. The first is that the symptoms are often poorly defined and vague, and they are only experienced when the arm is placed in certain positions. The second is that the nerves can be compressed at the spine, elbow, or wrist level, making the precise location of the compression difficult to define. The physician should be aware of the patient who has had an elbow and wrist release and continues to experience problems. The compression may have been at the level of the thoracic outlet in the neck all along.

TREATMENT. If a cervical rib or other structural problem is present, surgery is indicated. In other patients, better posture, exercises to strengthen the neck musculature, and the avoidance of provocative positions during sleep and at other times may be helpful. If conservative measures fail, surgery is indicated. The most effective operation is resection of a portion of the first rib, which relieves the pressure on the nerves.

Cubital tunnel syndrome. This syndrome arises from compression of the ulnar nerve as it passes through the osseofibrous canal around the medial epicondyle at the elbow (cubital tunnel).

ETIOLOGY. In most individuals, the ulnar nerve is protected as it lies between the medial epicondyle and olecranon. Sometimes, though, the pressure within the cubital tunnel increases with marked flexion of the elbow. Elbow flexion also stretches the ulnar nerve in this region, and the nerve can be further aggravated when the area is constantly leaned on. Many workers keep their elbows flexed for hours on end. Some examples are telephone operators, watchmakers, electronic assembly workers, pianists and other musicians, and others who do fine manipulative work. Many hours of constant flexion and extension of the elbow against resistance can cause inflammation on the medial aspect of the elbow. Shoveling, digging, and use of hand saws or large power machinery are examples of activities that can produce this result. A myriad of activities within the scope of daily life stress the ulnar nerve as the elbow flexes and extends repetitively. If an individual has an abnormally mobile ulnar nerve that snaps over the medial epicondyle, constant irritation can produce cubital tunnel syndrome.

CLINICAL PRESENTATION. The sensory symptoms include pain and paraesthesias in the elbow and forearm that radiate into the ring and small fingers. The patient complains of an aching discomfort in this region that is often aggravated by elbow flexion or leaning on the elbow. Such aggravation may occur when the patient drives their car, reads a newspaper, or holds a phone for a long period of time. Motor problems include difficulty with fine manipulation and clumsiness caused by involvement of the intrinsic muscles of the hand. The physical signs consist of decreased sensation in the small finger and ulnar aspect of the ring finger. The methods used to assess this condition are similar to those used to evaluate carpal tunnel syndrome. The palmar cutaneous branch of the ulnar nerve, as well as the dorsal branch that supplies the dorsal and ulnar aspect of the hand may be affected; if so, abnormal sensation occurs in these regions. A positive Tinel's sign is elicited by tapping over the ulnar nerve in the region of the cubital tunnel or, frequently, within 5 to 10 cm proximal or distal to this area. Weakness of the FDP to the small and ring fingers may occur, and paralysis of the intrinsic muscles may cause clawing of the ring and small fingers. There is also weakness of grip strength, weak abduction of the fingers against resistance, and weak adduction of the thumb. These features may be severe in chronic and advanced cases. Patients usually present with pain and other sensory symptoms long before motor features or paralysis occurs, and the condition must be treated at an earlier stage.

TREATMENT. Cubital tunnel syndrome should initially be treated nonoperatively, and, as with the entrapments already described, careful analysis and modification of the patient's work habits and home activities are essential. Night splinting of the elbow in a soft splint that holds the joint extended will decrease both the pressure in the cubital tunnel and the stretch of the ulnar nerve in that region. Reducing inflammation with rest, oral antiinflammatory medication, or cortisone injection may help. Care should be taken that cortisone not be injected directly into the nerve. It is used to reduce inflammation and swelling around the nerve. Electrodiagnostic testing is done for those patients in whom the diagnosis is uncertain. The persistence of severe symptoms despite adequate conservative treatment for 2 to 3 months is usually indication for surgical release and transposition of the ulnar nerve at the elbow. Several surgical methods can be used to transpose the ulnar nerve. The nerve may be placed in a subcutaneous position or submuscularly, beneath the flexor pronator muscle group. This procedure requires detachment of the muscle group from the medial epicondyle, replacement of the nerve in its new location beneath the muscle, and reattachment of the muscle group. Some surgeons advocate either simple release of the fascia or medial epicondylectomy. I have found that submuscular transposition is the most reliable procedure for most patients.

Ulnar tunnel syndrome. As the ulnar nerve courses through the ulnar tunnel (Guyon's canal), the ulnar nerve lies on the radial side of the pisiform bone and then on the ulnar side of the hook of the hamate. The nerve lies on the capsule of the wrist joint, the pisohamate and pisotriquetral ligaments, and is covered superficially by the volar carpal ligament. This is superficial or volar to the transverse carpal ligament and the carpal tunnel. The ulnar nerve travels with the ulnar artery, with the nerve lying on the ulnar side.

ETIOLOGY. No tendons travel with the nerve and artery through the ulnar tunnel. However, swelling can produce increased pressure in this canal, as can space-occupying lesions or tumors, and cause compression of the nerve. Swelling can be produced by repeated trauma, either blunt or direct, or repetitive flexion and extension of the wrist.

CLINICAL PRESENTATION. Most often, patients with entrapment in this region primarily experience sensory symptoms, but they may have motor symptoms in addition or motor symptoms alone. The sensory symptoms include paraesthesiae, pain, and numbness in the small finger and the ulnar aspect of the ring finger. In the region of the ulnar tunnel, the ulnar nerve divides into sensory and motor branches. If the deep motor branch is affected as it travels deeply between the abductor digiti minimi and the flexor digiti minimi muscles, motor problems such as weakness, poor coordination, and weak thumb adduction will result. As with other nerve entrapment syndromes, electrodiagnostic studies across this region may be helpful, but false negative and false positive results are not unusual.

TREATMENT. Treatment is similar to that of the other neuropathies described previously, with surgery reserved for those situations in which conservative measures have failed.

Radial nerve

Radial tunnel syndrome. The radial nerve may be injured in fractures of the radius, in blunt trauma to the upper arm, elbow, or forearm, and in crush injuries. More frequently, it is affected by entrapment at the elbow or proximal forearm, which causes what is known as radial tunnel syndrome.

The radial nerve can be compressed in the upper arm, where it has a close relationship with the posterior aspect of the humerus in the radial groove. Fractures of the humerus may cause damage to it in this location. Symptoms may be caused by work positions that place constant pressure on the radial nerve, pressing it against the underlying bone. Just distal to the elbow, the radial nerve passes under a fibrous arch known as the arcade of Frohse, which is the proximal fibrous edge of the supinator muscle between the two heads of the supinator muscle.

Compression of the radial nerve in the region of the elbow causes pain in the forearm but usually without paralysis or weakness. The patient typically complains of an aching sensation on the extensor surface of the forearm that may radiate distally into the dorsum of the hand. Certain provocative tests are helpful in making the diagnosis. In one such test, the patient is made to forcefully extend the middle finger against resistance. Pain in the proximal forearm indicates entrapment of the nerve by the origin of the extensor carpi radialis brevis. Supination against resistance may also produce pain and indicates compression at the arcade of Frohse. The most consistent physical finding in radial tunnel syndrome is marked tenderness with pressure over the radial tunnel between the mobile wrist extensor muscle group and the extensor digitorum communis in the proximal forearm. This tenderness is 4 or 5 cm distal to the lateral epicondyle, and it sometimes coexists with lateral epicondylitis. Thus, it may sometimes be difficult to separate these two conditions, but it is important to do so.

TREATMENT. Initially, compression of the radial nerve in the radial tunnel should be treated conservatively. Changing the patient's activities, changing the way the extremity is used, and local cortisone injection are often helpful. When no relief is obtained with conservative measures, surgery is indicated. Release of the arcade of Frohse is performed, and the other sites where the nerve may be trapped are checked.

Case 2

A 41-year-old mill worker developed severe pain over the lateral aspect of his right elbow after a period in which he was required to lift heavy pieces of lumber for 4 hours straight—an intensive activity to which he was unaccustomed. From that time on, he noted increasing pain on the lateral aspect of his elbow with lifting and heavy use of his right arm. The pain became so severe he had to quit work for 3 weeks, and when he returned, he had a lifting limit of 30 pounds. However, his symptoms continued, and he was treated with local cortisone injections on several occasions. He worked intermittently over the next 6 months and at some point was diagnosed as having compression of the radial nerve at the level of the radial tunnel, just distal to the lateral epicondyle. This area was markedly tender. Injection into the region of the radial tunnel substantially reduced his symptoms, but they recurred each time he returned to work.

Eventually this patient underwent surgery to release the radial nerve and the common extensor origin at the elbow. Four months later his condition had improved substantially, and he was able to return to work, but with a permanent restriction against repetitive lifting.

Posterior interosseous nerve syndrome. Posterior interosseous nerve syndrome may also present with pain in the forearm that is poorly localized, but it is accompanied by progressive weakness and motor loss. There is loss of extension at the MCP joint and a loss of thumb abduction and extension.

The intrinsic muscles of the thumb extend the IP joint, especially when the thumb is held across the palm. These muscles are best tested with the hand lying palm down, flat on the examining table. If the patient elevates the thumb off the table, the extensor pollicis longus can be seen to contract. The extensor carpi radialis is supplied proximal to the elbow and is usually not affected.

Wartenberg syndrome. This syndrome arises from compression of the radial sensory nerve in the distal forearm. The nerve branches from the main trunk of the radial nerve before the deep branch of the radial nerve (posterior interosseous nerve) enters the supinator muscle. In the distal forearm and at the wrist level, the nerve is superficial and crosses the region of the radial styloid and anatomic snuffbox. It usually becomes symptomatic after a crush injury to the area with swelling, or following a laceration. Sensation on the dorsoradial aspect of the hand and the dorsal aspect of the first web space is decreased. However, if a neuroma develops, the patient will experience exquisite pain and sensitivity in that location. There is usually pain with a positive Tinel's sign over the nerve. This problem must be differentiated from de Quervain's synovitis. There is often inflammation in the entire area with a positive Finkelstein test, so these two problems may coexist. The provocative test for the Wartenberg syndrome is performed by placing the forearm in full pronation. This may cause the patient to experience burning paraesthesias on the radial aspect of the wrist and hand.

Tendonitis and synovitis

Tendonitis is a poorly understood condition in which there is pain and tenderness along the course of a tendon as a result of inflammation that is usually located at the origin or insertion of a muscle. It is typically caused by repetitive movement of the upper extremity, and, for that reason, is considered a cumulative trauma disorder. Sometimes, a single incident or short period of overuse can precipitate the symptoms, especially in individuals who are unaccustomed to the activity in which they have indulged. The repetitiveness of the task, the force required, and position of the joint are all factors in the pathogenesis of this problem. The anatomic site affected varies, as does the symptomatology and the patient's response to treatment. Often, tendonitis requires the patient to be off work for a significant amount of time, and it can even result in permanent disability.

The synovial sheath surrounding tendons consists of two layers connected at either end to form a closed space around the tendon. This anatomy promotes gliding and smooth movement. The synovial layer may become inflamed in the flexor tendons at the wrist or in the fingers, or in the extensor tendons in the region of the extensor retinaculum on the dorsal aspect of the wrist. In conditions such as rheumatoid arthritis, lupus erythematosus, and other collagen vascular diseases, this problem is secondary to the underlying systemic disease. Cumulative trauma may also produce inflammation and swelling of the synovial sheath, in which case the condition is referred to as synovitis. There are other causes of synovitis such as infection with bacteria, fungi, and other microorganisms, but these types of cases are beyond the scope of this chapter. Tendons and their synovial sheaths tend to become inflamed at certain sites more often than others.

Clinical presentation.   The overriding complaint of patients with tendonitis is pain, which is generally located near the region of the muscle origin or tendon insertion. A careful history of the patient's job and other daily activities is crucial to making the diagnosis. It is important to establish how the problem arose and whether it is improved by rest, stretching, warm-up exercises, or ice. The exact site of pain must be examined with specific reference to tenderness, swelling, crepitus, and the smooth movement of tendons as the joints are taken through an active and passive range of motion. Too often, vague pain in an area is attributed to tendonitis where no specific evidence for this

problem exists. To make the diagnosis, the physician should be able to identify the specific tendon and site affected. It is important to obtain an x-ray film in the region of a bony prominence to determine whether that bony prominance or some abnormal calcification has caused the problem. Although almost every tendon has been subject to tendonitis, the most common such problems are described below.

First compartment.   In 1895, de Quervain described an inflammation of the abductor pollicis longus and extensor pollicis brevis where they traverse the first dorsal compartment of the extensor retinaculum at the wrist. (In many individuals, the abductor pollicis longus is composed of more than one tendon slip, and the compartment is divided by an additional septum into two separate subcompartments.) The pain and swelling associated with this inflammation are localized over the compartment at the level of the radial styloid or just distal to it. Symptoms are caused by an activity requiring repeated ulnar deviation of the wrist and vigorous movement of the thumb. Local swelling and erythema may be present.

The Finkelstein test is performed by having the patient hold the thumb in the palm as the examiner gently ulnar deviates the wrist. This test must be done extremely gently because it can elicit severe pain in patients with this condition and even in patients who do not have inflammation in this location.

The differential diagnosis of pain in this region includes arthritis at the carpometacarpal joint of the thumb, tenderness or neuroma formation of the sensory branch of the radial nerve at the wrist, and scaphoid fracture.

Second compartment (intersection syndrome). The extensor carpi radialis longus and brevis can become inflamed at the point where the thumb muscles—the abductor pollicis longus and extensor pollicis brevis—cross over these wrist extensors. Therefore, this condition has been called intersection syndrome. It may be brought on by repetitive wrist flexion and extension, and it is characterized by pain, tenderness, and swelling about 4 or 5 cm proximal to the radial carpal joint. The presence of crepitus that can be palpated in the region as the patient moves the wrist and thumb is diagnostic. An audible creaking may accompany this movement.

Third compartment.   This is a much less common tendonitis that occurs where the extensor pollicis longus changes direction at the wrist as it curves around Lister's tubercle of the distal radius. It occurs in metabolic conditions such as rheumatoid arthritis but may also develop with overuse of the thumb. This tendon has a tendency to rupture when it is severely affected, so the diagnosis should be made early and the cause of the problem avoided. Cortisone injection into this tendon increases the risk of rupture and, in my opinion, should not be used in this area.

Fourth compartment. The extensor indicis proprius and extensor digitorum communis tendons may become inflamed within this compartment. Such inflammation is associated with repeated flexion and extension of the MCP joints or the presence of an aberrant muscle.

Fifth compartment. The extensor digiti minimi tendon may become inflamed as it travels over the head of the ulna, especially if the shape or size of the latter is abnormal.

Sixth compartment. The extensor carpi ulnaris tendon may become inflamed as it traverses the head of the ulna. This condition is usually associated with an abnormally mobile tendon subluxing over the head of the ulna as the patient brings the wrist from radial to ulnar deviation with pronation and supination of the forearm. It may be caused by a single traumatic episode.

Flexor carpi radialis tendonitis. Chronic pain in the region of the distal extent and insertion of the flexor carpi radialis must be distinguished from the other causes of discomfort in this region. These include ganglion cysts, which are not uncommon, aneurysm or thrombosis of the radial artery, scaphoid wrist fracture, and trapeziometacarpal arthritis.

Synovitis of the digital flexor tendons. This problem occurs with synovitis at the wrist, which coexists with carpal tunnel syndrome. Metabolic causes such as rheumatoid arthritis must be ruled out. As the flexor pollicis longus traverses the tubercle of the scaphoid, it may rupture, especially if the cause of the inflammation is metabolic and associated with a severe chronic synovitis. Synovitis of the digital flexor sheaths occurs with repetitive action of the fingers against resistance—most often the index finger as it pinches or pulls on an activation device. Swelling must be differentiated from infections of the digital sheath.

Flexor carpi ulnaris tendonitis. Flexor carpi ulnaris tendonitis presents as pain over the region of this tendon and is caused by repetitive wrist flexion and ulnar deviation, especially against resistance. This problem must be differentiated from inflammation of the ulnar nerve or artery within the ulnar tunnel. Other problems within the wrist, such as a fracture of the hook of the hamate, fracture of the pisiform, or pisotriquetral arthritis must also be considered in the differential diagnosis.

"Trigger finger." Trigger fingers are common in people who are required to flex and extend their fingers frequently throughout the day. This problem may be associated with a synovitis of the flexor sheath. As the tendon passes through the A-1 pulley in the distal palm it becomes inflamed, and movement is painful. Actual hypertrophy of the flexor tendon is usually found. The thickening may result from repeated local trauma from instruments that cause pressure over the site. More commonly, though, no specific cause is evident. Ultimately, extension of the finger causes the flexor to catch on the pulley, which is known as triggering. In the most advanced stage, the finger remains locked in flexion.

Treatment of tendonitis and synovitis. Treatment begins with conservative measures to decrease the inflammation. The most effective anti-inflammatory medication is cortisone given by local injection. Most sites are amenable to injection, but caution should be exercised in some cases. In de Quervain's synovitis, dark-skinned individuals may develop atrophy and skin color change because some of the cortisone often ends up in a subcutaneous location. Also, one should avoid cortisone injection over a tendon that tends to rupture, such as the extensor pollicis longus. Injections are particularly helpful in de Quervain's synovitis, intersection syndrome, lateral epicondylitis, and trigger finger, where the injection is given just proximal to the A-1 pulley. When the injection is in the region of the synovium, the problem may resolve when the inflammation decreases. When the injection is in the region of the lateral epicondyle, the mechanism of action is less clear. Some tearing of the common extensor origin may occur with subsequent fibrosis that ultimately leads to a reduction in symptoms; alternatively, resolution may be achieved with the reduction of inflammation.

If conservative measures fail and debilitating symptomatology continues, surgical release is usually indicated. Some surgical considerations are important to bear in mind. When releasing a de Quervain's synovitis, it is essential to be aware of the superficial branch of the radial nerve. It may be injured or become symptomatic as scarring develops around it during the healing process. For this reason, we prefer a longitudinal incision in the region. The extensor pollicis longus may need to be rerouted on the radial side of Lister's tubercle, or an abnormally prominent Lister's tubercle may need to be removed to treat the inflammation. Occasionally, tendonitis of the fourth and fifth compartments can be released surgically. A snapping extensor carpi ulnaris tendon can be treated with reconstruction of the pulley to hold it in position. Flexor carpi ulnaris tendonitis and flexor carpi radialis tendonitis are generally treated by conservative measures. Surgical release is rarely indicated. Trigger finger usually responds to one or two cortisone injections; if this fails, however, simple release of the A-1 pulley under local anesthetic can generally correct the problem. Surgery for lateral and medial epicondylitis is controversial. Of the various procedures described, none is universally successful. Surgery should be reserved for cases in which severe debilitating symptoms have persisted for over a year despite adequate conservative measures.

SUGGESTED READINGS

Allen MJ: Conservative management of fingertip injuries in adults, *Hand* 12:257-265, 1980.

Armstrong TJ: Ergonomics and cumulative trauma disorders, *Hand Clin* 2:553-265, 1986.

Baylor C, Samuelson C, Sinclaire H: Treatment of grease gun injuries, *J Occup Med* 15:799-800, 1973.

Coonrad RW, Hooper WR: Tennis elbow: its course, natural history, and conservative and surgical management, *J Bone Joint Surg* 55A:1177-1182, 1973.

Fess EE: Rehabilitation of the patient with peripheral nerve injury, *Hand Clin* 2:207-215, 1986.

Gelberman R, Posch J: High-pressure injection injuries of the hand, *J Bone Joint Surg* 57A:935-937, 1975.

Gelberman RH, Aronson D, Weisman MH: Carpal tunnel syndrome: results of a prospective trial of steroid injection and splinting, *J Bone Joint Surg* 62A:1181, 1980.

Gelberman RH, Manske PR, Akeson WH et al: Flexor tendon repair, *J Orthop Res* 4:119-128, 1986.

Gelberman RH, Rydevik BL, Pess GM et al: Carpal tunnel syndrome: a scientific basis for clinical care, *Orthop Clin North Am* 19:115, 1988.

Gordon L: *Microsurgical reconstruction of the extremities: indications, technique, and postoperative care,* New York, 1988, Springer-Verlag.

Gordon L: Toe-to-thumb transplantation. In Green DP, editor: *Operative hand surgery,* New York, 1993, Churchill Livingstone.

Howard FM: Fractures of the basal joint of the thumb, *J Hand Surg* 12A:26, 1987.

Hunter JM, Cowan NJ: Fifth metacarpal fractures in a compensation clinic population, *J Bone Joint Surg* 52A:1159-1165, 1970.

Lane C: Therapy for the occupationally injured hand, *Hand Clin* 2:953-602, 1986.

Leddy JP: Avulsions of the flexor digitorum profundus, *Hand Clin* 1:77-84, 1985.

Lewis R: High-pressure injection injuries of the hand, *Emerg Med Clin North Am* 3:373-381, 1985.

Melone CP, Isani A: Fingertip injuries: a rational approach to management, *Orthop Rev* 14:83-93, 1985.

Thorson EP, Szabo RM: Tendonitis of the wrist and elbow, *Occup Med State Art Rev* 4:419-31, 1989.

Upton ARM, McComas AS: The double crush nerve entrapment and syndrome, *Lancet* 2:359, 1983.

Walker L, Meals R: Tendonitis: a practical approach to diagnosis and management, *J Musculoskel Med* 6:24-54, 1989.

Zook EG: Injuries of the fingernail. In Green DP, editor: *Operative hand surgery,* New York, 1982, Churchill Livingstone.

Shoulder and Elbow Disorders

Occupational disorders of the shoulder increasingly have become a problem in modern industry. Several recent studies indicate that shoulder complaints are second only to back claims in worker injuries in Australia[21,30] and Sweden.[13] The reason for the rise in shoulder injuries is unclear. Elbow injuries are much less common, but they constitute a significant cause of work-related injury to the upper extremity. This two-part chapter deals with injuries and disorders of both structures.

SHOULDER DISORDERS

Improved understanding of shoulder mechanics and pathologic conditions of the shoulder certainly has increased awareness of such injuries among health care practitioners. Another significant factor is the expanding use of computers in the workplace, requiring long hours of keyboarding. Performing repetitive light tasks, such as keyboarding, for prolonged periods may cause a type of repetitive stress injury often called *occupational cervicobrachial disorder (OCD)*.

Shoulder injuries in the workplace may be divided into four categories.

1. *Overuse injuries caused by repetitive light tasks (OCD).* These injuries are among the most common. The syndrome occurs mostly among keyboard operators and office workers and occasionally among musicians.

2. *Rotator cuff tendonitis.* This disorder is a more specific type of overuse injury that is most common in laborers whose work requires lifting, pushing, and pulling. Employees involved in overhead work are at particular risk.

3. *Traumatic injuries.* Traumatic injuries of the shoulder can occur in almost any occupational setting, although using heavy machinery definitely increases the risk. These injuries include fractures, rotator cuff tears, dislocations, and other types of injuries discussed later.

4. *Degenerative problems.* Degenerative shoulder problems may develop from many years of task-specific work, although the cause often is difficult to prove. A Finnish study found a higher incidence of radiographic evidence of osteoarthritis of the neck and shoulder in dentists than in farmers, possibly because of the sustained static loads required by dentistry.[17] Use of pneumatic drilling equipment also may predispose an individual to upper extremity arthritis.

To properly evaluate a patient's painful shoulder, the physician must understand both the anatomy and function of the shoulder.

Anatomy and biomechanics

Musculature. The shoulder actually consists of four joints: the glenohumeral articulation, the acromioclavicular (AC) articulation, the scapulothoracic articulation, and the sternoclavicular articulation (Fig. 9-1). All of these are involved in motion of the arm on the torso, and each can be a source of symptoms.

Glenohumeral joint. The glenohumeral (GH) joint has the greatest range of motion of any joint in the body. Although it is closest to a ball-and-socket joint, it differs from the hip in that the glenoid cavity is quite shallow, and most of the constraint of the joint comes from the surrounding soft tissue. Most of the joint's stability is provided by the capsule and its ligamentous thickenings. The bony glenoid provides little in the way of stability to the joint although the labrum, a fibrocartilaginous lip of tissue around the glenoid rim, effectively deepens the glenoid cavity and adds to the mechanical stability.

Three major ligamentous thickenings of the capsule of the GH joint are considered the main stabilizers of the shoulder. The most important is the inferior glenohumeral ligament (IGHL). This structure is shaped somewhat like a pouch or hammock with an anterior and inferior band that attaches from the anterior surface of the humerus to the anterior glenoid rim, where it becomes confluent with the labrum (Fig. 9-2). The ligament tightens with internal rotation and is the main stabilizer of the GH joint in abduction and external rotation (the throwing position). Most cases of clinical instability are due to stretching of this ligament or detachment from the glenoid rim, usually detaching the labrum along with it. Posterior translation of the humeral head is also increased with sectioning of the inferior glenohumeral ligament (GHL),

125

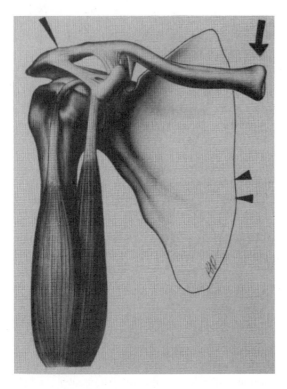

Fig. 9-1 The shoulder is made up of four separate joints: the glenohumeral joint *(wide arrowhead);* the acromioclavicular joint *(long arrowhead);* the scapulothoracic joint *(double arrowhead);* and the sternoclavicular joint *(full arrow).* (Modified from Neer CS: *Shoulder reconstruction,* Philadelphia, 1990, WB Saunders.)

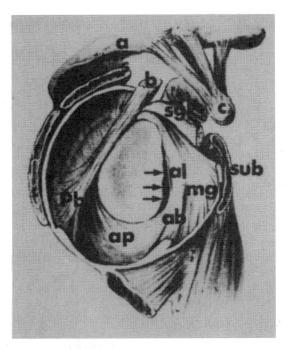

Fig. 9-2 Ligaments of the anterior aspect of the shoulder. Note the anterior band *(AB)* of the inferior glenohumeral ligament.

and surgical tightening of this ligament is one approach to treatment of posterior and anterior shoulder instability.

The middle glenohumeral ligament is a smaller thickening of the capsule that crosses beneath the subscapularis muscle and is thought to contribute to shoulder stability at the clinically less significant range of 45 degrees of abduction.

The superior glenohumeral ligament is a variable structure in the vicinity of the biceps tendon usually spanning from the superior tubercle of the glenoid to the superior anterior aspect of the lesser tuberosity. It has recently been demonstrated in cadaver studies as contributing to inferior joint stability, but this is not believed to be clinically significant.

Labrum. The glenoid labrum is a thin flap of fibrous tissue that attaches circumferencially to the glenoid rim through a transitional fibrocartilaginous zone. The labrum serves to increase the depth of the concavity of the glenoid and is the attachment site for the glenohumeral ligaments anteriorly, and the biceps tendon superiorly. This struc-

ture is significant because of its frequent involvement in pathologic shoulder conditions. Traumatic dislocations of the shoulder usually involve detachment of the labrum along with the IGHL from the anterior glenoid rim. Tears of the superior or anterior labrum can cause catching and pain similar to a torn meniscus in the knee, without symptoms of instability. A wide spectrum of abnormalities may occur at the junction of the biceps tendon attachment to the labrum, including detachment and tearing of the labrum, or splitting and degeneration of the biceps attachment. Since the advent of shoulder arthroscopy, this entity has become recognized more frequently as a common cause of shoulder pain. Subtle erosion of the labral surface occurs with all forms of instability as the humeral head displaces over the glenoid rim, and can often be a clue to direction of instability.

Rotator cuff. The deepest layer of muscles around the shoulder is a group of four muscles called the rotator cuff. These muscles are the ball bearing of the shoulder and stabilize the glenohumeral joint while the power muscles (deltoid and pectorals major) do their job. The rotator cuff is made up of the supraspinatus, infraspinatus, teres minor, and subscapularis muscles (Fig. 9-3, *A* and *B*). The infraspinatus and teres minor muscles are primarily external rotators of the humerus; the

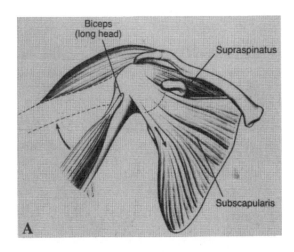

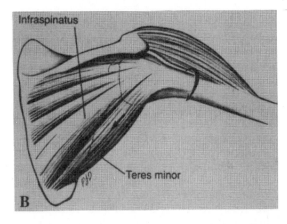

Fig. 9-3 Components of the rotator cuff. **A,** Anterior subscapularis and supraspinatus muscles. **B,** Posterior infraspinatus and teres minor muscles.

subscapularis muscle is an internal rotator; and the supraspinatus muscle is an elevator (abductor). One of the major functions of the rotator cuff is to depress the humeral head against the strong superior pull of the deltoid and prevent upward migration of the head. This maintains the proper fulcrum for elevation of the arm. In patients with a deficient rotator cuff, the humeral head will migrate upward against the acromion, resulting in weakness and pain (Fig. 9-4). Using selective nerve blocks, the supraspinatus and infraspinatus muscles have been found to provide 45% of abduction and 90% of external rotation strength.[7] In another study, the supraspinatus muscle was found to contribute 50% of the torque in forward elevation, the remainder coming from the anterior deltoid muscle.[15]

The supraspinatus and infraspinatus tendons are the most commonly involved structures in rotator cuff tendonitis. The etiology of this tendonitis is believed to result from impingement or pinching of the tendons against the overlying acromion and coracoacromial ligament. The acromion is a bony projection from the scapula that forms an arch over the rotator cuff tendons. Anteriorly the coracoacromial ligament attaches from the anterior edge of the acromion to the coracoid bone. Together the acromion and its continuation as the coracoacromial ligament create a wide arch and underlying passageway, through which the supraspinatus tendon travels. This passageway has been called the supraspinatus outlet.

The shape of the acromion differs among individuals, and it has recently been found that those with a curved or hook-shaped acromion are more prone to rotator cuff tears.[3] Based on cadaver studies, acromial shape has been divided into three types, depending on the extent of the curve: type 1 is flat and creates a spacious supraspinatus outlet; type 2 is gently curved and occasionally may result in impingement of the rotator cuff; type 3 is sharply curved or hooked and is most likely to cause impingement of the rotator cuff tendons (Fig. 9-5). These acromial shapes are congenital. Occasionally a patient may develop calcification along the coracoacromial ligament. This is a developmental problem and is more accurately called a spur than a curved acromion.

Factors other than the shape of the acromion may contribute to rotator cuff tendonitis. An area of relative hypovascularity at the attachment site of the supraspinatus tendon[26] is also the most common site for inflammation and tearing of the rotator cuff.[26] Some believe that the tendonitis begins as a primary tendonopathy and that impingement occurs secondarily with swelling and inflammation of the tendon and bursa. Other patients develop rotator cuff inflammation from direct trauma to the shoulder, and throwers sustain traction injuries to the rotator cuff. Whatever the initiating event, the shape of the acromion most likely influences the outcome.

The subacromial bursa is located between the rotator cuff and the overlying acromion and usually is continuous with the more anterior subdeltoid bursa. Its purpose is to facilitate movement between these structures. The bursa becomes inflamed in the early stages of rotator cuff inflammation and later may become fibrotic and scarred. An inflamed thickened bursa takes up space in the supraspinatus outlet and adds to the potential for impingement.

When patients with prolonged symptoms from rotator cuff tendonitis do not improve with conservative care, surgical modification of the shape of the acromion often is very helpful, along with removal of the nonfunctioning coracoacromial ligament and resection of the inflamed bursa.

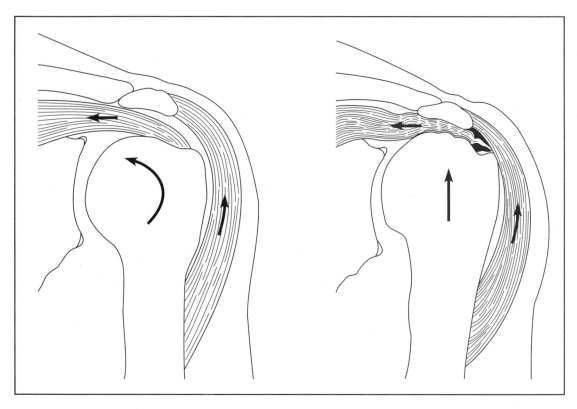

Fig. 9-4 A deficient rotator cuff results in unopposed proximal pull of the deltoid muscle.

INNERVATION. The innervation of the rotator cuff is clinically relevant, and palsies are not uncommon. The supraspinatus and infraspinatus muscles are innervated by the suprascapular nerve. This nerve is subject to compression neuropathy as it passes through the suprascapular notch of the scapula to innervate the supraspinatus muscle, and more rarely at the spinoglenoid notch, through which it passes to innervate the infraspinatus muscle (Fig. 9-6). A patient with marked rotator cuff weakness may have a suprascapular nerve injury.

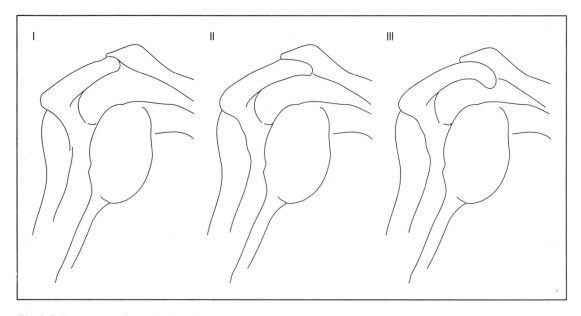

Fig. 9-5 Three types of acromial morphology.

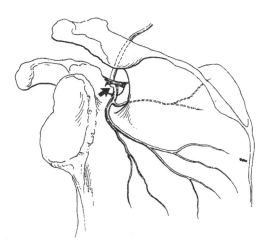

Fig. 9-6 The suprascapular nerve passes through the suprascapular notch, where it is subject to compression. (Modified from Rockwood CA, Matsen FA: *The shoulder,* Philadelphia, 1990, WB Saunders.)

The teres minor muscle is innervated by a branch of the axillary nerve and may be involved in a lesion affecting the axillary nerve. The subscapularis muscle is innervated by the upper and lower subscapular nerves.

Biceps tendon. The biceps tendon has two proximal attachments at the shoulder (Fig. 9-7). The tendon of the short head attaches to the coracoid process and is rarely involved in pathologic shoulder conditions. The tendon of the long head runs in the bicipital groove between the lesser and greater tuberosities passing under the transverse humeral ligament. It then penetrates through the rotator cuff between the supraspinatus and subscapularis tendons (the rotator cuff interval) and attaches to the glenoid at the supraglenoid tubercle or to the adjacent superior labrum. The tendon is stabilized in the groove by the transverse humeral ligament, the depth of the groove, and other surrounding soft tissue structures. Dislocation of the tendon usually occurs with rupture of the subscapularis muscle, although it is possible to have a subluxing tendon with a shallow groove and a deficient transverse ligament. This should be considered in a patient who complains of a clicking in the anterior aspect of the shoulder. A dislocating tendon may be diagnosed with the instability test described by Abbot and Saunders. With the patient's arm abducted in the plane of the scapula, the physician palpates over the bicipital groove while gently rotating the arm from a position of external rotation to one of internal rotation. A painful, palpable clunk should occur.

Tendonitis of the biceps tendon usually occurs in association with inflammation of the rotator cuff. This is due to impingement of both structures

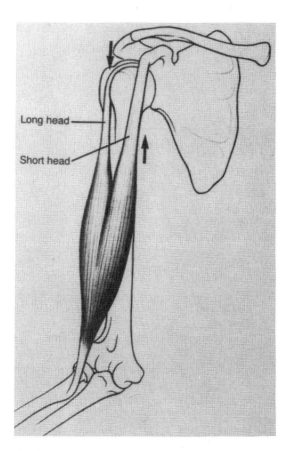

Fig. 9-7 The biceps tendon has both a long head and a short head. The long head, which enters the joint through the rotator cuff interval, is often involved in impingement syndrome. (Modified from Neer CS: *Shoulder reconstruction,* Philadelphia, 1990, WB Saunders.)

by the overlying coracoacromial arch and in rare cases as a clinically separate entity. Isolated bicipital tendonitis is caused by narrowing of the bicipital groove by a bony spur or a thickened transverse humeral ligament. Rupture of the biceps tendon is not uncommon in cases of long-standing impingement syndrome.

The intraarticular portion of the proximal biceps tendon probably functions as a weak humeral head depressor and adds some stability to the glenohumeral joint. Because of its frequent attachment to the superior labrum, it may be the cause of traction tears to this portion of the labrum, particularly in throwing athletes, where the biceps acts as a strong decelerator of the arm.

Acromioclavicular joint. The acromioclavicular (AC) joint, a common source of symptoms caused by arthritic changes or trauma, is a diarthrodial joint with an intervening fibrocartilaginous meniscus or disk. The entire joint space is only 1 to 2 mm wide and can only accommodate 1 to 2 ml of fluid. The direction of the joint is oblique, with the end of the clavicle facing inferiorly, posteriorly, and laterally.

The main anatomic features are the ligaments surrounding this joint. Three ligaments stabilize the AC joint. The conoid and trapezoid ligaments, which are the coracoclavicular ligaments, stabilize the distal end of the clavicle by attachment to the coracoid. The acromioclavicular ligament is a thickening of the superior capsule of the AC joint and resists primarily anteroposterior motion. One or all of these ligaments are disrupted with an AC separation, which commonly occurs with a fall on the shoulder.

Sternoclavicular joint. The sternal articulation of the clavicle is rarely involved in clinical complaints. Similar to the acromial articulation, the sternoclavicular (SC) joint has a meniscus. The joint is stabilized on all four sides by ligamentous attachments. Traumatic disruption of this joint is rare and most often is caused by motor vehicle accidents or sports injuries. Displacement may occur either anteriorly or posteriorly, either from direct impact or secondary to shoulder impact with transmission of abnormal forces across the clavicle. It is important to be mindful of posterior dislocation, which, although rare, can compromise the underlying pulmonary and vascular structures.

Scapulothoracic joint. The scapulothoracic articulation consists of the thin, concave, triangular-shaped scapula and its matching convex thoracic surface. The anterior surface of the scapula is covered by the attachments of the subscapularis and serratus anterior muscles. Bursae are found between these two muscles and between the serratus anterior muscle and the chest wall. The latter is the true articulating surface at which scapulothoracic motion occurs. The bursae may become inflamed and fibrotic, leading to pain and snapping.

The scapulothoracic joint is important because the scapula connects the axial skeleton on the upper extremity, and normal shoulder motion depends on scapulothoracic motion. It is generally accepted that elevation of the arm involves a combination of glenohumeral and scapulothoracic motion in the overall ratio of 2 to 1.[16] During specific phases of arm elevation, however, this ratio ranges from 1 to 1 to 4 to 1.[25] Patients with impaired motion of the glenohumeral joint due to adhesions or pain tend to compensate by increased scapulothoracic motion, often leading to periscapular muscle spasm and scapulothoracic bursitis.

Neurovascular structures

Brachial plexus. Stretch injuries to the brachial plexus often occur with dislocation of the glenohumeral joint (10% to 25%). Careful neurologic evaluation should be performed in the patient with a dislocation prior to relocation to document neurologic status. The most commonly injured nerve is the axillary nerve that runs immediately inferior and anterior to the joint, followed much less commonly by the radial, musculocutaneous, median, and ulnar neuropraxias.

Isolated neuropraxias can occur about the shoulder and most commonly involve the dorsal scapular nerve (serratus anterior muscle) and the suprascapular nerve (supraspinatus or infraspinatus muscle, or both). Although these may be traumatic in nature or secondary to anatomic impingement, spontaneous palsy may occur as well.

Thoracic outlet syndrome. The subclavian artery and brachial plexus pass between the scalenus anterior and scalenus medius muscles. Compression of these structures by the overlying clavicle may occur due to anomalous fibrous bands or the presence of a cervical rib. Patients usually have complaints similar to those for ulnar nerve compression, but any combination of vascular or neurologic symptoms may exist.

Evaluation and diagnosis of a painful shoulder

History. As in the evaluation of any ailment, a detailed medical history can provide important and helpful information for a patient with shoulder pain.

Location. To most people, "the shoulder" means anything from the neck to the elbow. The practitioner can obtain the most important piece of initial data by asking the patient to point directly to the area of discomfort.

Patients with rotator cuff symptoms most often localize the pain to the outer deltoid region. This pain pattern is caused by referred pain from the supraspinatus muscle and is most likely caused by the common nerve root origin between the axillary and suprascapular nerves (C5-6). Patients with primarily infraspinatus involvement of rotator cuff tendonitis may complain of more posterior pain.

Patients with a primary cervical pathologic condition usually point to the posterior paracervical musculature or the trapezius muscle for a muscular strain, or down the arm for radicular symptoms from a herniated disk. Depending on the level of disk involvement, cervical radiculopathy may also manifest as medial scapular pain along the rhomboids. Unfortunately, these findings may be misleading, because shoulder pain from almost any origin may cause secondary cervical spasm or rhomboid symptoms. Often this is due to a compensatory increase in scapulothoracic motion to minimize motion at a painful or stiff glenohumeral joint. This is thought to lead to a disruption in normal shoulder biomechanics (scapulothoracic rhythm), with increased strain on the periscapular and cervical muscles.

A patient with primarily acromioclavicular joint symptoms usually complains of anterosuperior pain and points to the joint area. Biceps tendon pain, anterior and inferior, often occurs in conjunction with rotator cuff symptoms. Glenohumeral pain from arthritis, trauma, or labral lesions often is difficult to localize, but the patient typically points anteriorly and describes the pain as deep.

Duration. An important point is whether the symptoms are acute (less than 2 weeks' duration) or chronic. This is very helpful in differentiating certain conditions and in determining the appropriate treatment. Chronic problems often are related to the work environment and may require ergonomic modification as well as medical treatment. Acute injuries, such as an acute rotator cuff tear or glenohumeral dislocation, may require immediate intervention.

Activity. It is helpful to determine what brings on the pain. Rotator cuff tendonitis is aggravated by overhead activities such as hanging a coat, combing the hair, and painting the ceiling. It is also quite common to have night pain with rotator cuff tendonitis and to be unable to sleep on the affected side. It has been hypothesized that the increase in pain at night may be due to the supine position. This eliminates the positive effect of gravity, (which in the upright position exerts an inferior pull on the arm, opening up the subacromial space. Patients often are less symptomatic when sleeping in a recliner chair in a semiupright position. AC joint pain is worst with motion across the chest, abduction past 90 degrees, and with certain specific exercises such as the bench press. Shoulder instability is most symptomatic with abduction–external rotation motions of the arm, such as throwing a baseball. Radicular pain often is constant and unremitting, although complete bed rest may help. Abduction and external rotation of the arm also decreases tension on the brachial plexus and may relieve radiculopathy by relaxing the involved nerve root where it is tented by the herniation. The patient may actually come into the office in the abducted position, with his hand on his head. Patients with adhesive capsulitis frequently have a loss of internal rotation first and have pain with activities requiring internal rotation, such as hooking a bra or reaching into the back pocket.

Sounds. One of the most common complaints heard from patients is that the shoulder makes noise—clicks, pops, clunks, or snaps. This can be a helpful diagnostic finding. Patients who complain of snapping and cracking under the acromion with forward flexion or arm rotation probably have chronic subacromial bursitis. With repeated impingement of the rotator cuff, the subacromial bursa becomes inflamed and thickened. The thickened bursa snaps back and forth across the greater tuberosity of the humerus, making a sound like chewing on rubber. A similar phenomenon occurs in the area of the scapulothoracic bursa. When this area becomes inflamed, the patient reports snapping as he protracts and rotates the scapula. The exact area of bursitis can be localized by placing the hand lightly over the suspected area of involvement and asking the patient to recreate the sound. For patients with loud and painful scapulothoracic snapping, it is important to rule out a scapular osteochondroma or rib exostosis, which can cause symptoms similar to scapulothoracic bursitis but more severe. These cases often require removal of the offending bony prominence.

Patients with a labral tear may complain of a clunk rather than a snapping sound. This is a loud, lower-pitched sound caused when a torn flap of labrum is caught between the glenoid and humeral head. As the flap is displaced from between the articular areas of contact, it makes a loud clunk similar to a McMurray test in the knee. If the patient cannot recreate this himself, the examiner sometimes can elicit it with a provocative test. The patient's arm is lifted passively in abduction with axial compression, and the examiner attempts to catch the torn superior labrum (the most common site) between the abducting humeral head and the stationary glenoid.

Another sound it is helpful to elicit is the grinding noise that is heard with degenerative arthritis of the glenohumeral joint; this is as much a tactile sensation as a sound. Starting with the patient's arm at his side, the examiner gently places her hand over his shoulder and carefully moves the arm through a passive range of internal and external rotation. A gritty, sandpaper vibration and often a grinding noise can be sensed in a patient with arthritis of the GH joint. Arthritis of the acromioclavicular joint causes a similar sensation, but it occurs superiorly at the AC joint with shoulder abduction and cross-chest motion.

Another pathologic shoulder sound is that of a subluxing biceps tendon, which causes a snap over the anterior aspect of the shoulder with external rotation of the arm in the transverse humeral ligament area. A loose body in the shoulder may cause a loud clunk or catching sensation similar to a torn labrum, but occurs with less predictable arm positions.

PAIN-FREE SOUNDS. Not all shoulder sounds are abnormal or need to be investigated; sounds that are nonpainful and otherwise asymptomatic are common. These may be caused by a mobile labrum, a synovial ledge, or by a tendinous structure snapping over a bony prominence.

Physical examination

Inspection. A common error clinicians make in examining the shoulder is failing to undress the patient. Special gowns are available that allow exposure of both shoulders but maintain modesty. Even regular gowns can be applied in a toga or chest-tie position so that complete bilateral evaluation of the shoulders can be performed.

The examiner begins by comparing both shoulders. A difference in shoulder heights may be caused by scoliosis or a congenital deformity. In a patient with chronic symptoms, it commonly is due to drooping of the symptomatic shoulder girdle caused by hypotonic musculature.

The physician should look for evidence of clavicle deformity from an old fracture or prominence of the AC joint due to degenerative hypertrophy or traumatic separation of the joint. The two sides are compared to detect evidence of atrophy. Deltoid atrophy may occur from disuse, axillary nerve injury, or postsurgical avulsion. Supraspinatus and infraspinatus muscle atrophy may be seen with severe rotator cuff tears or suprascapular nerve injuries. The chest contour will be altered with rupture of the pectoralis major muscle, an injury that can occur in heavy laborers. The patient should flex his biceps; the presence of a balled-up, "Popeye" muscle indicates a proximal rupture of the biceps tendon usually associated with a chronic pathologic condition of the rotator cuff. Scapular winging may be seen with scapulothoracic nerve palsy (Fig. 9-8). The winging usually can be made more prominent by having the patient push against a wall. Injury to the sternoclavicular joint may manifest with a prominence of the clavicle as it sits in a subluxed position at the sternum.

Palpation. Due to the relatively large soft tissue bulk of the shoulder, palpation may not be as rewarding as in other more subcutaneous areas of the musculoskeletal examination. However, specific, anatomically directed palpation should be performed.

Cervical spine. A proper evaluation of the shoulder should always begin with an examination of the cervical spine and a neurologic examination of the upper extremities. A cervical pathologic condition can often mimic a shoulder disorder. Many patients have been treated unsuccessfully for long periods for a suspected shoulder problem, when they actually had a cervical disorder.

Patients with a cervical origin of pain often have obvious spasm and even torticollis of the neck. Unfortunately, shoulder pain can cause sec-

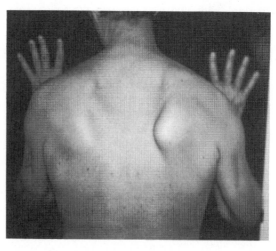

Fig. 9-8 Patient with scapular winging on the right.

ondary cervical spasm as well. The paracervical musculature should be palpated for spasm, fibrosis, and trigger points. A trigger point is identified as a very localized area of tenderness that recreates the patient's symptoms with palpation.

The patient's range of motion must be checked. A patient with cervical spasm often has decreased forward cervical flexion and decreased oblique forward bending. Palpation is performed along the levator scapula for spasm of this muscle. Isolated involvement of this structure (levator scapula syndrome) is an often-missed diagnosis.

A neurologic stress test is performed by applying axial loading to the top of the head or by extending the patient's neck posteriorly and laterally. Both of these maneuvers close down the neural foramina and elicit radicular pain in an inflamed nerve root.

Neurologic evaluation of the upper extremities should be done routinely to pick up subtle deficits. Motor strength of nerve roots is assessed by isolating muscles: the deltoid, the biceps, the triceps and wrist flexion, finger flexion and wrist extension, and hand intrinsics. Sensory testing should be done by dermatomal levels. Reflex testing of the biceps, triceps, and brachioradialis should be performed. Patients with shoulder or neck pain often demonstrate reduced grip strength on dynamometer testing as well. This should be performed as part of any upper extremity evaluation in an injured worker.

If thoracic outlet syndrome is suspected, Adson's test is performed. The patient holds the involved arm in 90 degrees of abduction and turns his head to the involved side. A loss or reduction of radial pulse suggests the syndrome (this finding may be subtle). In the test described by Roos, the patient actively opens and closes his hands for 3 minutes with the arms abducted 90 degrees. Ischemic pain indicates thoracic outlet syndrome. Other maneuvers that compress the thoracic outlet have been described, including the position of "military attention," with the shoulders held back and down while the examiner listens for a bruit. Occasionally a bruit may be heard over the supraclavicular area with compression of the subclavian artery. Even an experienced examiner can find this a difficult diagnosis to make, but it should be considered in any patient with medial cord (ulnar nerve) symptoms. Although not typically a work-related problem, posttraumatic compression of the thoracic outlet is possible after a work injury as a result of clavicular or proximal rib fracture or fibrosis of the scalenus muscles.

Acromioclavicular joint. The subcutaneous and prominent AC joint usually is tender to palpation if it is symptomatic. This is an area often missed on the cursory examination. Palpation will reveal any step-off or deformity of the AC joint following a separation or fracture through this joint, or any osteophytes in an arthritic joint. Tenderness is the most common finding.

The AC joint is most easily identified by walking the fingers along the clavicle toward the acromion until the prominence of the joint is felt. It is important to remember that the AC joint lies in an oblique plane, facing somewhat anterior and superior from the sagittal plane. To examine the joint, the examiner has the patient perform a cross-chest motion (passive adduction across the chest) while the examiner palpates the joint, feeling for crepitus, which often accompanies osteoarthritis of the AC joint. This maneuver also will cause pain in a symptomatic joint.

Rotator cuff. The rotator cuff cannot be palpated, but very often there is tenderness along the anterior edge of the acromion in a patient with rotator cuff tendonitis caused by impingement against the acromial arch (impingement syndrome). To better isolate the anterior acromion, distal traction is applied to the arm. This displaces the humeral head inferiorly and allows easier access to the anterior acromion.

The examiner also can palpate along the course of the supraspinatus and infraspinatus tendons above and below the spine of the scapula. In a patient with rotator cuff inflammation, one or both of these are often tender. The most effective test for diagnosing rotator cuff tendonitis is the impingement test. Passive rotation of the arm in 90 degrees of abduction also may reveal crepitus in the subacromial bursa as the rotator cuff is rotated internally and externally under the acromion.

Biceps tendon. The biceps tendon cannot be directly palpated proximally because of the bulk of the deltoid. However, the vicinity of the tendon can be easily isolated as it courses between the greater and lesser tuberosities. First, the patient relaxes his arm to diminish the bulk of the deltoid. With the arm in neutral rotation at the patient's side, the examiner palpates the anterior aspect of the shoulder while gently rotating the arm internally and externally. The groove between the tuberosities should be palpable. Tenderness in this area suggests an inflamed biceps tendon.

If doubt exists, the patient should hold his arm at his side with the elbow flexed to 90 degrees and the palm up. The examiner grasps the patient's hand as though for a handshake and has him perform a resisted supination maneuver (Yergeson's test). This strains the biceps tendon and in a patient with biceps tendonitis should cause anterior shoulder pain in the bicipital groove area. Speeds test is performed by having the patient hold the involved arm in 90 degrees of forward elevation and supination while the examiner provides resistance. Bicipital pain indicates tendonitis.

Function. The patient should always be asked to perform active motion, so that the examiner can assess function, and passive motion, to assess range of motion. Because the shoulder has such an expansive range of motion, it is practical to test it only in the most functional positions. Most daily activities require forward elevation in front of the body, and internal and external rotation. Pure abduction is used less commonly, and extension is rarely necessary. At the very least, the patient's active range of motion to forward elevation, external rotation, and internal rotation should be recorded for every shoulder examination. If the patient's job requires extension or abduction, those should be assessed as well.

External rotation should be measured with the patient's arm at his side and at 90 degrees of abduction (Fig. 9-9). Internal rotation is best measured by having the patient place his thumb behind his back; the highest spinous process reached (e.g., T-10) should be recorded. The disability guidelines of the American Medical Association (AMA) suggest measuring internal rotation at 90 degrees of shoulder abduction. Forward elevation is recorded simply on a scale of 0 to 180 degrees.

Adhesive capsulitis. Some patients' complaints are caused solely by restricted range of motion. This is most commonly seen in diabetic patients, who are prone to developing adhesive capsulitis, or "frozen shoulder" syndrome. The syndrome is a primary disease of the shoulder capsule that can mimic a number of other, more common disorders, such as rotator cuff tendonitis. Restricted range of

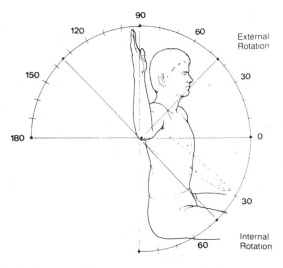

Fig. 9-9 Measuring external rotation of the shoulder at 90 degrees of abduction. (Modified from Neer CS: *Shoulder reconstruction,* Philadelphia, 1990, WB Saunders.)

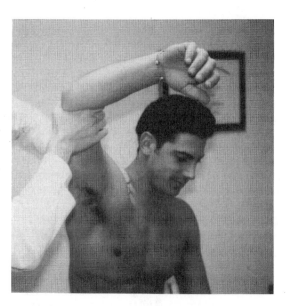

Fig. 9-10 To perform the impingement test, the patient's shoulder is internally rotated and then flexed forward against a stabilized acromion.

motion, especially in a patient with diabetes, should alert the examiner to think of adhesive capsulitis.

Specific evaluations

Rotator cuff. If the history and clinical findings indicate that the rotator cuff may be the source of the patient's pain, the examiner should perform additional tests.

Impingement Test. In the impingement test, the examiner attempts to pinch the rotator cuff between the humeral head and the acromion. If the cuff is inflamed, this test causes severe pain. The most effective way to perform the test is to stabilize the scapula from behind with one hand, and then forcefully elevate the internally rotated arm until the greater tuberosity strikes the anterior edge of the acromion (Fig. 9-10). Internal rotation of the arm is important, because this moves the prominent greater tuberosity anteriorly. Likewise, if the scapula is not stabilized, it will rotate as the arm is elevated, and true impingement will not occur. This test should cause pain in the lateral or anterolateral aspect of the shoulder. Occasionally it causes pain at an inflamed AC joint because of uncontrolled acromioclavicular motion.

Most pathologic conditions of the rotator cuff involve the supraspinatus and infraspinatus tendons. These tendons can be isolated on physical examination and tested for strength. To do this, the examiner has the patient elevate his arm in 90 degrees of abduction, 30 degrees of forward flexion, and maximum internal rotation to isolate the supraspinatus tendon (Fig. 9-11). Patients with rotator cuff tendonitis experience pain and weakness with resisted strength testing.

The infraspinatus muscle cannot be isolated from the teres minor muscle, but these two external rotators can be tested together. The patient holds his arms at his sides with the elbows against the body and flexed 90 degrees. External rotation

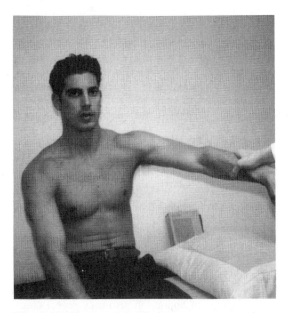

Fig. 9-11 The supraspinatus tendon is isolated and tested with the arm forward flexed, slightly abducted, and internally rotated.

is tested against manual resistance. With rotator cuff tendonitis, the involved side almost always is weak, and the maneuver causes pain along the infraspinatus muscle proximally.

Lidocaine Test. Weakness of the rotator cuff may indicate either tendonitis or possibly a torn tendon. The lidocaine test is a diagnostic procedure in which the rotator cuff is first anesthetized to eliminate pain and then tested for strength. If strength improves after lidocaine is injected into the subacromial space, chances are good the cuff is intact and the weakness was caused simply by pain. Persistent weakness after the injection suggests a torn rotator cuff. This test also is useful for verifying the diagnosis in a patient with equivocal or multiple findings. A patient often has some component of AC joint pain as well as the rotator cuff symptoms. The lidocaine test can help the physician determine the percentage of symptoms accounted for by each location.

TECHNIQUE. For practical purposes, the lidocaine may be combined with a long-acting steroid (Depo-Medrol) to achieve some therapeutic benefit as well as diagnostic information. The usual mixture is 2 ml of Xylocaine 2% with 1 ml of Depo-Medrol (40 mg).

The lidocaine-steroid mixture is injected into the subacromial space (bursa). This can be done in a number of ways. Because the subacromial bursa is an anterior structure, an anterior approach would seem most logical. However, the acromion slopes anteriorly, especially in patients with impingement syndrome and a hooked acromion, making access from the front difficult. This approach works best if an assistant applies distal traction on the arm to open up the subacromial space.

The posterior approach is the easiest but the least sensible. Because the bursa and the usual area of impingement are so far anterior, a very long needle must be used, and it is easy to miss the target.

We prefer a lateral approach with the patient sitting. Gravity provides some traction, and the anterolateral aspect of the bursa is easily accessible through an area of relatively low sensitivity (Fig. 9-12).

Acromioclavicular joint. The AC joint is difficult to examine. The most helpful test usually is simple palpation of the joint, as discussed previously. Pain sometimes can be elicited only with forced cross-chest adduction of the arm, and crepitus often can be felt with this maneuver as well.

The most definitive diagnostic test for a painful AC joint is a lidocaine injection. Although the joint is subcutaneous, this injection can be difficult. The joint is extremely small and obliquely

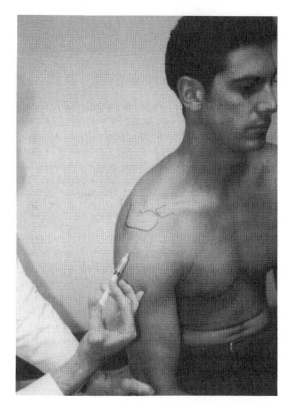

Fig. 9-12 Lateral approach for subacromial injections (author's preferred approach).

oriented. The total capacity of a normal joint is only about 1 to 2 ml and is even less in an arthritic joint. Furthermore, if the needle penetrates the inferior aspect of the joint, some of the lidocaine will seep into the subacromial space, obscuring the results.

The best way to perform this test is to use a $\frac{1}{2}$ inch, small-gauge needle (25) and to walk the needle along the acromion until the AC joint is felt. Pressure buildup is felt almost immediately, and only 1 ml of lidocaine can be injected.

Diagnostic studies

Clinicians are fortunate to have at their disposal an array of "high-tech" diagnostic tests. However, fiscally responsible clinicians must realize that a test is beneficial only if it will alter the course of treatment. Most diagnoses can be made by a skilled clinician using the history, physical examination, x-ray films, and the lidocaine injection test. In enigmatic cases, the most helpful test to be tried next depends on the suspected diagnosis.

X-ray films. Our standard shoulder series consists of a true anteroposterior (AP) view in internal and external rotation of the humerus, an axillary view, and a lateral scapular view with a 10-degree

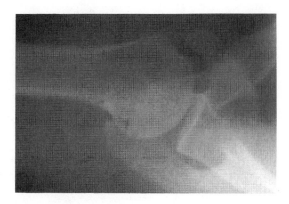

Fig. 9-13 Axillary view of the shoulder showing a large os acromiale.

caudal tilt. These four views should be enough for the standard shoulder evaluation. The 10-degree caudal tilt view has proved invaluable in assessing the shape of the acromial arch in patients with impingement syndrome. The axillary view is best for evaluating the integrity of the glenoid rim and for detecting an os acromiale (which we found in 4% of the population in our series) (Fig. 9-13).

Special x-ray views occasionally are necessary. For a suspected AC joint separation, an AP view of both AC joints with 10-pound weights suspended from the arms helps demonstrate the injury (Fig. 9-14). Stress films can be done to demonstrate subtle instabilities (Fig. 9-15).

Arthrography is a relatively accurate means of evaluating the integrity of the rotator cuff and is still used when magnetic resonance imaging (MRI) units are unavailable. However, an MRI scan is far superior to an arthrogram in sensitivity and accuracy, is noninvasive, and has all but replaced the arthrogram in the United States.

Ultrasonography.   Ultrasound examinations have been touted as an accurate, inexpensive method for evaluating the rotator cuff. However, it generally is acknowledged that interpretation of the results is highly dependent on the evaluator. In addition, ultrasound scans are less useful for evaluating other shoulder abnormalities, such as disorders of the labrum and biceps tendon. This procedure is not recommended because of its generally poor availability and limited scope.

Computed tomography.   CT is still the most accurate technique for evaluating bony lesions, and it is helpful in evaluating intricate fractures about the shoulder. Studies also support its use (with a simultaneous arthrogram) for evaluating labral tears, although this requires the invasiveness of the arthrogram, and the results are no better than those from an MRI scan. CT scans are rarely necessary

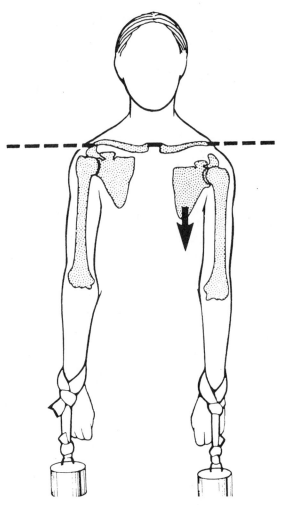

Fig. 9-14 Illustration showing separation of the acromioclavicular (AC) joint. (Modified from Neer CS: *Shoulder reconstruction,* Philadelphia, 1990, WB Saunders.)

and should be limited to preoperative planning of a complex fracture, or possibly to imaging of a tumor to evaluate the integrity of the cortex.

Magnetic resonance imaging.   The MRI scan has greatly improved the diagnosis of shoulder disorders. Intratendinous changes can be seen in rotator cuff tendonitis, and the actual size of a rotator cuff tear can be evaluated, including which tendons are involved. MRI can disclose tears of the labrum, disruptions of the biceps tendon, avascular necrosis of the humeral head, and glenoid cysts. However, most of these conditions can also be adequately diagnosed through the history, physical examination, and x-ray films. In addition, MRI often cannot differentiate partial tears from small complete tears, and it is inaccurate in the evaluation of articular cartilage.[12] Many patients

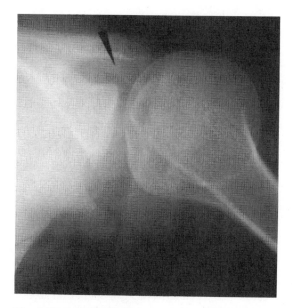

Fig. 9-15 Posterior stress x-ray film of the shoulder showing posterior instability.

with symptoms severe enough to warrant an MRI scan are candidates for surgery and are best evaluated by arthroscopy. MRI scans should be reserved for the enigmatic cases.

Arthroscopy. Arthroscopic evaluation of the shoulder, although invasive, is the "gold standard" diagnostic test. It can now be done in the office using local anesthesia and a miniature arthroscope (Fig. 9-16).[12] This has greatly reduced the risk and morbidity of the procedure and decreased its cost to one half to two thirds that of an MRI scan. Arthroscopy has proved invaluable in the definitive evaluation of injured workers with subjective complaints that are disproportionate to the clinical findings.

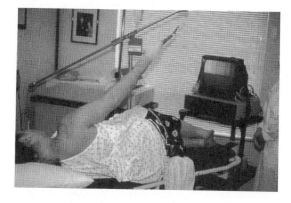

Fig. 9-16 Diagnostic arthroscopy of the shoulder can be done in the office using local anesthesia.

Common injuries and disorders

Rotator cuff. Injury to the rotator cuff is by far the most common shoulder injury seen in the workplace. Usually the onset of pain is insidious, and the injured worker typically is involved in a job that requires static loading with the arm in an overhead or reaching position (e.g., hanging clothes on a rack, working with a vacuum cleaner, or painting ceilings). Occasionally the injury is traumatic, the result of a fall directly onto the shoulder, or of a sudden distraction force on the arm (e.g., wheeling a heavy handtruck that slips, attempting to pull a person from a wreck, or even pulling aggressively on a stuck drawer).

Etiology. "Impingement syndrome," a term commonly used for chronic rotator cuff tendonitis, is quite descriptive. The acromion and anteriorly attached coracoacromial ligament form an arch over the rotator cuff. The shape of the arch and the thickness of the ligament determine how much space is available below for the rotator cuff tendons to pass. Anatomic studies indicate there are three basic acromial shapes: flat (type 1), curved (type 2), and hooked (type 3) (see Fig. 9-5). People with type 2 and type 3 shapes have less subacromial space and are more prone to impingement of the rotator cuff. The initiating insult that leads to tendonitis is still unclear. Most likely a worker may strain the rotator cuff, which causes inflammation and swelling. If the acromion is hook-shaped, the rotator cuff is more likely to be impinged, leading to a continuing cycle of pain and irritation to the cuff.

Clinical presentation. An acute rotator cuff injury is marked by severe pain in the shoulder and inability to lift the arm because of pain. In this case the cuff has suffered either a contusion from a direct blow or a partial tear (strain) from a distraction injury. The examination often reveals tenderness to palpation over the greater tuberosity and severe pain on attempts to actively elevate the arm. Passive elevation is more comfortable, until the greater tuberosity abuts the anterior acromion (the impingement sign). The rotator cuff is weak from pain. In these patients it is very helpful to perform a lidocaine test. With pain relief from the anesthetic, function usually improves dramatically, and a tear of the cuff can be ruled out.

A worker with insidious onset of shoulder pain usually has somewhat different complaints. Early on, the pain may arise while the patient is at work or immediately afterward. This progresses to night pain or pain during recreational activities involving the shoulder. These patients rarely complain of rest pain until late in the course. The cause of the night pain is unclear, but it may be simply that in a recumbent position, gravity effects on the arm are eliminated, allowing the humeral head to ride superiorly and forcing the inflamed rotator cuff up against the overlying acromion.

On examination, a patient with chronic rotator cuff tendonitis usually is not tender over the greater tuberosity, but he may have tenderness at the undersurface of the anterior acromion. The impingement test result is positive, and supraspinatus or external rotation resistance testing reveals pain or weakness of the rotator cuff. The patient often points to the lateral aspect of the shoulder at the deltoid insertion as the location of the pain, since pain from the rotator cuff often is referred to this location. When the infraspinatus muscle is primarily involved (much less often than the supraspinatus muscle) the patient usually points to the posterior aspect of the shoulder.

Differential diagnosis. Although impingement syndrome is the most common cause of rotator cuff tendonitis, a patient with an unstable glenohumeral joint can develop similar symptoms. When the humeral head is unstable, there are fewer restraints on superior migration, which allows the humeral head to slide up and pinch the rotator cuff against the acromion. This diagnosis is very difficult to make, even for an experienced shoulder surgeon. A patient with shoulder laxity who complains of symptoms similar to impingement syndrome should be referred to a specialist. Techniques that can aid in correct diagnosis are: a negative lidocaine test result, evidence of apprehension, and instability, as measured by examination under anesthesia.

It is important to carefully examine the adjacent AC joint as well. It is easy to mistake AC joint pain for rotator cuff pain, and problems in both may exist simultaneously. When this occurs, it is thought that altered scapular mechanics caused by weakness of the rotator cuff result in compensatory abnormal motion at the AC joint, which leads to pain. When doubt exists, the lidocaine test can be done on the AC joint to determine if or how much this joint is contributing to the patient's symptoms.

Biceps tendonitis often occurs in association with long-standing rotator cuff tendonitis, but it is rare as an isolated entity. These patients have tenderness in the bicipital groove and a positive result on Yergeson's test.

Other disorders that can cause shoulder pain and mimic rotator cuff tendonitis are polymyalgia rheumatica, cervical disk disease, Pancoast's tumor, and thoracic outlet syndrome. The pain of polymyalgia rheumatica is usually bilateral, is associated with headaches, and is not aggravated by impingement testing. Pancoast's tumor causes vague, more medial shoulder pain and usually is associated with Horner's syndrome and lung symptoms. A herniated cervical disk typically causes radicular-type, radiating pain and neurologic findings and is exacerbated by neck extension and axial compression of the cervical spine. Thoracic outlet syndrome causes medial, not lateral, arm pain and yields a negative result on impingement testing and a positive result on Adson's test.

Treatment. The goal in treating rotator cuff tendonitis is to reduce the inflammation, strengthen the rotator cuff, and prevent recurrence.

ACUTE INJURY. Initial treatment for an acute rotator cuff injury is strict rest, antiinflammatory medication, and ice. This injury is a contusion or strain and should be treated in the same way as any other acute injury of this type. The patient must be off work for at least 2 to 4 weeks to allow healing; a gradual return is allowed as motion and strength return. These patients often can tolerate an accelerated exercise regimen as soon as the symptoms subside.

CHRONIC DISORDERS. Patients with chronic rotator cuff symptoms are managed somewhat differently. Treatment commonly is divided into three phases.

Phase 1. In the initial evaluation, the physician should ask the patient specific questions about his job activities, and she should recommend ways to modify injurious work habits. For example, a pharmacist who was short in stature began having shoulder pain when high shelves were built in the pharmacy. His symptoms improved after his employer was asked to provide him with a footstool, which eliminated the need for constant overhead reaching. In another case, a hotel maid's shoulder pain subsided after she was told to alternate the arm she used to push the vacuum cleaner and to hold the machine closer to her body, thus avoiding a prolonged outstretched position.

Patients with chronic symptoms rarely need to be taken off work initially. Treatment should begin with a 2-week course of nonsteroidal antiinflammatory agents and an exercise regimen. The exercises strengthen the rotator cuff, which stabilizes the glenohumeral joint and helps keep the humeral head depressed. Although the supraspinatus tendon is the portion of the rotator cuff most often involved in rotator cuff tendonitis, the exercises are meant to strengthen the remaining cuff muscles, leaving the supraspinatus alone. The infraspinatus, teres minor, and subscapularis muscles act primarily as external and internal rotators of the arm. However, because of their oblique insertion on the humeral head, they also can act as depressors. Improving the tone of these muscles helps depress the humeral head and increase internal and external rotational strength. This helps increase the space available under the acromial arch and reduces the chance of impingement.

In the early phases of treatment, the patient should not perform any exercises that directly work the inflamed supraspinatus muscle; abduction exercises that work the deltoid muscle also should be avoided. The deltoid muscle crosses the subacromial space and attaches at both the acromion and the humerus. When this muscle contracts, the humeral head is lifted against the acromion, causing further impingement of the intervening rotator cuff.

To reiterate: The initial phase of exercise should be limited to internal and external rotation to strengthen the infraspinatus, teres minor, and subscapularis muscles. After the tendonitis symptoms have resolved, exercises to strengthen the supraspinatus and deltoid muscles may be appropriate. Scapular exercises may be started early if scapular mechanics are judged to be altered.

Phase 2. If the patient does not respond to phase 1 measures, a long-acting corticosteroid is injected into the subacromial space, and the patient is kept off work for 1 to 2 weeks. (At this stage the patient usually is referred to a specialist.) Depending on the job requirements, his return to work begins with restricted duties (i.e., no overhead activities and no lifting of more than 10 pounds). The injection may be repeated once, usually after 3 months. In rare cases a third injection is offered after a similar interval. If the patient's symptoms still

have not resolved and the physician suspects a rotator cuff tear rather than tendonitis, she should consider ordering an MRI scan or proceeding to surgery.

Phase 3. A patient who reaches phase 3 usually has had 3 to 6 months of severe symptoms, including night pain, inability to work, and difficulty going about the activities of daily living. Surgery involves expanding the subacromial space by resecting the acromial hood, the coracoacromial ligament, and the subacromial bursa; this creates more room for the rotator cuff tendons and prevents impingement (Fig. 9-17).

Arthroscopic techniques have greatly reduced the morbidity associated with this surgery. Arthroscopic treatment of impingement syndrome is done as an outpatient procedure and takes about 1 hour. The patient can begin physical therapy within a few days and usually can return to limited duties after 6 to 8 weeks. The surgery is successful in 80% to 90% of cases.

Calcific tendonitis. Calcific tendonitis appears to be distinct from rotator cuff tendonitis, although the presenting symptoms are similar and the two can overlap. The incidence of calcium deposits in painful shoulders is quite small (less than 10%), and the exact cause of the calcification is unclear, as is the reason why some individuals with rotator cuff tendonitis develop calcification and others do not.

The most common location for calcification is the supraspinatus tendon. Calcific tendonitis is be-

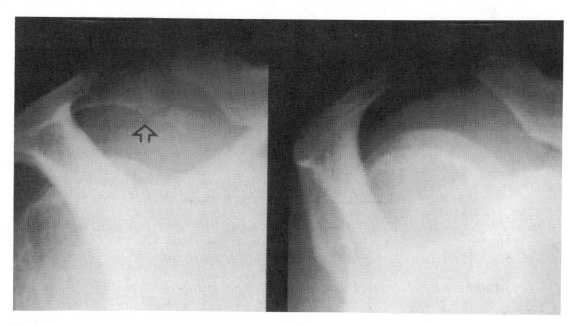

Fig. 9-17 Preoperative and postoperative x-ray films of the supraspinatus outlet after removal of a subacromial spur.

lieved to be a self-healing process that goes through formative and resorptive phases. The presence of calcium does not always correlate with pain.

Clinical presentation. The patient typically has an acute onset of extreme pain. The distribution is similar to that for rotator cuff tendonitis, but the pain is much worse. X-ray films show calcification, usually in the supraspinatus tendon. The pain severely limits range of motion. Dense calcification marks the formative phase, whereas fluffy calcification indicates the resorptive phase.

Differential diagnosis. Other causes of calcification around the shoulder include loose bodies, osteochondromatosis, osteoarthritis, gout, pseudogout, neuropathic joint conditions, and tumors with calcific foci. These disorders usually can be ruled out by their different appearance and location on multiple x-ray films of the shoulder.

Treatment. When calcification is found without associated pain, no specific treatment is required. Severe acute pain usually is best treated by injecting Xylocaine and cortisone into the subacromial space. Attempts can be made to simultaneously needle the involved area to break up the calcification, but this may be very painful. For a patient with chronic or resolving symptoms and fluffy calcification on the x-ray film, the disease is most likely in the resorptive phase and should respond to nonsteroidal antiinflammatory drugs (NSAIDs), exercise, ice, and activity modification. Resistant cases respond very well to arthroscopic removal of the calcium deposit; the pain is relieved immediately, and the patient is not kept off work for long.

Biceps tendonitis. Inflammation of the biceps tendon usually occurs in conjunction with rotator cuff tendonitis, because the biceps tendon enters the glenohumeral joint through the rotator cuff interval between the supraspinatus and subscapularis tendons. Isolated bicipital tendonitis is possible but rare; it may occur in an employee who does repetitive overhead work, as the tendon rubs back and forth over the lesser tuberosity.[23] Traumatic injury of the biceps tendon also is uncommon. Degenerative tears occur proximally, are more common than distal ruptures, and are almost always associated with chronic rotator cuff disease. Acute ruptures usually occur at the distal attachment at the radius.

Shoulder instability. Shoulder instability may be thought of in terms of direction (anterior, posterior, or multidirectional) or severity (subluxation, dislocation). The most common type of instability by far is anterior dislocation.

Dislocation. An injured worker with an acute shoulder dislocation usually reports having sustained a sudden force on the arm in an abducted and externally rotated position (the throwing position). If the shoulder has not spontaneously reduced, the diagnosis usually is easy. The patient holds the arm at his side in severe discomfort. The acromion appears prominent because of the displacement of the humeral head, which most often is lying anteroinferiorly, creating a sizeable bulge. If the shoulder has spontaneously reduced, diagnosis may be difficult. On examination the patient resists any attempts at abduction and external rotation (an apprehension sign) and is tender over the anterior shoulder. Spontaneous reduction is more common in a patient with a history of recurrent dislocation, and the history makes the diagnosis easier.

EXAMINATION. X-ray films should be taken before any attempt is made to reduce the dislocation, either to rule out associated fractures or to document that they existed before the examiner performed the reduction. Four views should be taken: an AP in internal and external rotation, a lateral, and an axillary. These views should be sufficient to determine the direction of dislocation (lateral view); to detect any fractures, including a Hill-Sachs defect (AP); and to assess the integrity of the anterior glenoid rim (axillary). The Hill-Sachs defect is an impaction fracture of the posterior aspect of the humeral head, which is caused by the glenoid rim as the shoulder dislocates.

A thorough neurologic examination is also essential because of the high incidence of neuropraxia associated with dislocations. Posterior dislocations are rare but can easily be missed. In these cases, the patient usually has suffered a blow to the anterior aspect of the shoulder, an electric shock, or a seizure, and he holds his arm internally rotated against his body. Because diagnosis is difficult on AP views, a good quality lateral x-ray film is required.

TREATMENT FOR ACUTE DISLOCATION. An acute dislocation is reduced after the patient has been sedated, which usually is done in the Emergency Room. The safest method of relocation involves applying distal traction on the arm with the patient supine and the torso stabilized. After reduction, the arm is supported in a sling or immobilizer. With an acute dislocation, healing may occur, and immobilization is recommended for about 3 weeks. (In individuals who suffer from recurrent dislocation, the duration of immobilization does not seem to matter; thus it should last only a few days.) After the immobilization period, the patient should begin an exercise program to regain range of motion and strength. However, he should avoid the position of abduction and external rotation. The patient may return to work for light duty after the pain subsides and motion returns. He should avoid heavy lifting until his strength returns.

TREATMENT FOR RECURRENT DISLOCATION. A patient under 30 years of age who has suffered a shoulder dislocation has a 50% to 90% chance of a recurrence. (The rate declines with age.[28]) Surgical reconstruction can reduce the chance of redislocation to less than 10%.[29] Surgery is recommended for a young laborer to allow him to return to heavy work and to prevent recurrence. Arthroscopic techniques now are used to stabilize many of these shoulders. The typical arthroscopic procedure takes 1 to 2 hours and is done on an outpatient basis. The patient usually may return to full duties by 3 months.

With a first-time dislocation in an older worker, whose chance of recurrence is less than 50%, a strengthening program and avoiding the abducted, externally rotated position are recommended.

Subluxation. Subtle shoulder instability allows the head of the humerus to slide over the glenoid rim, but no frank dislocation occurs. This condition is more common in a flexible, hyperelastic woman or a nonmuscular man. Often the patient has had at least one previous episode of true dislocation. The diagnosis is much more difficult to make than with dislocation.

EXAMINATION. With the patient standing, the examiner looks for asymmetry of the shoulder mass. Occasionally a patient has a disuse atrophy. The examiner should check for generalized hyperelas-

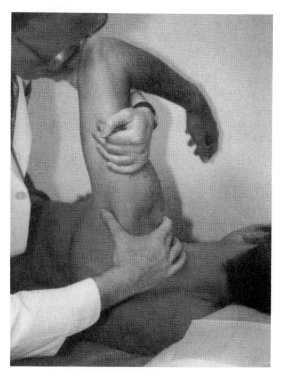

Fig. 9-19 Lateral decubitus method of testing for shoulder instability.

ticity, which is characterized by elbow, finger, and knee hyperextension (Fig. 9-18).

Testing for shoulder instability often is difficult because of the patient's apprehension and splinting. The examiner should passively abduct and externally rotate the arm, placing an anterior force on the shoulder from behind; this causes severe apprehension in a patient with instability, although true subluxation may not occur. Subluxation occasionally may be reproduced by examining the patient in the lateral decubitus position (Fig. 9-19). The patient relaxes and flexes his arm 90 degrees, and then lets the arm rest on the examiner's arm. At the same time, the examiner stabilizes the scapula with her opposite hand. She then attempts to translate the humerus anteroinferiorly and compares the two shoulders, checking for any difference.

Another test is the relocation test. The patient lies on his back, and the examiner abducts and externally rotates the arm while applying a posterior force to the anterior aspect of the shoulder (this contains any attempts at subluxation of the humeral head). The examiner then releases the posterior pressure, allowing the head to sublux. This recreates the patient's symptoms if the arm is subluxing anteriorly (Fig. 9-20).

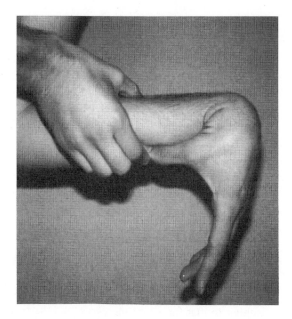

Fig. 9-18 Hyperelasticity is a risk factor for shoulder instability.

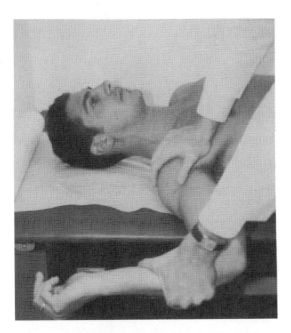

Fig. 9-20 Relocation test for anterior shoulder subluxation.

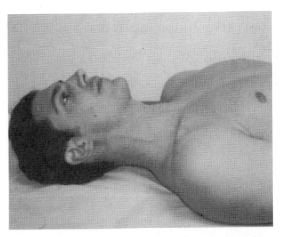

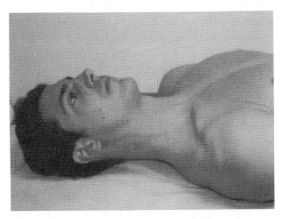

Fig. 9-21 Top, Normal appearance of shoulder before axial distraction force is applied. **Bottom,** Sulcus sign.

Posterior subluxation is tested differently. The patient's arm is abducted across his chest, and the examiner applies a posterior force along the axis of the arm while stabilizing the glenoid. This should cause posterior translation of the humeral head out of the glenoid, and recreate the patient's symptoms if the shoulder is subluxing posteriorly. In the Fukuda test, the patient relaxes his shoulders, and the examiner grasps them from behind, placing her thumbs on the scapular spine and wrapping her fingers anteriorly around the shoulder. She then applies a posterior force to the humeral head by flexing her fingers. The amount of posterior translation of the involved side is compared to that of the normal side. Normal translation is less than 50% of the diameter of the head.

Some patients are lax in more than one direction, a condition called multidirectional instability. These patients may have the findings of both anterior and posterior instability, and they usually have inferior instability as well. True superior instability does not occur because of the overlying bony acromion. Inferior instability is diagnosed from the presence of a sulcus sign. To elicit this sign, the examiner pulls inferiorly on the patient's relaxed arm as it lies at his side. If the humeral head can be subluxed inferiorly, a sulcus is created beneath the acromion because of a vacuum effect (Fig. 9-21).

Despite the tests described above, diagnosis is difficult in these patients, who usually need to be referred to a specialist. Often the correct diagnosis can be made only by examining an anesthetized patient. This allows careful examination of both shoulders with complete muscle relaxation and eliminates patient apprehension as a variable.

Labral tears. The labrum can tear without disrupting the attachment site of the inferior glenohumeral ligaments. Often this is a flap or buckethandle tear of the superior labrum, although the anterior labrum may be involved as well. The patient usually complains of a painful click in his shoulder. A provocative test that may be helpful is the abduction compression test. The examiner stabilizes the patient's scapula with one hand and uses the other to passively abduct the involved shoulder while applying an axial compression force. If the superior labrum is torn, the flap should be caught between the abducting humeral head and the superior rim of the glenoid, producing a clunk and pain. The treatment of this lesion is similar to that for a torn meniscus, and the flap usually requires arthroscopic removal. Recovery and return to work are rapid.

Other diagnostic tests. Imaging studies for shoulder instability occasionally are helpful, and MRI scanning currently is considered the procedure of choice if imaging is indicated. For an obvious dislocation, MRI can be used to determine the cause of the dislocation. This most commonly is a detachment of the inferior glenohumeral ligaments from the glenoid (Bankart lesion). Occasionally instability is caused by stretching of these ligaments, and true detachment does not occur. In rare cases the ligaments may be detached from their insertion on the humerus. For subluxators, a lax capsule may be the only disorder that is hard to detect on an MRI scan. For these reasons, MRI may not be the best choice. The most reliable diagnostic method is examination of the shoulder using anesthesia, along with shoulder arthroscopy.

Shoulder arthroscopy allows the physician to inspect the glenohumeral ligaments directly for detachment or stretching and to evaluate the glenoid and humeral surfaces for subtle signs of damage caused by subluxation. This often can be invaluable in determining the direction of instability.

Fractures. Fractures in the shoulder area typically are the result of a fall directly onto the shoulder or of direct trauma to the shoulder caused by a piece of heavy equipment or from a motor vehicle accident.

Initial management. Evaluation of a fractured shoulder should include a thorough history, a neurovascular examination, and x-ray films. Because shoulder fractures usually are caused by severe trauma, the physician should check for other injuries as well. Pain often makes these patients uncooperative for x-ray evaluation. The basic views that are necessary and require little if any motion by the patient are AP and scapular lateral views. Additional views may be necessary, including axillary or clavicle views. With severe fractures, CT scanning is helpful for evaluating comminution. After the fracture has been identified, the arm usually is most comfortable internally rotated against the body in an immobilizer (the most stable arrangement) or sling.

Displaced shoulder fractures often require surgical reduction and fixation. Standard orthopedic textbooks discuss the various techniques available for surgically treating these injuries. Fractures take an average of 6 to 8 weeks to heal, followed by an additional 2 to 3 months of rehabilitation. The injured employee can expect to be out of work for 4 to 6 months unless light duties that do not require use of the shoulder are available.

Prognosis. Treatment of a fracture in an injured worker is similar to that for any individual. For heavy laborers, however, strong consideration should be given to immediate surgical fixation to allow early joint motion and return of function. With surgical treatment the patient often returns to work sooner than with nonsurgical treatment because of the quicker mobilization and reduced muscle atrophy. Fractures of the shoulder require 6 to 8 weeks for bony healing and 2 to 3 months of rehabilitation before any return to work can be considered.

Common types of fractures. FRACTURES OF THE CLAVICLE. Fractures of the clavicle are among the most common injuries seen in workers. Most of these involve the middle third of the clavicle and have an excellent prognosis. The patient usually has an obvious deformity in the relatively subcutaneous clavicle. The examiner should carefully check for neurovascular injury because of the nearness of the brachial plexus and subclavian vessels. Fortunately these complications are rare. Treatment with a sling or figure-eight bandage for 6 weeks or until union occurs usually is adequate. Surgery is very rarely indicated.

Fractures of the lateral third of the clavicle are more complicated because of the presence of the coracoclavicular ligaments and the articulation with the AC joint. Careful x-ray evaluation is necessary to determine the stability of the fracture and to detect intraarticular involvement. Surgery may be necessary for these injuries to stabilize the joint or the fracture, or both. Referral to a specialist is recommended.

FRACTURES OF THE PROXIMAL HUMERUS. Fractures of the proximal humerus are classified according to the number of displaced fragments (Fig. 9-22). The four main potential fragments are the humeral head, the shaft, and the greater and lesser tuberosities. A fragment is considered significant if it is displaced more than 1 cm or 45 degrees. The more fragments present, the more likely it is that the blood supply to the humeral head will be disrupted, resulting in avascular necrosis.

The diagnosis is made by x-ray films. These patients have pain and swelling of the shoulder. Occasionally the fracture occurs with a dislocation, and x-ray films are essential to make the correct diagnosis.

Nondisplaced fractures are simply immobilized until bony union occurs. A significantly displaced fracture in a worker usually warrants adequate reduction. If this cannot be accomplished by closed methods of manipulation, surgical reduction and internal fixation may be indicated (Table 9-1). If the blood supply to the humeral head has been sufficiently compromised, replacement of the humeral head with a prosthesis may be indicated. Any fracture should be referred to a specialist for treatment.

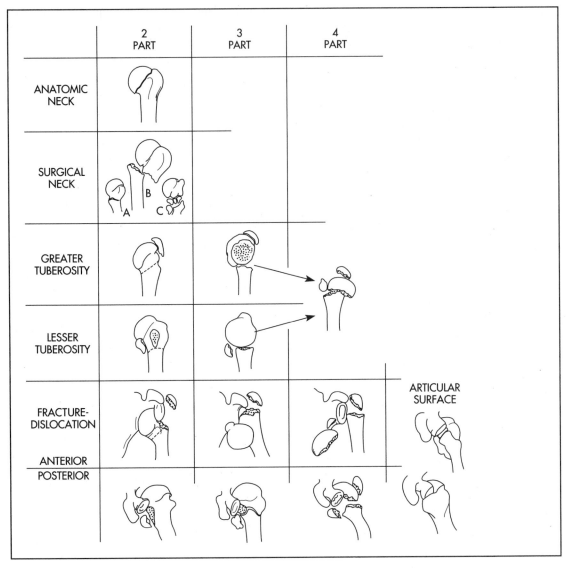

Fig. 9-22 Classification of fractures. (Modified from Neer CS: *Shoulder reconstruction,* Philadelphia, 1990, WB Saunders.)

OCCULT FRACTURES. Isolated fractures of the greater tuberosity are not uncommon; they often occur in conjunction with an anterior shoulder dislocation. Occasionally these fractures are not displaced, which makes them difficult to see on plain x-ray films. If a worker has persistent pain in the greater tuberosity area after a fall on his shoulder, a number of occult fractures can be identified by MRI scan. These patients often have been misdiagnosed as having a rotator cuff strain and treated with exercise; they actually need to avoid activity until the bone heals.

"Keypunch" syndrome. Keypunch syndrome is more properly known by the name occupational cervicobrachial disorder (OCD). OCD is actually a symptom complex of generalized shoulder and neck pain that usually affects the posterior paracervical musculature, the periscapular musculature, and the rotator cuff. The basic pathologic condition is intermittent muscle myalgia, and the disorder usually is associated with pain that radiates into the upper arm.

It should be kept in mind that OCD is not a specific diagnosis; rather, it is a description of a symptom complex of industrial origin.

The incidence of OCD among keypunch operators has been reported as somewhere between 16% and 28%.[18] A number of surveys have reported a much higher incidence of symptomatic individuals (70% to 80%), although most of these did not seek medical care.[23,31] People who work at a cash register seem to have even more trouble than keyboard

Table 9-1 Treatment according to four-segment classification*

	Incidence† (1%)	Problem	Author's treatment
Minimal displacement	80	Adhesions	Passive exercises progressing to active exercises as continuity permits
Two part	10	Usually amenable to closed reduction	Closed treatment, except for greater tuberosity and some shaft displacements
Three part	3	Rotary forces of muscles prevent accurate closed reduction	Open reduction, internal fixation, and cuff repair, except prosthesis is now preferred in older patients and greater tuberosity three-part displacement with frail head attachments
Four part	4	High incidence of avascular necrosis or posttraumatic arthritis	Prosthesis to replace the head with accurate fixation of the tuberosities and cuff repair
Articular surface fractures "Impression"	3		
Under 20%		Stable	Closed reduction, immobilization in external rotation
20% to 40%		Often unstable after closed reduction	Transplant lesser tuberosity if unstable
Over 50%		Redisplace into head defect	Prosthesis
"Head-splitting"		Articular surface crushed	Prosthesis

* These generalizations apply only to active patients who are good surgical risks and have good motivation and reasonable life expectancy.
† Expressed as a percentage of all upper humeral fractures and fracture-dislocations.
Modified from Neer CS: Fractures about the shoulder. In Rockwood CA Jr and Green DP, editors: *Fractures in adults,* ed 2, Philadelphia, 1984, JB Lippincott.

operators, possibly because they work standing up and frequently must twist to face customers.

Etiology. The most likely explanation for OCD involves static muscle loading. Keyboard operators and other repetitive-task workers often must hold their shoulders in a static posture of forward flexion and slight abduction while performing repetitive, fine manual tasks with the distal extremity. A typical keyboard operator may type as many as 80,000 strokes a day.[21] Values have been determined for the endurance limit of a muscle in static contraction, and these values vary between 8% and 15% of the maximum voluntary contraction (MVC).[5,27] Based on these values, it is commonly recommended that static muscle loads be maintained at less than 5% of the MVP.

Other factors have been proposed as contributing to OCD. Increased scapular elevation, as a result of stress or keyboards of improper height, leads to increased strain on the trapezius muscle.[10,24] Physiologic changes, such as interstitial myofibrositis, may interfere with adequate blood flow, leading to ischemia and fatigue.[2] A number of studies have demonstrated elevated muscle enzymes in workers with shoulder and neck complaints.[4,11] The contribution of psychosocial factors must also be considered.[18]

Diagnosis. It should be emphasized that OCD is mostly a diagnosis of exclusion. The differential diagnosis should include all specific causes of shoulder pain common to workers, such as rotator cuff tendonitis, cervical radiculopathy, scapulothoracic bursitis, arthritis of the AC or glenohumeral joint, and thoracic outlet syndrome.

Luck and Andersson[19] have divided OCD into three stages, based on pathophysiology. These stages are helpful in discussing the diagnosis and treatment of the condition with the patient.

Stage 1: The patient typically has diffuse complaints that arise only while he is working. The physical examination often is normal.

Stage 2: The patient usually has some tenderness along the trapezius muscle and rhomboids. The attachment site of the levator scapula muscle also may be tender.

Stage 3: The patient has had chronic symptoms for some time, with palpable myofibrosis, several areas of muscle tenderness, and pain with the extremes of shoulder range of motion. Weakness may be present, mostly from disuse.

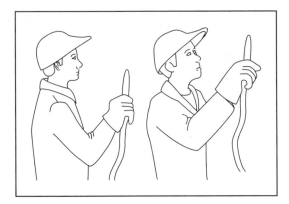

Fig. 9-23 Reducing the weight of hand tools and holding the hand close to the body reduces strain on the rotator cuff. (Modified from Rockwood CA, Matsen FA: *The shoulder,* Philadelphia, 1990, WB Saunders.)

As mentioned previously, rotator cuff tendonitis is a possible alternative diagnosis. However, tendonitis is much more likely with heavy labor than with light office or assembly line work (a 1984 study found an 18% incidence of supraspinatus tendonitis in welders[14]).

The factors that contribute to rotator cuff tendonitis are sustained forward elevation of the arm and use of heavy hand tools. For individuals with a hook-shaped acromial arch, forward elevation may result in greater impingement of the rotator cuff tendons between the humeral head and the acromion, leading to inflammation and eventual degeneration. Even with less direct impingement, sustained contracture of the supraspinatus muscle may result in reduced blood flow to a tendon that normally has areas of avascularity. Impingement of the rotator cuff tendons in an elevated arm also may occur at a hypertrophied coracoacromial ligament, an osteophytic AC joint or, with internal rotation, even at the coracoid.

Rotator cuff strain can be reduced by keeping the arm as close to the body as possible and minimizing the weight of hand tools. No muscle fatigue was found in welders who worked with the arm in less than 30 degrees of flexion (Fig. 9-23).

Treatment. A primary care physician involved in the treatment of an injured worker should develop an understanding of the patient's work environment, so that she can make appropriate treatment recommendations.

Patients with early OCD (stage 1) usually require only ergonomic modifications in the work position, scheduled breaks for stretching and rest, and instruction in a proper exercise program for range of motion and strengthening. Increased baseline muscle tension of the shoulder girdle is thought to predispose a person to OCD, and relaxation techniques, including biofeedback, may be helpful.[19]

The same measures are used to treat patients with stage 2 symptoms, but these employees may require time off work, and antiinflammatory drugs frequently are prescribed for them.

Workers with chronic OCD (stage 3) often require job retraining.

Prevention. The health care practitioner can contribute as much to preventing work-related shoulder injuries as she can to treating them. The physician often can suggest ways to reduce shoulder strain at work (Table 9-2). For example, individuals who work at keyboards should take several 5- to 10-minute active breaks during the day[19] (because the muscles recover quickly from this sort of work, a longer break is not needed[6,9]). "Micropauses" should be taken every 10 to 15 minutes.

The general rule is to keep the reach target low and close to the body to reduce forward flexion and abduction of the shoulders. The time to muscle fatigue falls markedly as the arm is extended (forward flexion of the shoulder). See Chapter 22 (Cumulative Trauma) for further discussion.

ELBOW DISORDERS
Anatomy and biomechanics

The elbow joint is both a hinge joint and a pivoting joint, which makes it capable of flexion, exten-

Table 9-2 Parameters influencing shoulder load and methods to reduce loads

Parameter	Load-reducing factor	Examples
Moment arm	Reduce horizontal distance	Move work closer; stand or sit close to workplace; slope work surface
	Adjust vertical height	Adjust table height; adjust chair height; slope work surface
External load	Reduce load magnitude	Divide into several loads; choose light tools; use tool balancer
	Provide arm support	Armrests; balance slings

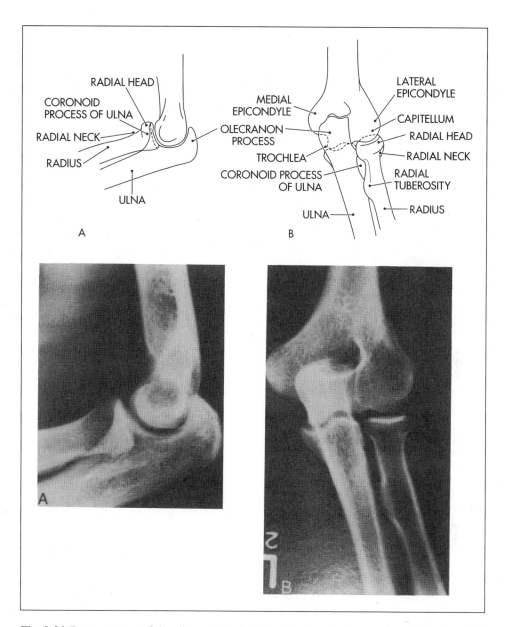

Fig. 9-24 Bony anatomy of the elbow. (Modified from Neviaser R: *Emergency orthopedic radiology,* New York, 1985, Churchill Livingstone.)

sion, and rotation. Normal range of motion is from 0 to 145 degrees of flexion and from 75 degrees of pronation to 85 degrees of supination. Functional motion usually requires only 30/130 degrees of flexion/extension and 50/50 of pronation/supination.[22] The elbow is strongest at 90 degrees of flexion. Supination is 15% stronger than pronation, and the dominant extremity normally is 5% to 10% stronger than the opposite side.[1]

The elbow joint is relatively constrained and is formed by the articulation of the distal humerus with the radial head and the olecranon (Fig. 9-24).

The normal elbow joint is in approximately 6 degrees of valgus relative to the humeral shaft because of a valgus angulation of the distal humerus. Significant bony landmarks are the medial and lateral epicondyles, the radial head, and the olecranon.

Musculature

Elbow flexion. The biceps muscle crosses the anterior aspect of the elbow overlying the brachialis muscle and attaches to the posterior aspect of the radial tuberosity. The tendon also has a broad aponeurosis that extends medially to attach to the fascia of the forearm. The medial edge of this aponeurosis (called the lacertus fibrosus) can be a site of impingement of the median nerve. The biceps muscle functions as both a flexor and a supinator of the arm. The brachialis muscle, the other major flexor of the elbow, runs deep to the biceps along the anterior capsule of the joint and inserts primarily into the coronoid process. Because of its proximity to the capsule, the brachialis muscle is believed to be a primary culprit in myositis ossificans of the elbow. The brachioradialis muscle forms the lateral border of the antecubital fossa and attaches at the radial styloid, quite distal from its broad humeral origin.

Elbow extension. The main elbow extensor is the large triceps muscle. The three heads of the triceps converge into a tendinous attachment to the olecranon process of the ulna. Tendonitis and rupture of this tendon can occur but are rare.

The anconeus muscle is a small muscle that extends from the lateral epicondyle to the lateral aspect of the proximal ulna. Its function is still debated, but it serves as a landmark for needle aspiration and surgical approaches to the elbow.

Wrist/finger extensors. The extensor mass originates at the lateral epicondyle of the humerus and includes three wrist extensors (the extensor carpi radialis longus, the extensor carpi radialis brevis, and the extensor carpi ulnaris), as well as the extensor digitorum communis, which provides finger extension. Inflammation and tendinous degeneration at the origin of the extensor carpi radialis brevis is thought to be the cause of tennis elbow.

Flexor/pronator group. The medial epicondyle of the humerus gives origin to the flexor carpi radialis and the flexor carpi ulnaris, which provide wrist flexion, as well as to the pronator teres, which is the major pronator of the forearm. Inflammation at the attachment site of these muscles produces the symptoms of medial epicondylitis (golfer's elbow).

Neurovascular structures. The brachial artery and vein, along with the median nerve, cross the elbow overlying the brachialis muscle medial to the biceps tendon and deep to the lacertus fibrosus. Their location is important when considering injections about the elbow. The radial nerve passes through the lateral intermuscular septum in the arm, crosses the elbow, and descends along the anterior aspect of the lateral epicondyle beneath the brachioradialis muscle. The nerve then divides. Part continues anteriorly to terminate as the sensory superficial radial nerve; a posterior (deep) branch swings back around the radial neck, penetrates the supinator muscle, and descends as the posterior interosseous nerve. This latter portion of the nerve is subject to entrapment in the radial tun-

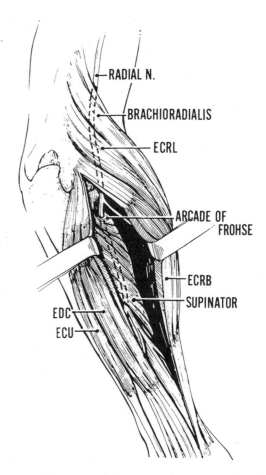

Fig. 9-25 The radial nerve can be compressed at the arcade of Frohse. (Modified from Green DP: *Operative hand surgery,* New York, 1993, Churchill Livingstone.)

nel, causing symptoms that mimic lateral epicondylitis (Fig. 9-25).

The ulnar nerve derives from the medial cord of the brachial plexus; this is why compression of the medial cord (such as occurs in thoracic outlet syndrome) may produce complaints characteristic of an ulnar nerve disorder. The nerve penetrates the medial intermuscular septum, crosses the elbow, and courses superficially in the cubital tunnel on the medial aspect of the elbow, where it is vulnerable to blunt trauma. The nerve is in intimate contact with the ulnar collateral ligament and the posterior portion of the flexor pronator muscle mass, which explains the ulnar nerve symptoms that frequently accompany disorders of these structures (e.g., medial epicondylitis and ligament instability). See Chapter 8 (Hand and Wrist Disorders) for further discussion.

Physical examination

Inspection. The patient should be inspected with the entire upper extremity exposed. Symptoms ascribed to the elbow may arise either proximally or distally, and the entire extremity, including the cervical spine, should be examined in any patient who complains of elbow pain. Cervical radiculopathy, thoracic outlet syndrome, and carpal tunnel syndrome all can manifest as elbow pain. Because the radius and ulna are intimately related along their entire course by the interosseous membrane, injuries at the wrist can lead to late sequelae at the elbow (the proximal radioulnar articulation). The elbow should always be examined in a patient with a wrist injury.

The alignment of the elbow should be evaluated, including range of motion. The angle formed by the humeral articulation with the ulna and radius is called the *carrying angle*. An abnormal carrying angle, which may be the result of a growth disturbance from a childhood fracture, can lead to delayed secondary problems, such as stretching of the ulnar nerve in an excessively valgus elbow (an example of an underlying condition for which apportionment would be indicated).

The patient should be asked to flex and extend his elbow, and the examiner should compare its range of motion to that of the opposite side. Regardless of the cause, a stiff elbow by itself can cause symptoms and needs to be addressed. Pronation and supination also should be measured and compared to those actions on the opposite side. The patient should pronate and supinate with his arm against his side (neutral abduction); this prevents the shoulder from abducting to accommodate for the stiff elbow, which would produce a false measurement.

The examiner should look for obvious abnormalities, such as the irregular "Popeye" bulge caused by a ruptured biceps tendon, or a large effusion of the joint, such as occurs with a fractured radial head. Olecranon bursitis, rheumatoid nodules, and gouty tophi also are easily recognized.

Palpation. The normal bony landmarks of the elbow that are commonly involved in injuries should be palpated. The examiner should look for tenderness, first over the lateral and medial epicondyles, which are easily located, and then over the attachment sites of the wrist extensors and flexors. These sites are tender in patients with tendonitis. In severe cases a gap may be palpable where the tendon has been disrupted. The physician should palpate for degenerative spurs, and over the olecranon process for bursitis or spurring.

Effusions of the elbow are best palpated over the anconeus muscle, in the triangle defined by the lateral epicondyle, the radial head, and the tip of the olecranon. The biceps tendon attachment also should be palpated (resisted supination can make this configuration more prominent). The examiner

should press the radial head with passive supination and pronation to evaluate for a fracture.

While ranging the elbow, the examiner should palpate the ulnar nerve in the cubital tunnel to check for subluxation of this structure. The examiner also should test for Tinel's sign by percussing over the nerve in the tunnel in an attempt to recreate the patient's symptoms.

Function. Because the forearm muscles attach at the elbow, grip strength should be tested in a patient with elbow pain. Strength, which is diminished in most elbow injuries, is a good guide in assessing the patient's recovery and readiness to return to work.

The patient should be asked to perform resisted wrist flexion and extension; with medial or lateral epicondylitis, these movements are weakened and painful. The forearm circumference can be measured to assess muscle atrophy.

The medial and lateral collateral ligaments are tested for instability by applying varus or valgus stress across the elbow, with the joint slightly flexed to unlock the bony articulation.

Common injuries and disorders

It is useful to divide work-related elbow injuries into two categories: *traumatic overuse* or *degenerative conditions.**

Overuse injuries account for the largest percentage of injuries on the job. These include primarily tendinopathies (medial and lateral epicondylitis, the most common elbow problems in the workplace) and neuropathies (radial tunnel syndrome, cubital tunnel syndrome).

Degenerative injuries (stiff elbow, arthritic elbow, or an elbow with a loose body) are more difficult to attribute to work-related causes because of their insidious onset. However, subtle evidence suggests that long-term, repetitive microtrauma can lead to degenerative changes.

Lateral elbow pain. Lateral epicondylitis is most common in middle-aged workers (the peak incidence occurs among individuals in their forties). The condition typically involves the origin of the extensor carpi radialis brevis tendon at the lateral epicondyle of the elbow.[8] Occupations that pose a particular risk are carpentry, plumbing, typing, writing, and other grip-intensive activities.

Diagnosis. The patient usually points directly to the lateral aspect of the elbow as the source of pain, although in advanced cases joint effusion may accompany the syndrome, making the pain more diffuse. In chronic cases a loss of motion

---

* Traumatic injuries (fractures, lacerations, dislocations) usually are not work-specific and are treated in much the same way as acute injuries from other causes.

may occur, and a 10- to 15-degree flexion contracture may be present. These patients are exquisitely tender directly over the lateral epicondyle at the origin of the extensor mass. In severe cases inflammation may lead to partial disruption of the tendon, and an actual small defect may be palpable, although this is rare. Bony changes may occur, creating a palpable spur at the epicondyle, but this, too, is rare.

Differential diagnosis. Radial tunnel syndrome is the only disorder that can easily be confused with lateral epicondylitis. Radial tunnel syndrome is caused by compression of the deep branch of the radial nerve approximately 3 to 4 cm distal and 1 cm anterior to the lateral epicondyle in the radial tunnel. Compression may be caused by the edge of the supinator (the arcade of Frohse; see Fig. 9-25), the tendinous margin of the extensor carpi radialis brevis, by the recurrent branch of the radial artery, or by a fibrous band in the area of the radial head. The tenderness usually is more distal than in lateral epicondylitis, and a nerve conduction test may show polyphasic potentials.

A subtle diagnostic finding is proximal forearm pain upon resisted extension of the middle finger. An injection of lidocaine into the radial tunnel can help confirm this diagnosis. Because this syndrome does not compromise the sensory branch of the radial nerve, there are no sensory deficits.

Nondisplaced fractures of the radial head and neck also can be misleading if they manifest as lateral elbow pain. However, unlike with lateral epicondylitis, the patient usually has a history of trauma, and he may have swelling and ecchymosis. In these cases tenderness is localized directly over the radial head, distal to the lateral epicondyle.

Treatment. If left untreated, lateral epicondylitis gradually resolves over a 2-year period. However, most patients cannot tolerate the symptoms this long, and most (95%) respond to conservative treatment. This treatment usually can be divided into three stages.

STAGE 1. Initial treatment consists of having the patient apply ice to the elbow, take NSAIDs for pain, and modify his activities. The patient should avoid gripping activities, particularly in pronation, to prevent continuous reinjury. If gripping is necessary for work, a compression tennis elbow strap is used to minimize repetitive trauma to the tendon insertion. It is thought that this strap works by functionally creating a more distal anchoring site for the extensor tendons and by reducing the load on the inflamed proximal tendon attachment. Electromyographic (EMG) studies using an inflatable elbow strap have shown reduced proximal muscle activity. Conditions resistant to these measures sometimes are relieved by deep friction massage or iontophoresis, although the latter treatment is expensive and not always effective.

Patients in this stage are allowed to continue working, but they should be taught ways to modify lifting and gripping techniques to prevent recurrence.

STAGE 2. In this stage, steroid injections around the extensor attachment are helpful, but repeated use has been associated with degenerative changes in the tendon. Injections generally should be reserved for cases in which stage 1 treatment fails. Two or possibly three injections are given at 3-month intervals.

Workers with a stage 2 condition usually are given 1 to 2 weeks of light duty and a wrist splint to forestall gripping activities. A progressive exercise program of isotonic wrist flexion and extension is then begun.

STAGE 3. If the condition resists conservative treatment for longer than 6 months, the patient is considered a candidate for surgery. If no spurring is seen on x-ray films and there is no palpable gap in the tendon, the patient may be able to undergo release of the extensor attachment in the office, a technique that is successful in more than 90% of cases. The procedure is performed in the examining room using local anesthesia. A Band-Aid is applied to the wound, and the patient is back at work in less than a week.[38] However, if bony excrescences are seen on the x-ray film at the lateral epicondyle, open release and debridement are recommended.

Medial elbow pain. When an injured worker complains of medial elbow pain, three basic diagnoses should be considered: medial epicondylitis, instability of the medial collateral ligament, or cubital tunnel syndrome.

Medial epicondylitis. Medial epicondylitis, which is much less common than lateral epicondylitis, is caused by a tendonopathy at the origin of the flexor carpi radialis or the pronator teres where they attach to the medial epicondyle of the elbow. Golfers, throwers, and workers who grip and lift heavy loads are at risk of developing the disorder.

The condition is diagnosed by palpating over the medial epicondyle, which should recreate the patient's symptoms. Resisted pronation and wrist flexion also should elicit pain. Grip strength is diminished on dynamometer testing, but usually less than with lateral epicondylitis.

TREATMENT. The treatment of medial epicondylitis is similar to that for lateral epicondylitis. Initial measures include applying ice, use of NSAIDs, and modifying activities. If the condition does not improve, the patient should be restricted to light duties or taken off work temporarily and given a cortisone injection. The injection should be given *around* the tendon, not directly into it. Care must be taken to avoid the adjacent ulnar nerve. Frequent injections are not recommended, because they can lead to rupture of the tendon; no more than two or three injections should be given over a year's time. In rare cases a patient will require surgical release and debridement.

Injury of the medial collateral ligament. A much less common cause of medial elbow pain is instability stemming from an acute or chronic injury to the medial collateral ligament. These patients are tender along the ligament, but this is difficult to differentiate from tenderness in the overlying flexor muscle mass or from medial epicondylitis. The diagnosis is made by demonstrating laxity to valgus stress on examination. A lidocaine injection to relieve pain may facilitate the examination. In severe cases laxity may also be demonstrated on x-ray films by having the patient hold his arm in maximum external rotation over the edge of the table. Gravity provides a valgus stress, and the x-ray film will show the medial joint space gaping open.

TREATMENT. Acute injuries of the medial collateral ligament are treated with rest and immobilization. In chronic cases with documented instability, surgical reconstruction of the ligament may be necessary.

Cubital tunnel syndrome. Cubital tunnel syndrome is treated with NSAIDs and protection of the nerve. Workers who lean on their elbows are given elbow pads. Night splinting of the elbow occasionally helps. A subluxing ulnar nerve or a true compression neuropathy may resist conservative treatment and require surgical neurolysis and transposition of the nerve to a protected submuscular position.

Anterior elbow pain. Distal biceps tendonitis is uncommon but may occur in a heavy laborer as a result of repetitive elbow flexion and heavy carrying. Tenderness is present over the tendon's insertion site at the radial tuberosity. The patient also may have a loss of terminal elbow extension. Treatment consists of applying ice, rest, and use of NSAIDs, followed by a stretching and strengthening program. Disability is rare unless rupture occurs.

Avulsion of the distal biceps attachment is rare and usually the result of a sudden heavy extension force on a flexed elbow. The patient may or may not have a prior history of tendonitis. The diagnosis is fairly obvious, with severe pain, swelling, ecchymosis, a palpable defect in the antecubital region, and a balled-up, contracted tendon. Surgical repair should restore strength and is recom-

mended, especially for laborers. A loss of extension is not uncommon.

Trauma. A fall onto the outstretched hand is the most common mechanism of fracture for the elbow, although a direct blow to the elbow occasionally occurs. In general, the occupational medicine practitioner is not asked to treat severe intraarticular fractures of the elbow; these are the purview of a specialist and are not discussed in this chapter.

Fractures of the radial head are common and also are caused by a fall onto the outstretched hand. These fractures often are difficult to visualize on the initial x-ray films, and follow-up films after 2 weeks or a bone scan may be needed to verify the break. Occasionally the only sign on a x-ray film is a prominent posterior fat pad, which indicates bleeding in the joint (Fig. 9-26).

The patient is tender directly over the radial head, effusion is palpable, and ecchymosis may be present. Range of motion is limited by pain and hemarthrosis. The diagnosis can be confirmed clinically by aspirating the elbow and verifying the hemarthrosis; this procedure may also significantly relieve the pain. The landmark for aspiration is the triangle formed by the lateral epicondyle, the tip of the olecranon, and the radial head. A needle inserted into this triangle enters the joint through the anconeus muscle.

If the fracture is only minimal or not displaced, it is best treated by aspirating the joint, injecting a local anesthetic, and having the patient begin range-of-motion exercises as soon as the pain al-

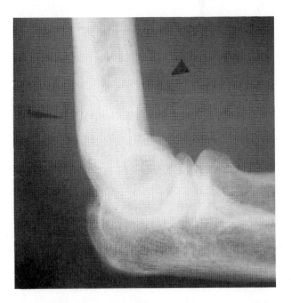

Fig. 9-26 Lateral x-ray film of the elbow of a patient with an occult radial head fracture, showing prominent anterior and posterior fat pads.

lows. He also should be given a sling for a few days for comfort. The most common complication of this injury is loss of motion. In more severe fractures, with significant displacement of fragments, surgical reduction and fixation are recommended. If reduction is impossible, excision of the radial head may be necessary.

Dislocation of the elbow is uncommon but quite dramatic in appearance. It usually results from a fall onto the outstretched hand with the elbow slightly bent. In the most common type of dislocation, the olecranon moves posteriorly, although other types are possible. Initial treatment requires an x-ray film and a careful neurovascular examination to rule out associated injuries. To reduce the dislocation, the patient is placed in the prone position, and traction is applied with the elbow bent 90 degrees off the end of a table. Immobilization at 90 degrees is enforced for 2 to 3 weeks, and then range-of-motion exercises are begun. Redislocation or residual instability is extremely rare, and an overall satisfactory result can be expected by 6 months. The patient may have permanent loss of terminal extension, but strength and function should otherwise allow him to return to work.

Degenerative disease. Degenerative elbow disease is difficult to attribute to a work-related injury, although acute trauma may exacerbate an underlying degenerative process, and therefore may be accountable to some degree by apportionment. Degenerative disease of the elbow is relatively rare and most often seen in patients with a history of previous trauma or excessive abuse of the joint from sports activities (e.g., baseball pitchers).

These patients usually have reduced range of motion in the elbow, but they often have no other symptoms until a loose body arises from the displacement of an osteophyte, which may be caused by acute trauma. Treatment usually involves removing the loose body arthroscopically and debriding the degenerative joint. The potential for return to work in this situation is good. Elbow replacement may be necessary for severe degenerative disease, but this is highly unusual.

Olecranon bursitis. Inflammation of the bursa of the olecranon may be acute or chronic and inflammatory or septic. It may be caused by acute trauma or repetitive stress, but a direct fall onto the elbow is the most common cause. Acute olecranon bursitis usually is marked by a swollen, erythematous, painful bursa and difficulty moving the elbow because of pain from stretching of the bursa. The elbow joint itself is not involved. Treatment consists of applying ice to the area, using NSAIDs, immobilizing the joint, and rest. A padded elbow brace also may be helpful.

Infectious bursitis may occur as a result of direct inoculation from a skin abrasion or from secondary hematogenous seeding. Occasionally it may be difficult to differentiate a severely inflamed, sterile bursitis from an early infection. When the diagnosis is unclear, the bursal fluid should be aspirated and cultured, and the patient should be treated with antibiotics and an antiinflammatory drug until the culture results are available.

Care should be taken to use meticulous sterile techniques, because iatrogenic infection of a previously sterile bursa is not uncommon.

A patient with septic bursitis is treated with antibiotics, and frequent follow-up visits are scheduled. If the condition does not resolve quickly, incision and debridement of the bursa is indicated.

Olecranon bursitis may also occur in conjunction with systemic inflammatory conditions such as gout and rheumatoid arthritis. A thorough history should reveal such an illness, and treatment should involve both the systemic and local disorders.

Loose bodies. Loose bodies in the elbow arise from one of three sources: osteochondral fragments produced by a fracture; displaced osteophytes or joint fragments caused by degenerative disease; and, in rare cases, synovial proliferation. Loose bodies are most commonly seen in the elbows of former pitchers, gymnasts, and other athletes who placed high demands on their elbows in their youth. Asymptomatic loose bodies are not treated. If the patient complains of loss of motion, catching, or pain, the loose bodies should be removed arthroscopically; the prognosis is excellent.

REFERENCES

1. Askew LJ, An KN, Morrey BF, Chao EY: Functional evaluation of the elbow: normal motion requirements and strength determination, *Orthop Trans* 5:304, 1981.
2. Awad EA: Interstitial myofibrosis: hypothesis of mechanism, *Arch Phys Med Rehabil* 54:449-453, 1973.
3. Bigliani LU, Morrison D, April EW: The morphology of the acromion and its relationship to rotator cuff tears, *Orthop Trans* 10:228, 1986.
4. Bjelle A, Hagberg M, Michaelson G: Occupational and individual factors in acute shoulder-neck disorders among industrial workers, *Br J Ind Med* 38:356-363, 1981.
5. Bjorksten M, Itani T, Jonsson B, Yoshizawa M: Evaluation of muscular load in shoulder and forearm muscles among medical secretaries during occupational typing and some nonoccupational activities. In Jonsson B, editor: *Biomechanics X,* Baltimore, 1987, University Park Press.
6. Chapman LJ: Work-rest schedules in light industrial and office work (contract no 86-71383), Cincinnati, 1986, National Institute of Occupational Safety and Health.
7. Colachis SC, Strohm BR: The effects of suprascapular and axillary nerve blocks on muscle force in the upper extremity, *Arch Phys Med Rehabil* 52:22-29, 1971.
8. Coonrad RW: Tendonopathies at the elbow, 40:Chapter 4 Vol XL American Academy of Orthopedic Surgeons, 1991.

9. Funderbunk CF, Hipskind SG, Welton RC, Lind AR: Development and recovery from fatigue induced by static efforts at various tensions, *J Appl Physiol* 37:302-396, 1974.

10. Hagberg M, Sundelin G: Discomfort and load on the upper trapezius muscle when operating a word processor, *Ergonomics* 29:1637-1645, 1986.

11. Hagberg M, Michaelson G, Ortelius A: Serum creatinine kinase as an indicator of local muscular strain in experimental and occupational work, *Int Arch Occup Environ Health* 50:377-386, 1982.

12. Halbrecht J, Wolf E: Office arthroscopy of the shoulder, *Orthop Clin North Am* 24(1):193-200, 1993.

13. Hammond G, Torgerson W, Dotter W, Leach R: The painful shoulder, *Instr Course Lect* 20:83-90, 1971.

14. Herberts P, Kadefors R, Hogfors C, Sigholm G: Shoulder pain and heavy manual labor, *Clin Orthop* 191:166-178, 1984.

15. Howell SM, Imobersteg AM, Segar DH, Marone PJ: Clarification of the role of the supraspinatus muscle in shoulder function, *J Bone Joint Surg* 68:398-404, 1986.

16. Inman VT, Saunders JR, Abbot LC: Observations on the function of the shoulder joint, *J Bone Joint Surg* 26:1, 1944.

17. Katevuo K, Aitasalo K, Lehtinen R, Piettila J: Skeletal changes in dentists and farmers in Finland, *Community Dent Oral Epidemiol* 13:23-25, 1985.

18. Kiesler S, Finholt T: The myster of RSI, *Am Psychol* 43:1004-1015, 1988.

19. Luck JV, Andersson GB: Occupational shoulder disorders. In Rockwood CA, editor: *The shoulder,* Philadelphia, 1990, WB Saunders.

20. Luopajarvi T, Kuorinka I, Virolainen M, Holmberg M: Prevalence of tenosynovitis and other injuries of the upper extremities in repetitive work, *Scand J Work Environ Health* (suppl) 3:48-55, 1979.

21. McDermott F: Repetitive strain injuries, a review of current understanding, *Med J Aust* 144:196-200, 1986.

22. Morrey BF, Askew LJ, An KN, Chao EY: A biomechanical study of normal functional elbow motion, *J Bone Joint Surg* 63A(6):872, 1981.

23. Ohara H, Aoyama H, Itani T: Health hazards among cash register operators and the effects of improved working conditions, *J Hum Ergol* 5:31-40, 1976.

24. Onishi N, Sakai K, Kogi K: Arm and shoulder muscle load in various keyboard operating jobs of women, *J Hum Ergol* 11:89-97, 1982.

25. Poppen NK, Walker PS: Normal and abnormal motion of the shoulder, *J Bone Joint Surg* 58A:195, 1976.

26. Rathburn JB, McNab I: The microvascular pattern of the rotator cuff, *J Bone Joint Surg (Br)* 52:540-553, 1970.

27. Rohmert W: Problems in determining rest allowances, *Appl Ergonomics* 4:91-95, 1973.

28. Rowe CR: Prognosis in dislocations of the shoulder, *J Bone Joint Surg* 38A:957-997, 1956.

29. Rowe CR, Patel D, Southmayd WW: The Bankart procedure: a long-term, end-result study, *J Bone Joint Surg* 60A:1-16, 1978.

30. Stone WE: Repetitive strain injuries, *Med J Aust* 2:616-618, 1983.

31. Taylor R, Pitcher M: Medical and ergonomic aspects of an industrial dispute concerning occupational-related conditions in data process operators, *Community Health Studies* 8:172-180, 1984.

10 Neck and Thoracic Spine Disorders

Occupational injuries to the cervical and thoracic region can vary from the most benign and self-limited soft tissue types to the truly serious, such as spinal cord and crush injuries. Fortunately, the relatively benign soft tissue injuries far outnumber the more serious ones. An important skill for the occupational medicine specialist is the ability to separate them on initial clinical examination; unfortunately, this is not always as simple as the physician would like.

ANATOMY
Cervical vertebrae

The cervical spine is designed to provide relatively extensive amounts of movement and positioning. The downside of such mobility is a lack of the more rigid structural support present in the thoracic spine. The head has been compared to a bowling ball sitting on top of the cervical spine bones, and therefore is highly vulnerable.

The cervical spine's unique bony configuration allows certain movements to be coupled with specific spinal segments. There is little rotation between the atlas and occiput; rotation takes place primarily between the atlas and axis (C1 and C2). Significant flexion and extension is allowed between the occiput and atlas and through the remaining cervical vertebrae below C2. This lower cervical spine region, however, has only minimal rotation. Approximately 80 degrees of cervical rotation in each direction and 200 degrees of flexion/extension motion are permitted.

The intervertebral discs in the cervical spine act as a shock-absorbing mechanism and a form of structural support. The soft intradisc nuclear fluid allows transition of compressive forces and displacement across the disc to reduce mechanical stress. Strong attachments between the vertebral body end plates and the annular disc fibers provide important structural support at each level. The alignment and pattern of attachment of these elastic disc fibers allows motion between segments.

Ligaments

Powerful ligamentous structures of the cervical spine act to permit and prevent motion in various planes. The anterior longitudinal ligament along the anterior aspect of the vertebral bodies resists hyperextension. The posterior longitudinal ligament and ligamentum flavum similarly act to prevent hyperflexion. The posterior longitudinal ligament also acts to protect the neural canal from encroachment by nuclear disc material. An associated complex of supra and interspinous ligaments posteriorly also act to provide structural support to the cervical spine.

Cervical joints

The cervical facet joints act to restrict lateral bending while permitting motion in other directions. A series of joints include the uncovertebral joints and the true cervical facet joints. The uncovertebral joints are not true synovial joints per se, but result from the shape of the vertebral bodies. The joints also provide a weight-bearing surface.

Spinal canal and cord

The spinal cord is well protected within the central portion of the cervical spinal canal. The cord itself normally occupies approximately one third of the available room in the central canal. It is important for the clinician to be quite familiar also with the various patterns of dermatomal distribution of the cervical nerve roots and the myotomal distribution. With the possible exception of the rhomboid muscles that appear to be primarily C5 innervated, the remaining upper extremity muscles involve innervation from two and typically three nerve roots. The innervation pattern follows general guidelines, but may vary from one individual to the next.

Brachial plexus

The brachial plexus is far more complex in terms of the overlapping patterns and distributions and alignment of the various neural elements. The upper trunk of the brachial plexus includes primarily the C5 and C6 nerves. The middle trunk involves primarily the C7 nerve. The lower trunk is a combination of primarily the C8 and T1 nerves. See Fig. 10-1.

Muscles

The superficial muscular structures (the rhomboids, trapezius, scalenes, and levator scapulae)

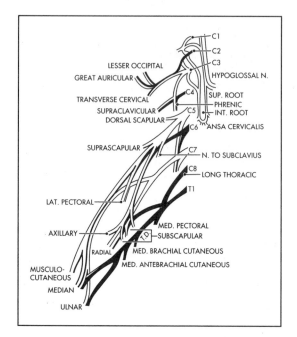

LESSER OCCIPITAL
GREAT AURICULAR
TRANSVERSE CERVICAL
SUPRACLAVICULAR
DORSAL SCAPULAR
SUPRASCAPULAR
LAT. PECTORAL
AXILLARY
RADIAL
MUSCULO-CUTANEOUS
MEDIAN
ULNAR

C1
C2
C3
HYPOGLOSSAL N.
C4
SUP. ROOT
PHRENIC
C5
INT. ROOT
C6
ANSA CERVICALIS
C7
N. TO SUBCLAVIUS
C8
LONG THORACIC
T1
MED. PECTORAL
SUBSCAPULAR
MED. BRACHIAL CUTANEOUS
MED. ANTEBRACHIAL CUTANEOUS

Fig. 10-1 Simplified scheme of cervical and brachial plexuses, showing the distribution of nerve fibers in the roots of origin. Brachial plexus based partly on Seddon; T. D., thoracodorsal. (Reprinted with permission from JE Rodriguez: Anatomy of the cervical spine. In J Regan, editor, *Spine state of the art reviews: cervical spine disease,* 1991, Hanley & Belfus, p. 162.)

are common sites of pain complaints. The deeper cervical spinal musculature includes the erector spinae, suboccipital, splenius, and other deep muscles. Injuries to these structures can occur acutely and chronically.

Thoracic spine

The thoracic spine, a rigid structure, is typically more resistant to injury. The very narrow neural canal in the thoracic spine, however, leaves little functional reserve for the spinal cord. Injuries here are far more devastating in terms of neurologic consequences should the spinal cord itself become compromised. The patterns of recovery and potential for significant recovery after thoracic spinal cord injury are generally considered quite poor.

The vascular supply to the spinal cord, particularly in the midthoracic region, is considered a watershed area with little collateral blood supply. This compounds the potential for devastating consequences when the spinal cord is damaged in this region.

The patient with persistent thoracic pain of an unexplained origin needs to be considered quite carefully because of the high frequency of more serious underlying medical problems. These in-

clude complaints of cardiac and pulmonary origins and metastatic disease to the spine. The individual nerve roots are well-protected in the thoracic spine and are rarely affected without significant injury to the thoracic region in general. The same holds true for the thoracic intervertebral discs. The ligamentous structures here have a great deal of support from the local bony structures and are less of a source of pain complaints in comparison to the cervical spine.

The thoracic spine is a major area for referral pain from the cervical spine in particular. The latissimus muscles, for example, from C5, C6, and C7 can often be a source of referred pain from the patient with cervical irritation. It is also quite common for the diffuse soft tissue/myofascial pain patterns of the cervical spine to be associated with thoracic involvement. Careful attempts should be made to reproduce thoracic pain by cervical maneuvers when the source of pain is unknown.

KEYS TO THE MEDICAL HISTORY

The specific mechanism of injury gives the clinician an early sense as to the underlying source of the patient's complaint. The patient who presents, for example, with a hyperflexion injury should be considered a candidate for possible discogenic injury due to the compressive loading of the disc during hyperflexion. In contrast, the patient with a hyperextension pattern of injury will often load the cervical facet joints. Obviously the patient with major traumatic injury needs to be considered for a more serious underlying process such as a fracture. The patient with more chronic, insidious complaints often will show findings of underlying degenerative disc disease, chronic facet joint changes and facet arthropathy, and significant soft tissue restrictions from loss of musculoligamentous flexibility. These are also the patients in whom a postural mechanism as a significant underlying source of pain needs to be evaluated carefully. Understanding the mechanism of injury, when possible, can focus the evaluation in many ways.

The severity of pain is often a poor indicator of the severity of the underlying injury, although the patient who presents with severe complaints needs to be taken seriously until proven otherwise. Multiple factors play into the patient's pain complaints: anxiety, cultural issues, the extent of the injury itself, or issues related to secondary gain. The examining physician therefore needs to assess the patient's subjective complaints with this in mind.

A key historical point in the cervical spine is the issue of radiating symptoms into the upper extremities. This is less a factor in thoracic spine injuries due to the lower likelihood of nerve root involvement. Pain can be referred on a neurogenic or sclerotomal basis, or in the typical diffuse patterns seen in myofascial pain complaints. The patient's complaints of referred pain must be carefully reviewed for the pattern.

Complaints of numbness, tingling, or weakness suggest a neurologic basis. This can be confirmed in some cases on the physical examination. The absence of objective findings on physical examination, however, does not disprove the possibility of referred neurologic complaints. The correlation between the objective findings and the subjective complaints is particularly important. In the patient with suspected spinal cord injury, any history of transient quadriparesis or quadriparesthesia is quite important. The patient who presents with complaints of lower extremity symptoms must be considered as potentially having spinal cord involvement.

A general review of systems can be valuable in assessing the extent and nature of the patient's complaints. Systemic complaints such as fever, chills, sweats, or weight loss may point to a medical source as a possible etiology. Particularly important in the patient with cervical and thoracic injury is the history of any bowel or bladder complaints, suggesting spinal cord injury. This includes not only incontinence, but particularly bladder frequency, urgency, hesitancy, or sense of incomplete voiding. A general review of possible associated risks factors would include a history of smoking, use of alcohol, and drug use. Alcohol and drug use are particularly important issues that need to be addressed when assessing potential for a work-related injury and the legal issues that might arise.

Psychosocial factors are also important in reviewing possible causes for patients' complaints of pain. A history of anxiety, low energy, poor appetite, sleep disturbance, early morning awakening, loss of interest in activities, and forgetfulness can all be associated with psychological factors that may play an important part in the patient's symptoms. Although a complete psychiatric history is not reasonable in this setting, basic screening for serious psychological risk factors should be included.

An important issue in the work setting relates to the presence or absence of similar complaints in the past. The patient, for example, who presents with a history of longstanding neck and upper back pain that is attributed to a work setting without a specific witnessed injury must also be looked at cautiously. This is not an uncommon problem. Such data can be valuable for the employer and workers' compensation carrier in assessing the acceptance of the claim as a valid workers' compensation injury. Oftentimes the medical history will change over time.

A review of the patient's work activities and job requirements can also be quite valuable, since a decision must be made about returning the patient to the work setting, either with full or restricted duty. Patients often are not the best historians when describing the nature of the demands of their job. When dealing with the patient on a long-term basis, a formal job description can often be of help, although the patient, in some cases, may provide more accurate information than the formal job description. Attempts to return a patient with neck and upper back pain to repetitive overhead lifting, frequent twisting and turning of the neck, or prolonged postural stress will often meet with a poor result. If modifications and adjustments can be made to allow the patient to work temporarily avoiding the deleterious activities, he can often be returned to the work setting much more quickly. The medical literature reports that the longer a patient remains out of work the less likely he is to return to his previous employment, or in many cases to any kind of reasonable employment. Early return to work promotes recovery, and attempts should be made to do so early with a comprehensive plan.

One problem that may arise in the medical/legal setting is a relationship between initial complaints and symptoms that appear later. It is not uncommon for the patient who presents with an initial neck injury to ascribe later complaints in other parts of the body to the original injury. The use of a pain drawing can be invaluable so that the patient has the opportunity to outline the nature of his complaints. It can also be helpful in expediting the history for the clinician, as it allows the examiner to focus more quickly on the nature of the patient's symptoms. Pain drawings are also beneficial when nonanatomical and nonphysiologic drawings suggest psychological factors or malingering.

One of the most valuable pieces of information that can be obtained is an assessment of the patient's job satisfaction. Probably no other single factor is associated with potential to return to work than the presence or absence of general job satisfaction.

When the patient is seen in the subacute or chronic setting, a review of past therapeutic efforts can also be helpful. Returning patients to unsuccessful treatment will, unless carefully reviewed with the patient as to the rationale, lead to dissatisfaction. This may push the patient toward doctor-shopping or noncompliance.

Without a history of major trauma, there is no great urgency in completing an extensive medical workup. The history is valuable in identifying those patients with potential neurologic complaints, particularly spinal cord involvement, and medical causes such as angina, or dissecting aortic aneurysm that can often be masquerading as a musculoskeletal problem. Finally, the medical history is valuable in identifying potential conflicts and starting the patient toward a program of treatment and early return to full function.

KEYS TO THE CLINICAL EXAMINATION

The physical examination is used to rule out or confirm diagnosis from the patient's history or to screen for more serious underlying pathology. The physical examination must be directed toward specific patient complaints and must follow a careful routine so that significant findings are not overlooked. The usual regimen should include inspection, palpation, range-of-motion testing, neurologic examination, and specific maneuvers to confirm the possibility of other clinical syndromes. See Table 10-1.

Inspection

The patient should be examined for body habitus, posture, and overall level of conditioning. This can be a tip-off to perpetuating or exacerbating factors that may be a component of the clinical complaints. The patient who sits with a slumped, head-forward posture and who is obese and deconditioned is at high risk for significant long-term problems. The patient also should be evaluated for specific structural abnormalities including scoliosis and kyphosis.

The patient's general behavior is an important key during a clinical examination. The patient who presents as anxious or depressed may require further evaluation of potential associated psychological factors. The patient's level of consistency in reporting complaints and behavior throughout the examination may point toward presence or absence of true organic pathologic conditions. Many patients, for example, appear to be able to move freely and look around the room when distracted, but on formal range-of-motion testing, show guarding that was not evident when casually observed. This must be taken into consideration when making a final assessment of the patient's condition. The patient who presents with a history of an acute traumatic injury should be carefully evaluated for such signs as swelling, bruising, or abrasions that may confirm the clinical complaints. Absence of such findings that otherwise are expected to be present also will alert the clinician to possible discrepancies.

Palpation

Palpation is specifically designed to evaluate areas of tenderness and muscle spasm. Tenderness is primarily subjective in nature, but hypersensitivity may be a tip-off to psychogenic factors that are in play. Palpation of painful areas can, of course, also be helpful in confirming possible specific sources of pain—the facet joints, occipital nerves, or spinous processes, for example. Muscle spasm provides strong confirmation as to the reliability of the patient's complaints. Muscle spasm, in itself, however, is relatively nonspecific; a variety of causes can lead to secondary muscle spasm. The palpation of the cervical, supraclavicular, and axillary areas for the presence of lymphadenopathy should be routinely included in examining the spinal patient. When part of the clinician's routine examination, palpation can be accomplished relatively quickly and can often identify more serious problems early on.

Range of motion

There is significant controversy regarding the clinical value of testing range of motion. There is little in the medical literature to suggest that changes in range of motion are reliable indicators of the severity of the patient's underlying complaints or indicative of any specific underlying disorder. Range-of-motion testing, however, is part of the assessment of disability rating in the medical/legal setting and should be part of the routine examination. Many states require range-of-motion testing for disability rating, and the American Medical Association (AMA) Guidelines for Evaluation of Permanent Impairment include range-of-motion loss as an important component in the disability examination.

Pain with various maneuvers on range-of-motion testing can be helpful in evaluating specific areas of discomfort and injury. The patient who has pain upon extension and rotation of the cervical spine in one direction may often have problems related to facet irritation or intervertebral canal narrowing in that region. A variety of more sophisticated methods other than simple visual examination and recording range of motion have been used. Some methods are more reliable than simple visual inspection, but all have potential problems in their reliability. A recent example is the use of inclinometers in determining accurate and reliable ranges of spinal motion. This is incorporated routinely now in the AMA guidelines, third edition.

Neurologic examination

The neurologic exam typically comprises motor, sensory, and reflex testing. Other special maneuvers are available as well in assessing neurologic function.

Motor testing relies, in part, upon the patient's cooperation, especially if accurate muscle-grading is to be accomplished. Some patients exhibit weakness secondary to anxiety, pain inhibition, or malingering. Weakness should be recorded as true weakness, or a thorough description of the weakness should be included. This might include such descriptions as "ratchety," "pain-inhibited," or "give-away" patterns of weakness. Visible muscular atrophy that is measurable (particularly if asymmetric) can be an important indicator of true muscle weakness. It is important to understand that significant neurologic loss can take place before clinical weakness is actually noted. It has been reported in some studies that up to 40% of axons must be lost before true clinical weakness is

apparent. For medical-legal purposes, recording of any atrophy in comparison to the opposite side, particularly in the extremities, should be noted. Visible fasciculations may also confirm neurologic involvement. These can be the result of either central nervous system (CNS) or peripheral nerve involvement. Patients with widespread muscular fasciculations may often have an underlying CNS disorder such as motor neuron disease. Abnormal muscle tone such as spasticity may also indicate CNS involvement. Familiarity with the pattern of the various nerve roots and innervation of individual nerves is essential.

Sensory testing can be carried out in a variety of ways to look for neural dysfunction. Pain reaction to sharp–dull testing, light touch, vibration, position sense, and heat and cold are all used. Typical clinical screening, however, involves the use of

---

Table 10-1 Classification of head and neck pain

I. Intrinsic causes of musculoskeletal pain

1. Skeletal abnormalities
   A. Fracture
   B. Neoplasm, primary or metastatic
   C. Infection, osteomyelitis
   D. Paget's disease
   E. Osteoporosis
   F. Endocrinologic, hyperparathyroidism
   G. Hematologic, sickle cell, multiple myeloma
2. Joint abnormalities
   A. Synovitis, capsulitis, discitis
   B. Joint effusion, hemarthrosis
   C. Osteoarthritis
   D. Rheumatic disease, rheumatic arthritis
   E. Disc derangements
   F. Joint instability, ligamentous laxity
   G. Neoplasms, primary or metastatic
3. Ligaments
   A. Trauma, sprains, rupture
   B. Chronic laxity
   C. Contracture
   D. Neoplasms
   E. Infection

4. Muscles, tendons, fascia
   A. Myofascial pain, fibromyalgia
   B. Trauma, strains, tears, ruptures
   C. Inflammatory conditions, polymyositis
   D. Infectious conditions, trichinosis
   E. Polymyalgia rheumatica
   F. Vasculitides
   G. Ischemic claudication, compartment syndrome
   H. Neoplasms
   I. Contracture, biomechanical abnormalities
   J. Overuse syndromes
   K. Nutritional avitaminosis
   L. Toxins, venom
5. Nerve structures (added for completeness)
   A. Entrapment, compression
   B. Trauma, stretch, laceration
   C. Deafferentation, neuromas
   D. Reflex sympathetic dystrophy, causalgia
   E. Neuritis, neuralgia, tics
   F. Peripheral neuropathy, diabetes, toxins
   G. Ischemia, vasculitis
   H. Infection, herpes, AIDS

II. Extrinsic causes of musculoskeletal pain

Other organs referring pain to the musculoskeletal system
A. Heart: myocardial infarction, angina
B. Lungs: pleuritis, tumors (especially Pancoast's tumor)
C. Eyes: infection, strain
D. Ears: infection, tumors
E. Nose and sinus: infection, abscess, tumors
F. Throat and teeth: infection, tumors
G. Central nervous system: syringomyelia, Arnold-Chiari syndrome, spasmotic torticollis, tumors (especially acoustic neuromas, neurofibromas, and other slow-growing tumors), infections, vascular abnormalities and accidents, supratentorial factors

---

From CD Schwab: *Musculoskeletal pain: physical medicine and rehabilitation: state of the art reviews. Referred pain syndromes of the head and neck.* S Gnatz, Hanley and Belfus, Philadelphia, 1991, p. 590, with permission.

light touch or sharp–dull sensation. Caution must be used with pinwheels that can potentially draw blood and transmit infectious disease. They pose no problem if run very lightly over the limb, and are disinfected between use. Use of a disposable sterilized needle is an alternative. A 25-gauge needle will usually suffice. Although largely subjective in nature, sensory testing has an important objective component: the correlation between the patient's symptoms and known anatomical patterns of sensory distributions. The patient, for example, with circumferential loss of sensation in one limb will typically represent a nonphysiologic pattern of loss.

Deep tendon reflexes should be evaluated for their absolute value also in comparison to the opposite side. Hyporeflexia typically represents involvement of a nerve root or peripheral nerve; hyperreflexia suggests central nervous system involvement. Babinski, Hoffmann's, and clonus testing should also be routinely included in evaluating the cervical and thoracic patient. Asymmetry of reflex changes or the presence of long tract signs is far more reliable than a generalized mild increase or decrease in reflexes. Reflex examination is one of the few truly objective findings to rely on.

The patient with cervical and thoracic complaints should also routinely undergo a screening examination of both shoulders. It is not at all uncommon for shoulder pain to be referred from the cervical or thoracic spine. Early identification of shoulder involvement can be helpful in preventing long-term complications and confusion about the nature of the clinical diagnosis. Range-of-motion testing of the shoulder, actively and passively, and palpation over the primary shoulder structures should be carried out. When doubt arises, a more thorough shoulder examination can then be undertaken. (See Chapter 9 on the shoulder.)

Other more specialized cervical and thoracic examinations include Adson's maneuver for evaluation of thoracic outlet syndrome, evaluation of the scapula for winging or asymmetry of motion, testing for Tinel's sign or tenderness over specific peripheral nerves such as at the carpal tunnel or ulnar groove, and the use of Waddell's sign for assessment of patient reliability, in terms of psychogenic factors or malingering. (The association, however, between Waddell's findings and long-term functional outcome such as return to work remains controversial.)

In recent years the area of functional assessment, particularly of the injured worker, has received particular attention. The key to carrying out a good clinical examination is to develop a routine that is relatively quick, easily repeated, and thorough. This needs to be combined with a careful understanding of CNS and peripheral nerve anatomy to allow a careful and reliable neurologic examination. The major concern in the patient with cervical and thoracic complaints other than serious associated medical illness is a neurologic syndrome that goes undiagnosed. The examiner who develops such a routine quickly becomes familiar with variations from the normal that suggest possible serious problems. A routine also allows comfort with findings that are suggestive of nonorganic processes such as psychogenic factors and malingering.

LABORATORY AND IMAGING STUDIES

Although great advancement has been made in diagnostic testing options available to the clinician, the value of such tests in evaluating the cervical and thoracic region is controversial. The true clinical value of some tests is also uncertain. The clinician must be familiar not only with the types of tests available and their relative indications, but also with their relationship to a given problem.

There is great controversy around the relative value of standard, plain x-rays. Such tests are routinely ordered in the occupational and emergency room setting. In an acute setting, absent suspicion of spinal fracture, tumor, or infection, there is little to suggest, however, that they are of any value in initiating a treatment program. Further controversy exists over the types of films to order, with the suggestion that simple anterior and posterior (AP) and lateral views will often provide much of the essential diagnostic information. The patient who presents with a history of significant traumatic injury requires careful radiologic evaluation, however. AP, lateral, and oblique films are all valuable in assessing for potential fracture. Oblique films particularly screen for a facet fracture. An odontoid view may be helpful in more thoroughly assessing the upper cervical levels.

Occasionally in fairly significant, traumatic injuries involving the cervical spine, flexion/extension films allow for assessment of ligamentous instability in cases where no obvious fracture is identified. Severe ligamentous disruption can lead to serious spinal instability and this may not be seen on static films. These films are more commonly obtained in the subacute phase when the anticipated course of recovery from cervical trauma is not taking place.

Where there is a history of thoracic trauma, AP and lateral films will usually suffice, although a chest x-ray can be of value in assessing pulmonary involvement. Rib films show potential rib fractures with greater specificity than does routine chest radiography. The vast majority of rib fractures, however, are treated symptomatically, and unless there is something to suggest a severe rib fracture, such films are often of little clinical value.

Computed tomography (CT) scans can be valuable when more extensive assessment of the bony anatomy of the spine is desired. This is particularly important when trying to ascertain the degree of potential instability in the patient with evidence of a spinal fracture. These studies allow evaluation of the bony anatomy and the integrity of the spinal canal itself. A herniated disc may also be seen on such films. A major problem with the use of CT scanning as a diagnostic tool is a high degree of false positive findings. Studies have shown as many as one third of asymptomatic patients to have abnormal CT scan findings. CT scanning does allow evaluation of the spinal cord to some degree, but does not allow the degree of evaluation available through the use of magnetic resonance imaging (MRI).

CT myelography is used in selected cases, but it has been relegated to a secondary role, given the widespread availability of MRI. CT myelography does have some clinical value, however, particularly in the postoperative patient where metallic fusion may distort the MRI, in the evaluation of spinal tumors, and in the evaluation of a syrinx. Multiplanar CT scanning with three-dimensional views is of particular value in assessing the integrity of the intervertebral canal and the foraminal openings for compression of individual nerve roots. This may not be seen on many currently available MRI scans. Some of the higher quality MRI scans, however, are more than adequate in that regard. The referring physician should understand that the quality of CT and MRI scans for spinal imaging often varies greatly.

The ability to evaluate the spinal cord, intervertebral disc, and associated soft tissues has been dramatically improved through the availability of high-quality MRI scans. MRI has also been invaluable in detecting spinal tumors and in assessing bony anatomy as well. Spinal infections such as discitis or local abscesses can often be well-identified through the use of MRI scanning. One of the major controversies, as with the CT scan, however, is the issue of false positive findings. Numerous studies suggest that asymptomatic individuals will have a high percentage of so-called abnormal findings on MRI.

When more extensive diagnostic imaging such as CT or MRI is indicated on a clinical basis, it is important to choose the tests wisely. If the test is being done simply to take a look, it is likely not indicated. There should be specific reasons why the scan is being ordered, with a clear understanding of how it will affect treatment choices. MRI scanning is of greater value for most indications in spinal imaging. CT is most useful for specific bony abnormalities such as stenosis in the central or intervertebral canals; for fractures; and for situations such as claustrophobia or metal implants where MRI is not tolerated. When doubtful about the proper procedure, consultation with the radiologist can be valuable in assessing the appropriate choice for the questions that are to be answered.

There is little to support the usefulness of CT or MRI in the acute setting unless serious spinal pathology is suspected. In most cases, the study will not change the early treatment and may mislead the clinician and patient because of the high percentage of false positives. We tend to reserve such imaging studies for concerns about fracture, tumor, infection, or where significant neurologic objective changes are present at the initial clinical examination. The patient with neurologic symptoms, but without obvious neurologic findings, does not often require early diagnostic testing of this type. This patient can often be managed conservatively initially and tested later, depending on the extent of progress.

When patients present with neurologic complaints, electrodiagnostic testing, including electromyogram (EMG) and somatosensory evoked potentials (SSEP), can be of great clinical value. This allows evaluation of the nervous system physiology for comparison with the nervous system anatomy obtained through imaging studies. When done by a trained clinician, the percentage of false positives with electrodiagnostic testing tends to be fairly low. There is a somewhat greater percentage of false negatives when these tests are done early. The findings in the first 10 to 21 days postinjury tend to be fairly subtle and are often missed by all but the most experienced electrodiagnosticians. The individual performing such testing should be capable of carrying out a good clinical exam since electrodiagnostic testing is an extension of the clinical examination. Laboratories where such tests are done by technicians and not under the guidance of a directly-involved physician should be avoided, if at all possible. In many cases, the test, like the physical examination in the office, is altered as one goes through the procedure to focus in on a particular problem as it arises. The examining physician's skill is a major limiting factor in obtaining thorough and properly done electrodiagnostic tests. Clinicians who order such tests regularly should become familiar with physicians who are well-trained in performing the test and capable of evaluating the clinical situation independently.

A common pitfall in the clinical evaluation of cervical and thoracic injuries is the overlap between referred central nervous system, or nerve root pain, and peripheral nerve entrapment. These findings are often subtle. Electrodiagnostic testing can be particularly valuable in helping the primary care physician make a decision about surgical consultation.

Somatosensory evoked potentials (SSEPs) can be used to evaluate the integrity of the central nervous system and individual nerve roots in many cases. EMG and nerve conduction studies, commonly available in most areas, are valuable for assessing the peripheral nervous system and for radicular findings. The patient who presents, for example, with complaints of numbness and weakness in an extremity, may simply have nerve root irritation and pain inhibition with a sense of weakness and no significant nerve injury. The presence of electrodiagnostic changes does not necessarily mandate surgical referral; most radiculopathies improve quite well with aggressive conservative care. However, such patients should be watched more closely since the long-term prognosis may be more guarded.

Routine screening for signs of infection with complete blood count (CBC) and sedimentation rate, liver and thyroid function assessment, and glucose testing are of particular value in the patient for whom there is suspicion of an associated medical finding as a source of complaints. Such routine screening for all patients is not of any proven clinical value and is not cost-effective. Since the yield is simply too low to justify such testing without some clinical suspicion to suggest other possible medical problems.

Bone scans are not routinely used in the occupational setting and are usually valuable in assessing more complicated medical causes for pain. The scan is of particular value in the medical/legal evaluation of possible bony injury. It is not uncommon for patients to have bony changes on films that may, in fact, represent old traumatic injuries that are not the result of the specific event for which the patient is being evaluated. When there is such doubt, bone scanning can help the clinician gauge more accurately the chronicity of the bony changes. The patient who presents, for example, with a wedge compression fracture in the thoracic region with some mild generalized osteopenia may not always have a new fracture. This fact has important ramifications in relationship to potential issues of compensation and disability.

COMMON INJURIES
Radiculopathies

Patients presenting with radiculopathies from cervical and thoracic injuries in the occupational setting are uncommon. They are among the most challenging patients, but also among the most rewarding to treat. The number of disc herniations in the cervical spine far outweighs those seen in the thoracic spine, due to the anatomical reasons outlined earlier. Because of the difficult nature of treating the thoracic spinal cord, significant thoracic herniations leading to cord or nerve root involvement are probably best referred immediately to the specialist. Many patients with cervical disc herniation without the associated features of myelopathy will do quite well with conservative care, particularly if initiated early and aggressively. Such patients usually manifest early more extreme complaints of axial skeletal pain along with associated complaints of radiating pain, numbness, tingling, or weakness. The early evaluation should be focused on identifying the patient with radiculitis; that is, the patient with patterns of nerve root irritation versus radiculopathy by objective clinical signs of neurologic impairment. A careful motor, sensory, and reflex examination is essential. Some patients will present with nerve root irritation without hard neurologic findings, and these patients are usually managed quite well conservatively. See Table 10-2.

The patient with radicular pain should also be screened for myelopathy with Babinski, clonus, and Hoffmann's tests. Alteration of gait or loss of balance can also be an early tip-off to a myelopathic component. In the patient who is in the subacute or chronic phase, measurement for atrophy can also be a sign of nerve root involvement. Many patients with myofascial patterns of pain or secondary shoulder involvement will also have extremity symptoms requiring careful clinical examination to separate them from those with true radiculopathy. Occasionally patients with traumatic injuries to the neck will also have a peripheral nerve injury masquerading as a radiculopathy. Familiarity, therefore, with the various motor and sensory patterns in the upper extremities is essential in making an accurate early diagnosis.

Unless medical causes or fractures are suspected, plain x-rays are not helpful. Cervical myelography and myelogram followed by CT scan may be used, but MRI scan is essentially the state-of-the-art when more extensive diagnostic testing is undertaken. Unless they present with a significant motor weakness or myelopathic component, however, most patients can be treated conservatively and followed closely before such testing be-

Table 10-2 Physical examination abnormalities in cervical radiculopathy

Root	Absent or diminished reflex	Decreased sensation	Muscle weakness
C5	Biceps (?)	Lateral arm	Deltoid, infraspinatus
C6	Biceps, brachioradialis	Lateral forearm–thumb	Biceps, wrist extensors, pronator teres
C7	Triceps	Middle finger	Wrist extensors, triceps, pronator teres, long finger flexors
C8	Triceps (?)	Medial forearm–little finger	Long finger flexors, thenar, hypothenar, intrinsics

From I MacLean, editor: *Physical medicine and rehabilitation clinical of North America. Electromyography: a guide for the referring physician.* HA Spindler and G Felsenthal, *Electrodiagnostic evaluation of acute and chronic radiculopathy,* WB Saunders, Philadelphia, p. 55, with permission.

comes necessary. If the patient is recovering quickly, more extensive diagnostic testing is unnecessary. When the patient is not improving over a reasonable course of time, however, more extensive testing is warranted. This is particularly true in patients where neurologic complaints and objective findings are deteriorating in the face of aggressive intervention. An MRI and electrodiagnostic testing to ascertain the extent of neurologic involvement become essential.

Typical early intervention approaches include a restrictive cervical collar such as a Philadelphia or other rigid cervical orthosis. Soft collars for this type of injury usually do not provide enough restriction of motion. The patient should be started on antiinflammatories. If objective neurologic changes are noted, a tapering course of oral prednisone is an inexpensive and very effective means to reduce the inflammatory reaction quickly. A typical dose would be 20 mg 3 times a day for 3 days followed by 20 mg twice a day for 2 days and 20 mg once a day for 2 days. Such short-term courses of corticosteroids in patients otherwise medically cleared for its use can be a very powerful and effective means of early intervention. For less severe cases such as the mild objective changes of radiculitis, oral nonsteroidal antiinflammatory drugs (NSAIDs) are usually quite satisfactory. Icing for spasm several times a day over the upper back and cervical region can do much to improve the secondary associated muscular discomfort that accounts for a good deal of the overall pain. Ergonomic changes to avoid heavy mechanical forces on the neck during treatment are also of great value. Postural stress, such as prolonged sitting, can be as devastating as frequent twisting, turning, or overhead lifting for such patients. As the patient recovers, work activity can again be increased. A more protracted course of

recovery is expected in these cases, given the severity of injury. One would like to see, however, that with initial intervention, the patient is improving from visit to visit. Patients with objective neurologic change should be followed at least weekly until it is clear they have stabilized. When patients are not improving with aggressive intervention over a period of 2 to 4 weeks, referral to a consulting spine specialist (such as a physiatrist or orthopedist) should be considered. Such patients do not necessarily require surgical intervention; many do well with more extensive intervention such as cervical epidural and selective nerve root blocks and other methods of controlling the pain and inflammatory response during the healing phase.

Early physical therapy to work on strengthening, to prevent deconditioning, and to start the patient on active exercise and self-managed techniques for pain control can be of great value. Such patients are typically referred 3 times a week for the first 2 to 3 weeks and their response monitored. The goal is to get the patient on an independent program as quickly as possible. Physical therapy, though one of the mainstays of treating cervical and thoracic pain, also has the potential for developing a patient dependency that can rival even the use of narcotic medication. Emphasis must be placed on exercise and not on passive modalities after the first several weeks.

Narcotics may have some value in short-term use, but beyond 7 to 10 days typically become counterproductive and other measures should be undertaken. The use of a tricyclic medication to help with sleep and stabilize irritable nerve pain should be considered as an alternative along with an antiinflammatory medication.

The patient with radiculopathy and neurologic change who is not improving should be referred for specialist consultation and/or further diagnostic testing. It should be remembered that the natural course of recovery, even for herniated discs and radiculopathies, is good without surgical intervention. Close monitoring of the patient's neurologic status, combined with aggressive conservative care, can keep many patients from potentially unnecessary surgery. There is certainly a role for surgery, however, and a small percentage of patients will eventually come to surgical intervention. Patients with one-level cervical involvement tend to do quite well surgically and patients with two or more level involvement, such as multilevel degenerative disc disease and multilevel stenosis, tend to do rather poorly. When surgery is planned, a careful explanation of what is being attempted and why the surgical approach is being undertaken should be requested from the surgical consultant. Given the severity of the underlying condition, these patients have a higher risk than typical for development of long-term chronic pain problems and, therefore, early aggressive intervention and evaluation of any psychological risk factors is important. This is not a situation where benign neglect lends itself to a positive long-term outcome.

Whiplash syndrome

A common presentation is the patient with a whiplash injury from a motor vehicle accident. These have been described by many practitioners as subjective soft tissue injuries. Typically, x-rays are taken to rule out the possibility of fracture, given the potential forces involved. Most patients, however, will have benign, self-limited conditions that will improve over a course of approximately 4 to 6 weeks with or without intervention. A reasonable percentage of patients, however, will have legitimate long-term complaints, and these patients need to be identified and approached in a more aggressive fashion.

The G-forces involved in a whiplash injury can be quite substantial. Anatomic studies have shown significant association of such injuries with disruption of the ligamentous complex in the cervical spine including micro-tears, frank ligamentous disruption, and facet capsular injuries. Typically, the patients are forced into a hyperextension and then hyperflexion posture, causing irritation to the facet capsules with extension, and on flexion to the posterior ligamentous structures, and potentially to the disc during flexion and loading. X-rays tend to be of little diagnostic value, but are done because of the traumatic nature of the situation, to rule out a serious bony injury, and for medical/legal purposes. Initial evaluation should seek to identify the patient with serious bony injury or any neurologic involvement. Patients with

tenderness over bony areas or visible bruising or discoloration suggesting direct blow to the skeleton should have x-rays taken. A careful neurologic examination allows screening for any associated injury.

Treatment includes icing, NSAIDs, and short-term immobilization with a soft collar, which acts primarily as a reminder and support to the patient rather than providing any true significant restriction of spinal motion. Prolonged immobilization, however, can make the patient anxious about beginning to use her neck and encourages deconditioning and stiffness of cervical musculoligamentous tissues. Typically, 3 to 5 days of immobilization will suffice. The patient should be encouraged to ice the area several times a day and to slowly increase her activity level as tolerated. In more severe cases, early intervention with physical therapy to restore mobility and reduce soft tissue swelling can be of help. Early exercise can include isometric exercises with the use of pressure by the patient against her hand to encourage strengthening without forcing range of motion.

Such patients usually can return to most work activities, except for the most strenuous activities, within 24 to 48 hours, as the soft tissue swelling subsides. When they are taken off work, they should be examined in 2 to 3 days to verify their status, should any longer term disability be anticipated. When such patients are not improving after 10 to 14 days, referral to physical therapy for more active intervention is indicated. They should then be followed every 1 to 2 weeks during the early phase to monitor the recovery process and assess potential return to function. Narcotics are best avoided in these patients. Muscle relaxants are of dubious clinical value, and if pain relief is required, then pain medication should be considered. Sleep disturbances may be treated with one of the tricyclic medications. Muscle spasms are managed by local application of ice rather than the use of pills.

More sophisticated diagnostic testing has limited value in the whiplash patient unless clear suspicion exists that a more serious underlying process is present. The patient with axial, primarily soft tissue, pain without radiating symptoms and negative plain x-rays is unlikely to have a serious underlying process and early extensive diagnostic testing has a fairly low yield. Given the high percentage of false positives with such testing, treatment is often not affected by the test results.

If such patients continue to experience symptoms at 6 weeks, the clinician should become more seriously concerned about long-term recovery. This is the point where patients start to settle into the chronic phase of such soft tissue injuries. Unfortunately, in spite of our best efforts, some patients do not improve in such a timeframe. Litigation may be a barrier to the patient's recovery period. Absent the mechanical factors involved, most physicians see far more patients who have been rear-ended than who admit to having hit someone else and developed resultant neck and upper back complaints. On the other hand, studies have suggested that, absent secondary gain factors, reasonable percentages of patients with such soft tissue injuries do not improve. Evaluation of the patient's compliance with treatment and other factors must be taken into consideration when assessing such issues. Referral to a spine specialist who routinely deals with such patients may be of value, and other means of assessment may sometimes be undertaken. These include surveillance of the patient at the request of the insurance company, participation of a rehabilitation nurse to monitor the treatment and patient recovery process through more direct involvement with the patient, or possibly a psychological evaluation. These patients can be truly challenging.

Myofascial pain

Much attention has been drawn in recent years to the diagnosis of myofascial pain as a common form of persistent symptoms in patients with few objective findings. It is characterized by trigger points, areas of tenderness that result in distal referral of symptoms in relatively predictable patterns. Like many other areas of spinal medicine, the concept of myofascial pain is controversial. Little objective data support the existence of structural abnormalities. Some recent studies have suggested alteration of the cellular makeup of tissues involved in patients with myofascial pain. Others have termed it simply a wastebasket for nondefinable diffuse spinal pain.

Essentially, it is a diagnosis of exclusion with no particular confirmatory tests. Many such patients tend to have a fairly chronic pattern of pain. The clinician should rule out psychogenic and secondary gain factors as the primary cause of symptoms. Certainly, stress and psychological factors, if not the primary cause, seem to be factors in perpetuating myofascial pain patterns. Others have shown a correlation between the presence of myofascial pain and sleep disturbance. Such patients may have radiating patterns of symptoms; for example, pain in the neck, trapezius, and over-the-shoulder region, but not in a strict dermatomal fashion. No objective neurologic findings are to be noted. Subjective patterns of symptoms will tend to vary and, as noted above, are related to multiple factors including stress, posture, and activity level. Diagnostic testing, except to rule out other causes, is of no known clinical value.

Treatment should generally be oriented toward promoting activity and mobilization of the tissues that are involved. Active programs of stretching, strengthening, teaching proper body mechanics, and changing the patient's ergonomic set-up when appropriate, should all be encouraged. A great mistake is to allow the patient to fall into a pattern of treatment with passive modalities such as massage and ultrasound without becoming involved in an active exercise program. This is clearly one condition where patients need to learn self-management of their problem, not only due to the difficulties in effective treatment, but also due to the chronicity of the syndrome. Such patients will not typically tolerate early aggressive exercise, but must be encouraged to work through discomfort to improve their overall level of flexibility and strength. Aerobic conditioning also plays an important part in treatment. Short-term use of antiinflammatories for patients who present with an acute flare may be of some benefit. Medications on a long-term basis are not indicated. Trigger point injections have been used with some effectiveness, as has the spray and stretch technique. There is not much to support the use of steroid injections, and there is some concern that such parenteral medications have detrimental side effects. Local anesthetics such as xylocaine and marcaine have been used. Dry needling or acupuncture may be equally effective. Sleep disturbance and possible associated depression, not uncommon, may be effectively treated with low-dose tricyclic antidepressants. Tricyclics are one of the mainstays of treatment for such patients, at least in the early phases.

It is important to reassure the patient that she does not have a serious life-threatening or potentially progressive disease. After an appropriate workup and examination have been undertaken, reassure the patient that she can feel hurt without necessarily experiencing harm. Typically, the use of immobilization with soft collars is not indicated, because this not only feeds into the soft tissue restriction pattern, but fosters a sense of dependency.

Patients not improving with 2 to 3 months of conservative care should be referred. They are managed best by a nonsurgical spine specialist, such as a physiatrist or rheumatologist, or when other concerns are present, by referral for psychological evaluation.

Thoracic outlet syndrome

Thoracic outlet syndrome, like myofascial pain, tends to be a clinical diagnosis. Typical presentation may include neck and upper back symptoms, but primarily radiating symptoms of numbness, tingling, and pain into one or both upper extremities. Pain in the forearm and hand tends to be more in an ulnar distribution involving the C8 and T1 dermatomes, likely due to the greater susceptibility of the lower cervical trunks to compression from thoracic outlet mechanisms.

The most common clinical explanations are either compression from a cervical rib (a large transverse process at C7, with resultant local neural compression) or from entrapment as the neurovascular structures pass through the scalene muscles. For those reasons, surgical procedures have included the removal of cervical ribs or scalenectomies.

The differential diagnosis includes ulnar neuritis with associated neck or upper back pain, cervical radiculopathy, or myofascial pain. Clearly, the more serious neurologic abnormalities among these need to be ruled out prior to diagnosing thoracic outlet syndrome.

The mere absence of a cervical rib and such a pattern of symptoms do not suggest a thoracic outlet syndrome. This condition, like the bulging disc syndrome, presents high potential for overly aggressive surgical approaches when a patient is not improving. Although there are some fairly extensive reports in the literature, surgical intervention rarely should be required.

The most effective forms of treatment tend to be short-term use of antiinflammatories and physical therapy approaches. Some short-term physical therapy modalities (ice, electrical stimulation, or ultrasound) for the patient with significant neck and upper back pain may be of help. The mainstay, however, should be a program of postural reeducation and exercise. Exercise should focus on stretching the cervical and upper thoracic region. Many of these patients are simply too short anteriorly in the cervical and upper thoracic region, leading to soft tissue restrictions and resultant secondary thoracic outlet syndrome patterns. This is not at all uncommon, particularly for the patient who is slumped forward many hours a day doing computer or clerical work. Work on proper posture and adaptations to the ergonomic environment are of particular value. These will take care of the vast majority of patients. It is rare for thoracic outlet syndrome to result in a true period of disability, except among the most severe cases. Patients taken off work for thoracic outlet syndrome should be seen by a spine specialist, unless they are rapidly improving with appropriate physical therapy and exercises. Anything beyond 1 to 2 weeks of severe symptoms suggests a more serious underlying problem or secondary factors. The long-term prognosis tends to be quite good, particularly when postural reeducation and active patient involvement are encouraged.

The use of narcotic medication is to be avoided, and injections for thoracic outlet syndrome tend to have minimal value. Electrodiagnostic testing and scanning is of particular value to rule out other associated problems; in the more significant cases, electrodiagnostic testing can be useful to confirm the diagnosis of thoracic outlet syndrome. Again, however, it should be emphasized that thoracic outlet syndrome is largely a clinical diagnosis. See Chapters 8 and 22 for further discussion of thoracic outlet syndrome.

Cervical and thoracic facet pain

Like other true synovial joints, the cervical and thoracic facets may become pain generators. They are prone to loading in the cervical spine with extension or in the thoracic spine with shoulder retraction. In the aging degenerative spine, patterns of osteoarthritis can manifest as cervical facet pain. Patients are particularly aggravated by extension and extension/rotation maneuvers in the cervical spine. They tend to do better in flexion positions which unload the joint surfaces. Differential diagnoses include soft tissue and myofascial pain, cervical disc disease without significant neurologic complaints, and medical causes. Referred pain, in these patients, tends to be in a less strict dermatomal fashion and more proximal, typically not manifesting below the upper arm/elbow region of the cervical spine. Some referral may occur down into the interscapular region. In addition to the true facet joints in the thoracic spine, the costovertebral and costotransverse joint complexes may exhibit similar patterns.

The diagnosis can often be assisted by plain radiography where facet joint spurring and degenerative change are noted. Acute facet synovitis without the development of degenerative changes can be equally painful and may not be seen on plain films. More extensive testing (MRI, CT, electrodiagnostic) can be considered, but usually is not required in the early treatment unless a more serious problem is also suspected.

Treatment should focus on range of motion, strengthening and conditioning, postural reeducation, and ergonomics. Antiinflammatories rather than narcotics are usually all that are required. For more resistant cases, local corticosteroid injections, including facet joint and other joint blocks, can be considered. These tend to be quite effective in the more resistant cases and can usually move the patient along more actively in the rehabilitation process.

The pain complaints can typically become significant, particularly in the acute phases with serious facet synovitis. Modalities including icing, electrical stimulation for muscle spasm, ultrasound, and gentle mobilization can reduce the acute symptoms and allow the rehabilitation process to begin more aggressively. Failing this, blocks are considered.

Patterns of disability can vary, depending on the nature of the symptoms, but such symptoms decrease in 3 to 6 weeks. An MRI or CT scan, depending on the clinical situation, should then be considered before blocks are undertaken. This rules out a more serious pathology which can mimic facet pain.

On the long-term, patients tend to do quite well, assuming good compliance with a program as outlined above. As they get into the degenerative phase, however, such patient's symptoms tend to flare more quickly with various activities. Proper body mechanics and continued independent stretching and strengthening are required to avoid or reduce the frequency of flares. Short-term flares are usually treated best with antiinflammatories, icing, and avoiding heavy exacerbating activities. Patients then return to normal activity.

The syndrome most likely to mimic facet joint pain and facet synovitis in the cervical spine is spinal stenosis. Flexion-extension films may show significant narrowing of the intervertebral canal on extension, significant disc space narrowing, and bony foraminal narrowing. Oblique views can help to identify the potential for neural compression. The patient with significant spinal stenosis will often develop over time a more typical radicular pattern associated with neural compression. This does not occur in the patient with facet pain only. Patients with facet pain as a diagnosis who are not improving should be evaluated for possible spinal stenosis.

These patients are typically referred when they have not responded to treatment over 3 to 6 weeks or they begin to develop a neurologic involvement.

CASE STUDIES
Case 1

A 37-year-old software engineer complains of right shoulder pain and intermittent tingling and numbness in the first and second digits of the right hand. Symptoms have been increasing for approximately 6 months. He had originally been seen by his family physician and was treated with antiinflammatory medication without improvement. Because of concern on the part of the physician about a possible radiculopathy, he was referred to a neurosurgeon for consultation. The physician diagnosed a possible cervical radiculopathy and ordered an MRI scan which showed a small disc bulge at the C5-6 level. The patient was referred to physical therapy consisting of traction and hotpacks. During physical therapy, he began to experience the onset of neck pain and noted no relief. At the time of his follow-up visit with the neurosurgeon in 4 weeks, he reported he was beginning to have pain in the neck which was getting steadily worse with physical therapy and that he had not improved. The physician at that time recommended an anterior interbody infusion of the C5-6 vertebra for increasing complaints of neck pain and unresolving arm pain with conservative care.

The patient was then seen for a third opinion. Cervical motion was full and the neurologic examination was normal, except for a positive Tinel's sign at the right wrist. Shoulder motion showed pain on external rotation with abduction and laterally over the subacromial space. This reproduced typical shoulder pain, but not his new neck or old hand symptoms. A diagnosis was made of shoulder impingement syndrome secondary to an exercise program that included regular swimming 4 to 5 days a week, and carpal tunnel syndrome secondary to an overuse syndrome of the upper extremity. This was felt to be related to his work as a software engineer. The neck pain was resolving upon discontinuation of the traction.

In followup at 4 weeks, he was noted to be dramatically better and essentially had no shoulder symptoms and no longer reported any neck pain. Hand tingling and numbness was intermittent and he was started on night splints with complete resolution of his symptoms over the subsequent month. Ergonomic changes were made to assist in resolving the carpal tunnel problem.

In this example several mistakes occurred that could have been even more seriously compounded. The patient's overall history was not taken in enough detail to allow an understanding of other activities that might be feeding into his complaints; that is, his vocational requirements and his athletic endeavors. Additionally, based on pain in more than one portion of the upper extremity, a radiculopathy was quickly diagnosed when, in fact, a good examination of the peripheral nervous system and shoulder would have suggested other causes of his symptoms. Most important, a disc bulge that was probably asymptomatic was diagnosed as the probable source of his symptoms. He had essentially a normal neurologic examination, however, and the disc abnormality was a simple annular bulge without evidence of nerve compression or herniation. Diagnosis must be logical and based on a sensible correlation of the history, physical examination, and radiologic findings, as discussed previously. Additionally, less radical treatment such as exercise, ergonomic changes, and modification of certain lifestyle habits may have a dramatic effect and should always be approached first unless severe progressive and likely irreversible changes would be expected to occur.

Case 2

A 24-year-old woman seeks medical attention days after being rear-ended in a motor vehicle accident while delivering a bank deposit for her employer's store. The car sustained mild denting but no severe damage. The patient presents with complaints of neck and diffuse upper back pain that appears to be getting steadily worse. She had been seen in the emergency room immediately post-accident and x-rays taken reported to be unremarkable. She was given codeine, muscle relaxants, and a soft collar. She was advised to return to the occupational health clinic for followup should she not be improving. She denies any other associated symptoms including radiating extremity symptoms and any loss of consciousness or direct blow to the body at the time of the accident.

Examination was remarkable for guarded cervical range of motion in all directions, all limited approximately 50%. There was diffuse tenderness over the cervical paraspinals, trapezius, and in the interscapular regions bilaterally. Neurologic examination was normal, and no long tract signs were noted. The patient works as an assistant manager at a local supermarket and has been out of work since the accident.

The patient was first taken off all narcotic and muscle relaxant medications and started on an antiinflammatory. She was advised to start icing at home and to discontinue the use of the cervical collar. She was then referred for physical therapy to include soft tissue mobilization, ultrasound, muscle stimulation, instruction in body mechanics, and a home exercise program with emphasis on stretching and posture. She was given a slip at that time to remain off work for another week. At the follow-up examination, she reported some resolution of symptoms, but persistent pain, again primarily in the cervical and, to a lesser degree, in the upper thoracic region. The neurologic exam remained normal. Cervical range of motion was mildly improved.

She was seen 1 week later and was advised at that time that she was cleared to return to work, provided she did not have to do any repetitive overhead lifting that was likely to aggravate the symptoms. The pain was reproduced by cervical extension and rotation, suggesting a posterior element pain pattern. When seen 1 month post initiation of therapy there were mild persistent complaints of pain and no spasm was noted. Neurologic exam remained normal. Cervical range of motion was mildly limited, about 10 to 20% in all directions, primarily due to voluntary guarding. At that time, she was advised that some individual symptoms may persist, but that there was no significant evidence of any serious long-term complications. She was advised to continue with an independent exercise program and to use over-the-counter antiinflammatories only should she experience a significant flare-up.

This case is a typical presentation of a person after a motor vehicle accident whiplash injury. The neck and upper back are involved secondary to lack of support of these areas during the accident itself. The mechanisms involved injure the posterior cervical ligamentous structures. In addition, hyperextension will often lead to an acute facet synovitis that is likely to refer into the upper thoracic and interscapular region and lead to secondary muscle spasm. These patients typically have tenderness over the cervical facets and pain with facet loading maneuvers.

Potential problems in this patient would be the early emphasis on immobilization and use of narcotic medications rather than active mobilization and antiinflammatory measures. Fortunately, this was corrected fairly quickly. It was important to get the patient back to work and activity, with reassurance that she was not likely to do any major long-term harm, provided reasonable guidelines were followed. The patient who is involved in potential litigation often becomes trapped in the cycle of pain and disability. Early return to work, whenever possible, should be encouraged. When the patient is in significant pain during the acute phase, however, limited rest or avoidance of aggravating activities is quite reasonable.

The other important issue is the persistence of long-term symptoms after such injuries. Such problems have been well-documented to occur in a nonlitigation setting after motor vehicle accidents. When patients present with such persistent symptoms, emphasis on self-treatment and self-management techniques and reassurance are extremely important. A longer therapy course may be considered, but caution must be exercised to avoid dependence on physical therapy. Therapy should move from the passive to the active approach fairly rapidly. Occasionally patients require more aggressive intervention over time: local injections, more extensive therapy including joint mobilization, or potentially a trial of other measures such as acupuncture. Such approaches, however, should be undertaken primarily in the patient who is also involved in an active approach to managing her own symptoms. Preferably, the patient is off narcotic medications and appears to be trying to avoid a pattern of chronic passivity and disability. Using aggressive measures of intervention may only perpetuate the cycle and need to be considered carefully before being undertaken. They are particularly valuable as adjuncts to active treatment. Further diagnostic testing in this case, such as an MRI scan, in spite of persistent symptoms, is unlikely to change the clinical recommendations.

Case 3

A 57-year-old warehouseman goes to the physician about 24 hours after being struck by a falling box at work. The accident was witnessed. The patient reports pain in the neck, upper back, and radiating down the right arm. He describes a general sense of weakness in the right arm and pain with use. He is uncertain about any numbness and denies any bowel or bladder changes. He is otherwise in his usual good health and denies any past similar problems other than occasional stiffness and tightness with heavy lifting or sleeping in awkward positions.

On examination, there is significant guarding in all directions and range of motion is difficult to adequately assess secondary to pain. There appears to be some pain-inhibited give-away type of weakness in the wrist extensors and biceps of the right arm. There is a patchy loss of sensation in a vague distribution over the lateral forearm and back of the right hand, thumb, and index *finger regions. Reflexes are 1+ and symmetric. Cervical paraspinal and trapezius spasm and diffuse tenderness are noted. Cervical x-rays show mild anterior spurring from C4 through C7 with mild disc space narrowing.*

The patient is started on a course of antiinflammatories, is given a soft collar, and is taken off work for 3 days. On follow-up examination, clinical findings are essentially unchanged, except for reports of some increasing numbness in the right arm and feelings of increased pain. He describes sleep as poor. After checking the patient's vital signs and going over a review of systems again concerning his general health, he is started on a low-dose tricyclic antidepressant, 10 mg a night, with instructions to double the dose after 3 days if necessary. He is advised to ice, to stay off work, and is referred to physical therapy to include modalities and stretching with review of posture and body mechanics.

On follow-up examination in a week, there is some improvement in his sleep, but only minimal overall improvement in pain. Therapy is reported to give good temporary relief. The NSAIDs are discontinued and the patient is started on a course of oral prednisone, tapering over one week. The physical therapy is continued, and the patient is advised to remain off work as no light duty is available.

The patient is seen in 1 week and notes that although he initially felt better during the first few days on prednisone, his symptoms once again increased as he tapered down. Neurologic exam remains remarkable for some weakness and sensory loss, as noted previously, with persistent guarded range of motion. At this point, an MRI scan is ordered and shows multilevel degenerative disc disease, two-level spinal stenosis, and disc bulges at multiple levels. He is then referred on to a consultant for further evaluation and treatment.

This type of patient, referred because of failure to progress, presents a long-term management problem. Fortunately, he was treated early and aggressively with active measures, including avoidance of narcotics, active early intervention, and antiinflammatory measures. Unfortunately, the extent of the underlying problems were such that he was not making the anticipated progress. The imaging studies revealed preexisting pathology. A single event in a long course of mild degenerative changes can initiate a long-term problem. These patients need to be treated aggressively to avoid such long-term complications. Because of the multilevel problems involved, surgical interventions are not likely to meet with major success, in spite of the severity of the symptoms. He probably is a candidate, however, for a trial of cervical blocks, potential work-hardening ap-

proaches, and other rehabilitation measures. Patients with this picture are best referred to a consultant early rather than letting the clinical course progress too far because of the high risk for prolonged disability. It is crucial to act early and aggressively and to avoid passive approaches that make patients dependent.

SUGGESTED READINGS

Cady LD, Bischoff DP, O'Connell ER et al: Strength and fitness and subsequent back injuries in firefighters, *J Occup Med* 21:269-272, 1979.

Cailliet R: *Neck and arm pain,* ed 2, Philadelphia, 1981, FA Davis.

Deyo RA: The role of the primary care physician in reducing work absenteeism and cost due to back pain, *Spine: State of the Art Reviews* 2:17-30, 1987.

Frymoyer JW, Newberg A, Pope MH et al: Spine radiographs in patients with low back pain, *J Bone Joint Surg* 66A:1048-1055, 1984.

Haldeman S: The electrodiagnostic evaluation of nerve root function, *Spine* 9:42, 1984.

Hall FM: Back pain and the radiologist, *Radiology* 137:861-863, 1980.

Hollinshead WH, Jenkins DB: *Functional anatomy of the limbs and back,* ed 5, Philadelphia, 1981, WB Saunders.

Keane GP: The history and physical examination in spine care. In White AH, editor: *Total spine care: the spine care approach,* St Louis, (in press).

Keane GP, Saal JA: The sports medicine approach to occupational low back pain, *West J Med* 154:525-527, 1991.

Mayer TG, Gatchel RJ, Kishino ND et al: Objective assessment in spine function following industrial injury: a prospective study with comparison group and one-year follow-up, *Spine* 10:482-493, 1985.

Mayer TG, Gatchel RJ, Mayer H et al: A prospective two-year study of functional restoration in industrial low back injury, *JAMA* 258:1763-1767, 1987.

Saal JA, editor: Neck and back pain: state of the art reviews, *Phys Med Rehab,* 1(4), 1987.

Saal JA, editor: Sports injuries: state of the art reviews, *Phys Med Rehab* 1(4), 1987.

Saal JS, Saal JA: Electrophysiologic evaluation of lumbar pain: establishing the rationale for therapeutic management in lumbar spine surgery techniques and complications. In White AH, editor: St Louis, 1987, Mosby.

Saal JS, Keane GP, Lerman RJ: Objective assessment in lumbosacral spine function, *Crit Rev Phys Med Rehab* 2:25-28, 1990.

Teresi LM, Lufkin RB, Reicher MA et al: Asymptomatic degenerative disc disease and spondylosis of the cervical spine: MR imaging, *Radiology* 164:83-88, 1987.

Wiesel SW, Tsourmas N, Feffer HD et al: A study of computer-assisted tomography: the incidence of positive CAT scans in an asymptomatic group of patients, *Spine* 9:549-551, 1984.

11 Low Back Disorders

Low back pain is the most common cause of disability in individuals under 45 years of age and the third most common cause in the 45 to 64 age group.[4] Currently 2.6 million Americans are temporarily disabled by chronic low back pain.[11] Approximately 2% of all workers injure their back annually.[3] The majority of injured workers return to work within 60 days, yet 2 to 3% develop chronic disabling complaints.[9] Low back disability from 1960 to 1980 increased 14 times faster than the actual population growth.[6] Social security disability awards from 1957 to the mid 1970s increased 347% for all conditions, yet increased 2680% for back pain.[8] Incredibly, 10% of all low back injuries accounted for 80% of the total cost.[13] It is estimated that 50% of individuals disabled due to low back pain have absolutely no objective findings.

Fig. 11-1 illustrates that as the length of time off work for a low back injury increases, medical, legal and disability costs accelerate. This increasing expenditure does not result in improved outcome (return to work), and might actually contribute to prolonging the disability. The ability to ever work again decays rapidly after 6 months. If an injured worker has not returned to work within two years of the injury, he will most likely never work again.[5]

ANATOMIC CAUSES OF LOW BACK PAIN
Discogenic pain

The majority of occupational low back injuries involves the lumbovertebral disc, the diarthrodial facet joint, and/or lumbar nerve root. The lumbar spinal column is composed of five lumbar vertebrae stacked on top of each other with the intervertebral disc between each bone (Fig. 11-2). The intervertebral disc is composed of the outer fibrous ring called the anulus fibrosus and a gelatinous center called the nucleus pulposis. Torsional and repetitive flexion loads to the lumbar spine cause anular injury that progresses to disc degenerative changes.[7] Lifting is a significant cause of anular tears and disc derangement resulting in herniation of the nucleus pulposis. The L4-5 and L3-4 discs are at increased risk for torsional injury as they lie above the intercristal lines (above iliac crests). The

L5-S1 disc is at increased risk for axial loading and repetitive flexion injuries.[2] Kirkaldy-Willis described the degenerative process starting with anular tears, progressing to herniations of the nucleus pulposis, and resulting in degenerative disc disease with spinal stenosis.[16]

The most common description of an acute low back injury is a lumbar sprain or strain. Presumably a ligament or muscle is stretched causing injury and pain. Anatomic dissections support the proposition however that the anulus fibrosis and facet joints are actually injured resulting in characteristic pain syndromes.[16] Low back injuries are described on the basis of an injury to the disc, facet joint, or nerve root, rather than a muscle or ligament. Injury to a disc, facet joint, or nerve root often results in secondary muscle spasm. A direct blow to the spinal musculature, however, can certainly cause local muscle injury and spasm.

Patients with discogenic injuries can present with back pain only, back pain and leg pain without a neurologic deficit, or back pain with leg pain and a neurologic deficit. In the middle age to older population one is often faced with an occupational injury to a lumbar motion segment superimposed on a preexisting degenerative segment. It is essential to understand the natural history of degenerative disc disease to adequately evaluate and treat these injuries.

Facet pain

There are two lumbar facet joints for every intervertebral segment. These joints are diarthrodial in nature and have articular cartilage, synovium, and a capsule. The lumbar facet joint is placed under increased load with extension or torsional maneuvers.[1] The degenerative process involves not only the intervertebral disc but also the facet joint. Facet sclerosis, arthropathy, and enlargement can result in foraminal narrowing that can also cause radicular leg symptomatology.

Facet injuries often present with back pain or with back pain and referral to the buttock or upper leg. It has been reported that facet pain can refer pain as low as the foot although this is rare. An effused facet can also cause radicular leg pain with neurologic deficit.

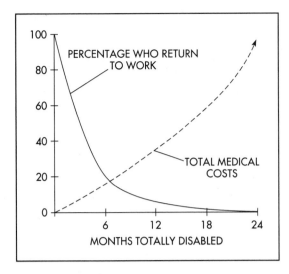

Fig. 11-1 Return to work and total costs in relationship to length of total disability.

Spinal stenosis

A subset of patients have congenitally small central canals. The majority of patients with spinal stenosis present following the onset of degenerative deterioration of the spine resulting in bony osteophytes from the intervertebral end plates or the

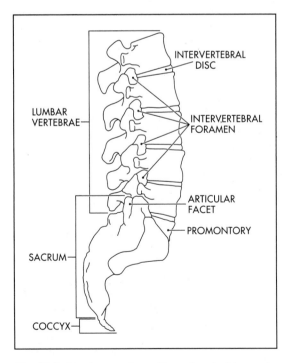

Fig. 11-2 Lumbar vertebrae. (Reproduced with permission from White AH, Anderson R: *Conservative care of low back pain,* ed 1, Baltimore, 1991, Williams and Wilkins, p 46)

facet joints. The osteophytes can cause foraminal or central stenosis with resulting radicular or cauda equina compression. The level of spinal stenosis can often be determined by the radicular pattern of sensory, myotonal, or motor deficit (Fig. 11-3).

Generally, spinal stenotic patients present in their middle to advanced ages. It is important to include vascular claudication leg pain in the differential diagnosis, as this is common in that age set also.

Radiculopathy

An intervertebral disc herniation compressing a spinal nerve root often presents with leg pain in association with sensory and motor deficit. Foraminal narrowing secondary to arthritic bony changes can cause static or dynamic nerve root compression in the foramina. A congenitally small spinal canal can also cause radicular leg pain. Mechanical trauma or sudden traction to the nerve root can also cause injury.

The majority of occupationally related back and leg pain patients present without a true neurologic deficit. It has been well established, however, that an injury to the intervertebral disc can cause leakage of inflammatory chemicals resulting in a chemical radiculitis (noncompressive radiculopathy).[10] Fig. 9-3 is helpful in understanding the possible lumbar motion segment that might be involved in the area of leg discomfort. For instance, a lateral L4-L5 disc herniation into the L4 foramina would classically present with anterior leg pain, an L4 sensory deficit, and weakness in the L4 innervated muscles. A paramedian L4-L5 disc herniation would affect the L5 nerve root, and a central L4-L5 herniation might affect the S1 root, each with a unique clinical presentation.

Nonmechanical low back pain

There are numerous nonmechanical sources of low back pain. A traumatic injury to the spine can result in a vertebral body fracture, particularly if there is underlying osteoporosis. Rarely a pars interarticularis fracture will occur acutely, though more often this is a congenital problem that develops in teenage years. Rheumatologic conditions (including rheumatoid arthritis) and seronegative arthropathies can present with low back pain. A careful history will often elicit systemic manifestations or other joint involvement which will suggest a rheumatologic entity.

Primary or metastatic tumors can present with low back pain, although this is uncommon in the younger population. Uterine fibroids, endometriosis, and prostatitis can also cause low back pain. Osteomyelitis and disc space infections should be considered when a patient presents with low back

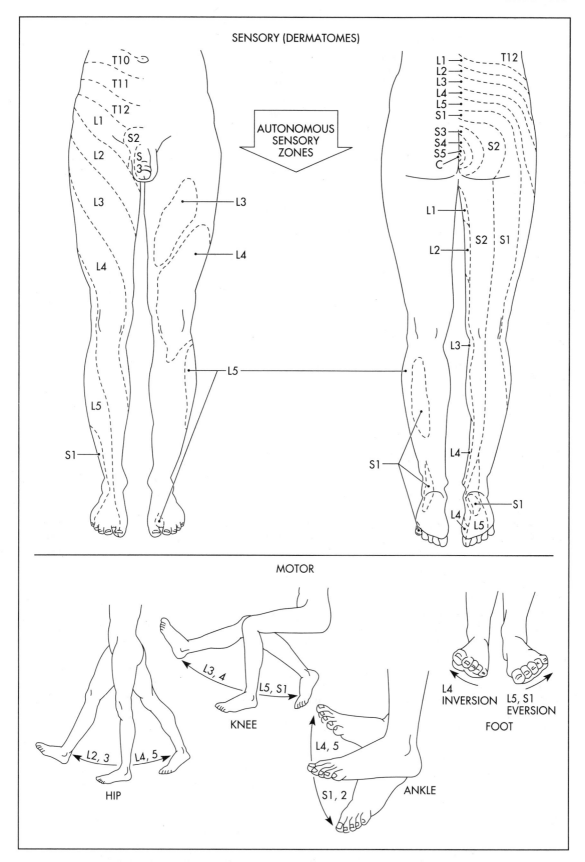

Fig. 11-3 Sensory and motor innervation of lower limb. (Reproduced with permission from Keim HA, Kirkaldy-Willis WH: *Clinical symposia*, vol 36, no 6, 1987, Ciba-Geiby, p 7.)

pain in association with a fever, although a fever is not always a presenting symptom or sign. In the older population an abdominal aortic aneurysm is a consideration for back pain, particularly in association with claudication leg discomfort.

MEDICAL HISTORY
Chief complaint

It is extremely important to ascertain the injured worker's chief area of pain. The location of the pain is the clinician's first insight into the pathophysiologic sources of pain. Equally important is having the patient diagram his areas of pain. A pain diagram (Fig. 11-4) enables the patient to illustrate the area of pain as well as the nature of the pain. This provides valuable insight into the clinical problem; for example, an S1 radiculopathy will present with a classic distribution of pain down the leg. This also enables the clinician to monitor the resolution or advancement of the pain syndrome. There are physiologic presentations of pain, and there are also nonorganic illustrations of pain that often suggest psychologic or functional issues. The pain diagram serves as a document in the medical chart for future reference.

Nonoccupational problems are often lumped together with occupational injuries. A careful monitoring of the pain diagram will facilitate attention to only the occupational problems.

History of current illness

Ninety percent of musculoskeletal diagnoses can be obtained by an accurate history. The date and place of injury (occupational or nonoccupational), mechanism of injury, and temporal nature of the pain are important. An inquiry as to the location, frequency, and severity of the pain is necessary. Documenting how the pain affects functional tasks at work, home, and recreational activities is essential.

Aggravating and relieving factors will enable the clinician to distinguish mechanical versus nonmechanical pain and what the pain's actual source. A careful detailed history of similar past pain will provide insight into previous disability and whether this might represent an ongoing degenerative process. The treatment for an initial anular tear with no previous history of back pain versus the twentieth episode of back pain will obviously affect management. An inquiry into prior surgical history and its relationship to the chief complaint is necessary. An occupational history documenting the individual's type of work and length of time on the job and in the career is important. Specific physical demands of the work including lifting, pulling, squatting, and hand use enable the clinician to make an informed decision about the patient's ability to return to that work. An inquiry

about the length of sitting, standing, and walking is also important. One should also determine recreational activities or household activities that are limited due to the pain. One must also specifically inquire about nonoccupational sources of injury or aggravation. Job satisfaction and pending litigation need to be determined.

A comprehensive medical history and past surgical history not related to the chief complaint is necessary. Careful documentation of the treatments for the current occupational problem or injury is necessary. Current and previous medications and their potential side effects need to be reviewed. Finally, all pertinent outside records and imaging studies need to be reviewed prior to reaching a clinical impression.

Using a visual analog scale from 0 to 10 will quantify subjective pain complaints sequentially. Documenting the percentage of back pain versus leg pain is particularly important when surgical considerations are considered.

CLINICAL EXAMINATION

A comprehensive evaluation of the lumbar spine patient involves an assessment while standing and walking, sitting, lying supine, and then prone.

Standing and walking

The low back pain patient is initially observed while walking into the exam room and during removal of his shoes or socks. His level of comfort while sitting or standing is noted.

The lumbar spine is inspected for scoliosis, kyphosis, lordosis, or an unusual shift. Increase in lumbar lordosis can suggest a spondylolisthesis. Decreased lumbar lordosis might reflect paravertebral muscle spasms.

The patient is asked to forward flex as far as is comfortable. The range of motion is documented in degrees and pain complaints are recorded. One observes if there is any list while moving forward or backward that might suggest a true pain generator. Lumbar extension, lateral bending, and rotation are similarly observed, and the range of motion and pain complaints are recorded.

Typically pain with lumbar extension would suggest a facet syndrome, lateral disc or large central disc abnormality, or stenosis. Typically, pain in flexion would suggest a discogenic injury.

Sitting

The bilateral patellar and Achilles reflexes are obtained. Babinski and clonus testing is performed. While the patient is distracted, straight leg raising while in a sitting position is performed, and the patient is carefully observed for grimacing or description of back or leg discomfort.

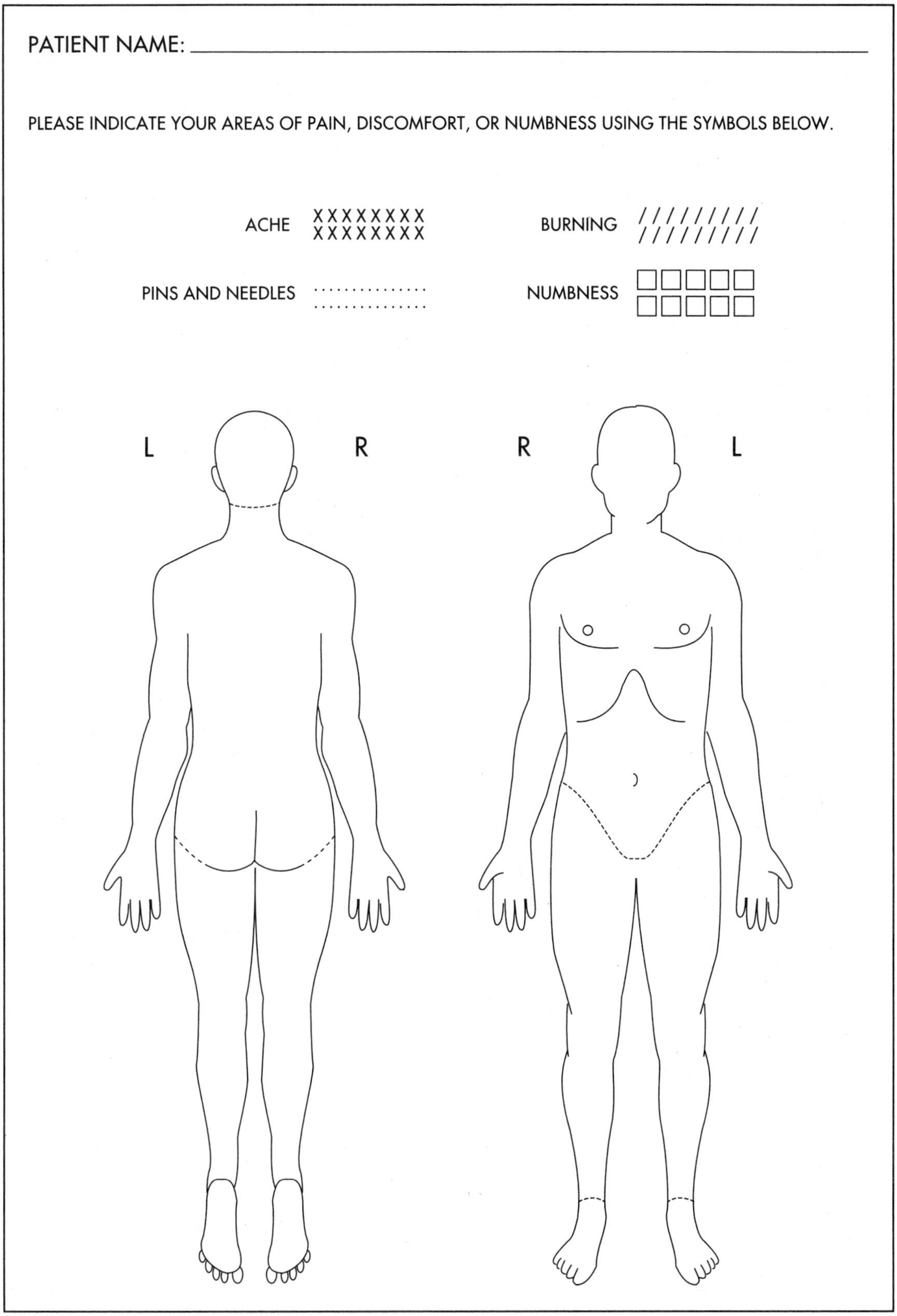

PATIENT NAME: _____

PLEASE INDICATE YOUR AREAS OF PAIN, DISCOMFORT, OR NUMBNESS USING THE SYMBOLS BELOW.

ACHE   X X X X X X X X
        X X X X X X X

BURNING   / / / / / / / / /
           / / / / / / / /

PINS AND NEEDLES   · · · · · · · · · · · · · ·
                    · · · · · · · · · · · · · ·

NUMBNESS   ☐☐☐☐☐
            ☐☐☐☐☐

L   R   R   L

Fig. 11-4 Pain diagram.

Supine

The bilateral iliopsoas, quadriceps, tibialis anterior, extensor hallucis longus, peroneus longus, and posterior tibialis muscle strength is assessed. True neurologic weakness is noted. Cogwheel weakness or breakaway weakness (nonphysiologic response) is also noted. Legs are observed for atrophy. Maximum thigh and calf circumference is measured. Sensory examination involving pinprick is obtained with special attention paid to a possible peripheral neuropathy or a distal nerve entrapment syndrome.

Straight leg raising in supine is performed. Dorsiflexion and plantar flexion of the ankle are assessed. Dorsiflexion of the ankle will increase dural tension, often increasing or causing back pain or leg pain. Plantar flexion of the ankle will reduce dural tension and thus should reduce back pain or leg pain. Knee flexion also reduces dural tension and would be expected to reduce back pain and leg pain.

Hip internal and external rotation is assessed for limitation and pain. Patricks maneuver (hip flexion and abduction) is also performed. Pain in the groin infers intraarticular hip pathology; pain in the buttock suggests spinal or sacral iliac dysfunction. The femoral nerve is palpated in the groin. The bilateral femoral, popliteal, dorsal pedis, and posterior tibial pulses are assessed.

The patient is then asked to bring his knees to his chest. This will further assess if there is a consistent pain response with lumbar flexion that causes reversal of the lumbar lordosis.

Prone

Quadricep flexibility is assessed. Femoral stretch sign (patient prone, knee flexed at 90 degrees, the leg is lifted off the table) is performed to assess if this causes leg discomfort in the anterior thigh suggesting an L3 or L4 nerve root problem. The femoral stretch maneuver also causes lumbar spine extension, which will often recreate low back pain in facet and stenotic patients.

Nonanatomic or superficial skin tenderness is assessed, (Waddell sign).[14] The spinous processes, interspinous ligament, and soft tissues overlying the lumbar facet joints are palpated to determine if there is localized sensitivity. The paraspinal muscles are palpated to assess if there is muscle spasm. The bilateral sciatic notches and sacroiliac joints are also palpated for pain. Finally the patient is asked to perform a press-up involving extension of the lumbar spine. Press-ups often reduce discogenic pain, and increase facet and stenotic pain.

During the examination, one tests for nonorganic physical signs (Waddell signs) that suggest psychological factors contributing to perceived pain and dysfunction. There are five types of physical signs Waddell has described: tenderness, simulation, distraction, regional, and overreactions.[14] Nonorganic tenderness can be either superficial or nonanatomic. Simulation tests involve axial loading and rotating the spine, movements that should not cause lumbar pain. Straight leg raising while sitting (flip test) is the most useful distraction test. Cogwheel (giving way) weakness and nonphysiological sensory disturbances are effective regional tests. Overreaction during the examination (such as disproportionate verbalization, facial expression, collapsing, etc.) is also a nonorganic sign.

DIAGNOSTIC STUDIES

Although a comprehensive history and physical examination will determine the source of spinal pain in 95% of the injured workers seen, laboratory or imaging studies may be necessary to confirm the diagnosis, and occasionally to determine the diagnosis.

Imaging studies

Lumbar x-ray films. Occupationally related back pain without traumatic etiology, history of back pain or injuries, and a normal neurologic examination does not require lumbar x-ray films initially. On follow up however, if there is no improvement with a conservative care program that will be outlined later, then lumbar x-ray films should be obtained within 2 weeks of initiating treatment.

Individuals who present with traumatic injury, a history of back complaints, neurologic deficit, or a clinical suspicion of spondylolisthesis or osteoporosis should have lumbar x-ray films obtained on the date of initial evaluation.

Individuals who have had traumatic acceleration deacceleration spinal injuries that could result in ligamentous injury and subsequent instability should have flexion and extension x-ray films. Individuals with spondylolisthesis or spondylolysis should also have flexion and extension x-ray films if they do not respond to a conservative care program.

Magnetic resonance imaging versus computed tomography. MRI imaging has provided anatomic detail of the lumbar spine including the vertebral bodies, intervertebral discs, facet joints, thecal sac, and spinal nerve roots. MRI scans are indicated for the nonoperated spine patient who presents with a true neurological deficit or has failed a conservative care plan after 4 weeks. The advantages of MRI include precise soft tissue detail and no ionizing radiation.

CT scans are indicated for individuals suspected to have bony changes resulting in stenosis or fracture. Postoperative patients tend to require CT scan since often the reason for a failed back surgery is missed stenosis not appreciated on pre-operative MRI scan.

MRI scan with metrizamide is indicated in post-operative patients in whom one suspects postoperative scarring or arachnoiditis. Myelography is rarely required if sophisticated MRI and CT technology is available.

Electromyography and somatosensory evoked potentials. Neurophysiologic assessment of the spinal nerve root and peripheral nerves often is necessary for definitive diagnosis and for assessing the prognosis. If a diagnostic question arises about a radiculopathy, such as whether it is peripheral nerve entrapment or peripheral neuropathy syndrome, electromyography (EMG) nerve conduction study can distinguish the problem. This study is also valuable in individuals who present with subjective complaints of leg pain yet have no objective evidence of neurologic dysfunction and are not improving with appropriate treatment.

EMG is a valuable tool in monitoring neurologic recovery or deterioration through time in an objective manner. The EMG nerve conduction study primarily is an effective tool for monitoring motor radiculopathy and peripheral motor and sensory neuropathies. The somatosensory evoked potentials (SSEP) test is effective, however, in monitoring sensory radiculopathies that cannot be adequately assessed with the EMG nerve conduction study. A patient with leg pain and numbness with a normal EMG nerve conduction study would benefit from an SSEP study to assess the possibility of a sensory radiculopathy.

Discogram. Discograms involve placing a needle into the disc to record the amount of dye received, the pain that is recreated, and the image on x-ray film. Lumbar discograms are valuable in diagnosing internal disc disruption syndrome. This syndrome is characterized by an axial load to the spine with severe pain in sitting yet often normal neurologic exam and normal MRI and CT imaging. A discogram will often show small fissures in the injured disc that are painful.

Discograms are also effective in preoperative planning to assess if a disc is the source of pain. It is unadvisable to fuse into an apparently benign-appearing disc on MRI scan that is actually painful on discogram. Discograms are also valuable in delineating the actual source of pain in individuals who have multilevel degenerative disc disease. Often painful anular fissures not appreciated on conventional MRI or CT imaging are detected on discograms.

Triple-phase bone scans are helpful in ruling out fractures, metastatic spread to the spine, and rheumatological syndromes. It is occasionally important to determine whether a spondylolysis is new or old.

Laboratory tests

Rheumatologic screens including sedimentation rate, rheumatoid factor, ANA, HLA, B27 are important when a systemic rheumatologic process is suspected. There is no clearly established role for thermography in the assessment of spinal pain syndromes.

EVALUATION AND MANAGEMENT OF MECHANICAL LOW BACK PAIN

Assuming a nonmechanical source of back pain has been ruled out by appropriate history, physical exam, and (if needed) imaging studies, three major categories of mechanical back pain can be analyzed. The majority of occupational injuries to the low back result in pain syndromes secondary to the intervertebral disc, facet joint, or spinal stenosis. Any of these three categories can result in radicular leg pain or true radiculopathy (motor loss, reflex changes, or sensory loss)

Discogenic pain

Table 11-1 summarizes each of these three pain syndrome subsets. Discogenic pain syndromes occur often following a bending, lifting, or twisting episode. Sitting aggravates the pain while standing or walking relieves the pain.

On physical examination there is increased pain with flexion and often reduced pain with lumbar extension. Lumbar x-ray films can show disc space narrowing or degenerative disc changes. An MRI scan will often show the intervertebral disc abnormality. A treatment program emphasizing a maximum of 2 days of bedrest, antiinflammatory medications and acetaminophen, and a physical therapy or chiropractic rehabilitation program is necessary. Essential to the rehabilitation process is education about the nature of the injury as well as discussion of ergonomic risk factors. The therapy program initially can involve pain-relieving modalities such as ice, electrical stimulation, and deep heat. Immediately, spinal range of motion is assessed and advanced. Abdominal, trunk, and lower extremity strengthening exercises are initiated. A McKenzie extension program will often provide pain relief. Lumbar traction is often an effective means of reducing back and leg discomfort.

Facet pain

Facet injuries in the occupational setting often involve a twisting or axial load injury. Standing and walking tend to aggravate the pain while sitting relieves the pain. On physical examination, lumbar extension tends to increase the pain while lumbar flexion relieves the pain. On x-ray films there is often facet sclerosis and narrowing noted. MRI scan or a CT scan are effective for imaging these joints.

Table 11-1 Categories of lumbar pain and their characteristics

	Discogenic pain	Facet pain	Spinal stenosis
Mechanism of injury	Bending, lifting, twisting while leaning forward	Twisting, axial load	Any
Aggravating factors	Sitting	Standing, walking	Walking
Relieving factors	Standing, walking	Sitting	Sitting
Physical examination	Pain with flexion	Pain with extension	Pain generally with extension
X-ray films	Disc Space narrowing, DJD	Facet sclerosis narrowing, DJD	Bony osteophytes
Imaging study	MRI	MRI or CT	MRI or CT
Physical therapy prescription	Traction, extension program	Flexion program, facet gapping, joint mobilization	Flexion program, cycling

The acute treatment will also involve bed rest, not beyond 2 days, antiinflammatory medications in conjunction with acetaminophen, and initiation of a therapy program. Therapy will emphasize a flexion program that tends to unload the facet joints. Lumbar facet gapping (opening the facet joint) or mobilization (moving the facet joints) is often effective in relieving pain. All occupational low back patients require education and ergonomic assessment.

Stenotic pain

Spinal stenotic patients can injure themselves in virtually any manner. Walking tends to aggravate the back pain and cause leg pain, whereas sitting provides relief. Generally they will note increased back pain and leg pain with extension, some relief with flexion. Lumbar x-ray films will often show bony osteophytes consistent with degenerative changes. CT scan tends to be more specific in identifying bony changes.

The initial management of a stenotic back injury includes bedrest no longer than 2 days, antiinflammatory medications in conjunction with acetaminophen, and a rehabilitation program. Stenotic patients tend to respond better to a lumbar flexion program. Bicycling is often better tolerated than walking.

Aerobic conditioning

All occupationally injured patients should be encouraged to maintain aerobic conditioning three times a week. Generally, swimming is the least stressful activity to the lumbar spine. Discogenic patients tend to respond well to a walking program, whereas facet and stenotic patients do well with a bicycling program.

Medications

For individuals who present in severe pain, particularly if they have a neurologic deficit, consideration for a 1-week course of oral prednisone should be entertained. There is little role for narcotic medications in the management of mechanical low back pain. Occasionally, muscle relaxants are necessary during the acute stages of low back pain management. Tricyclic antidepressants are very valuable in acute and chronic back pain management. Aspirin, nonsteroidal medications, and acetaminophen are the primary medications used.

TREATMENT PLAN FOR SPINAL PAIN

An algorithm for managing occupational low back pain and disability is outlined in Table 11-2. The acute patients present with pain less than 4 weeks, subacute patients with pain greater than 4 weeks, and chronic patients with pain greater than 3 months.

Any occupational back patient presents in one of three manners: low back pain only, low back pain with leg pain and a negative neurologic examination, and finally low back pain, leg pain, and a positive neurologic examination. The four potential treatment steps would include (1) reducing pain and restoring function, (2) establishing a definitive diagnosis, (3) resolution of the pain and workers' compensation claim, and (4) surgical consideration.

All occupationally related back patients will undergo Step A. This step ensures that every patient has a clinical diagnosis based on a thorough history and physical exam, often supplemented with routine lumbosacral x-ray films. Intervention is aggressive and timely emphasizing early activity (maximum of 2 days of bedrest), exercises specific

Table 11-2 Algorithm for managing low back pain and disability

Duration of pain	Low back pain only	Low back, leg pain; negative neurologic test	Low back, leg pain; positive neurologic test
<4 weeks	Step A	Step A	Steps A and B
>4 weeks	Step B	Step B	Steps B and D
>3 months	Step C	Step C	Steps C and D

Step A: Reduce pain and restore function

1. Obtain an accurate working diagnosis based on the history, physical examination, and x-ray films.
2. Start treatment early (exercise depends on diagnosis).
3. Instruct the patient in proper back techniques and ergonomics.

Step B: Establish a definitive diagnosis

1. Perform advanced diagnostic tests.
2. Administer diagnostic and therapeutic injections.
3. Start advanced stabilization training.

Step C: Resolve pain and workers' compensation claim

1. Emphasize the function, not the pain.
2. Perform a functional or work capacity evaluation.
3. Return to work, permanent and stationary (maximum medical improvement); vocational rehabilitation; and/or independent medical examination.
4. Recommend a psychologic evaluation.

Step D: Consider surgery

1. Consider for progressive neurologic deficiency or intractable pain

---

for the injury, limited passive therapy modalities, and immediate back education and ergonomic instruction. The therapy should be directed at reducing pain and inflammation, restoring spinal function, eliminating obstacles to returning to work, and targeting a realistic return to work date.

If after 4 weeks the injured worker is not able to return to work then Step B begins. The clinician now must definitively establish a diagnosis using all the sophisticated diagnostic tools now available. At this point, the clinician needs to focus on the legitimately injured worker and identify the malingerer or patient motivated by secondary gain. Advanced diagnostics including imaging studies, MRI and CT scan, bone scan, flexion and extension x-ray films, discograms, nerve physiologic studies (EMG, SSEP), and laboratory studies should enable the clinician to isolate a specific pathophysiologic pain generator. Diagnostic and therapeutic injections (epidural, facet injection, selective nerve root injections) can isolate the actual pain generator, particularly when sophisticated diagnostic studies have identified many abnormal structures (such as multilevel degenerative disc protrusions). The cortisone injections will often provide symptomatic relief that can facilitate rehabilitation, restore function, and contribute to return

to work. They also provide an insight into pain tolerance, pain behavior, and nonphysiologic responses. Often, additional lumbar spine stabilization therapy is required for the more seriously injured worker. Spinal stabilization involves strengthening spinal trunk and extremity muscles statically and dynamically.

At 12 weeks postinjury, Step C, resolution of the injury and workers' compensation claim must be insight. California state law mandates that at 90 days postinjury the clinician must consider if the worker will return to his regular and customary work or is a candidate for vocational rehabilitation. At 12 weeks postinjury off work, the injured worker is now considered a chronic pain patient. The rehabilitation of a chronic pain patient is completely different from that for an acutely injured patient. Assuming the patient has received appropriate treatment through Steps A and B, ongoing hands-on therapy to reduce pain will not be beneficial in altering eventual outcome and actually might contribute to ongoing disability.

The emphasis in the chronic pain patient is focused on an independent aerobic exercise program emphasizing functional goals, such as increased lifting capacity or sitting tolerance, in order to facilitate return to work. Occasionally a functional work capacity evaluation and work hardening program might facilitate return to work.[12] Psychologic evaluations at this point might be necessary to identify psychosocial barriers to recovery. Vocational guidance and resolution of outstanding lawsuits will also help facilitate return to work.

At 3 months postinjury, the injured worker has either returned to work, entered vocational rehabilitation, or has been deemed capable of working despite subjective complaints that are not substantiated by objective findings or diagnostic tests. Occasionally an independent medical examination is necessary to force closure of claims involving individuals who have not responded to appropriate treatment in a reasonable manor.

Rarely will an occupationally injured worker require surgical intervention, Step D. Individuals with a progressive neurologic deficit that correlates with anatomic imaging studies should undergo prompt surgical intervention (cauda equina syndrome). The majority of spinal surgery, however, is performed on the basis of subjective pain complaints. Only those individuals who have a definitive pathophysiologic pain generator that is repetitively alleviated temporarily with diagnostic injections and who have no major psychologic risk factors, who have not responded to Steps A, B, and C above, should be considered for spinal surgery. The outcome with spinal surgery in the workers' compensation population is historically very poor. The spinal literature supports the previously mentioned conservative approach to nonmalignant mechanical spinal pain syndromes. Weber's classic study has demonstrated that lumbar disc herniations with radiculopathy have a better long-term outcome without surgery than with surgery.[15]

SUMMARY

Occupational low back injuries are the most frequent problem faced by occupationally oriented physicians. A careful history and physical examination with judicious use of diagnostic studies will provide a diagnosis in the majority of these patients.

An aggressive rehabilitation approach emphasizing reduction of pain, restoration of function, and return to work will facilitate better outcomes and reduce medical legal costs. An algorithm of treatment that has been successful in a busy occupational medicine clinic has been presented.

REFERENCES

1. Adams MA, Hutton WC: The mechanical function of the lumbar apophyseal joints, *Spine* 8:326-330, 1983.
2. Adams MA, Hutton WC: The relevance of torsion to the mechanical derangement of the lumbar spine, *Spine* 8:241-248, 1981.
3. Alston W et al: A quantitative study of muscle factors in chronic low back syndrome, *J Am Geriatr Soc* 14:1041-1047, 1966.
4. Anderson GBJ: Low back in industry, *Spine* 6:53-56, 1981.
5. Beals RK, Hickman NY: Industrial injuries of the back and extremities: comprehensive evaluation—an aid in prognosis and management, *J Bone Joint Surg (Am)* S4A:1593-1611, 1972.
6. Cats-Baril WL, Frymoyer JW: Identifying patients at risk of becoming disabled because of low back pain, *Spine* 16:605-607, 1991.
7. Farfan HF et al: The effects of torsion on the lumbar intervertebral joints: the role of torsion in the production of disc degeneration, *J Bone Joint Surg* 52:468-497, 1970.
8. Fordyce W: Back pain. In Rosen J, Solomon L, editors: *Compensation and public policy prevention in health psychology*, Hanover Vt, 1985, University Press of New England.
9. Frymoyer JW: Back pain and sciatica, *N Engl J Med* 318:291-300, 1988.
10. Marshall LL, Trethewie ER, Curtain CC: Chemical radiculitis: a clinical, psychological, and immunological study, *Clin Orthop Rel Res* 129:61-67, 1957.
11. National Center for Health Statistics: Prevalence of selected impairment: United States—1977, PHS series 10 no 134, Hyattsville, Md, 1987, Department of Health and Human Services.
12. Sontag MJ: Functional assessment of the spinal pain patient, *Neck and Back Pain State of the Arts Reviews*, Philadelphia, 1990, Hanley & Belfus.
13. Spengler DM: Back injuries in industry: a retrospective study, *Spine* 11:241-245, 1986.
14. Waddell G et al: Nonorganic physical signs in low back pain, *Spine* 2:117-125, 1980.
15. Weber H: Lumbar disc herniation: a controlled prospective study with 10 years of observation, *Spine* 8:131-140, 1983.
16. Yong-Hing K, Kirkaldy-Willis WH: The pathophysiology of degenerative disease of the lumbar spine, *Orthop Clin North Am* 14:491-504, 1983.

12 Knee Disorders

The past decade has seen dramatic changes in orthopedics concerning the natural history, diagnosis, and approach to treatment of injuries to the knee. The development of the arthroscope and surgical techniques to treat these conditions with significantly less morbidity than the traditional open means has enabled orthopedic surgeons to accelerate healing and the return to employment of injured workers. It also has been a significant aid in evaluating patients with chronically painful conditions of the knee, formerly not amenable to traditional treatment and/or diagnostic tests.

The majority of knee conditions can be treated conservatively, however, especially those seen in a work environment. Determining which patients require additional care necessitates an adequate knowledge of anatomy, proper physical examination techniques, and the ability to make a differential diagnosis.

Compared with many other joints in the body, the knee is relatively subcutaneous, and most of the bony landmarks can be palpated. On physical examination a number of tests that are predictable, are reproducible, and can objectify the patient's complaint of pain can be performed. This is not like the lower back or neck where pain can be a predominant feature and objectifying an injured worker's complaints can often be difficult. A careful history and physical examination can provide an accurate diagnosis in most cases so that a specific treatment plan can be developed to minimize the length of time that the injured worker is disabled and return the employee to gainful activity and employment.

ANATOMY

Knowledge of the knee anatomy is essential to understanding and diagnosing the various disorders that involve the knee joint. Although radiographs are essential to the establishment of a diagnosis in any joint, the knee, with its multiplicity of soft tissue components, requires an adequate knowledge of the structure and function of not only the skeletal system but the ligamentous, capsular, musculotendinous, and intraarticular structures as well.

Skeleton

The femur, tibia, and patella comprise the skeletal components of the knee joint. All three surfaces are covered with articular cartilage that allow frictionless gliding as the knee moves through a range of motion. Degeneration of the articular cartilage narrows the space between the femur, tibia, and/or patella with subsequent radiographic changes and symptoms. Normally, articular cartilage is white, smooth, and glistening; as early degeneration occurs, fraying of the articular cartilage can occur (chondromalacia), causing crepitations and grinding as the knee goes through a range of motion. Further degeneration and wear of the articular cartilage leads to the development of exposed bone that produces the more apparent radiographic abnormalities generally associated with degenerative joint disease (Fig. 12-1). Articular cartilage loss can be focal, such as one sees in trauma, or diffuse, which is more consistent with the aging process and chronic conditions.

The knee functions like a hinge joint but physiologically is a gliding joint that actually goes through rotation, especially in the last 15 degrees of extension. This is due to the shape of the femoral condyles, proximal tibia, and the structure of the medial and lateral meniscus. Interruption of this normal screw home mechanism of the knee, whereby the knee rotates as it comes into full extension, can be caused by injuries to the anterior or posterior cruciate ligaments or the meniscus.

The patella, a sesamoid bone located within the structure of the quadriceps mechanism, functions to improve the extensor moment of the knee. It improves the ability of the quadriceps to elevate the tibia from a fully flexed position by improving the moment arm, a common concept in physics. The distal femur has a groove, the trochlea, in which the patella glides. The shape of this femoral groove varies from individual to individual. A centered patella offers the best biomechanical advantage for extension of the knee without symptoms. Malalignment of the patella in the femoral groove is caused by congenital factors or trauma from previous dislocations. Stretching of the medial

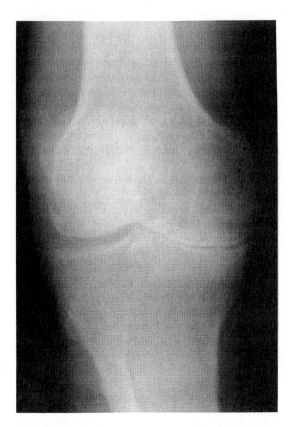

Fig. 12-1 X-ray film of right knee depicting complete loss of medial joint space articular cartilage.

structures or a tight lateral retinaculum can cause the patella to track laterally, causing increased pressures under the patella and subsequent symptoms.

Although changes in the articular cartilage can give rise to symptoms, the etiology of pain in patients with disorders of the articular cartilage is not known.

Extraarticular structures

Anterior structures. The quadriceps muscles covering the front of the thigh converge to attach to the patella through a thick tendon with contributions from the vastus medialis obliquus (VMO), vastus lateralis (VL), rectus femoris, and vastus intermedius. The convergence of these four muscles onto the patella provides stability for the patellofemoral joint and powerful extension for the knee. The quadriceps expansion continues over the patella and extends distally to form the patellar tendon. Lateral expansions of the quadriceps mechanism over the medial and lateral aspect of the patella (medial and lateral retinaculum) provide additional coverage and support to the anterior aspect of the knee. These structures cover the capsule of the knee joint and synovium. Two fat

pads that fill the space between the lower portion of the patella and the joint are visible just medial and lateral to the patellar tendon, especially with the knee in flexion (Fig. 12-2).

Damage to the quadriceps tendon or patellar tendon can cause dramatic loss of extensor power and major disability to the knee. Injuries to the medial or lateral retinaculum (primarily medial) can cause recurrent dislocations or recurrent tracking problems involving the patellofemoral joint. Inflammation at the site of attachment of the quadriceps to the patella or of the patellar tendon to the patella can be caused by repetitive overuse and chronic tendonitis can result.

Lateral structures. The lateral side of the knee contains a series of tissue layers that provide ligamentous support and stability to the lateral portion of the knee (Fig. 12-3). The major ligamentous structure is the fibular collateral ligament, which courses from the lateral femoral epicondyle distally to attach to the fibular head. This short, stout ligament provides lateral ligamentous support. The popliteus tendon courses up from the posterior inferior aspect of the knee joint, coming around the posterolateral corner of the knee, and attaches anterior and under the fibular collateral ligament near the lateral femoral epicondyle. The popliteus provides rotational stability and resistance to external rotation because of its role as an internal rotator. The arcuate ligamentous complex is located posteriorly and provides support to the posterolat-

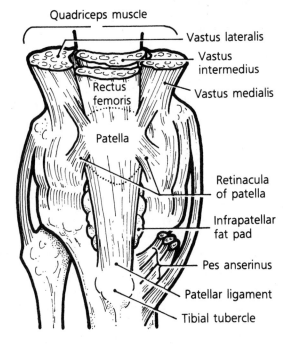

Fig. 12-2 Anterior knee musculature (from Aaos: *Athletic training and sports medicine,* ed 2, 1991).

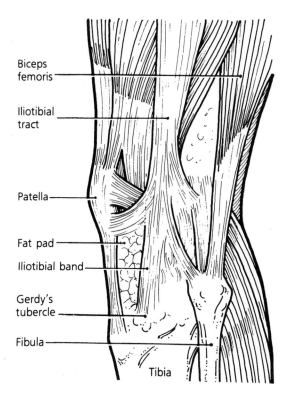

Fig. 12-3 Lateral knee musculature (from Aaos: *Athletic training and sports medicine,* ed 2, 1991).

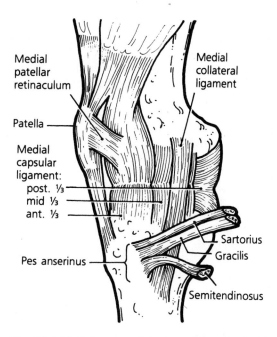

Fig. 12-4 Medial aspect of the knee (from Aaos: *Athletic training and sports medicine,* ed 2, 1991).

eral corner of the knee joint. These structures are damaged in patients with varus or lateral instabilities.

These structures are covered by the iliotibial band, a broad band of fasciae that arises from the tensor fasciae latae and the anterior superior iliac spine. It courses distally over the greater trochanter and ends in a wide band that attaches to Gerdy's tubercle on the proximal tibia. This thick investing fascia aids in extension of the knee through the terminal 30 degrees. The fact that the iliotibial band glides anteriorly in extension and posteriorly in flexion can give rise to bursitis or inflammation where the iliotibial band glides over the prominence of the lateral femoral epicondyle. The biceps tendon posteriorly attaches to the fibular head with the peroneal nerve, exiting under the biceps tendon and coursing superficially around the posterolateral corner of the fibular head and diving into the lateral compartment before it divides into the superficial and deep peroneal branches.

Medial structures. The major anatomic structure on the medial side of the knee is the medial collateral ligament. It originates from the medial femoral epicondyle and attaches on the proximal tibia distally. It is a thin broad ligament and provides restraints to valgus deformation of the knee

(Fig. 12-4). A deep portion of the medial collateral ligament attaches to the meniscus and capsule and provides additional medial support. Coursing superficially to the distal portion of the medial collateral ligament is the pes anserinus, the distal insertion of the sartorius, gracilis, and semitendinosus tendons. A number of bursa surrounding these tendons can occasionally give rise to symptoms. At the posteromedial corner of the knee is an expansion of the posterior capsule, with the semimembranosus tendon inserting distal to the medial joint line at the posteromedial corner. The complex interplay of the ligamentous complex on the medial side of the knee combines to provide excellent stability to valgus stress in the knee.

Coursing with the saphenous vein on the posteromedial aspect of the knee joint, is the saphenous nerve that gives off an infrapatellar branch at the level of the semimembranosus. Injuries to this nerve can occur causing sensory changes around the knee. The nerve has also been implicated in causing some of the more chronic nerve pain syndromes, especially following blunt trauma or surgical procedures.

Posterior structures. The posterior aspect of the knee contains the major neurovascular structures supplying the lower leg and foot. The popliteal vein and artery lie deep in the popliteal fossa, covered by the medial and lateral head of the gastrocnemius muscles. A tiny sesamoid bone called the fabella lies in the lateral head of the gastrocnemius, is frequently seen on x-ray film, and can occasionally be mistaken for a loose body. The posterior capsule can become weakened, giving rise to a popliteal cyst (Baker's cyst) that can extend out underneath the medial head of the gastrocnemius, causing fullness and swelling in the popliteal fossa.

Intraarticular structures

Suprapatellar and medial plicae. The knee joint is lined by a synovial membrane that extends above the superior pole of the patella, forming a large bursa, or suprapatellar pouch. This space allows for fluid motion of the knee in flexion and extension and allows for smooth gliding of the patella in the femoral groove. Embryologic remnants can occur within the knee and form intrasynovial folds or plica that can occasionally cause symptoms. The suprapatellar plica courses transversely across the suprapatellar pouch and may be complete or incomplete. The medial plica (medial synovial shelf) courses from the fat pad inferiorly, attaching to the medial capsule, extending superiorly just to the level of the superior pole of the patella. Both of these plica are normally small and thin and do not cause symptoms. Occasionally, following repetitive trauma or blunt trauma these

can thicken and hypertrophy and cause snapping and pain within the knee joint.

Medial and lateral menisci. The medial and lateral menisci are two horseshoe or C-shaped fibrocartilaginous discs that lie between the femur and tibia, provide shock absorption and lubrication, and enhance stability of the knee. These relatively avascular structures have minimal blood supply except in the outer 3 to 4 mm near the periphery. This is why most meniscal tears do not heal. However, there is an excellent supply of capillaries to the peripheral 3 to 4 mm of the meniscus so that tears in these locations can be repaired successfully (Fig. 12-5). Absence of an entire meniscus will lead to decompensation of the affected compartment over time and is well known to cause degenerative arthritis.[5,7,16] The absence of normal ligamentous stability in the knee will accelerate this abnormal wear if the meniscus has been surgically removed.

Anterior and posterior cruciate ligaments. The anterior and posterior cruciate ligaments are the major restraining ligaments in the knee to anterior and posterior translation of the tibia on the femur, respectively (Fig. 12-6). The anterior cruciate ligament originates from the posterior aspect of the

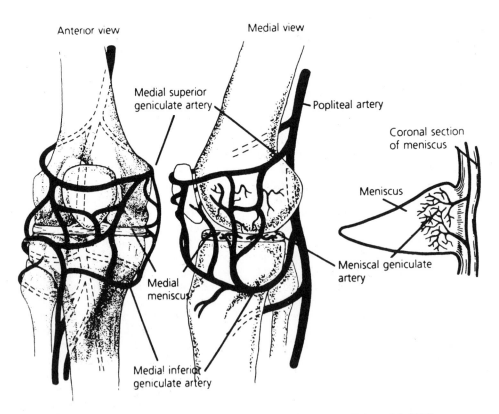

Fig. 12-5 Blood supply of the knee (from Aaos: *Athletic training and sports medicine,* ed 2, 1991).

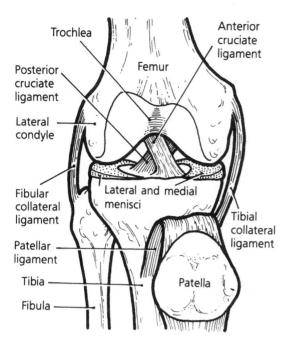

Trochlea

Anterior cruciate ligament

Posterior cruciate ligament

Femur

Lateral condyle

Fibular collateral ligament

Lateral and medial menisci

Patellar ligament

Tibial collateral ligament

Tibia

Fibula

Patella

Fig. 12-6 Ligamentous structures of the knee (from Aaos: *Athletic training and sports medicine,* ed 2, 1991).

lateral femoral condyle in the intercondylar notch and attaches just lateral to the medial tibial spine on the proximal tibia anteriorly. The posterior cruciate ligament originates from the medial aspect of the distal femur in the intercondylar notch anteriorly and inserts a broad thick band on the proximal tibia posterolaterally. The posterior cruciate ligament is much less frequently injured than the anterior cruciate ligament, with the most common injury being a direct blow to the anterior proximal tibia with the knee in flexion, driving the tibia posteriorly and tearing the posterior cruciate ligament. The anterior cruciate ligament is most commonly torn in higher velocity injuries either through hyperextension or a rotational valgus injury of the knee joint. Loss of either ligament can cause major decompensation of the knee and pivoting and twisting is impaired. Absence or tearing of the anterior and/or posterior cruciate ligament often leads to a high percentage of progressive meniscal and articular cartilage defects that can accelerate the rate of degenerative arthritis in the knee.[6,9,10,11,13]

HISTORY

Obtaining an accurate history pertaining to injuries of the knee is essential to establish a clear diagnosis. Most knee disorders can be diagnosed on the basis of a specific and accurate history. In the work-related injury, the mechanism of the injury,

the circumstances under which it occurred, and the amount of initial impairment is critical in establishing a diagnosis. It will also help validate the consistency of the claim with the level of disability that the patient may allege.

It is particularly important to obtain as specific a mechanism of injury as possible. How the injury occurred—whether it was involved with a twist, a fall, a direct blow—provides important clues about the nature of the injury itself. The presence of immediate impairment, inability to bear weight, or whether the patient was able to continue working will also frequently support or controvert the severity of the initial difficulties. The presence of immediate versus delayed swelling and the location of the swelling are particularly important in determining whether significant intraarticular damage has occurred. For example, the presence of immediate swelling, especially in the suprapatellar area, would signify intraarticular bleeding and probable significant damage to intraarticular structures. Delayed swelling (over 24 hours) is usually considered a reactive effusion; it is a reaction of the synovial lining to a traumatic incident to the joint. The fluid is generally blood tinged or yellow and is frequently seen with articular cartilage injuries, meniscal tears not involving the capsule or the periphery of the meniscus, or inflammatory synovitis. The presence or absence of heat should also be noted in assessing the quality of an effusion. Heat associated with effusion can be seen in patients with inflammatory arthritis, such as gout, rheumatoid arthritis, or Reiter's syndrome, or in infectious processes as well.

Extraarticular swelling is generally localized to the area where the injury occurred and is often associated with ecchymosis and specific point tenderness. Swelling in the prepatellar bursa is usually localized just anterior to the patella or patellar tendon and is not associated with intraarticular swelling. It often follows either direct trauma or repetitive kneeling or abrasions to the area. Patients complaining of swelling inferior to the lower pole of the patella in the fat pad area should not be confused with those presenting with actual intraarticular effusion or prepatellar bursitis (Fig. 12-7). Hoffa's syndrome, an uncommon inflammation of the fat pads, can cause localized tenderness and swelling in this area and is usually a self-limited process responsive to the usual antiinflammatory modalities.

The duration of symptoms is an important indicator of the severity of symptoms. Immediate impairment with inability to walk clearly accompanies more serious intraarticular or extraarticular injuries. A patient who is able to continue working for several weeks following a minor injury to the

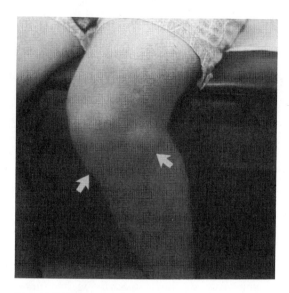

Fig. 12-7 Hoffa's syndrome. Note the enlarged fat pads medial and lateral to the patella.

knee, not accompanied by objective physical findings or symptoms, such as effusion, buckling, or giving way, will be much less likely to have a significant intraarticular problem than a patient who has symptoms immediately. Patients with chronic knee pain following a rather insignificant injury should be carefully questioned about preexisting difficulties, such as one might see in the case of degenerative arthritis aggravated by some form of work injury. Questioning the patient about whether they have ever received medical care concerning the knee, x-ray films, or previous treatment is important. In younger patients there will often be a history of a remote injury associated with sports that was minimally treated but may be a significant contributing factor to the current disability. For example, many young adult patients may have had a seemingly minor knee sprain playing football or skiing. Many of these patients may have had an injury to the anterior cruciate ligament that was later aggravated by some form of work activity. Specific detailed questioning about the previous injury is necessary to ascertain whether any preexisting condition existed.

The location of pain in patients with knee injuries is a helpful indicator of pathology and can often lead to a specific diagnosis. For example, the patient should be questioned as to whether the pain is localized over the medial joint line, the medial femoral epicondyle, medial collateral ligament, or along the medial retinaculum. Anterior knee pain, described as an aching pain in the front of the knee, is most often associated with patellofemoral disorders such as chondromalacia

and is less likely associated with mechanical problems such as meniscal tears or ligament injuries.

The presence or absence of mechanical symptoms within a knee joint should be carefully ascertained. The presence of locking, such as, difficulty fully extending the knee from a flexed position after a squat or a momentary catching in the knee where the knee is unable to move followed by a release, usually signifies significant intraarticular derangement such as meniscal tears or loose bodies. These symptoms are occasionally associated with episodes of giving way or buckling where the muscle control to the knee is lost. Some patients, however, will report giving way which is actually related to weakness of the quadriceps. Specific mechanisms for the giving-way episode should be investigated. For example, the patient should be asked if the knee gives way when they turn a corner or pivot (as seen in meniscal tears or ligament instabilities) or whether the giving-way occurs when they are standing and the knee buckles backwards. Backward buckling or buckling forward is often seen in muscular weakness rather than actual mechanical difficulties within the joint. Many patients will state that the knee gives way when they go up or down stairs, and this may be due less to a mechanical derangement within the joint than to quadriceps weakness or pain. Other causes of knee joint buckling include chondral injuries (irregular flaps of articular cartilage that catch while the knee is being brought through a range of motion), (Fig. 12-8), as well as ligament instabilities, loose bodies, or meniscal tears. Episodes of recurrent

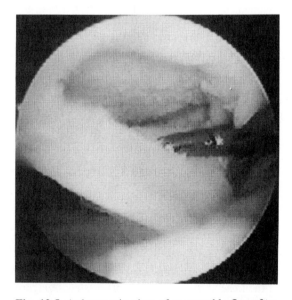

Fig. 12-8 Arthroscopic view of an unstable flap of articular cartilage held down with a probe exposing underlying bone.

patellar subluxation can also cause a patient to complain of giving way, but generally the patients will be pivoting or twisting and will feel their kneecap pop out.

As with any orthopedic disorder, the patient should be questioned as to whether they are having symptoms in the joint above or below the affected joint in question. Specifically, hip pain or hip pathology is notorious for referring pain to the anterior aspect of the knee and can occasionally be seen in degenerative arthritis of the hip, avascular necrosis, or tumors of the femur. Patients should be questioned about any associated groin or night pain that can often give clues to other occult nonindustrial causes of knee pain.

Past medical history in all patients with knee injuries should also be evaluated. Remote injuries to the knee joint not considered significant may play a role in the pathogenesis of meniscal tears in young active patients. In addition, in older patients who present with evidence of degenerative arthritis, a history of symptoms in the knee or care will obviously play a role in whether apportionment may become an issue as their claims develop.

PHYSICAL EXAMINATION

In general, the physical examination should confirm the diagnosis that one suspects on the basis of an accurate history. The general principles of observation, palpation, examination for range of motion, stability, and special mechanical tests should be followed routinely.

Careful observation of the patient not only during the exam but also before the examination starts is critical, especially in workers' compensation cases, for validating the severity of the patient's complaints. Physicians should observe if the patient is using crutches properly or, if only using a cane, it is used in the proper hand (the hand opposite the affected leg). Whether the crutches or immobilizer or braces are worn and used or appear to be clean and recently purchased are also important. The patient should be observed for a limp not only in the examining room but also as he enters the room. Especially after leaving the office, the occasional patient can be seen to have a marked improvement in their gait pattern. The patient's knee should be examined for the presence or absence of abrasions, visible areas of ecchymosis, intraarticular or extraarticular swelling, or deformity.

With the patient in the standing position, alignment of the extremities should be observed. A valgus (knock kneed) (Fig. 12-9) or varus (bow-legged) (Fig. 12-10) disposition to both legs is documented, especially if there is asymmetry. Observation of patellar tracking should be docu-

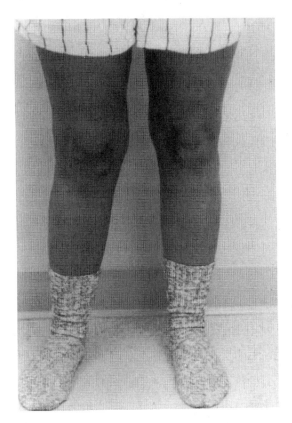

Fig. 12-9 Valgus knee. Right knee of patient with lateral compartment arthritis in abnormal valgus alignment.

mented. The patient sits with the leg hanging at 90 degrees over the edge of the table and is asked to extend the leg through a range of motion. The position of the patella in the femoral groove should be observed and often subtle patellar tracking problems can be determined by watching the patella slide laterally out of the femoral groove as the knee comes into full extension (the J sign). The presence or absence of an extensor lag—the inability to hold the leg in full extension against gravity—is one of the earliest clues to a quadriceps tendon or patellar tendon rupture.

Palpation of the various bony landmarks around the knee can often give clues about the area of the greatest pathology. Palpation of the patella with the patient sitting and extending the knee against gravity often gives information about the quality of the articular cartilage under the patella. Palpable and occasional audible crepitations of the patella articular cartilage can be felt. This may be normal in an older individual and not necessarily the cause of symptoms. Comparison with the normal side is important and asymmetry should be noted. A history compatible with anterior knee pain and crepitations are probably significant. In

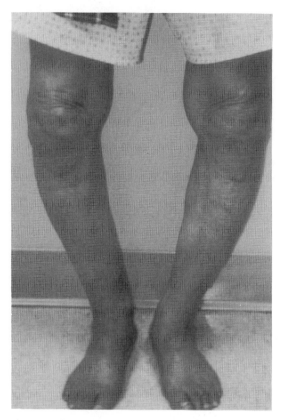

Fig. 12-10 Severe varus deformity of the knees in an 89-year-old man with medial compartment arthritis.

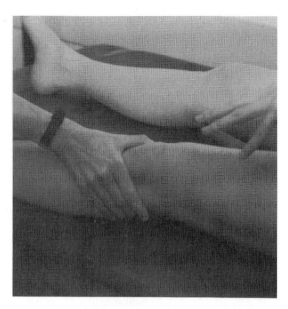

Fig. 12-11 Apprehension sign. Passive lateral glide of the patella will cause the patient discomfort and will result in reflex contraction of the quadriceps, indicating instability.

addition, alignment of the patella can also be palpated with the knee in full extension or slight flexion to 10 degrees. Assessment of patellar tilt is performed by placing the thumb and index finger on the edges of the patella. In addition, the patella should be passively slid medially to test the tightness of the vastus lateralis. It should also be passively slid laterally to assess excessive mobility of the patella in the femoral groove. Pain reported by the patient or apprehension of the patient when the patella is passively slid laterally in full extension is known as the apprehension sign and is often pathognomic of recurrent patellar dislocations or subluxation (Fig. 12-11).

Stability assessment is carried out with the patient in the supine position. It is imperative that the physician perform the examination with the patient relaxed. A cooperative patient who is not anxious or concerned about severe pain during the examination will be able to relax the quadriceps and hamstrings about the knee, allowing a much better ligament exam. Excellent assessment of knee stability can be obtained with gentle rather than forceful manipulation.

The collateral ligaments are assessed with the knee in full extension and secondarily with the knee in 30 degrees of flexion. With the examiner's hand resting proximal to the popliteal fossa to support the thigh with the palm on the lateral side, the other hand grasps the patient's ankle and gently lifts the leg. A lateral force is directed against the medial ankle, which will open the medial side of the knee. Patients with medial collateral ligament injuries will report pain, and opening of the joint at 30 degrees of flexion will be noted (Fig. 12-12). Comparison to the opposite side is mandatory, especially in the individual with ligamentous laxity. A medially directed force (varus stress) at the ankle will assess the lateral collateral ligaments and lateral ligamentous structures.

Complete ligament tears will offer minimal resistance at the end of stressing the joint and will often feel as a mushy or soft endpoint. A firm endpoint signifies partial injury. Patients with complete ligament tears often have little pain with this maneuver because the two ligament ends are no longer in contact and there is less feedback inhibition from overstretching the collagen fibers. Conversely, mild sprains of the medial collateral ligament can often produce severe pain with this maneuver, but the patient will have good joint stability and no abnormal opening with valgus stress.

Evaluation of the anterior and posterior cruciate ligament is critical to assess major stability to the knee. The anterior cruciate ligament is damaged in more than 95% of all cruciate injuries. Less than 5% of cruciate injuries are to the posterior cruciate

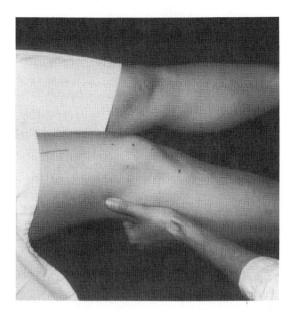

Fig. 12-12 Collateral ligament testing. Laterally and medially directed force is placed at the ankle with the fulcrum at the knee to stress the medial and lateral collateral ligaments.

ligament. The anterior cruciate can be evaluated even in the acutely swollen and tender knee in most patients. The patient's knee should be observed at 90 degrees of flexion from the side and a telltale hint of a posterior sag of the tibia on the femur can be often seen (Fig. 12-13). This posterior sag is a primary finding in posterior cruciate liga-

ment injuries. This often may not be seen in the acute phase, but in the chronic patients it can often be easily visible.

The Lachman's test is the most accurate test for detecting anterior cruciate ligament injuries, especially in the acutely injured knee. The patient's knee is flexed to 20 degrees and supported by the hand underlying the thigh. The femur is fixed with the upper hand and is used as a fulcrum. The tibia is grasped proximally, with the foot resting still on the table, and the tibia is then brought forward on the femur as the femur is gently pushed posteriorly (Fig. 12-14). This push/pull test is positive in patients with torn anterior cruciate ligaments and can be done even in the acutely swollen knee. The anterior drawer test is done with the knee at 80 to 90 degrees of flexion to assess the competency of the anterior and posterior cruciate ligaments. The examiner sits on the patient's foot to stabilize it, the knee is flexed to 90 degrees, the examiner's hands are placed behind the knee in the proximal tibia, making sure that the hamstring tendons themselves are relaxed, and the tibia is then gently pulled forward on the femur (Fig. 12-15). In patients with an absent anterior cruciate ligament the tibia can translate anteriorly 1 to $1\frac{1}{2}$ cm. The amount of translation of the tibia is graded. One plus (1+) signifies 5 mm of anterior translation, 2+ (10 mm), and 3+ (1.5 cm) if one compares the knee with the normal side. Examining the tibia's translation posteriorly (posterior drawer) can also be done in the same position. In the acutely injured knee this test can often be difficult because

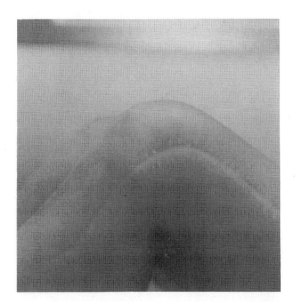

Fig. 12-13 "Posterior sag" sign. The tibia is subluxed posteriorly on the femur as a result of a tear of the posterior cruciate ligament.

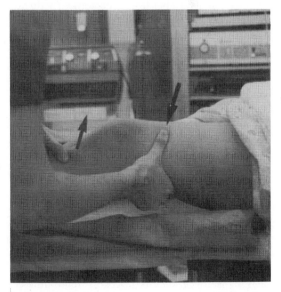

Fig. 12-14 Lachman's test. The thigh is stabilized with a posteriorly directed force, and the tibia is subluxed anteriorly.

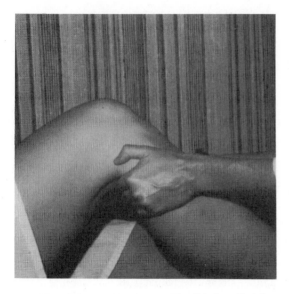

Fig. 12-15 Anterior drawer test. The tibia is pulled forward with the knee at 90 degrees, and excessive translation on the femur confirms tear of the anterior collateral ligament.

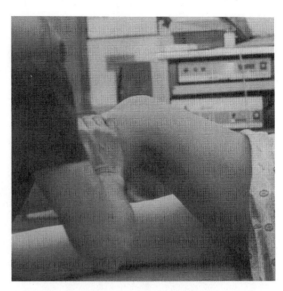

Fig. 12-16 Pivot shift test. Abnormal anterior and lateral rotation of the tibia on the femur indicates severe ace injury.

of the presence of an effusion, making knee flexion to 90 degrees difficult and because the patient is apprehensive. In the acute knee, therefore, the Lachman's test is a more sensitive indicator of anterior cruciate ligament competency, whereas in the chronic knee both tests are used in combination to assess the anterior cruciate ligament.

The pivot shift test is a maneuver designed to test the competency of the anterior cruciate ligament in rotation. This test is performed with the patient supine as the examiner stands on the lateral side of the involved extremity. With the knee extended, one hand grips the heel and rotates the foot internally while the other hand applies a valgus stress to the proximal tibia with the palm of the hand just posterior to the fibular head (Fig. 12-16). If the tibia subluxates anteriorly, the test is positive and it reduces with a palpable and visible shift or jerk at about 30 to 40 degrees flexion. A positive pivot shift implies serious instability of the knee.

Two primary tests assess meniscal integrity. McMurray's maneuver is performed with the patient supine, with the patient's foot cupped in the palm and forearm of the examiner to allow comfortable manipulation of the knee. The examiner's opposite hand is placed with the thumb and forefinger on the medial and lateral joint line of the patient's knee. The knee is flexed to approximately 110 to 115 degrees of flexion, the foot is rotated, the tibia is then rotated on the femur into external rotation, and the knee is passively extended. The

examiner listens and feels for an audible click or pop over the medial meniscus (Fig. 12-17). This maneuver traps the torn meniscus under the femoral condyles and as the leg is extended the meniscus often reduces, producing the characteristic click. The lateral meniscus is assessed by flexing the knee and internally rotating the tibia to determine the presence of a click over the lateral meniscus. Pain accompanied by a click can be seen in condylar disorders as well as meniscal

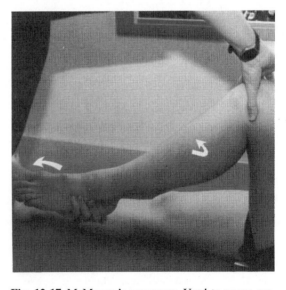

Fig. 12-17 McMurray's maneuver. Used to assess medial and lateral meniscal tears.

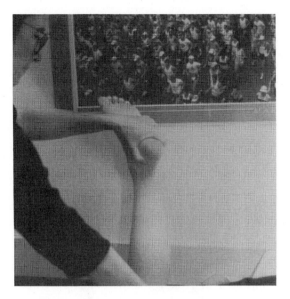

Fig. 12-18 Apley's test. A downward pressure, with rotation of the femur on the tibia of a patient in the prone position, causes pain in a patient with meniscal pathology.

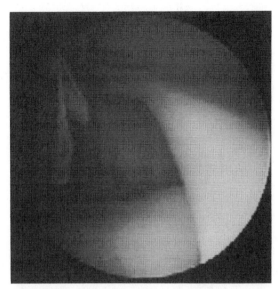

Fig. 12-19 Hypertrophied plica covering the medial femoral condyle as seen arthroscopically.

tears, but the presence of a click between 90 and 40 degrees of flexion often signifies meniscal pathology. The Apley's test is done with the patient prone and the knee flexed to 90 degrees. The examiner puts pressure on the patient's foot and rotates the tibia on the flexed knee and femur. If pain is produced, this is significant for possible meniscal pathology as well (Fig. 12-18).

In addition, the patient should be asked to fully squat or duck walk, which tests the competency of the posterior horns of the meniscus. Difficulty doing so may imply a posterior horn meniscal tear.

Pathologic plicae can occasionally produce a characteristic click over the medial side of the knee with flexion and extension. A plica can often be palpated as a thickened band just medial to the patella and superior to the fat pad and cause soreness to the patient as it is rubbed over the condyle (Fig. 12-19). Infiltration of the area with 1% xylocaine and reduction of symptoms can often confirm the diagnosis.

DIAGNOSTIC TESTS
X-ray films

Standard x-ray films of the knee should be obtained in all patients having undergone any significant acute trauma. In the acutely injured knee, the presence or absence of fractures, loose bodies, effusion, and preexisting difficulties should be assessed. This is especially important in the injured worker who may have had some preexisting difficulties with the knee that need to be documented

at the time of the original work injury. Anterior and posterior (AP), lateral, tunnel, and merchant (30-degree tangential view of patella) views are performed. Weight-bearing x-ray films should be obtained in patients more than 50 years old who have pain in their knees associated with walking and recurrent effusions. Weight-bearing x-ray films are much more sensitive to assess any actual articular cartilage loss in the joint, whereas non–weight-bearing x-ray films (routine AP films) do not assess the joint dynamics when the joint is loaded. Tunnel views are also helpful in determining the presence of any loose bodies and looking at the more posterior aspect of the femoral condyle, especially in chondral lesions.

Arthrograms

The popularity of arthrograms has diminished in recent years with the increased popularity of magnetic resonance imaging (MRI). The radiographic exposure and the invasive nature of the procedure with a needle to inject dye and air into the joint has been a drawback for some patients. Arthrograms, however, are still indicated and useful in patients who have peripheral tears of the menisci that often cannot be adequately imaged with MRI. In addition, pathologic plicae, popliteal or Baker's cysts, and occasional chondral lesions can often be seen by a skilled radiologist performing arthrograms when MRIs cannot disclose these as well (Fig. 12-20). Arthrograms are useful in patients with persistent pain following partial meniscectomy. The procedure is used to assess whether any residual mechanically unstable meniscal fragments

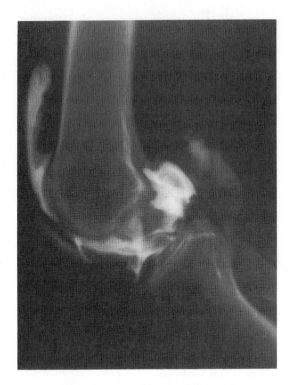

Fig. 12-20 Arthrogram of the knee disclosing a popliteal or Baker's cyst.

remain. As will be noted later, MRIs occasionally are not as helpful in this regard.

Magnetic resonance imaging study

The use of MRI has gained increasing popularity over the last 5 years as a diagnostic tool in assessing derangements and injuries to the knee joint. The ability to image soft tissues and bony and articular cartilage defects has allowed the radiologist to assist the orthopedic surgeon and primary care physician in determining accurate diagnoses in the knee. MRI is particularly helpful in assessing ligamentous injuries, meniscus injuries, and intraosseous problems. Studies have shown a high correlation between MRI findings and arthroscopic results (in the 85% to 90% range).[2,8,15] The lack of radiation and noninvasive nature of the procedure make it an attractive alternative for patients. There may be a tendency to overutilize MRI, however, in patients rather than performing an adequate detailed physical exam and history. MRI is an adjunctive aid to the diagnosis of knee pathology and is, in and of itself, not diagnostic alone. The findings on MRI must continue to correlate with the subjective and objective findings of the examiner.

Difficulties may arise in interpreting MRI findings, especially in regards to meniscus tears. Radi-

ologists have traditionally described meniscal pathology by placing the findings on MRI into various grading patterns.[2,8,15] Grade I lesions signify mild intrameniscal degeneration that is not associated with objective pathology. Grade II intrameniscal degeneration is a term frequently used in describing MRI findings. This is not associated with tears, but is primarily seen in the aging process where the internal matrix of the meniscus has developed fluid and some degeneration (Fig. 12-21). In most cases, these do not cause significant symptoms and are often interpreted as actual meniscal tears. Grade III lesions are consistent with tear patterns; that is, at arthroscopy pathology in the meniscus can be identified. The signal within the meniscus must reach the articular surface to correlate with visually identified pathology (Fig. 12-22). The practitioner should once again be reminded of correlating the MRI descriptive findings with physical examination and historical information.

For example, a 60-year-old patient who has struck her patella against a blunt object at work and has early degenerative changes seen on x-ray films may have an MRI that shows a Grade II intrameniscal degeneration. Obviously, the meniscal degeneration preceded the contusion injury to the patella and would not have correlation with the current symptomatology. Surgery in these patients would not be indicated unless physical findings were consistent with meniscal pathology (McMurray's, specific joint line tenderness, recurrent effusions, locking, giving way).

The use of MRI in patients who have previously undergone meniscectomy also has drawbacks in interpretation.[1,8] MRI is so sensitive that following successful meniscectomy removing the major me-

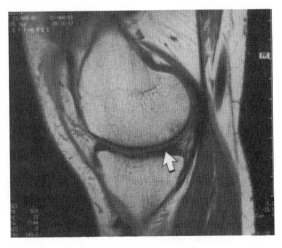

Fig. 12-21 Grade 2 intrameniscal degeneration. Note that the signal does not contact the articular surface.

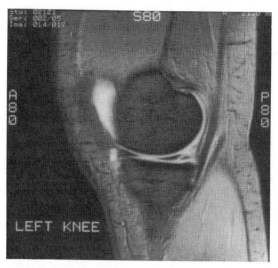

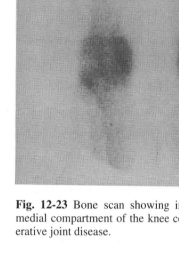

Fig. 12-22 Medial meniscus tear. The signal reaches the articular surface and signifies an actual tear that can be identified at arthroscopy (grade 3).

Fig. 12-23 Bone scan showing intense uptake in the medial compartment of the knee consistent with degenerative joint disease.

chanical portion of the meniscus, some remaining degeneration in the meniscus may be imaged by MRI. Arthroscopists will always try to retain as much stable meniscal tissue as possible so that the joint will not decompensate and develop progressive arthritis. This may mean that some remaining abnormal meniscal tissue is stable to probing and is not mechanically unsound but is clearly not normal visually or pathologically. MRIs in these patients will continue to show abnormal meniscal signal, and this may not in fact correlate with their current pathologic complaints.

Bone scans

Bone scans can be used to assess the painful knee when definite diagnosis cannot be established. Obviously, in a patient who complains of severe unremitting knee pain associated with a negative MRI and bone scan, it would be difficult to support the presence of significant joint pathology. Functional overlay or secondary gain factors may be a consideration in these types of patients. Bone scans are useful in determining the presence or absence of degenerative arthritis, as they can often localize degenerative changes to a specific condyle or compartment of the knee (Fig. 12-23). In addition, chondral lesions occasionally will show an abnormal uptake in the affected condyle or patella. Other traditional modalities such as MRI and arthrogram may fail to show these. Therefore, bone scan can be not only a confirmatory test but also an excellent assessment of specific intraarticular pathology.

EVALUATION AND TREATMENT OF COMMON KNEE INJURIES
Contusions

Contusions about the knee involve a direct blow to areas around the knee joint. Contusions may be associated with local soft-tissue swelling and/or ecchymosis, specific tenderness at the area of the impact, and, in most cases, short-term symptoms. Because the knee bones are subcutaneous they are susceptible to direct injury. Periosteum covering the bones are richly endowed with nerve fibers and occasionally can be quite tender for several weeks. Direct blows not associated with twisting or significant velocity or force rarely cause any long-term impairment in the knee. Treatment generally consists of ice to the area, use of short-term antiinflammatory agents, elevation, occasional short-term use of immobilization, or assistive devices if the patient has difficulty bearing weight.

Most commonly involved in contusions is the prepatellar area. Some of these patients may go on to long-term anterior knee pain syndromes, which are often not associated with significant intraarticular pathology. The exact etiology of the pain has remained a mystery, and it is important in these particular cases to document the presence or absence of atrophy, effusion, subpatellar crepitations, and patellar tracking. An occasional case may develop posttraumatic chondromalacia behind the patella, but these patients usually have a fairly significant mechanism of injury, such as falling from a height onto a directly flexed knee, with the force directly onto the patella. These patients generally present symptoms and develop subpatellar crepitations and initially show evidence of significant trauma. These particular cases are difficult in patients with no objective findings who continue to complain of intractable anterior knee pain made worse with squatting, stooping, and climbing stairs. In these cases it is often extremely helpful to get a bone scan to document whether any change in the bony homeostasis of the knee (such as seeing an area of focal increased uptake correlating with the area of pain). In patients with positive scans, arthroscopy may be indicated from a diagnostic standpoint, although the long-term benefits are somewhat variable.

Prepatellar bursitis

Prepatellar bursitis, or housemaid's knee, is a condition commonly affecting workers who spend a great deal of time on their knees, such as housekeepers, carpenters, floor layers, or religious people. The bursa covering the patella is generally very thin but with chronic irritation can be thickened and even following minor trauma can fill with fluid, causing an unsightly mass. Many of these fluid-filled sacs are actually minimally symptomatic. It is primarily a cosmetic problem for the patient. When associated with heat and other objective signs of inflammation, occasionally it can be painful.

Treatment consists of ice, occasional mobilization of the joint in the acute setting, and aspiration if the bursa is quite distended. Careful, aseptic technique is necessary to avoid infecting the bursa. The technique of aspiration of a prepatellar bursa involves a sterile, thorough cleansing with betadine solution of the entire area surrounding the anterior knee. The most prominent area of fluid is infiltrated with 1% lidocaine with a 30-gauge needle, and a small wheal is developed. Then, with an 18- or 20-gauge needle, using sterile technique, the bursa can be aspirated and the fluid milked into the syringe. Cultures should be obtained routinely, especially if the fluid is cloudy. Once aspiration of the bursa is completed, a sterile compression dressing is applied, and the knee is often immobilized for a few days. When the worker returns to her previous position, protection with a firm knee pad is strongly recommended whenever kneeling is performed. Septic bursitis can frequently follow blunt trauma to the knee, especially if there is an abrasion. It must be vigorously treated with antibiotics and aspiration for culture and occasionally incision and drainage.

Recurrence is not common, and if the condition becomes chronic it may be necessary to formally excise the bursa surgically.

Lacerations

Lacerations about the knee in the industrially injured patient commonly involve high-speed injuries. The use of a saw or sharp object for cutting is a common mode of injury to the soft tissues about the knee itself. It is important in obtaining a history from these patients to ascertain the position of the knee at the time of the injury. The tendinous structures can be torn or lacerated when the knee is flexed, although when the knee is examined in the emergency room in full extension these areas may not be completely visible in the wound. The knee should be put in the same position at which the injury occurred so that deeper anatomic structures can be assessed.

Careful and thorough cleansing of the wound with copious irrigation of saline solution and removal of all foreign tissue should be done. A high index of suspicion for either intraarticular extension of the wound or tendinous injury should also be kept in mind. Radiographs of the knee should be performed routinely if the laceration is through to the subcutaneous tissues. X-ray films can often disclose air within the joint, indicating an open knee laceration, and immediate orthopedic consultation should be obtained. The presence of blood with fat droplets in the wound would also hint of an intraarticular injury. Again, injuries to the medial and lateral side of the knee can easily enter the joint because of the lack of muscle between the skin and the capsule. If any question arises as to the integrity of the joint capsule or patellar or quadriceps tendon, orthopedic consultation should be obtained.

Extensor mechanism injuries

Injuries of the extensor mechanism take many forms and involve the quadriceps tendon, patellar fractures, patellar tendon ruptures, patellar dislocations or subluxations, and posttraumatic chondromalacia. Less disabling but equally frustrating and with the possibility of chronic symptoms include patellar tendonitis and chronic anterior knee pain syndromes.

Rupture of the quadriceps tendon. Quadriceps tendon ruptures may be complete or incomplete. These usually occur by a fall on the flexed knee in a middle-aged or older individual. The classic presentation of a patient with a quadriceps tendon rupture would be inability to fully extend the knee or hold the knee at full extension with the hip flexed 30 degrees. A lag would be present; the thigh could be lifted through the use of the hip flexors but the knee could not be maintained in full extension or held against resistance. In general, a palpable defect can be felt and tenderness superior to the pole of the patella should again alert the examiner to a possible injury to the quadriceps tendon. Lateral radiographs of the knee will show a patella baja: a low-lying patella compared to the normal side. In patients with a question of partial ruptures, MRI has been useful in determining the location and extent of the defect (Fig. 12-24). Occasional patients have incomplete or partial tears of the quadriceps (rectus femoris only). The medial and lateral retinaculum is still intact and the patients can straight-leg raise. Therefore, tenderness superior to the pole of the patella with the presence of any defect and any weakness of the quadriceps should lead one to have a high index of suspicion for quadriceps tendon ruptures.

Immediate surgical repair and consultation with an orthopedic surgeon is advised. Local treatment with ice and immobilization is mandatory until surgical repair can be performed. As the repair often tightens the quadriceps significantly, disability following quadriceps tendon ruptures is prolonged, with frequent difficulties obtaining full flexion. One would expect the disability to last a minimum of 6 months because of the extensive nature of the rehabilitation required following surgical repair. Workers involved in repetitive squatting activities, climbing, or power lifting may have chronic difficulties, and job retraining may be indicated.

Ruptures of the patellar tendon. Patellar tendon ruptures present in a fashion similar to those with quadriceps tendon ruptures. Tenderness at the inferior pole of the patella following a fall on the flexed knee or a jump and the inability to hold the leg in full extension are all clues to this diagnosis. X-ray films will disclose a patella alta or a high-riding patella. Comparison views are always helpful if any question exists as to the location of the patella on lateral views. There may be a preexisting history of pain in the patellar tendon area or a previous history of patellar tendonitis in some of these patients. Predisposing factors include previous surgery in the area of the patellar tendon (old reconstruction of the anterior cruciate ligament with patellar tendon), previous steroid injections for recurrent tendonitis, and a history of gout. Treatment consists of surgical repair and prolonged disability can be expected similar to quadriceps ruptures.

Patellar dislocation and subluxation. Dislocations of the patella can be acute or recurrent and chronic. Acute patellar dislocations are generally the result of a twisting injury with the foot planted or due to a direct blow on the medial aspect of the knee. Nearly 100% of patellar dislocations are lateral and are often spontaneously reduced by the time the patient comes to the emergency room. Reduction is effected by extending the knee so that the patella then slips back into the femoral groove. In the injury, the medial capsule tears, the vastus medialis may stretch or also be torn, and osteochondral fractures of the undersurface of the patella or the superior portion of the lateral femoral condyle can occur (Fig. 12-25).

Referral to an orthopedic surgeon is indicated. Immobilization for 3 to 6 weeks is generally recommended unless evidence of osteochondral frac-

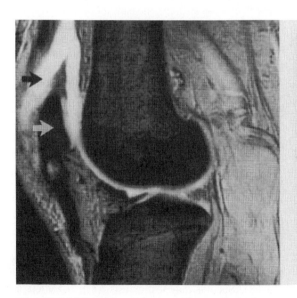

Fig. 12-24 Magnetic resonance image disclosing a complete quadriceps tendon rupture. Black arrow, normal tendon; white arrow, fluid in the tear.

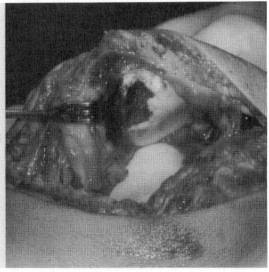

Fig. 12-25 Osteochondral fracture of the patella in patient with acute dislocation. The displaced fragment was replaced and subsequently healed.

tures and loose bodies are seen on x-ray film. Recurrence is likely in the younger patient and repetitive dislocations require surgical correction.

Subluxations of the patella can also occur acutely or chronically. Subluxation or a partial dislocation occurs with a similar mechanism to that seen in patellar dislocations. Predisposing factors to this condition must be sought so that proper treatment can be rendered. Patients with recurrent subluxation or dislocation of the patella often have mechanical malalignment of the lower extremities. A patient often has a valgus knee with pronated feet and a lateral patellar tendon insertion that causes increased disposition of the patella to subluxate laterally as the knee is brought through a range of motion, hence an increased Q angle (Fig. 12-26). Patients may also have inpointing patellas, with a slightly varus tibia, but an increased Q angle due to the medial location of the patella in respect to the distal femur. These are generally congenital conditions and will predispose the patient to recurrent subluxation (Fig. 12-27). The addition of a flat femoral groove, patella alta, or tight lateral retinaculum combined with an atrophic vastus medialis are all predisposing factors for patients with recurrent subluxation of the patella.

The history is usually one of repetitive giving-way of the knee with rotational injuries, and the patient often complains of the knee popping out. Symptoms are momentary, with rapid resolution by full extension of the knee. Swelling may or may not be present; in general, a small effusion is present but may not occur for 24 hours. Following the acute event, tenderness along the medial retinaculum and along the medial border of the patella

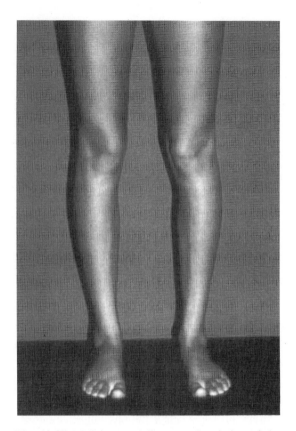

Fig. 12-27 Malicious malalignment. Inpointing of the patella, with tibia vara and pronated feet predisposed to patellar tracking problems.

can often be felt, but a careful patellofemoral examination is also mandatory. Measurement of the quadriceps for atrophy, measurement of the Q angle, assessment of the femoral groove and lateral retinacular structures of the patella are necessary. The usual ligamentous and meniscal tests are also performed to rule out any underlying or concomitant intraarticular pathology. Following repetitive episodes of subluxation, the undersurface of the patella may become roughened and cause post-traumatic chondromalacia. Crepitations of the knee brought through a full range of motion can be palpated, and symmetry with the other knee should be assessed. Patellar apprehension sign is usually positive following an acute episode, while this may or may not be present in the chronic patient.

Again, radiographs are critical to establishing the diagnosis. The Merchant or tangential view is necessary to assess the location of the patella in the femoral groove at 20 degrees of flexion (Fig. 12-28). Special diagnostic tests such as MRI or arthrography are not usually necessary unless one wishes to rule out other intraarticular pathology that may confuse the diagnosis.

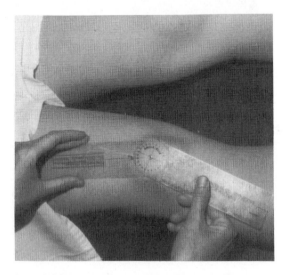

Fig. 12-26 Measurement of the Q angle. The angle formed between femur, center of patella, and tibial tubercle (nl ≤ 15°).

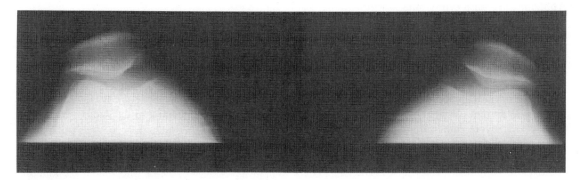

Fig. 12-28 Bilateral subluxation of patella seen on Merchant's view.

Following the initial acute subluxation, treatment should consist of a carefully supervised strengthening program of the quadriceps combined with stretching of the hamstrings, quadriceps mechanism, and lateral retinacular structures. Patellar taping has been recently used by many physical therapists to try to improve the function of the knee's medial structures and patella tracking. Braces with lateral restraining pads often give the patients an increased sense of security but do nothing in the long run to correct the deformity. They may be helpful, however, following an acute episode to facilitate improved function of the quadriceps mechanism during the rehabilitative phase. Hot packs, ultrasonography, and massage are minimally effective and these patients should be actively rehabilitated with a therapist skilled in patellofemoral mechanics. All exercises should be done in a pain-free range; staight-leg-raising to strengthen the quads and strengthening of the abductors, adductors, hamstrings, and hip flexors are critical to the success of the rehab program (Fig. 12-29). The use of Cybex or leg-extension exercises from 90 degrees often cause irritation of the patellofemoral joint and should not be performed. Increased popularity of closed chain exercises that employ the use of quarter squats, stairmaster, have been effective in later phases of rehabilitation to improve quadriceps function as well. Stationary bicycle, swimming, and treadmill are also excellent adjuncts.

Patients with recurrent subluxation of the patella should have an orthopedic evaluation to determine if surgery is indicated. Indications for surgery in patients with recurrent subluxation are significant radiographic findings of subluxation combined with subpatellar chondromalacia not improved with traditional rehabilitative methods. A cooperative patient able to participate in the postoperative program is essential for success of any surgical procedure, but particularly so in the patellofemoral disorders. Surgery consists of primarily arthroscopic methods that would consist of a lateral release (releasing the lateral retinaculum) to allow the patella to obtain a more centralized position in the femoral groove and occasionally proximal realignment of the vastus medialis, transferring this distally. Transferring the patellar tendon medially is done if the Q angle is excessively large. Determining which surgical procedure should be performed is based on careful history, physical and radiographic criteria with the surgeon trying to correct the underlying mechanical predisposing factor.

Surgery is not without risks, however, especially in patients with patellofemoral disorders, and is more successful in those with evidence of recurrent dislocation or subluxation compared with those with chronic anterior knee pain syndromes, which will be discussed subsequently.

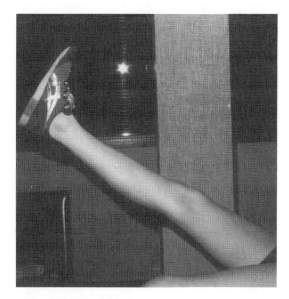

Fig. 12-29 Straight leg raising exercise to strengthen the quadriceps. Patient is partially sitting to reduce strain on lower back.

Anterior knee pain syndromes

The complex family of syndromes involving pain in the anterior aspect of the knee is generally one of the most frustrating treatment areas for orthopedic surgeons. The etiology of these painful states has not been clearly delineated. Many patients with pain in the anterior aspect of the knee have minimal to normal physical examinations but may experience severe unremitting pain. Likewise, many patients have severe chondromalacia with subchondral crepitations and loss of joint space and experience no pain (Fig. 12-30). The exact etiology of pain is not clear, and these patients must be examined carefully with a specific program of rehabilitation and treatment outlined, especially before any surgical intervention.

Often the history in these patients is that of a previously asymptomatic knee that sustains some form of minor trauma, be it a direct blow, twist, or fall. The patient will complain of severe pain around the anterior aspect of the knee that is worse with stair-climbing, squatting, or sitting with the knee flexed (theater sign). Relief of pain by extending the knee will often be seen. There are minimal symptoms with walking on level ground; however, walking down hills or stairs is often worse. There is usually no history of swelling or locking. The pain is generally described as a generalized ache that is under the patella and occasionally in the popliteal area as well. Sporting activities such as running and aerobics often exacerbate symptoms.

Physical examination should focus on assessment of the extensor mechanism. Measurement of the quadriceps for atrophy, malalignment in the standing position with a valgus recurvatum knee, or conversely inpointing of the patellas can lead to possible congenital etiology of the pain. Generally, there will be symmetric findings but with only one symptomatic knee. Assessment of the retinaculum for tightness and position of the patella (whether it is alta or baja) should also be performed. Frequently, there is tenderness along the medial retinaculum of the patella or the undersurface of the lateral facet of the patella. Subpatellar crepitations are palpated as the leg is brought through full extension and lateral tracking or a J sign should be observed as the knee comes into full extension. Chondromalacia, or softening of the undersurface of the patella, is often due to a combination of these findings. The vastus medialis should be observed for its point of attachment to the patella as patients with high insertions of the vastus medialis often cannot effect adequate medial forces to stabilize the patella in the femoral groove. Ligamentous examination will generally disclose either a normal ligament exam or some generalized ligamentous laxity. This can be assessed by the thumb-to-forearm test or assessment of hyperextension of the elbows. Patients with generalized ligamentous laxity often have a shallow femoral groove and instability of the patella as it tracks from flexion to extension. Absence of physical findings in patients with anterior knee pain should alert the physician to proceed slowly in terms of any surgical intervention. Prolonged conservative treatment is indicated in these particular patients.

Radiographic assessment again is mandatory to assess the position of the patella in the femoral groove and the presence or absence of any other intraarticular bony pathology. MRIs in general are not helpful and are usually normal. Bone scans do have some effectiveness in assessing the patient with chronic patellofemoral pain. Occasionally, patients may have a mild reflex sympathetic dystrophy of the patella that would be characterized by intense pain, hypersensitivity to touch, coolness of the patella, and even possibly osteopenia by x-ray. Many times these physical findings are absent, and the only complaint is severe pain. Occasionally, the three-phase bone scan can be helpful in seeing if increased vascularity of the patella is consistent with a dystrophic process or a localized chondral injury that may not be present by any other radiographic means (Fig. 12-31). A normal bone scan in a patient with intense pain and normal physical findings may still be seen, but it should also alert the physician to possible secondary gains or other nonanatomic causes.

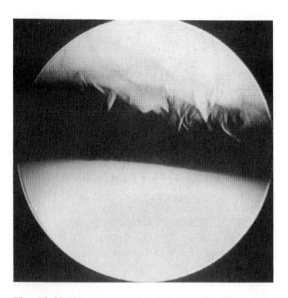

Fig. 12-30 Chondromalacia of the patella. The irregularity of the articular cartilage will give rise to audible or palpable crepitations.

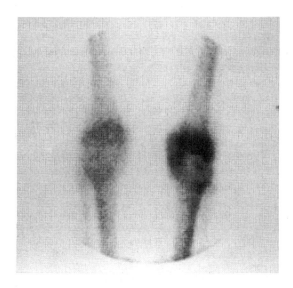

Fig. 12-31 Bone scan in patient with reflex sympathetic dystrophy showing diffuse uptake in the entire knee on blood pool and 3-hour delay.

Treatment of the anterior knee pain syndrome is primarily conservative. The principles of rehabilitation previously outlined in the section on subluxation should be followed. The results of physical therapy should be assessed every month. Patients who will be responsive to conservative treatment will do so within the first month. An additional approximately 4 to 6 weeks of therapy following may be useful in bringing the patients into the more advanced phases of rehabilitation so that they may be able to function in their work activities, especially if they involve stair-climbing, squatting, or heavy lifting. Prolonged physical therapy (greater than 3 months) has not been shown to be an effective, cost-effective means to management of these patients. Pain that persists and is unchanged following 8 to 12 weeks of supervised physical therapy should be a red flag for other possible functional or nonanatomic causes for pain or other sources of intraarticular pathology. It is at this point that bone scan or MRI may be indicated to try to confirm or deny the presence of true anatomic causes for pain.

Patient education is key in this group of patients. Activity modification may be necessary if an underlying cause is established that is not responsive to conservative treatment rather than surgical intervention. For many patients in our active society, however, this is not an acceptable option, and arthroscopic surgery should be a last resort in the assessment of these patients. Improvement following arthroscopic surgery is not as predictable in this group of patients (70% or less) as in those with radiographic or physical evidence of recur-

rent subluxation, tilt of the patella, or recurrent dislocation.

One group of patients who have chronic anterior knee pain syndromes, however, benefit from surgical intervention: those with lateral patellar facet compression syndromes. These patients will have no history of subluxation or dislocation, but on physical exam will have definite evidence of tilting of the patella, a tight lateral retinaculum, and radiographic evidence of narrowing of the lateral portion of the patellofemoral joint. These patients often have concomitant chondromalacia or softening of the undersurface of the patella. These patients may be excellent candidates for arthroscopic lateral release if they fail the standard rehabilitation protocols.

Iliotibial band syndrome

Iliotibial band syndrome is a bursitis or inflammation of the iliotibial band in its distal portion as it crosses the lateral femoral epicondyle. With repetitive flexion or extension of the knee, such as often seen in bicycle riding or running, inflammation can occur at the point where the iliotibial band rubs against the lateral femoral epicondyle. Bursitis can form accompanied by pain; inflammation, and occasionally local swelling and heat. It is usually described as an aching pain that is specific and localized to the lateral femoral epicondylar area.

Differential diagnosis includes lateral meniscus tears, popliteus tendonitis, and/or lateral compartment arthritis. Diagnosis is established by locating specific point tenderness not over the lateral joint line but over the lateral femoral epicondyle in both flexion and extension of the knee. Local infiltration with 1% xylocaine with relief of the patient's symptoms confirms the diagnosis.

Treatment consists of ice, oral anti-inflammatory agents, stretching of the hamstrings and iliotibial band, and cessation of the activity that caused it for short periods. Local injection with corticosteroid can be performed as a last resort and surgery is only rarely performed. In the recalcitrant case, orthotics are occasionally helpful.

Popliteal (Baker's) cysts

Baker's cysts or popliteal cysts are an outpouching of the synovial membrane in the posterior aspect of the knee. Seventy percent of patients who present with popliteal cysts have concomitant intraarticular pathology, most specifically meniscal tears. The cyst is usually a secondary symptom and the focus of the evaluation should be on establishing a treatable intraarticular problem such as a medial meniscus tear. Once the meniscus tear is treated arthroscopically, most of the symptoms from popliteal cysts resolve. Removal of the cyst is rarely indicated, but is done if the patient has recurrence of swelling that is localized and requires repetitive aspirations. Diagnosis is confirmed by physical examination and ultrasonography, a less expensive imaging mode than an arthrogram or MRI. Excision of a popliteal cyst is occasionally performed for the recurrent chronic cases that are causing neurovascular compromise (rare) or severe pain that cannot be treated conservatively. Recurrences can occur following surgical excision. Popliteal cysts may rupture and when this occurs, patients present with severe calf pain of acute onset that usually mimics a deep vein thrombosis. The diagnosis in these cases again can be confirmed by ultrasound or arthrogram. Symptoms generally resolve with rest, antiinflammatories, and heat alternating with ice.

Meniscal injuries

Meniscal tears. Injuries to the menisci occur in a variety of ways, most commonly with a twist, pivot, squat, or valgus injury to the knee. The shape of the meniscus as well as its relationship to the femoral condyles make the usual mechanism of injury through shear and rotation or direct compression through squatting. Patterns of tears often differ based on the patient's age and produce symptoms characteristic of the various tear types. Tear patterns are characterized into longitudinal (Fig. 12-32), horizontal (Fig. 12-33), or transverse (Fig. 12-34). Although it is not necessarily critical for the primary care physician to understand the various tear types, symptoms do correlate directly with these types of patterns.

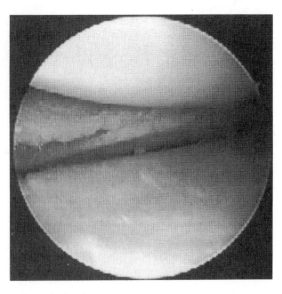

Fig. 12-33 Horizontal tear of the meniscus.

The longitudinal tear (more commonly known in the more extensive types as a bucket-handle tear) occurs in younger individuals. The history is that the knee undergoes a sudden twist, often associated with a squat, that tears the meniscus parallel to the free edge of the margin of the meniscus. In the more extensive tears, the patients may complain of acute locking with inability to extend or flex the knee, pain directed over the meniscus involved, and giving way. An effusion usually follows. Function is often normal in between episodes of acute locking if the meniscus spontaneously reduces.

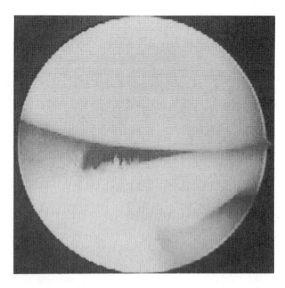

Fig. 12-32 Longitudinal tear of the medial meniscus seen arthroscopically.

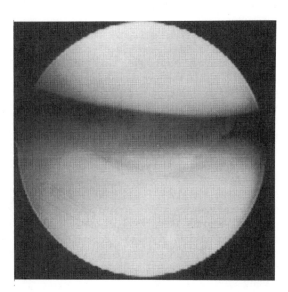

Fig. 12-34 Radial or transverse tear of the lateral meniscus.

Physical examination is characterized by atrophy of the quadriceps, presence of an effusion in many cases, tenderness over the involved meniscus, a positive McMurray's maneuver, and Apley's maneuver. A characteristic click associated with the McMurray's maneuver usually confirms the diagnosis. Pain alone associated with McMurray's maneuver, not associated with a click, may or may not be consistent with meniscal damage.

As a result of an inherent lack of blood supply to the majority of the meniscus, meniscal tears in general do not heal spontaneously. Surgical treatment is usually indicated. If possible, tears near the periphery should be identified early via either MRI or arthrography so that early repair can be effected. Since the edge of the meniscal tear is rather sharp in longitudinal tears compared with the more degenerative type of tears, repair is often successful. Careful examination for cruciate instability must be performed in patients with longitudinal tears because underlying anterior cruciate ligament instability is often the cause of the meniscal tear. Treatment of the meniscus alone without treatment of the ligament instability will often lead to failure of the repair and certainly worsening of the instability if the meniscus is removed. In the era of cost containment, patients with classic findings of meniscal pathology, especially associated with locking, may or may not need further diagnostic testing. Obviously, confirmation via MRI or arthrogram is useful in convincing the patient of the necessity of surgery, but it is not always indicated if physical findings are consistent with the history and classic symptoms for meniscal or mechanical derangement.

Surgical removal of the meniscus is not without possible sequelae. It has long been shown that total meniscectomy is followed by degenerative changes in the affected compartment within 20 to 30 years.[5,16] With the advent and the use of the arthroscope, lesser portions of the meniscus are removed. Recent studies, however, have shown that degeneration of the affected compartments still can occur but at much reduced rate.[5] As mentioned previously, the presence or absence of cruciate instability will often affect the long-term prognosis of these patients.[9-11,13]

In general, disability following surgery lasts 6 weeks. Most patients can return to pain-free function in a work environment and sports with minimal impairment. Some patients report occasional soreness with full squatting for long periods of time and a slight lack of full flexion. Following a successful repair, full function of the knee should be expected. Patients undergoing meniscal repair will not have the usual 6-week rehabilitation process; it will be prolonged for a minimum of 3 to 4 months as a result of the need to protect the suture line from further compression or shear forces. In general, running, pivoting sports, or prolonged squatting are prohibited for 4 to 6 months.

Horizontal or cleavage tears were first described by Smillie in 1946.[14] The symptoms associated with cleavage tears are classic (Fig. 12-35). Generally, the patient is an older individual with gradual onset of pain. The patients classically complain of an ache in the affected side of the joint, classically on the medial side, with point tenderness over the affected meniscus. Pain at nighttime is common, with many patients reporting improvement of symptoms by placing a pillow between their knees. Symptoms are worsened with squatting and pivoting. Recurrent effusions and buckling are often common symptoms, although locking is usually not a predominant symptom of a horizontal cleavage tear. If the tear becomes unstable and a free flap forms, patients may then start complaining of giving-way episodes or clicking.

Physical examination reveals point tenderness over the affected meniscus, pain and resistance to deep flexion with a positive McMurray's, and occasional effusion. Ligament exam is generally normal. Radiographs are important to assess any underlying degenerative arthritis involving the affected compartment. These should be obtained in the weight-bearing position rather than non-weight-bearing to pick up subtle changes in the joint space itself. This will be important to the injured worker where documentation of preexisting degenerative joint disease will affect the prognosis and also apportionment.

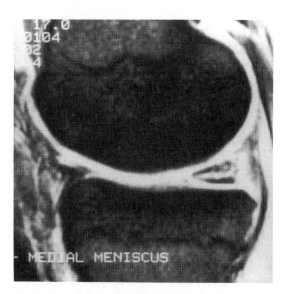

Fig. 12-35 Magnetic resonance image showing a horizontal cleavage tear of the medial meniscus.

MRI has been an excellent tool in diagnosing these tears. Confusion, however, has arisen in terms of the grading pattern often used in MRI. A degenerated meniscus may not be symptomatic but, because of the specificity of MRI, may be seen on the sagittal images as a Grade II intrasubstance degeneration. Although changes within the meniscus itself are not associated with mechanical derangement, the Grade III tears are significant.

The problem becomes more difficult in the patient with underlying degenerative arthritis of the knee, medial joint line pain, and an abnormal MRI. Arthroscopic resection of a degenerative meniscus may not help. In fact, symptoms may worsen with decompensation of the knee because of the removal of the remaining portion of the meniscus. As a result of an inherently poor blood supply of a degenerative meniscus, repair is not indicated. The presence of degenerative changes on the femur or tibia at arthroscopy portends a much poorer prognosis in patients undergoing partial meniscectomy.[4,12] These patients should be carefully counseled about the recurrence of symptoms. Laborers who perform heavy work activities should be advised that the prognosis for long term, complete relief of symptoms is guarded. Progression of the degeneration may be seen within 10 to 15 years or sooner, especially if ligament instability exists. The occasional preoperative use of bone scan in these patients is a helpful indicator to detect the presence of underlying degenerative changes so that careful patient preoperative education and postoperative care can be made.

Patients experiencing pain over the involved meniscus not associated with mechanical symptoms should be treated with antiinflammatory medications, ice, and short periods of restriction of activities, particularly squatting and pivoting. Many of these patients' symptoms will resolve within a number of weeks with conservative treatment. The role of physical therapy in treating these conditions is not clear except in the short term to help the patients rehabilitate their muscles and try to reduce inflammation and swelling. The benefits of long-term therapy have not been shown to affect the outcome in patients with degenerative meniscal tears. If symptoms persist for more than 4 to 6 weeks despite traditional conservative means, referral to an orthopedic surgeon should be considered. An MRI may be obtained if physical exam warrants it.

Other tear patterns exist, such as the parrot-beak tear or tear of a discoid lateral meniscus, and in general will present with similar symptoms as those discussed previously.

The important consideration in young patients with meniscal tears is assessment of whether re-

pair can be performed. In an older individual the important consideration is underlying degenerative arthritis that would affect the long-term prognosis.

A particular problem exists in middle-aged patients having undergone previous partial meniscectomy who continue to have persistent joint line pain. In the absence of true mechanical symptoms (swelling, atrophy, click, giving way, buckling) careful consideration of degeneration of the compartment rather than the meniscus versus possible secondary gain factors should be undertaken. As mentioned previously, MRI will often show persistent changes in the involved meniscus. Repeat arthroscopy in these patients does not disclose unstable fragments; rather, persistent degenerative changes are likely to be the cause of the patient's symptoms. In the patient with persistent pain following partial meniscectomy, use of bone scan and/or arthrography should be considered. Negative studies are helpful in distinguishing the possible functional pain component syndromes and nonanatomic pain syndromes from those having persistent or progressive degeneration of the affected compartment.

Meniscal cysts. Meniscal cysts are rarely seen in association with meniscal tears. In general, cysts are associated with a horizontal tear. The horizontal component extends to the periphery of the meniscus where an outpouching of the synovium occurs which can fill with joint fluid, producing a ganglion-type cyst right over the joint line (Fig. 12-36). Patients will complain of local swelling, pain, and tenderness over the involved meniscus and the cysts are confirmed via MRI or

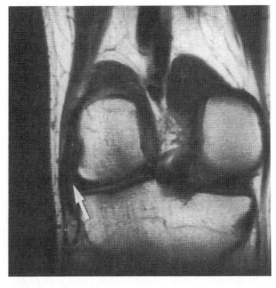

Fig. 12-36 Meniscal cyst involving the lateral meniscus.

arthrography. In most cases arthroscopic decompression and partial meniscectomy relieves patients of their symptoms. Open excision of the cyst is rarely indicated, especially if arthroscopic means fail.

Injuries of the ligaments

Ligamentous knee injuries can be classified as intraarticular or extraarticular. In general, extraarticular ligamentous injuries are not as severe nor do they cause as much disability or impairment as do the intraarticular type. The role of the primary care physician in assessing the acutely injured knee is to determine the difference between a potential intraarticular versus extraarticular injury and plan on early referral if a significant injury is identified.

Extraarticular injuries

Medial collateral ligament. Injuries to the medial collateral ligament are the most common ligamentous injuries to the knee. They are generally sustained as a result of a moderate force directed from the lateral aspect of the knee, stressing the knee into valgus and subsequent stretching or complete tearing of the medial collateral ligament. Collateral ligament injuries are graded as I (mild), II (moderate), and III (severe or complete). All have specific characteristics.

An example is that of a patient whose planted foot is struck from a laterally directed force with or without a twisting component. The knee is placed into valgus with progressive injury to the superficial and deep fibers. Patients report occasionally hearing a rip or pop accompanied by pain localized to the medial aspect of the knee. Immediate disability is usual but not universal, especially in patients involved in sporting activities who may not feel the full effects of the injuries for 1 or 2 hours later. A feeling of giving way or instability of the knee portends a more severe injury. Swelling is generally immediate and localized to the medial side of the joint, with pain at full extension or flexing past 90 degrees.

Physical examination for isolated medial collateral ligament injuries usually discloses soft-tissue swelling and/or ecchymosis over the origin or insertion of the medial collateral ligament. Point tenderness over the medial femoral condyle or proximal medial tibia should be elicited and will offer clues as to the location of the tear. Range of motion may be restricted, especially in extension. Extension often stretches the injured fibers, initiating a significant pain response. There will often be an absence of an effusion. Lachman's test and AP drawer are negative. Valgus stressing of the knee is accompanied by pain in the milder injuries and by significant instability in the more severe injuries. In Grade I sprains of the medial collateral ligament, the ligament fibers are only partially stretched and are still in continuity. The pain and initial disability are usually more severe in the Grade I sprains (lack of extension, pain with full flexion, and difficulty bearing weight). In Grade I injuries, the joint is stable to valgus stress at 0 and 30 degrees of flexion, but is usually accompanied by pain. Grade II, or moderate, medial collateral ligament injuries imply partial tearing of the ligament. There will often be pain and findings similar to Grade I but with valgus stress an increased opening will be noted of up to 5 to 10 mm. A firm endpoint is usually felt. In Grade III, or complete medial collateral ligament tears, the patients classically have little pain with valgus stress, and a soft endpoint to valgus stress is felt because of complete disruption of the fibers. These are usually accompanied by more ecchymosis and swelling medially. Careful assessment of the anterior and/or posterior cruciate ligament should be sought in these patients, because this implies a larger force necessary to tear the ligament completely.

Differential diagnosis includes patellar subluxation, medial meniscal tear, inflamed or hypertrophic plica, or chondral injuries on the medial side of the knee.

Treatment consists of immobilization for pain relief and ice. Grade III injuries are referred to an orthopedic surgeon for careful assessment for other intraarticular or cruciate injuries. Weight-bearing is prohibited only during the acutely painful phase. A knee immobilizer or, more recently, one of the commercially available splints with adjustable hinges generally affords the patient fairly good relief of pain, and many of these patients are then able to weight bear. Collateral ligament sprains usually resolve within 3 to 6 weeks in the milder injuries and 6 to 12 weeks in the more severe injuries. Physical therapy is useful in rehabilitating the quadriceps (if they are becoming atrophied), assisting in regaining range of motion, and reducing pain. Rehabilitation using a stationary bicycle or pool is often useful for regaining motion as well. The old adage of "do what doesn't hurt" is useful in progressing the rehabilitation of these injuries. Continued symptoms in spite of treatment after 6 to 8 weeks would indicate the possible need for MRI to rule out occult intraarticular pathology.

Acute surgical repair of Grade III medial collateral ligaments is no longer indicated; the results have been found to be identical to those treated conservatively.[3] Patients requiring surgery are those who have concomitant or associated cruciate ligament injuries and/or meniscal injuries.

Lateral collateral ligament. Isolated injuries to

the lateral collateral ligament (fibular collateral ligament) are rare. These injuries are usually associated with severe intraarticular injuries of posterior or anterior cruciate ligament. The presence of lateral instability with varus stress should alert the primary care physician to refer this patient for orthopedic consultation. For milder ligamentous injuries on the lateral side of the knee, the customary conservative treatment of ice, short-term immobilization while the leg is painful, and use of antiinflammatories is usually sufficient to allow these patients to return to useful employment. Continued symptoms after 4 to 6 weeks of conservative treatment would be indication for orthopedic consultation and possibly MRI.

Differential diagnosis includes lateral meniscus tears, popliteus tendon injuries, chondral injuries on the lateral femoral condyle, or occult tibial plateau injuries.

Intraarticular injuries

Anterior cruciate ligament. Anterior cruciate ligament injuries can cause significant disability and long-term impairments in the knee. Treatment considerations vary according to the patient's age, expected activity level, future employment needs, and ability to cooperate in a rehabilitation program. Whenever an anterior cruciate ligament injury is suspected, referral to an orthopedic surgeon is indicated, and careful assessment for meniscal damage that may be amenable to repair should be performed.

The patient generally has a history of a high-velocity injury such as skiing, a fall from a height, or an activity in which an object struck a planted leg. Hyperextension is a common mechanism of injury as well as a rotational injury. The patients will report hearing a pop (up to 70%) and immediate swelling is frequently seen. A history of immediate instability may or may not be elicited depending on associated soft-tissue injuries. In the acute setting, swelling is immediate; in the chronic setting a repetitive history of giving way or popping out is obtained. Patients with chronic instability of the anterior cruciate ligament will complain of difficulty stepping off a curb, turning corners, and the feeling as if their bones are shifting. This is often followed by a reactive effusion and indicates possible meniscal damage.

In the acute setting, physical exam will show a tensely swollen knee with a ballottable patella and variable joint line tenderness. Careful assessment of the collateral ligaments should be made in addition to the anterior cruciate ligament. There may be tenderness along the posterior lateral aspect of the lateral proximal tibia where capsular structures may have been damaged. Radiographs often show an avulsion of the capsule, a small fleck of bone

off the proximal tibia, called the lateral capsular sign or Segond's sign. A positive Lachman's test is nearly always seen, although a positive anterior drawer at 90 degrees may be difficult to elicit because of the patient's swelling. If the knee is aspirated, blood is usually encountered without presence of fat. A pivot shift may or may not be elicited in the acute setting, again due to patient pain and/or guarding.

Differential diagnosis in the acute hemarthrosis or acutely injured knee includes acute patellar dislocation, intraarticular fractures such as tibial plateau fractures, chondral injuries, or capsular tearing causing hemarthrosis.

Routine x-ray films should be obtained, looking closely for the presence of a Segond's sign or other associated bony injuries such as plateau fractures or loose bodies. Referral to an orthopedic surgeon in cases of anterior cruciate ligament injury should be performed early rather than late so that an accurate early plan of treatment can be made. MRI is a useful test to assess associated meniscal pathology or condylar injuries.

In the chronic setting, physical examination will demonstrate a positive Lachman's, positive anterior drawer, and a positive pivot shift if the instability is severe. If meniscal injuries have occurred, McMurray's maneuver and specific joint line tenderness are often found. Instrumented ligament tests, using mechanical devices that can quantitate the amount of abnormal tibial excursion, are also useful. These devices compare the normal with abnormal side with specific numbers. Radiographs are useful to assess any underlying degenerative changes which have already occurred in these patients, particularly in the chronic case. MRI again is a useful test to determine the status of the meniscus so proper surgical planning can occur.

Conservative treatment consists of rehabilitation of the hamstrings, quadriceps, and hip flexors in the sedentary patient not electing to undergo reconstruction. Many patients can function in their daily activities without episodes of instability if their knee is strong. The use of custom ligament braces can give many patients an increased feeling of security with activities involving pivoting and twisting, although these do not completely control the instability.

Surgical techniques have improved considerably over the last 5 years in orthopedics to allow arthroscopic insertion of ligaments through small incisions primarily for fixing the tendon to bone. Those rare acute tears that have a bone fragment attached to the cruciate stump may do well repaired primarily. Isolated primary repair of midsubstance anterior cruciate ligament tears has not been shown to be effective.[6] For these reasons, reconstruction with a substitute is almost universally recommended. Tissues to use in substitution include patellar tendon, the semitendinosus, and gracilis, and cadaveric allografts. Prosthetic ligaments may be used on the patient who has had previous knee reconstructions or other surgeries.

Untreated anterior cruciate ligaments in patients who are physically active have been reported to be associated with progressive tearing of the meniscus in 60% of patients, followed over 5 to 10 years.[6,11] For this reason, the progressive deterioration of the meniscus in patients with anterior cruciate ligament instability, surgical reconstruction is currently believed to be the optimum mode of treatment by many orthopedic surgeons. The issues of age and future activity level come into play, however, and careful decision making based on each individual patient needs to be made.

The issue in anterior cruciate ligament instabilities is not only the functional impairment it causes, but also that over time the menisci tear and removal will cause degenerative arthritis and long-term disability. These factors are often considered in determining the need for future medical care and prognosis in the industrially injured patient. Isolated anterior cruciate ligament injuries in patients with an intact meniscus who wish to restrict their activities will often do well without any surgical intervention.

The technique of ligament reconstruction has evolved over the years so that insertion can be done arthroscopically. Most of the intraarticular work is done via the arthroscope and one or two incisions are made over the proximal tibia and lateral distal femur for fixation of the graft once the holes have been drilled for the graft to pass through. Depending on the graft material selected, protection for 4 to 6 weeks is mandatory to allow ingrowth of the graft into the bone. Rehabilitation of the quadriceps and hamstrings following surgery usually requires 4 to 6 months for return to moderate work. In addition, the graft itself needs to be protected from undue torquing loads and stresses during the initial 6 to 12 months as revascularization of the graft occurs and it develops its own inherent strength. Adequate rehabilitation is the key to a successful functional and surgical result.

Posterior cruciate ligament. This rare injury usually occurs following fairly significant trauma to the knee. The usual mechanism is a direct blow to the flexed tibia, driving the tibia posteriorly and tearing the posterior cruciate. There continues to be some controversy as to the proper treatment of posterior cruciate ligament injuries in active young people and no universally accepted mode of treatment has been accepted.

As mentioned, the history in the acute setting is usually that of a direct blow anteriorly to the flexed knee. Often, there is not massive swelling or hearing of a pop as is so common in anterior cruciate ligament injuries. Diagnosis is often much more subtle and made in the chronic setting.

Diagnosis is suspected when an abrasion is present over the anterior proximal tibia, swelling in the knee occurs, and the patient has complaints of instability. In the more severe injuries, there are concomitant lateral side injuries as well, so combined ligamentous injuries are much more easily diagnosed than isolated posterior cruciate ligament injuries alone. There may or may not be a posterior sag on physical exam in the acute setting; this often appears in the more chronic setting as the soft tissues relax and the patient also becomes more comfortable during the examination. A posterior drawer is generally positive. In the chronic setting, patients may present with anterior knee pain syndromes. As the tibia subluxes posteriorly, the patella compresses on the anterior femur due to the fact that its attachment on the proximal tibia is more posteriorly directed (Fig. 12-37). The patients will often present with crepitations under the patella, wear over the medial femoral condyle, and only on physical examination or occasionally MRI will the diagnosis of posterior cruciate ligament injury be recognized.

Treatment consists of referral to an orthopedic surgeon as soon as a diagnosis is made. At this point, the determination of other concomitant ligamentous injuries, especially lateral and posterolateral, will be made and the issue of surgical inter-

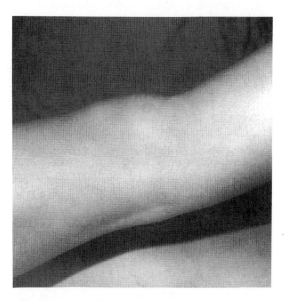

Fig. 12-37 Posterior sag of tibia on femur in patient with chronic posterior cruciate ligament instability.

vention will also be decided. Many orthopedic surgeons believe that in the isolated posterior cruciate ligament injury with normal menisci, conservative treatment affords an excellent result. There may be some work preclusions for working on heights and around moving machinery or heavy work, but in general these patients can function adequately in most other jobs.

Inflammatory conditions

Recurrent effusions in patients may be seen that are not due to actual industrial trauma but might well be due to manifestations of systemic illness, such as rheumatoid arthritis, gout, or gonoccal infections. In active young men with singular joint swelling unrelated to trauma, the diagnosis of Reiter's syndrome should be considered. The patients should be questioned for a history of back pain, conjunctivitis, urethritis, and an HLA-27-B may help confirm the diagnosis. Treatment is by injection of corticosteroids and antiinflammatory agents and is not surgical. Physicians should be aware of the possibility of patients presenting with Reiter's syndrome who are human immunodeficiency virus (HIV) positive. A careful history about possible exposure to various risk factors should be sought in this group of patients and an HIV test should be considered if not previously performed in patients with the diagnosis of Reiter's syndrome.

Industrial causation in the occurrence of these synovial conditions is somewhat controversial. The role of trauma or microtrauma in the onset of rheumatoid arthritis is a matter of debate. Acute gout is known to follow minor trauma and is a self-limiting process. A careful history of preexisting difficulties, as well as history of causative incident in the onset of symptoms, should be sought so that clarification of industrial causation can be made.

Knee aspiration: indications and technique

The decision to aspirate a knee is generally determined by the desire to make the patient more comfortable or to assist in the diagnosis. There are absolute and relative indications for knee aspiration. Absolute indications include the need to make a firm diagnosis if infection is suspected. Any knee that is hot, warm, and will not move should be aspirated to rule out acute bacterial infection. Acute gout can often appear like an infection with a hot, acutely painful knee. However, the reduced number of white blood cells, lack of bacteria on gram stain, and presence of crystals on microscopic examination will confirm the diagnosis. Other indications for aspiration of the knee are primarily relative. In patients with acute hemarthrosis the

diagnosis of anterior cruciate ligament tear, fracture, or acute patellar dislocation should be entertained. Examination of the blood should be performed to determine the presence of fat globules. The blood is placed in an emesis basin and this can be placed under light; fat will appear as a thin layer of oil on the surface of the blood and implies intraarticular fracture. Additional diagnostic testing such as MRI and immediate orthopedic referral at that point would be indicated if plain films do not disclose the source of the fracture.

Knee aspiration also is often performed in the chronically inflamed knee for diagnostic purposes. The fluid is sent for cell count, protein, glucose, and cultures. Knee aspiration for the purpose of instilling a small dose of steroids is occasionally indicated in the older patient whose only other option is surgical or in the patient with acute inflammatory arthritis (rheumatoid arthritis or Reiter's syndrome) for whom usual conservative measures have failed. Repetitive intraarticular injections of corticosteroids can cause significant articular cartilage damage and is not recommended in the young patient.

The technique for knee aspiration demands strict attention to sterile technique. The procedure should be done with sterile gloves, with a thorough sterile cleansing of the skin with a betadine or similar solution. The entire knee should be prepped, not just the small area where the needle is to be inserted. The patient should be given an informed consent that potential for infection, although small, is present.

Bony landmarks should be palpated prior to prepping the knee and the area just superior and lateral to the upper lateral pole of the patella is palpated. The knee is in full extension and should be relaxed. A small skin wheal is made using a 30-gauge or 25-gauge needle and then the deeper subcutaneous and fascial areas are also injected with the same needle with 1% plain xylocaine. This makes the patient much more comfortable during the actual aspiration itself. Relaxation is critical to entering the joint easily and without trauma to the cartilage surfaces. An 18-gauge needle (if aspirating blood) or 20-gauge needle (for regular joint fluid) can be used to enter the joint and should be attached to a 20 or 60 cc syringe depending on the size of the effusion. Once the needle is inserted into the joint, a pop is felt and the fluid is withdrawn. It may then be sent for cell count, culture, and sensitivities, protein, and glucose if infection is a concern, and it can also be observed for the presence of fat if one is concerned about intraarticular fractures. Once completed, the aspiration site should be covered sterilely for at least 24 hours to allow the puncture site to seal.

DIAGNOSTIC PEARLS

In evaluating the patient with the work-related injury, nonanatomic factors often come into play. Patients for a number of reasons may not desire to return to their previous employment, and may see the work injury as a way to be retired early from their job or be retrained into another line of work. This is especially true in California and many states where vocational rehabilitation is a ready option. Objectifying complaints of pain in these patients is extremely important to support the validity of claims. The following are a number of helpful guidelines in objectifying these complaints.

1. Substantiating the history through coworkers or witnesses is important in validating the diagnosis. Obtaining names of witnesses in the first visit for later reference is important.
2. Always check the wear in assistive devices. In a patient alleging an inability to walk, the recently purchased cane or crutches that are not soiled should raise one's index of suspicion about claim validity. Knee immobilizers should be stained and worn, especially if they have been used for awhile.
3. Check for the proper use of the cane or crutch. In general, a cane or a crutch when used singly should be used in the hand opposite to the affected knee, allowing for a more even gait pattern.
4. In patients alleging the inability to walk or who have alleged the use of crutches, there should be atrophy of the quadriceps present. Immobilization of a limb for even a week can cause a substantial amount of atrophy. The lack of atrophy often implies relatively normal function and use of the limb. It is one of the earliest indicators of internal pathology.
5. In patients stating an inability to bear weight or to walk without a severe limp, it is often suggested that the patient be asked to walk backward. Those with a truly antalgic gait will limp on the appropriate leg. Those who are amplifying their symptoms will often become confused, limping on the incorrect leg, tripping over their feet, and hesitating for a while to think before they do walk backward.
6. When injections are planned, either a joint aspiration, aspiration of prepatellar bursa, or trigger point injections, always use local anesthesia for infiltrating the skin. A 30-gauge needle is minimally painful and can provide the necessary anesthesia to the skin so that inserting larger needles is not bothersome to the patient. A comfortable procedure will instill confidence of the patient in the physician and will also tend to make the patient relax so a more detailed examination can be performed.
7. Always examine the joint above and below. In patients with atypical pain about the knee, x-ray films of the hip are mandatory to rule out occult hip disease, tumors, or degenerative joint diseases referring pain to the knee.
8. And for the most important pearl of all, in the age of sophisticated diagnostic tests such as MRI, do not forget the age-old adage, "if all else fails, examine the patient."

CASE STUDIES
Case 1

A 54-year-old man was seen for a second opinion for proposed arthroscopy of the knee. He complained of lateral knee pain with an inability to walk following a twisting injury at work. Pain had been present for 4 weeks and an MRI of the knee disclosed a degenerated lateral meniscus. When seen in the office, the patient presented with a flexed hip and knee with inability to bear weight. Passive rotation of the hip caused severe knee pain. Radiographs of the hip joint revealed a pathologic fracture through an acquired immunodeficiency syndrome (AIDS)-related lymphoma of the proximal femur (Fig. 12-38). The patient never had an HIV test and the diagnosis of AIDS had never been entertained or made until testing was done. Obviously, arthroscopic surgery was not performed.

Case 2

A 58-year-old ironworker developed medial knee pain, clicking, and giving-way episodes following a twisting injury at work. X-ray films on the initial examination showed mild to moderate degenerative changes of the medial compartment. Physical examination showed tenderness over the medial meniscus, a small effusion, and a positive McMurray's sign and a stable ligamentous exam. MRI disclosed a degenerative meniscus tear involving the posterior horn of the medial meniscus. Surgery included a partial medial meniscectomy leaving a stable rim and showed some moderate degenerative changes of the medial femoral condyle and medial tibial plateau.

The patient did well for approximately 3 months, then presented with continued pain and aching in the medial aspect of his knee; the pain was worse with weight-bearing. He did not have any associated giving-way or buckling episodes. It was his physician's opinion that he was having pain associated with degenerative arthritis of the medial compartment of his knee. The patient sought a second opinion as referred by his attorney, who obtained a second MRI scan that showed continued degenerative changes with abnormal Grade III signal in the posterior horn of the medial meniscus of a horizontal nature. It was the second physician's opinion that the medial meniscus was again torn and that the patient required a second arthroscopy. At the time of the second arthroscopy performed by the second physician, the me-

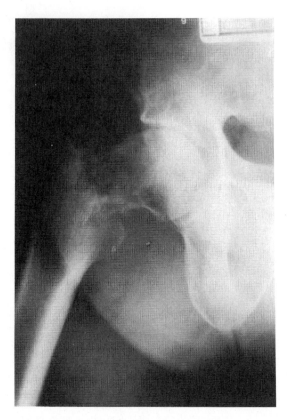

Fig. 12-38 Osteolytic defect in proximal femur with pathologic fracture in HIV-positive patient with lateral knee pain. Patient denied hip pain.

ative component. This can be managed conservatively rather than arthroscopically unless the symptoms become intractable. Certainly, following partial meniscectomy, patients may persist with medial compartment symptoms, but they are probably not due to recurrent meniscal tears but to the residual degenerative changes in the knee.

dial meniscus was stable, although degenerated, but had no unstable fragments. It was clear that the patient's pain was coming from degenerative changes in the medial compartment as there was a mild synovitis, but the findings were not so severe that any further surgery had to be done.

This case shows that in the older patient with radiographic findings consistent with degenerative arthritis, MRI may in fact show a degenerative meniscal tear. If there are no associated mechanical symptoms, such as locking, buckling, giving-way, or recurrent effusions, symptoms are in all likelihood coming from the degener-

REFERENCES

1. Bronstein R, Kirk P, Hurley J: The usefulness of MRI in evaluating menisci after meniscus repair, *Orthopedics* 15(2):149-152, 1992.
2. Crues JV III et al: Meniscal tears of the knee: accuracy of MR imaging, *Radiology* 164:445, 1987.
3. Indelicato PA: Nonoperative management of complete tears of the medial collateral ligament, *Orthop Rev* 18:947, 1989.
4. Jackson RW, Rouse DW: The results of partial arthroscopic meniscectomy in patients over 40 years of age, *J Bone Joint Surg* 64:481-485, 1982.
5. Johnson R et al: Factors affecting late results after meniscectomy, *J Bone Joint Surg* 56A:719-729, 1974.
6. Johnson RJ et al: Current concept review: the treatment of injuries of the anterior cruciate ligament, *J Bone Joint Surg* 74A:140-149, 1992.
7. Krause W et al: Mechanical changes in the knee after meniscectomy, *J Bone Joint Surg* 58A:599-604, 1976.
8. Mink JH et al: MR imaging of the knee: technical factors, diagnostic accuracy, and further pitfalls, *Radiology* 165(P):175, 1987.
9. Noyes FR et al: The symptomatic anterior cruciate–deficient knee. I. Long-term functional disability in athletically active individuals, *J Bone Joint Surg* 65A:154, 1983.
10. Noyes FR et al: The symptomatic anterior cruciate–deficient knee. II. The results of rehabilitation, activity modification, and counseling on functional disability, *J Bone Joint Surg* 65A:163, 1983.
11. Pattee GA et al: Four- to 10-year follow-up of unreconstructed anterior cruciate ligament tears, *Am J Sports Med* 17:430, 1989.
12. Rand JA: Arthroscopic management of degenerated meniscus tears in patient with degenerative arthritis, *Arthroscopy* 1:253-258, 1985.
13. Sherman MF et al: A clinical and radiographical analysis of 127 anterior cruciate–insufficient knees, *Clin Orthop* 227:229, 1988.
14. Smillie I: *Injuries of the knee joint,* Edinburgh, 1946, E & S Livingston.
15. Stoller DW et al: Meniscal tears: pathologic correlation with MR imaging, *Radiology* 163:452, 1987.
16. Tapper E, Hooper N: Late results after meniscectomy, *J Bone Joint Surg* 51A:517-526, 1969.

13 Foot and Ankle Disorders

The foot and ankle are frequently involved in occupational trauma. Twisting injuries in workers getting on and off trucks, walking on uneven ground, or tripping over objects are commonly seen in the occupational medicine clinic. Crush injuries from dropping objects onto the foot or rolling objects over the foot are also seen.

More recently static problems within the foot are becoming a concern. Workers such as bellmen or doormen who stand, walk, and carry for 8 hours daily, day after day, can develop more chronic injuries such as plantar fasciitis or neuromas. Even these indolent problems can result in lost worktime for those whose jobs demand long hours on their feet. One hotel in San Francisco, the Westin St. Francis, through early intervention with proper footwear and shoe inserts, has significantly reduced lost worktime from foot problems in bellmen and food servers.

A working knowledge of the anatomy, physiology, and function of the foot and ankle is necessary to evaluate and treat these individuals. Evaluation must include the soft tissue and osseous structures.

ANATOMY

The ankle joint is a hinge joint composed of an articulation of the lower end of the tibia including the medial malleolus, the lateral malleolus of the fibula, and the articular portion of the body of the talus. The fibula extends more distally on the lateral aspect of the joint than does the medial malleolus on the medial aspect of the joint. This gives greater lateral osseous support to tilting of the talus within the ankle mortise itself. The superior surface of the talus is wider anteriorly than posteriorly. This accounts for a widening of the ankle mortise in dorsiflexion and a narrowing in plantar flexion.

Because of this increased osseous support on the lateral aspect, the lateral ligaments are smaller and do not lend the same support to the ankle joint as do the medial collateral ligaments (Fig. 13-1). The lateral ligaments are composed of three distinct structures. The anterior talofibular ligament blends with the anterior portion of the capsule. The posterior talofibular ligament, the strongest of the three lateral ligaments, attaches to the posterior process of the talus. The calcaneofibular ligament, a cord-like structure that crosses both the ankle joint and the subtalar joint, is found deep to the peroneal tendons.

The medial collateral ligament is also known as the deltoid ligament. It is a strong fanlike structure that is composed of one deep component and three superficial components. Because of the structure of the osseous and ligamentous system, the lateral portion of the joint is more prone to ankle sprains with any type of twisting or inversion motion. The worker who is constantly getting on and off a truck or working on uneven ground is especially susceptible to these injuries.

Just proximal to the ankle joint is a strong syndesmosis between the distal portion of the tibia and fibula. This syndesmosis is maintained by a series of ligaments both around the area and within the confines of the syndesmosis known as the interosseous membrane. These ligaments can be torn in an ankle injury, especially with an external rotatory component. This area is usually compromised with more severe fractures and dislocations.

The subtalar joint, also known as the lower ankle joint, is an articulation between the talus and the calcaneus. It is actually three separate joints that work together in concert. The largest of the joints is formed by the posterior facets of the talus and the calcaneus. The anterior and middle facets are formed by the sustentaculum tali of the calcaneus and a corresponding area on the head of the talus. These are most injured in crush-type injuries as encountered in the worker falling from a height with resultant fracture of the calcaneus.

The area between the posterior facet and the anterior and middle facet is the sinus tarsi. This is filled with the thick interosseous ligament that holds together the talus and calcaneus. The main blood supply to the body of the talus is located in the sinus tarsi. An injury to this area may result in an avascular necrosis of the body of the talus. This occurs most commonly with fractures of the neck of the talus caused by dorsiflexion injuries, as in car accidents. The motions allowed around the subtalar joint include pronation, a combination of

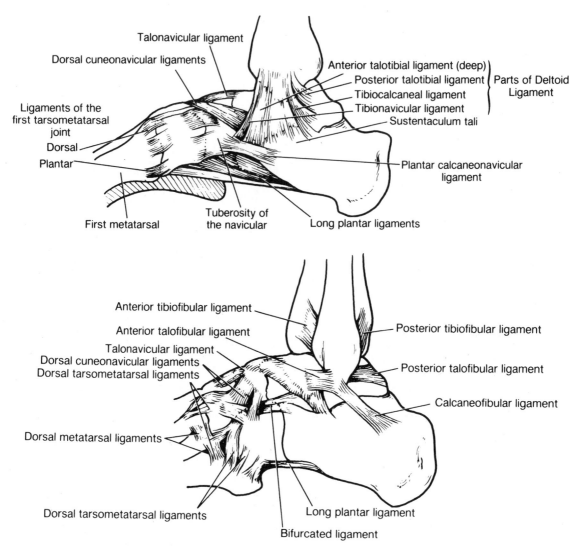

Fig. 13-1 Soft tissue structures of the foot and ankle.

dorsiflexion, eversion, and abduction, and supination, a combination of plantar flexion, inversion, and adduction. Injuries to these structures become important in the case of plantar fasciitis, heel spurs, or neuromas seen in the worker who is always on his feet.

The midtarsal joint is composed of the talonavicular joint and the calcaneocuboid joint. These structures are most injured along with the subtalar joint in a fall from a height or in crush injuries. Ligaments support the various articulations within the mid-tarsal joint.

The tarsometatarsal joint, also known as Lisfranc's joint, consists of the first three metatarsals articulating with the corresponding cuneiform. The fourth and fifth metatarsals articulate with the cuboid. This joint (Lisfranc's) is usually disrupted with a dorsiflexion force to the anterior portion of the foot. Note that the second metatarsal is locked between the first and third metatarsocuneiform articulations, acting as a keystone to stability. The remaining portions of the various aspects of the joint are supported by a series of ligaments between the metatarsals and cuneiforms or cuboid.

The five individual metatarsophalangeal joints are supported by a series of collateral ligaments allowing motion mainly in the dorsiflexion direction. The tibial and fibular sesamoids are located plantar to the first metatarsal head. The sesamoids are invested within the muscle belly of the flexor hallucis brevis. They are most commonly injured with direct trauma to this area as in any force to the ball of the foot.

HISTORY

As in all aspects of medicine, the history gives the initial hints to the injury. The key question is the mechanism of injury. The physician is then able to focus the examination on certain specific areas. For example, jumping onto the foot may result in injuries caused by dorsiflexion forces. This would include direct trauma to the sesamoids or metatarsal areas, dislocations around Lisfranc's joint, or injuries to the head and neck of the talus in the mid-tarsal area. One may also see soft-tissue injuries including stretching or rupturing of the plantar fascia as well as injuries to the Achilles tendon.

Twisting motions may cause sprains or fractures of the ankle or avulsion fractures from the peroneus brevis (base of the fifth metatarsal). Soft tissue or osseous injuries depend on the degree of force. Direct blows to the foot may cause localized injuries to the area that was traumatized.

It is also helpful to know the type of injury and any treatment between the injury and when the patient is seen. Often, because of the shock of the injury, pain is not immediately discerned. There may be a delayed onset of the pain as swelling takes place. The pain may become more severe with continued weight-bearing and activity on the extremity. If one uses heat during the initial period, the swelling may be more severe and the pain greater than one would expect. If one uses ice immediately, the swelling and pain may be kept to a minimum. Radiating, electrical type pain will usually indicate injury to a nerve either by direct blow or compression from an osseous part or from swelling. One must always be aware of trauma to the neurovascular system.

EXAMINATION

The evaluation begins with observation of the injured part. Swelling, erythema, or disfigurement should be noted. If not seen initially, ecchymosis may be noted around the area or distal to the injured area. Often ecchymosis is noted distal to the area because gravity allows the blood to pool distally. The dorsalis pedis and posterior tibial arteries should be palpated to ascertain the circulatory status (Fig. 13-2). The capillary return of the digits should also be assessed. This is performed by applying pressure to the distal end of the digits and then releasing the pressure. The return should be within 1 to 3 seconds. Any longer is a sign of vascular embarrassment.

A neurologic assessment is then performed (Fig. 13-3). This is usually done by using a pin to assess sensation in specific areas. The superficial peroneal nerve innervates the dorsolateral aspect of the foot and medial aspect of the hallux. The deep

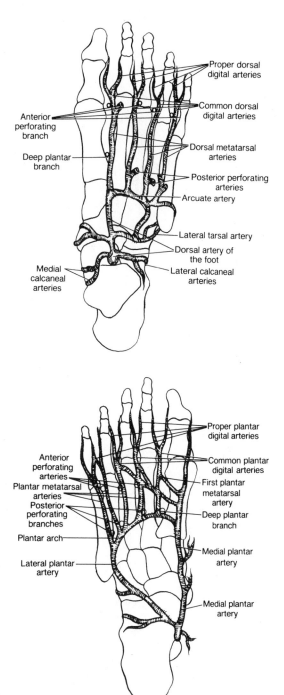

Fig. 13-2 Vascular supply to the foot.

peroneal nerve innervates the area between the hallux and the second toe. The intermittent dorsal cutaneous nerve innervates the lateral aspect of the second digit. The sural nerve innervates the lateral aspect of the fifth digit. The saphenous nerve is responsible for the medial aspect of the rear foot and ankle. The plantar aspect of the foot is innervated

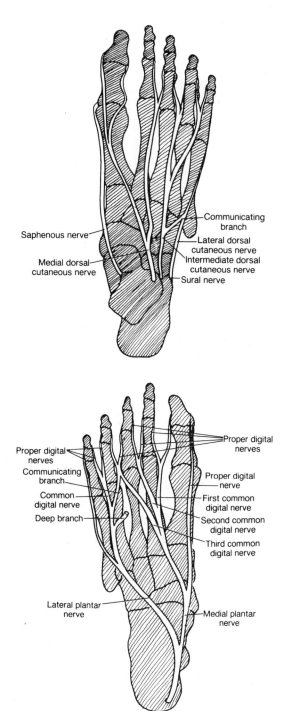

Saphenous nerve

Medial dorsal
cutaneous nerve

Communicating
branch

Lateral dorsal
cutaneous nerve
Intermediate dorsal
cutaneous nerve

Sural nerve

Proper digital
nerves
Communicating
branch
Common
digital nerve
Deep branch

Proper digital
nerves

Proper digital
nerve
First common
digital nerve
Second common
digital nerve
Third common
digital nerve

Lateral plantar
nerve

Medial plantar
nerve

Fig. 13-3 Neurologic supply to the foot.

by the lateral plantar nerve predominantly as well as the medial plantar nerve. The medial calcaneal nerve innervates the heel.

Palpation is the next step in evaluation. One emphasizes the maximum area of pain on examination, but should also be aware of other injuries that may occur with specific mechanisms of trauma. An example is a twist of the ankle that will usually cause a rupture of the ligaments or a fracture of the ankle. However, one must also consider the possibility of an osteochondral fracture of the talar dome, a fracture of the lateral process of the talus, or a fracture of the base of the fifth metatarsal. By palpating the specific ligaments around the ankle and the bony elements one can usually determine a ligamentous injury versus an osseous injury.

Depending on the problem, muscle testing should be performed. These tests should include the anterior tibial tendon, the extensor hallucis longus tendon, and the extensor digitorum longus tendon on the dorsum of the foot. The peroneal tendons are tested on the lateral aspect of the ankle and foot, and the posterior tibial tendon is tested on the medial aspect of the ankle and foot. The Achilles tendon should also be tested posteriorly.

The specific joints are then put through a range of motion. One should observe not only the degree of motion but also the quality. Crepitus should also be noted. The range of motion of the ankle joint in dorsiflexion averages approximately 10 degrees, whereas plantar flexion is approximately 55 degrees. The total range of motion of the subtalar joint is approximately 30 degrees. One notices the quality of motion through the midtarsal joint as well as metatarsophalangeal joints.

IMAGING STUDIES

Standard x-rays are still the hallmark in diagnosing most injuries to the foot and ankle. When a fracture or dislocation is suspected, a non–weight-bearing film is ordered. Because of the overlap of various bones and joints, three views should be obtained: an anterior-posterior, an oblique, and a lateral projection. These views give good visualization of the bones and major joints.

Subtle dislocations may be difficult to identify on non–weight-bearing films. A film with partial to full weight bearing may be more useful to determine these subtle changes. This is especially true through the midportion of the foot. Weight-bearing films are also helpful with more insidious problems of the foot and ankle such as plantar fasciitis and heel spur syndromes. One may visualize the important relationships of bones and joints as they would approximate the mid-stance phase of gait in a weight-bearing attitude to correlate structure to function.

Stress x-ray films of the ankle are extremely helpful in determining the integrity of the collateral ligaments once the possibility of fracture is eliminated. These are considered when one suspects complete rupture of the ligaments. Stress x-ray films are taken in both a lateral projection (anterior drawer sign) and an anterior posterior projection (inversion stress). A stress x-ray film is always read in comparison to the uninjured ankle. A value of at least 10 degrees difference between the two sides indicates ligamentous instability. If there has been previous injury to either ankle, the results may not be valid. Ankle arthrography could be utilized in those instances to ascertain the integrity of the ankle joint. A magnetic resonance imagining (MRI) scan is now often used in these instances as an alternative.

When an occult fracture or dislocation is suspected but not visualized on plain radiographs, one may order a computed tomographic scan of the foot and/or ankle. It would be preferable over an MRI in these instances. However, if soft tissue problems are suspected, such as ruptured tendons and nerve entrapments, an MRI would be most useful. A bone scan may be useful if one suspects a stress fracture (although an MRI could also be used in these instances) or to identify any areas of acute inflammation.

COMMON INJURIES

The ankle is among the most common joints injured by workers. It is difficult to assess the extent of injury solely by the amount of swelling. It is extremely important to note any immediate treatment such as ice or heat to a part. This would have significant effects on the amount of swelling and would account for varying amounts of pain that the patient is experiencing. The patient must be questioned as to the mechanism of injury. This will alert the physician to certain areas to examine. Palpation is performed to the osseous structures, such as the medial and lateral malleolus as well as the base of the fifth metatarsal. The proximal portion of the fibula should also be palpated as this may be injured in certain types of ankle fractures although not commonly. One should also assess the soft tissue elements including the collateral ligaments both medially and laterally.

Ankle sprains

Ankle sprains are common in the active worker. Once a fracture is ruled out, one must assess the extent of ligamentous damage. Ankle sprains are usually graded as to the degree of instability of the ankle joint. A grade I sprain would have minimal talar tilting and be considered a stable joint. A grade II sprain involves greater instability of the ankle and greater damage to the ligaments. A grade III sprain would show complete instability of the ankle and a greater than 10 degree difference on a positive stress test. It is important for the future considerations of the patient to determine

this degree of instability. It is often difficult initially to determine this by physical examination. The patient is usually in a significant amount of pain and may use the peroneal tendons to splint the area to limit the motion. This compensatory mechanism, however, hinders the examination. A common peroneal block at the neck of the fibula can be utilized to relieve peroneal spasm to allow a proper examination.

Once the degree of damage is ascertained, treatment may then be given. Grade I sprains are usually treated symptomatically with ice and Unna boots or posterior splints to reduce the swelling. An Unna boot is an excellent bandage initially for the first week of therapy to reduce a significant amount of swelling. After this, elastic supportive bandages may be used. Physical therapy and mobilization are begun during the first 2 to 3 weeks to allow early motion and ambulation. Treatment would continue for approximately 4 to 6 weeks until resolution.

Grade II and III sprains that show joint instability should be treated more aggressively. A below-knee walking cast may be used for 4 to 6 weeks. This gives the ligament a chance to heal in a stable position. In grade II sprains the casting period may be decreased to 3 weeks and, with the use of an ankle immobilizer, dorsiflexion and plantar flexion exercises are begun. The immobilizer will protect the patient from inversion and eversion. Surgical repair of the ligaments may be contemplated in the young athletic individual. However, this is usually confined to the top flight amateur or professional athlete. Casting is necessary after these procedures for a minimum of 4 to 6 weeks. After immobilization, physical therapy is used to encourage motion, ambulation, and help rebuild proprioceptive senses.

Sinus tarsi syndrome

An entity known as sinus tarsi syndrome may be seen after ankle sprains. This is usually first noticed at approximately 6 to 8 weeks after the injury. There would be pain to palpation to the area of the sinus tarsi and not to the ligamentous complex around the ankle. The symptoms, however, may mimic that of a patient with an ongoing ankle sprain. An injection of xylocaine to the sinus tarsi with complete relief is considered to be diagnostic. Cortisone injections may be attempted to relieve the discomfort. If chronic pain continues in this area, surgical evacuation of the sinus tarsi may be contemplated.

Standard x-ray films of the foot and ankle should be obtained if there is a possibility of fracture or significant ligamentous disruption. With an inversion ankle injury specific areas must be examined in addition to the traditional malleolar areas. An osteochondral fracture of the dome of the talus (Fig. 13-4), lateral process of the talus, and anterosuperior beak of the calcaneus, as well as fractures of the fifth metatarsal (Fig. 13-5), may occur with this mechanism. If a fracture is identified, care must be taken to identify other injuries that may not be apparent. This includes a diastasis of the tibia and fibula and possible rupture of the deltoid ligament. These may cause a widening and instability of the ankle joint. One must accurately assess the length of the fibula in relation to the medial malleolus. One of the major reasons for a poor result following treatment of an ankle fracture results from a shortening of the fibula. Most ankle fractures are repaired surgically with internal fixation.

Talar fractures

As mentioned previously, inversion ankle injuries may lead to more uncommon but serious injuries, including a transchondral fracture of the dome of the talus. When on the medial aspect of the dome, the fragment usually involves the posterior third of the dome. The mechanism of injury is inversion and plantar flexion. When involving the lateral aspect, the fragment usually appears in the middle third of the dome. The mechanism for this injury is inversion and dorsiflexion. When these injuries are present, the fragment's position within the ankle joint must be assessed. Open reduction and fixation or excision is usually necessary. If no displacement is identified, a below-knee cast is used for 6 to 8 weeks.

Calcaneal fractures

A fracture of the anterior superior process of the calcaneus may also occur with an inversion ankle injury. A key point in the examination is palpating this process, which is found just superior to the midpoint of a line drawn from the tip of the lateral malleolus to the styloid process of the fifth metatarsal and situated just distal to the sinus tarsi. It rarely involves the joint and is actually an avulsion fracture of the bifurcate ligament. This injury is best treated in a short-leg cast.

Fifth metatarsal fractures

A common injury that occurs as a result of an inversion injury is a fracture at the styloid process of the fifth metatarsal. This usually is the result of an avulsion of the peroneus brevis tendon. Assessment must include the specific location on the base of the metatarsal and whether the tendon is intact and the fifth metatarsal cuboid articulation is involved. Fractures of the process will usually heal

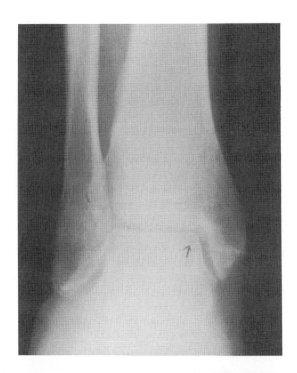

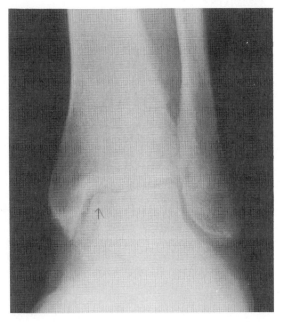

Fig. 13-4 Osteochondral fractures of the dome of the talus.

well with conservative treatment. Depending on the symptoms, this may include an Unna boot, elastic ankle strapping and surgical shoe, or a plaster cast immobilization. Fractures at the junction of the base and shaft are often repaired with internal fixation to prevent a nonunion. Those involving the joint should have an accurate reduction

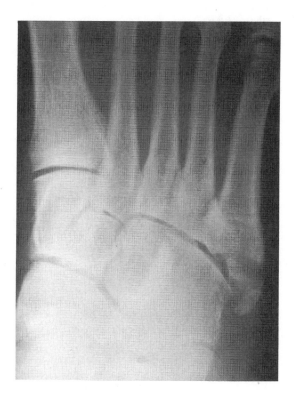

Fig. 13-5 Fractures of the fifth metatarsal.

and internal fixation to prevent future arthritic changes.

Cuboid/cuneiform fractures

Fractures of the cuboid (Fig. 13-6) and cuneiforms are much more uncommon and usually result from a moderate to severe amount of force. Displacement must be identified. These injuries are usually more severe in nature and should probably be referred. If there is no displacement and no joint involvement, cast immobilization would be necessary. If displacement or joint involvement is identified, open reduction to an anatomic position and fixation should be performed.

Tarsometatarsal dislocation

In assessing fractures of the foot, one must always be aware of a tarsometatarsal dislocation (Lisfranc's dislocation). These lesions are commonly missed because of the subtle nature of the dislocation and will usually be identified by x-ray evaluation. They involve mainly the first and second metatarsocuneiform joints or the entire metatarsocuneiform complex. There is usually significant edema and ecchymosis present. In reviewing the x-ray films, cortical avulsion fractures of the first or second metatarsals or a complete diastasis of

the first and second metatarsal may be present. This should alert the physician to ligamentous instability. Closed reduction may be attempted but usually fails because of the unstable nature of the injury. Open reduction and internal fixation will be necessary for most of these injuries.

Metatarsal fractures

Fractures of the metatarsals may result from direct trauma such as an object falling on the foot or striking the foot against an object. They may also occur from various twisting mechanisms. There is usually swelling specifically over the involved metatarsal with pinpoint pain to palpation. X-ray films show the nature of the injury. In many cases of a nondisplaced fracture, a weight-bearing short-leg cast may be applied. If there is displacement of the segments so that they overlap one another or a dislocation at the metatarsophalangeal joint, an open reduction is required.

Sesamoid fractures

One must also be aware of sesamoidal fractures. The sesamoids are in grooves on the plantar aspect of the first metatarsal. The dorsal aspect of the sesamoid is contained within the first metatarsophalangeal joint. Therefore, an injury to the sesamoid often causes pain with any movement

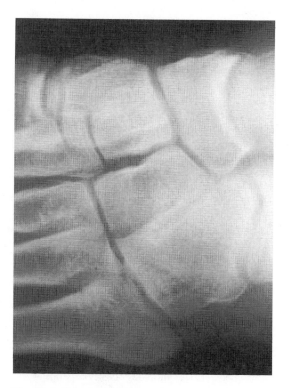

Fig. 13-6 Cuboid fracture.

of this joint. They can cause an irregularity in the joint that will lead to metatarsal sesamoid arthritis. Differentiating these fractures from a bipartite sesamoid may be difficult at times. The fractured sesamoid will usually have irregular edges and an irregular space between the two pieces of bone. A bipartite sesamoid will usually have rounded edges with a uniform space between the portions of the sesamoid. Conservative care is usually sufficient to take care of these injuries including accommodating padding, an Unna boot, or at times a plaster cast depending on the symptoms. One must remember that the sesamoid most always heals by a fibrous union, and only rarely will one see a bony union of the sesamoid.

Digital fractures

Digital fractures are quite common (Fig. 13-7). Accurate diagnosis is necessary to properly treat the injury. An x-ray film should be obtained to determine malalignment problems. If there is significant displacement of the fragments, reduction (whether open or closed) should be performed. If not, future problems may result that will have to be repaired surgically. If a distal tuft fracture is identified, reduction is usually not possible or necessary and the worker is treated symptomatically. If the fracture involves a joint, accurate reduction is necessary.

Dislocations of the interphalangeal joint are fairly common. Often these can be reduced under a local anesthetic digital block. This is usually performed as a field block at the base of the digit. Digital fractures or dislocations are usually bandaged by splinting the involved toe with an adjacent digit, sometimes known as buddy taping. A piece of gauze or cotton between the digits should be used to prevent maceration. This procedure will usually give proper stability to the fracture.

Stress fractures

The physician must also be aware of stress fractures of the foot. They most commonly involve the metatarsals and occur in people who are on their feet constantly or starting active jobs after being sedentary. The onset of pain is usually more insidious than that of an acute injury. Pinpoint pain to palpation will be positive over the involved shaft. X-ray films will probably be negative in the first 2 weeks after the incident. One may then see a fracture line with healing bony tissue around it. Bone scans or an MRI will usually be positive. Treatment is usually supportive including strapping, an Unna boot, or a short-leg cast, depending on symptoms.

Crush injuries

Crush injuries to the foot and ankle may be difficult to assess with regard to diagnosis and extent of treatment. Often a fracture is not identified despite the fact that one is suspected because of the degree of injury. There may be significant damage to the soft tissue area, however, and the patient must be watched closely for increasing amounts of pain or swelling causing a compartment syndrome. The neurovascular status of the foot must be completely assessed after these types of injuries. Significant swelling should be the key to the physician to serious complication. Hospitalization should be contemplated for continuous observation. If not, the patient should be seen daily for 3 to 5 days until the risk of this complication is reduced.

Lacerations

Lacerations are also common injuries to the foot. Evaluation of vital structures must be made before repairing the laceration. Evaluation of the neurovascular status as well as the tendinous structures is necessary. Depending on the extent of the wound, a tendon laceration may not be identified by simply exploring the wound. It may be necessary to use specific muscle testing, or, in the case of a deep wound, it may be necessary to obtain an MRI. If the laceration occurs on the medial aspect of the foot or ankle, one must carefully evaluate the posterior tibial tendon. If this tendon laceration occurs and is not diagnosed properly and repaired, devastating consequences occur. It will cause a significant flatfoot deformity of the foot leading to early arthritis and eventually to a triple arthrodesis.

Achilles tendon ruptures

Achilles tendon ruptures are usually characterized by the patient feeling a pop behind his or her ankle. A gap in the tendon may usually be palpated. Squeezing the calf, which usually produces plantar flexion of the foot, will not produce any motion. This is known as Thompson's test. The patient will be unable to rise on his foot if this injury has occurred. Treatment for an Achilles tendon rupture includes either an equinus gravity cast or surgical repair.

Puncture wounds

Puncture wounds usually heal quickly and uneventfully. However, with the risk of infections, especially pseudomonas, the patient must be observed closely during the first 24 to 72 hours. Shoes that absorb moisture (tennis shoes) frequently predispose one to pseudomonas. Pseu-

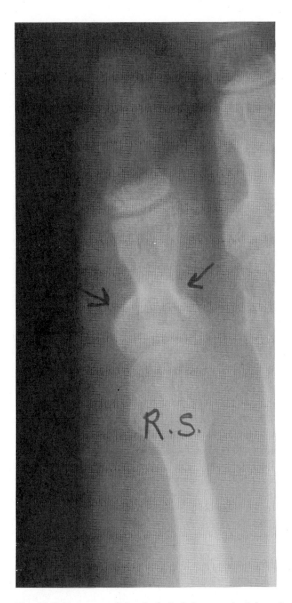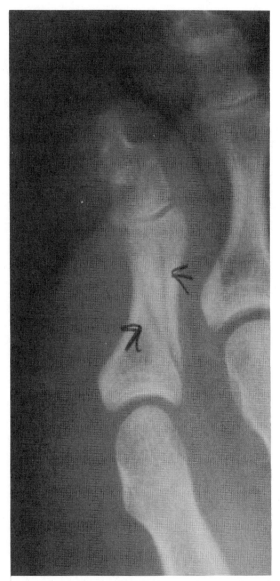

Fig. 13-7 Fractures of the shaft. *Left,* impacted; *right,* spiral.

domonas has a predilection for avascular areas such as cartilage and joint areas and then spreads to surrounding bone. Debridement of the wound edges and irrigation of the area are the hallmarks of treatment. The wound is left open and allowed to granulate. Tetanus prophylaxis should be considered. If one notes an infection or signs of infection during the first several days, aggressive therapy, including parenteral antibiotics to cover gram-positive and gram-negative organisms, is advocated to attempt to prevent the infection from spreading. Wide incision and drainage with irrigation and intravenous antibiotics would be neces-

sary to prevent a serious gram-negative osteomyelitis. Bone scans or MRI will be positive early in the course of osteomyelitis. X-ray films may not be positive for 10 to 14 days. This may occur in any area of the foot from seemingly simple puncture wounds. Serial x-ray films may be necessary since pseudomonas infections can literally dissolve a metatarsal head over the course of only a few days.

Nail injuries

Nail injuries can be seen in the worker from an object falling on the toe or from stubbing the toe.

These may cause a subungual hematoma that can be painful because of the collection of blood under pressure underneath the toenail. X-ray films should be obtained to rule out a fracture of the distal phalanx. It is not necessary in these cases, nor is it desirable, to remove the entire nail. Boring holes in the nail plate will be sufficient to release the trapped blood. A local anesthetic is usually not necessary in performing this procedure. A paper clip that is heated (red hot) at its tip usually works well. This melts the nail plate so that the blood trapped under the nail is released. It is important to remember that blood is under significant pressure so that when the clip is removed the blood will splatter. The physician must keep a gauze sponge over the area to prevent this from occurring. Depending on the size of the hematoma, several holes may be used for the evacuation. The patient is then placed on soaks and often the nail will eventually fall off and a new nail will grow. As the new nail begins to grow one may see the end of the nail or the side of the nail growing into the skin. A paronychia may result. A digital block at the base of the toe is used and the nail border must be avulsed (Fig. 13-8). The toe is soaked in normal saline solution or epsom salts and kept covered with a bandage. It is not usually necessary to administer antibiotics for this localized abscess.

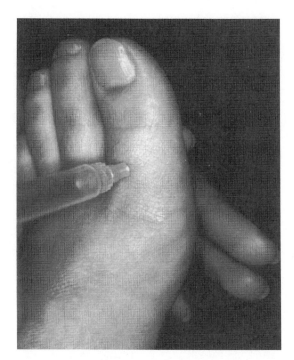

Fig. 13-8 Digital block position.

Plantar fasciitis

Another common problem is plantar fasciitis or a heel spur syndrome. This may present in employees who work on their feet or do a great deal of walking. It has also been seen in bus drivers who have had to keep their feet in constrained positions because of the angle of the pedals of the bus. The main etiology of these problems is pronation of the foot. This causes an elongation of the plantar fascia and intrinsic musculature of the heel. Eventually the periosteum is pulled from the calcaneal tuberosity. New bone, known as the heel spur, is formed. The pain, however, is due to the stretching of the fascia and a bursitis and not to the heel spur that is present. It is not always necessary to visualize the heel spur on x-ray film. Although the spur on a weight-bearing x-ray film looks like a sharp point, it is actually a ridge that runs across the plantar aspect of the calcaneus.

Initial treatment consists of a plantar rest strap. Injections of cortisone are useful at times when the symptoms are severe. The injection may be given from the medial aspect of the heel; this is less painful than a direct plantar injection. The treatment of choice in 95% of the cases will be a functional orthosis. Taping relieves the initial discomfort and acts as a test as to whether an or-

thotic device will be successful (Fig. 13-9). The device relieves the pull of the plantar fascia and intrinsic muscles by limiting pronation. Physical therapy can be an added modality if the pain persists. If the problem remains and ambulation is still painful, surgical correction may be contemplated. This consists basically of a plantar fasciotomy to relieve the pull on the plantar aspect of the heel.

Neuromas

Neuromas (perineural fibrosis) may cause pain in the ball of the foot, especially when the worker stands or walks constantly for long periods. It is a nerve entrapment caused by the instability of the metatarsals and must be differentiated mainly from a stress fracture. The pain is reproduced by palpation of the intermetatarsal space from the plantar surface along with lateral compression of the metatarsal heads. Initial treatment may consist of strapping or injections. Orthoses may be helpful in approximately 70% of the cases. When pain continues to be a problem, surgical excision may be contemplated.

Many of the static problems are present in workers who stand all day, especially on hard surfaces. It is recommended that these people use stiffer shoes with good support in the shoe. They should use lace-type shoes which will support the foot in a better position. For these people orthoses

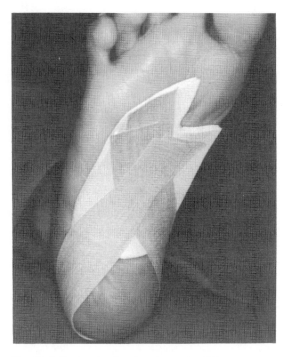
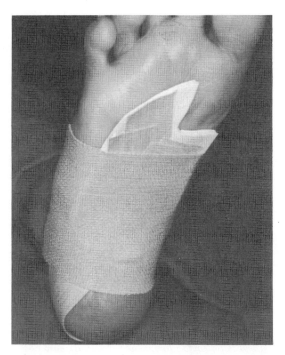

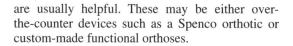

Fig. 13-9 Taping the foot for plantar fasciitis.

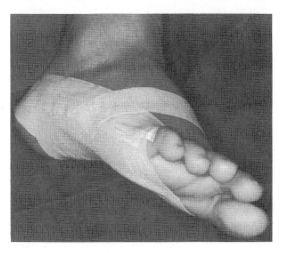

are usually helpful. These may be either over-the-counter devices such as a Spenco orthotic or custom-made functional orthoses.

ANKLE SUPPORT

Strapping with adhesive tape is not as prevalent as has been used previously. A common use of adhesive tape was to treat and immobilize foot and ankle disorders. With the advent of newer types of removable splints and ankle braces, such as the air cast ankle brace or the Sentek ankle brace, immobilization with compression can be obtained more efficiently. It also allows the patient to remove these so that physical therapy can be performed, enabling the patient to bathe in a normal fashion. Adhesive tape strapping is of benefit in treating a patient with an acute plantar fasciitis or heel spur syndrome as well as for neuroma pain. Strips around the heel crisscross on the bottom of the foot, tending to lock the subtalar and mid-tarsal joint to reduce the amount of pronation (Fig. 13-9). The effect is to reduce the stretch of the plantar fascia and reduce the symptoms. The disadvantage of the taping is that the patient must keep this area dry. It is used as a test for the benefits of an orthotic as well as providing temporary relief of symptoms.

When the taping is beneficial, a functional orthotic may be constructed to maintain relief of symptoms with a plantar fasciitis or with a heel

spur. They can also be effective in approximately 70% of the cases with a neuroma. The orthotic is made from a non–weight-bearing neutral position cast of the foot. The neutral position of the foot is that position in which the foot is neither supinated nor pronated. The device is then custom-made from this model of the foot to allow normal motion through the foot and eliminate abnormal pronation. In 95% of the cases plantar fasciitis and heel spur syndrome will be controlled and treated in a positive fashion.

An Unna boot is used to immobilize an ankle sprain that exhibits significant swelling. An air cast is an excellent device to stabilize the ankle externally. The patient is able to dorsiflex and plantar flex, but inversion and eversion are limited.

CASE STUDIES

Case 1

A 47-year-old hotel bellman complains of pain through his arch as well as his heel. The symptoms have been increasing over the previous 6 months and are becoming more severe. The patient states that he has significant pain when first getting out of bed in the morning and must limp to the bathroom. After walking on his foot for approximately 5 minutes, the symptoms begin to disappear and he is able to walk in a normal fashion. During the normal workday he begins to experience discomfort after he is on his feet approximately 3 hours. He then takes his lunch break and tries to elevate his foot. On getting up from his lunch break he also has a severe amount of pain which resolves within approximately 5 minutes of walking. He continues his normal activities and work and again has a moderate amount of foot pain and fatigue by the end of the day. Examination shows pain along the plantar fascia as well as the anterior medial aspect of the heel. Evaluation of gait shows that the patient is pronated throughout the stance phase of gait and pushes off on the medial aspect of the foot. X-ray films are taken that show a plantar calcaneal spur. The patient is placed into an adhesive tape strapping and is usually seen back in the office within 5 to 7 days. He reports that his symptoms were significantly reduced while the taping was on, and he was able to perform his normal job in a pain-free satisfactory manner. A plaster impression cast is taken of his foot and an orthotic is constructed. The patient reports complete relief of symptoms and a return to normal work activities as well as recreational activities.

Case 2

A 37-year-old newspaper deliveryman, who is constantly getting in and out of a truck on the job, twists his ankle and immediately feels pain over the lateral aspect of the ankle. He tries to continue working but has increasing pain and swelling over the area. He leaves work early, goes home, elevates the area, and puts ice on the ankle. The next day he seeks medical attention because of a continuing amount of pain. On evaluation a minimal amount of swelling and discomfort around the lateral aspect of the ankle is reported. No apparent instability can be assessed at this time. He is given an ankle support and a prescription for physical therapy. He attends a few sessions of physical therapy, which controls the swelling and his discomfort. He attempts to return to work and notices an increasing amount of symptomatology as well as swelling around the ankle. As this progresses for approximately 2 weeks, he has increasing difficulty in performing his normal duties of getting in and out of the newspaper truck. He again seeks medical advice and is referred for further evaluation. X-ray films show a transchondral fracture of the talar dome that occurred at the time of the initial injury. The patient is placed into a below-knee plaster cast for approximately 6 weeks to allow the area to rest and attempt to heal the lesion. On coming out of the cast he wears an ankle splint and is referred to physical therapy for range-of-motion and strengthening exercises. He is asymptomatic at this point and is allowed to return to work with the strapping. In this case the patient is asymptomatic and returns to all normal activities. It should be noted that there are times, especially with the transchondral lesion, that surgical treatment would be required.

CONCLUSION

Although foot and ankle injuries are among the most common type of problems encountered in workers' compensation cases, most injuries are fairly straightforward. The proper treatment is dictated by the extent of trauma. There are instances of more insidious problems, however, due to a patient's occupation and amount of time the patient is on his feet. A thorough knowledge of the anatomy, biomechanics, and function of the foot and ankle are required to ensure proper treatment and return the patient back to the workplace.

14 Mild Traumatic Brain Injury

The incidence of head injuries has reached epidemic proportions in industrialized nations. Traumatic brain injury is the leading cause of death in individuals under 40 years of age. Each year approximately 400,000 people are admitted to hospitals in the United States with a primary diagnosis of head trauma. Of these injuries, 80% are minor; however, even minor head injury can have major implications in terms of health care cost and time lost from work.

Generally, boys and men suffer head injury two to three times as often as girls and women. The peak age distribution is bimodal, with the highest peak occurring between the ages of 15 and 24. The second highest incidence occurs over 70 years of age. Motor vehicle accidents account for more than 50% of head injuries, and alcohol frequently is involved. A smaller number of head injuries are caused by assaults, falls, and sports-related accidents.

DEFINITION

The description "postconcussion syndrome" is being replaced by the preferred term "mild traumatic brain injury" (MTBI). The Head Injury Interdisciplinary Special Interest Group of the American Congress of Physical Medicine and Rehabilitation has proposed the following description of MTBI:

1. Any loss of consciousness
2. Any loss of memory of events immediately before or after an accident
3. Any change in mental state at the time of the accident (for example, feeling dazed, disoriented, or confused)
4. Any focal neurologic deficits; these may or may not be transient, but the severity of injury should not exceed the following parameters: (1) loss of consciousness for about 30 minutes or less; (2) after 30 minutes, an initial score of 13 to 15 on the Glasgow Coma Scale (GCS); and (3) posttraumatic amnesia for 24 hours[2]

Thus brain trauma can be caused by nonimpact injuries, and loss of consciousness is not a required element. However, the history usually shows some kind of change of consciousness, such as confusion or disorientation.

MECHANISM OF INJURY

MTBI can be caused in a number of ways: by the head striking a stationary object, such as the dashboard of a car; by a direct blow to the head; by a nonimpact acceleration-deceleration injury, commonly associated with whiplash. Rotational forces superimposed on acceleration and deceleration can result in shearing and stretching of axons and diffuse axonal injury, affecting the "transmission" lines of the brain and generally producing a diffuse pattern of microscopic involvement with limited or no focal injury. Focal injuries, if they occur, usually are confined to the areas of the cortex adjacent to bony prominences within the skull (most notably the prefrontal, temporal, and posterior occipital areas) and often are the result of coup or coup-contracoup injuries.[36]

CLINICAL EVALUATION

A good history is the cornerstone of evaluation of a patient with MTBI. The duration of loss of consciousness should be clearly defined. In addition, the periods of retrograde and anterograde amnesia should be assessed. Use of prescription or nonprescription (recreational) drugs, including alcohol, should be documented. The method of injury may have a bearing on subsequent medical and legal investigation and must be noted when this information is available, including whether passive restraint systems or helmets were used.

The physician must decide when computed tomography (CT) scanning or hospital admission is warranted. In his review of standard neurosurgical management following head injury, Andrews concludes that if no other injuries are present and the GCS is 15, the patient can be observed at home if a reliable adult is present.[3] Patients with a GCS score of 13 or 14 should be admitted to the hospital for at least 24 hours for hourly neurochecks. If abuse is suspected as the cause of injury, the patient should be admitted regardless of the severity of the injury.

Automatic CT scanning of all patients following MTBI is neither clinically warranted nor cost effective. A scan should be done if the patient shows focal neurologic deficits; worsening symptoms,

221

such as headache or nausea; persistence of altered consciousness; or deterioration in the level of consciousness. The incidence of neurosurgical intervention after MTBI has been estimated at only 1% to 3%.[44]

NEURODIAGNOSTIC STUDIES

Computed tomography and magnetic resonance imaging (MRI) are the imaging techniques most often used with MTBI. MRI offers greater resolution and superior visualization of white matter lesions.

In a recent study of 134 hospitalized patients with mild traumatic brain injuries, approximately 25% had demonstrable cortical or subcortical lesions on MRI within 3 days of injury.[43] However, the correlation between abnormalities found on MRI and neuropsychologic performance is weak at best.[40,41] Some authors have found MRI scans to be virtually normal, even in the acute phase following mild head trauma.[8]

Electroencephalography (EEG) may show mild, generalized slowing or low voltage, but as a rule a standard EEG is normal.[35] Even abnormal EEG findings have not been found to correlate with the reported symptomatology.

"EEG brain mapping" is a term used for quantitative EEG techniques that analyze data spatially and temporally and produce a numerical representation of the data rather than a waveform.[38] Subtle features that may elude detection in a routine EEG may become apparent with EEG brain mapping. Thatcher demonstrated the ability to differentiate between quantitative electroencephalograms of normal controls and those of individuals with MTBI with 90% accuracy.[37] However, as yet no standard, firm database describing MTBI has been universally accepted. EEG brain mapping is susceptible to what would appear to be statistically significant yet false-positive results. Currently quantitative EEG data should be used cautiously.

Single photon emission computed tomography (SPECT) can detect regional blood flow abnormalities. However, a significant limitation of this technique is that it measures relative, not absolute, blood flow[40]; therefore a region that appears to show increased blood flow may be hyperemic or may be surrounded by areas of decreased perfusion. SPECT images should not be interpreted without reference to MRI. Serial SPECT studies may be useful when patients with suspected MTBI are followed up. Currently, although SPECT findings are pathognomonic for Alzheimer's disease, findings with concussion are less consistent.

The neuropsychologic impairments documented after head trauma do not always correlate closely with SPECT abnormalities.[11] Positron emission tomography (PET) shows regional brain metabolism and may correlate with neuropsychologic testing after head injury.[34] Humayan demonstrated a difference in the cerebral glucose metabolic rate in parts of the temporal and frontal lobes between control individuals and a small number of cognitively impaired patients with head trauma who had normal EEG, MRI, and CT studies.[20]

Evoked potential testing offers little corroboration of MTBI. Even shortly after injury, the results are likely to be normal.

PATHOLOGY

Although gross anatomy, as shown by neuroimaging studies, may appear normal, postmortem microscopic pathologic investigation has shown evidence of neuronal damage. Oppenheimer[29] studied 59 patients with minor head trauma who had been unconscious for less than 5 minutes and who had died of pulmonary embolus or pneumonia. Autopsies showed autopsy microglial clusters associated with degenerating axons. In a study by Jane and colleagues,[22] monkeys were subjected to nonimpact acceleration-deceleration forces that caused mild head injuries and loss of consciousness for approximately 3 minutes. On gross examination, the brain appeared normal; however, the brainstem showed microscopic evidence of axonal degeneration.

Immunochemical tracer techniques have shown that axons throughout the brain usually are stretched, not torn, although secondary wallerian degeneration ultimately may ensue.[30,31] The process takes up to 24 hours in animal studies. Hayes, Povlishock, and Singha[17] have reviewed the proposed mechanism of traumatically induced neurotransmitter release and postsynaptic abnormalities, which may account for the clinical characteristics of patients who have experienced MTBI.

The symptoms that follow MTBI may be somatic, cognitive, or psychosocial in nature. Most patients appear to recover fully within 3 months of the date of injury. However, a significant number of patients are left with persistent, lingering symptoms. The wide range of symptoms and the variability of onset and duration have led many clinicians to suspect that persistent symptoms are produced by interaction of organic and psychosocial factors.

The most frequently reported symptoms are headache, dizziness, and impaired memory. Alves and colleagues studied more than 800 adults at the time of injury and at 3, 6, and 12 months. Most patients had no symptoms; of those who did, most had only one symptom. Although the incidence of headaches declined over time, other symptoms were reported with greater frequency at 3 months from the date of injury. Thereafter symptoms gradually began to improve. Individuals with more symptoms at 3 months tended to have more persistent problems.[1]

SYMPTOMS
Headache

In the study by Alves, about one third of all patients suffered headache at the time of injury.[1] By 3 months after injury, approximately 20% still complained of headache. If no intracranial pathologic condition is the cause (such as intracerebral or subarachnoid hemorrhage), most posttraumatic headaches are extracerebral in origin.[44] Musculoskeletal dysfunction is the most common cause of headache following MTBI.[21] Generally, the patient feels a pressure sensation involving the entire head.

Headache may be associated with whiplash and consequent muscle spasm. Spasm may produce muscle ischemia and trap the occipital nerves. The greater occipital nerve is especially susceptible because it emerges through the splenius capitis muscle. Occipital neuralgia is associated with a headache that radiates from the back of the head forward and sometimes into the eye.[5,6]

Musculoskeletal headaches are treated with physical therapy, trigger-point injection, transcutaneous electrical nerve stimulation (TENS), and biofeedback to reduce anxiety and muscle spasm. Nonsteroidal antiinflammatory agents should be used as first-line drugs. Narcotic analgesics should be avoided because their sedative side effects can further compromise cognitive function; this class of drugs should be used for short-term management only if absolutely necessary. Low-dose tricyclic antidepressant drugs can be a useful adjunct in the treatment of headaches. Injecting steroids or a local anesthetic (or both) into the greater occipital nerve as it emerges through the splenius capitis may help alleviate the symptoms of occipital neuralgia. Reassuring the patient that most headaches improve over time is also important.

Vascular headaches are less common. The patient may describe typical migraine symptoms, and individuals with a family history of the condition are thought to be predisposed to the development of these headaches.[16] Vascular headaches rarely occur alone after trauma. Treatment should be directed at both musculoskeletal and vascular sources. In addition to the treatment measures already described, calcium channel blockers and beta-blockers have been tried, with varying success. Temporomandibular joint (TMJ) dysfunction is a controversial cause of posttraumatic headache.

Dizziness

The dizziness that follows MTBI often is described as a sense of dysequilibrium or unsteadiness. Sometimes rapid head movements precipitate the sensation that objects in the room are moving.

The workup of a patient with dizziness should include an audiogram and complete otologic and neurologic examinations. Brainstem auditory evoked potential testing can provide objective evidence of dysfunction of the cochlear nerve or brainstem. Electronystagmography records spontaneous and induced nystagmus and can differentiate between central and peripheral causes of vestibular dysfunction. Peripheral causes are most common.

Acute auditory and vestibular injury can occur as a result of fracture of the temporal bone or microscopic injury to the cochlea or vestibular labyrinth.[18] Longitudinal fractures of the temporal bone may result in a conductive hearing loss. Transverse fractures of the temporal bone are much less common and are associated with fractures through the labyrinth, which disrupt the vestibular system and cochlea and can result in complete hearing loss. A vestibular-cochlea concussion can result in mild sensorineural hearing loss and labyrinth dysfunction associated with positional vertigo.[12]

The most common neurootologic cause of dizziness after MTBI is benign paroxysmal positional vertigo. Moving the patient quickly from a sitting to a supine position, with the head 30 to 45 degrees below horizontal and the affected ear turned down, induces nystagmus with a latency of 5 to 10 seconds and a duration of 10 to 15 seconds. This maneuver also reproduces the patient's symptoms of vertigo. Often patients note dizziness with any movement of the head, including rolling in bed. Benign paroxysmal positional vertigo is self-limited and usually lasts 6 to 12 months.

If the symptoms are disabling, meclizine and calcium antagonists may be useful. Physical therapy for vestibular habituation training may offer improvement to some patients.[19,28] Surgical intervention, such as vestibular nerve sectioning, may be effective for patients with chronic, persistent vertigo.

A perilymphatic fistula develops when an abnormal communication exists between the middle ear and the inner ear's perilymphatic space. Symptoms include fluctuating hearing loss, tinnitus, nausea, and dizziness. After MTBI these patients may experience a sense of dysequilibrium with complex visual stimuli, such as walking on a patterned carpet.[13] Bed rest often is recommended. If symptoms persist, surgery may relieve the dizziness but is less likely to restore hearing.

Individuals with jobs that require rapid changes of position, use of power tools, or work performed at heights should be cautioned not to return to work until symptoms have subsided completely.

COGNITIVE SYMPTOMS AND NEUROPSYCHOLOGIC ASSESSMENT

Cognitive impairments after MTBI are directly related to the type of pathophysiologic changes in neuronal structure and function that result from the physics and mechanics of impact and the secondary consequences of injury. The precise manner in which organic, or neurologically based, changes interact with personality variables and secondary emotional responses to trauma is still unclear. Cognitive processes may be influenced by a complex array of organic, psychologic, and personality variables, which typifies MTBI.[1]

Information processing ability

The application of a common heuristic analogy to the brain is undoubtedly useful, even if somewhat risky. Most recently we have attempted to understand its operations through the information processing model, with concepts borrowed from computer science. With the use of this model, the most common cognitive change resulting from diffuse axonal injury is in information processing ability, which is the brain's moment-to-moment capacity to take in information and perform various mental operations on it.

A limitation in information processing ability has repercussions on a number of other cognitive functions. The loss of information processing capacity and other, related cognitive problems primarily stem from deficits in the brain's attentional system.[10] Mental slowness, forgetfulness, distractibility, and inability to sustain attention are all by-products of attentional weakness.[15] Specific attentional skills affected by MTBI may include selective attention, sustained and divided attention, and concentration.

Memory

Memory problems are the third most common postconcussive complaint, after headaches and dizziness.[1,33] However, what most individuals refer to as "memory" most often is a problem stemming from impairment of attentional processes, which affects the brain's ability to selectively attend to, integrate, and store relevant information. Many individuals complain of "short-term" memory problems. These problems often are attentional in nature and bear little or no resemblance to the type of memory dysfunction seen in other organic mental disorders, such as dementia.

Many individuals do well on "memory" tests, because *they are aware their memory is being tested* and the confines of the testing environment are relatively well regulated.[27] Yet, in the course of their daily lives, they may not know *what is relevant* and *what should be remembered*. Their ability to selectively attend to relevant stimuli is weak, causing them to retain less information and to report that they cannot "remember." This problem usually is a weakness in *incidental memory,* or memory for unselected or uncued information (that is, the person was not cued ahead of time to selectively attend to the relevant stimuli).

Executive function

Problems with executive function may also occur with MTBI. Executive functions are largely subsumed by the frontal lobes and include self-awareness or "insight," self-monitoring ability, planning ability, organizational skills, initiation or "motivation," pacing of performance, self-correction, and efficient execution and completion of tasks ("task overview").

Executive functions also may be influenced by the individuals' psychologic and affective state, partly mediated by limbic-temporal connections (in some cases involving coup-contracoup injuries of the temporal lobe).

Unfortunately, to date few tests can adequately assess the often subtle yet profound changes that may ensue with impaired executive function in MTBI. This problem currently is receiving more attention from researchers, and some new assessment approaches are evolving.[26] Traditional frontal lobe testing was typified by the Wisconsin Card Sorting Test and the Stroop Test, both of which have some applicability to MTBI, but which may fail to discriminate more subtle executive problems.[27]

Traditional neuropsychologic tests have been recognized for their ability to localize specific lesions. Most of these tests were not designed to assess information processing efficiency, the cognitive ability most often impaired by diffuse brain damage caused by minor traumatic brain injury.[39]

In most individuals with MTBI, information processing deficits typically are evident immediately after injury and may persist for many weeks; in a small but clinically significant minority of individuals, these deficits may be permanent. As a measurement of improvement, test scores may not equate with recovery. Deficits may remain despite improved scores on some tests.[14]

The neuropsychologic tests that effectively measure cognitive problems are those capable of tapping into the subtle attentional and executive changes often associated with MTBI.[25] The Halstead-Reitan Neuropsychological Test Battery is recognized for its ability to elucidate the cognitive deficits more typically seen in moderate to severe head trauma, but it also has shown some applicability to MTBI, particularly with regard to reasoning, sustained attention, and processing speed.[4,32]

The Digit Symbol Subtest of the revised Wechsler Adult Intelligence Scale (WAIS-R), which has been recognized for years as a sensitive indicator of general cerebral dysfunction,[32] also has been shown to apply to MTBI.[27] In fact, Mateer's research, which used matched controls and two levels of brain injury (mild and severe), showed no difference between the two brain-injured groups (both did equally poorly). However, significant differences between the brain-injured and control groups were evident on a number of key tests, including the WAIS-R Digit Symbol Subtest, which measures sustained attention, speed of processing, and rate of learning—factors known to be affected by MTBI. Other tests shown to have some discriminatory ability with MTBI patients include the Wisconsin Card Sorting Test (loss of mental set), the Symbol Digits Modalities Test, the WAIS-R Performance IQ, the Auditory Verbal Learning Test, the Selective Reminding Test, the Controlled Oral Word Association Test, and the Complex Figure Test.[25]

The Paced Auditory Serial Addition Task (PASAT) was developed to assess changes in information processing speed and sustained attention more accurately.[14] Research has shown that this test is useful in determining the degree to which processing speed has been affected. Gentilini and colleagues[10] found that patients with MTBI differed from normal controls on all measures of attention (selective, sustained, divided, and distributed), even though the two groups showed no significant differences on selected neuropsychologic tests in an earlier study by the same authors. This finding reinforces the importance of selecting tests sensitive to attentional deficits and other subtle cognitive changes associated with MTBI.

A neuropsychologic evaluation goes far beyond "testing"; it encompasses a number of important areas and components, including careful clinical evaluation of personality and emotional and behavioral functioning; developmental history; premorbid psychologic, social adjustment, and substance abuse history; premorbid academic and vocational performance; neurologic risk factors; family perceptions; behavioral and process observations; objective findings from medical tests (such as EEG, CT, and MRI); type of injury; and reaction to litigation.[24,25] The neuropsychologist faces the difficult task of weaving clinical, behavioral, medical, historical, and cognitive/mental status information into an accurate, realistic, and sensitive portrait of the individual affected by MTBI.

PSYCHOSOCIAL PROBLEMS AND BEHAVIORAL CHANGES

Research seemed to indicate that most individuals who suffered minor head trauma recovered within 3 to 6 months without any apparent, lasting effects.[33] However, evidence is accumulating that the sequelae of MTBI may be more prevalent and may last longer in a higher percentage of victims than previously thought.[7] Alves has concluded the following:

There appears, at least, to be sufficient evidence to challenge the clinical view that the failure of postconcussive symptoms to resolve completely within 3 months provides clear evidence for neurosis, malingering, and other disparaging descriptors. At 3 months postinjury, the incidence of postconcussive symptoms varies from 24% to 84% in a relatively unselected sample, and there is evidence that a significant proportion of patients may exhibit symptoms for 1 year or beyond.[1]

Alves estimates that as many as half of MTBI patients are at risk of symptoms (two or more) *sometime* after their injury, and he recommends early intervention and follow-up.[1] Rimel and colleagues[33] found that one third of those who worked before the injury had not returned to work by 3 months after injury.

The patient's reaction to injury depends on a myriad of factors, including the time since injury, preexisting personality adjustment, individual coping skills, psychosocial supports, level of social-occupational functioning, willingness to receive feedback about the injury (presence or absence of "denial"), and motivation for improvement. The clinician must carefully weigh these variables in planning a treatment program.

Emotional and behavioral changes may include increased anger and irritability, depression, impulsivity, fatigue, loss of libido, poor tolerance of frustration, loss of motivation, increased anxiety, increased mistrust of others, and withdrawal or isolation. Suicidal ideation and suicide attempts may occur.[23] The patient may attempt self-medication through increased use of alcohol or drugs, or existing substance abuse tendencies may be exacerbated.

Kay[23] describes both "functional" and "dysfunctional" responses to MTBI. Functional outcomes include uncomplicated recovery, with only minor problems and limited conscious adaptation, and spontaneous accommodation in which impairment is dealt with through more specific compensatory strategies. Dysfunctional or maladjustive scenarios are classified into four groups: (1) failure, depression, and fear of insanity; (2) conditioned anxiety; (3) rigid denial; and (4) psychiatric imbalance.

Each scenario, which has important implications for psychologic adjustment, potential for intervention, and long-term adjustment, is determined by the nature of the deficits, expectations for recovery, social supports, and social and vocational demands.

To account for the wide variations in response to MTBI, Kay has proposed the concept of "individual vulnerability."[24] With each factor likely to contribute to the presence or absence of postconcussive symptoms, individuals carry a level of risk or vulnerability, and their adjustment is determined by the interaction of these risk factors.

Unfortunately, many MTBI victims do not receive the benefit of early diagnosis, education, and treatment. They may not receive help soon enough to prevent deterioration of their self-esteem, which puts them on a downward spiral of declining adjustment. Many patients interpret their failure in highly personalized terms, including the fear that they are "going crazy."[24] Even more unfortunately for some, these emotional and behavioral responses are interpreted by others as hysterical "neuroticism" or "malingering," which only invalidates the deterioration they have undergone.[23,24] As a result, a genuine cognitive deficit may not be detected because it is masked by secondary emotional reactions. Unfortunately, this experience is all too real for many victims of MTBI. The immediate effects of the injury may resolve, leaving a person who outwardly looks the same but whose ability to function in the world has been drastically changed.

TREATMENT AND REHABILITATION

Successful intervention depends on accurately identifying and describing the patient's problems. A neuropsychologic evaluation specifically geared toward MTBI is recommended as the first step in the treatment process. A formal neuropsychologic evaluation may not be necessary immediately after injury, but a targeted screening of symptoms should be done, followed by a more formal evaluation 3 to 6 months later if early symptoms have not resolved.[24] The screening should be performed within the first 4 to 6 weeks after injury. Besides a survey of all postconcussive symptoms, it should include tests sensitive to attention, concentration, speed of mental processing, word fluency, and new learning ability. The patient's emotional functioning and psychologic response to injury should always be assessed in conjunction with the above. If significant findings are obtained and the problems fail to resolve, further screening or complete assessment, or both, may be indicated in 3 to 6 months. The practitioner must consider the level of premorbid adjustment to better understand treatment complications, emotional status, speed of recovery, and overall coping ability.

The treatment process must address the symptoms in an integrated fashion, including cognitive, psychologic, psychosocial, and vocational components. The availability of treatment resources (programs and specialists) for MTBI and funding for such services are serious and sometimes formidable barriers. Cicerone[7] and Mateer[27] have de-

scribed the delivery of these services and their usefulness in addressing MTBI-related problems.

The unique features of MTBI necessitate a well coordinated treatment plan. Mateer[27] describes success in early interventions to address cognitive deficits, including providing information in the emergency room, careful discharge planning, and telephone follow up. She also emphasizes the need for comprehensive, multidisciplinary treatment of pain, depression, and psychologic and behavioral reactions. Traditional approaches involving use of tricyclic antidepressants to treat depression may be inadvisable in some cases because of the anticholingeric nature of these drugs and their potential for interfering with memory rehabilitation. Similarly, traditional psychotherapeutic techniques should be supplemented by education of the patient and family to improve their understanding of the injury, and cognitive-behavioral strategies to improve coping skills, such as dealing with increased anger and anxiety.

Cognitive interventions should be designed or targeted to improve functions, such as attention and concentration and provide practical compensatory strategies, including self-pacing, self-monitoring techniques, organization and planning skills, and environmental considerations (that is, level of stimulation and presence of distractors). Decisions on the relative importance of remedial versus compensatory treatments depend greatly on the individual's overall objectives, the time available for treatment, and the patient's response to the approaches tried. Measuring a person's level of cognitive ability before and after treatment is an excellent way to document change and validate the effectiveness of treatment.[27]

Vocational considerations are enormous, given the statistics on the impact of MTBI on employment.[33,42] Fogel and Paul-Cohen[9] outlined an approach to vocational assessment that included goal identification (immediate, short, and long-term), analysis of job performance ability, and evaluation of job duties, responsibilities, and knowledge. The complex symptoms of MTBI require careful analysis of many factors affecting vocational outcome, as well as coordination of vocational counseling with the other treatment interventions discussed earlier. Occupational adjustment is determined by the subtle interplay of behavioral, psychosocial, and cognitive factors.

Rimel and colleagues[33] found that 34% of those employed at the time of injury were not working 3 months later (excluding students, retirees, and others not employed before they were injured). Several premorbid factors were found to be predictive of whether an injured person would return to work, including type of employment, age, socioeconomic status, education, and income. Involvement in litigation was not a significant predictor. Individuals working in executive and managerial positions were *more likely* to return to work than skilled or unskilled laborers.

Two hypotheses have been advanced to explain these findings. People employed in executive and managerial positions may have access to more supportive resources and benefits, allowing them to remain employed despite difficulties (the "buffer" hypothesis). On the other hand, skilled or unskilled laborers may not have the same degree of motivation or incentive to return to work (the "injured worker" or "sick role" hypothesis). The authors also suggest that the variations in employment rate may be due to levels of psychosocial stress *before injury*. It was found that those unemployed at 3 months after injury, in contrast to those employed, had reported a significantly higher level of stress in the 12 months *before* their injuries.[33]

CASE STUDIES
Case 1

A successful, high-achieving, 19-year-old male college student was unloading a truck at his part-time job. He slipped on some grease and fell 4 feet from the loading dock to the street. He was knocked unconscious for approximately 5 minutes. He was taken to the emergency room of a nearby medical center and hospitalized overnight. He complained of severe headache and nausea. The results of his neurologic examination were within normal limits, and a routine CT scan showed no abnormalities. The following day he was discharged.

The young man returned to his studies, only to find over the next few weeks that he had difficulty concentrating on class lectures. He began to fall behind and started failing some of his examinations. As a result, he dropped out of school and returned to live with his family. Six months later he became seriously depressed and attempted suicide.

A psychiatric evaluation was conducted, but the accident and concussion were not causally linked to his problems, and he was diagnosed only with major depression. He was placed in a psychiatric facility and transferred to a residential program treating the mentally ill. Two years later, on the recommendation of a social worker familiar with head trauma, he underwent neuropsychologic evaluation. For the first time since his injury, he was given information on the residual effects of severe concussions, taught how to cope with the cognitive weaknesses, and referred to a postconcussion support group. The patient is no longer depressed and is now working part time. He has successfully begun the long-delayed adaptation to his injury and is receiving needed supportive social services.

This case is not unusual in regard to the long-term psychosocial consequences of MTBI and the relative failure to identify and treat the underlying problems early on. As is unfortunately common,

the patient was not given information about MTBI until it was properly diagnosed a few years later, following the neuropsychologic evaluation. His precipitous decline after the injury, with loss of self-esteem and depression, stand out against his good premorbid history.

Case 2

A 46-year-old male truck driver working for an express delivery company was involved in a multiple-car accident in which he suffered a severe whiplash injury and cervical neck strain, as well as suspected acceleration-deceleration–induced MTBI. The patient's employer referred him to an occupational medicine clinic, where he was diagnosed with whiplash, posttraumatic headaches, and dizziness. He was referred for physical therapy, and Tylenol with codeine was prescribed for his headaches.

The patient was kept off work for 2 weeks, and when he returned on a part-time basis, he found that his ability to attend to the written details at work had been markedly impaired. He complained of "memory problems." He was no longer as fast in filling out forms and made errors of transposition and omission, often having to repeat his work. His headaches and dizziness persisted. He was referred to a physiatrist, who prescribed a nonsteroidal antiinflammatory medication for his headache and started meclizine for his vertigo. Recognizing the need for neuropsychologic consultation, the physiatrist referred the patient for a complete assessment.

Neuropsychologic assessment revealed attentional deficits involving complex verbal and written information, a reduction in mental processing speed, and mild impulsivity. Emotionally, the patient was dealing with the posttraumatic aftermath of the accident. He responded positively to early supportive counseling and was given information on MTBI. The neuropsychologist taught him compensatory approaches for the cognitive weaknesses, and a vocational rehabilitation counselor provided job task modifications that enabled the patient to deal with the same workload more efficiently. The patient was able to return to work full time in 2 months. His headache improved over this time, and he was able to discontinue the meclizine by 3 months after the injury, with complete resolution of the vertigo.

This case study, in contrast to the first, illustrates well coordinated delivery of services. Proper diagnosis, followed by specialized neuropsychologic assessment, supportive counseling, cognitive remediation, and vocational consultation enabled the patient to return to work sooner and prevented the development of undesirable, long-term psychosocial consequences.

REFERENCES

1. Alves W: Natural history of post-concussive signs and symptoms. In Horn LJ, Zasler ND, editors: *Rehabilitation of post-concussive disorders*, Philadelphia, 1992, Hanley & Belfus, p 21.

2. American Congress of Rehabilitation Medicine: Definition of mild traumatic brain injury, Chicago, 1991, American Congress of Rehabilitation Medicine.

3. Andrews BT: Initial management of head injury. In Kraft GH, Berrol S, editors: *Physical medicine and rehabilitation clinics of north america,* Philadelphia, 1992, WB Saunders, p 249.

4. Barth JT, Macciocchi SN, Giordani B, et al: Neuropsychological sequelae of minor head injury, *J Neurosurg* 13:529-532, 1983.

5. Bode D: Ocular pain secondary to occipital neuritis. *Ann Ophthalmol* April:589-594, 1979.

6. Calliet R: *Neck and arm pain,* Philadelphia, 1981, FA Davis, p 73.

7. Cicerone KD: Psychological management of post-concussive disorders. In Horn L, Zasler N, editors: *Rehabilitation of post-concussive disorders,* Philadelphia, 1992, Hanley & Belfus.

8. Cytowic R, Stump DA, Larned DC: Closed head trauma: somatic, ophthalmic, and cognitive impairments in nonhospitalized patients. In Whitaker HA, editor: *Neuropsychological studies of nonfocal brain damage,* New York, 1988, Springer-Verlag, p 226.

9. Fogel K, Paul-Cohen R: Vocational rehabilitation after concussion. In Horn L, Zasler N, editors: *Rehabilitation of post-concussive disorders,* Philadelphia, 1992, Hanley & Belfus, p 161.

10. Gentilini M, Nichelli P, Schoenhuber R: Assessment of attention in mild head injury. In Levin HS, Eisenberg HM, Benton AL, editors: *Mild head injury,* New York, 1989, Oxford University Press, p 153.

11. Goldenberg G, Podeka I: SPECT as a tool for exploring the localizing value of neuropsychological dysfunctions in diffuse brain damage. Proceedings of the International Neuropsychological Society, Thirteenth European Conference. Innsbruck, Austria, July 4-7, 1990.

12. Griffiths M: The incidence of auditory and vestibular concussion following minor head injury, *J Laryngol Otol* 7:253-265, 1979.

13. Grimm R, Hemenway W, Lebray P, Black F: The perilymph fistula syndrome defined in mild head trauma, *Acta Otolaryngol (Stockh)* 464(suppl):1-40, 1989.

14. Gronwall D, Sampson H: *The psychological effects of concussion,* Auckland, 1974, Oxford University Press.

15. Gronwall D: Cumulative and persisting effects of concussion on attention and cognition. In Levin HS, Eisenberg HM, Benton AL, editors: *Mild head injury,* New York, 1989, Oxford University Press.

16. Haas Q, Lourie H: Trauma-triggered migraine: an explanation for common neurological attacks after mild head injury, *J Neurosurg* 68:181-188, 1988.

17. Hayes RL, Polvishock J, Singha B: Pathophysiology of mild head injury. In Horn L, Zasler N, editors: *Rehabilitation of post-concussive disorders,* Philadelphia, 1992, Hanley & Belfus, p 9.

18. Healy G: Hearing loss and vertigo secondary to head injury, *N Engl J Med* 306(17):1029-1031, 1982.

19. Herdman S: Treatment of vestibular disorders in traumatically brain-injured patients, *J Head Trauma Rehabil* 5(4):63-76, 1990.

20. Horn L: Post-concussive headache. In Horn L, Zasler N, editors: *Rehabilitation of post-concussive disorders,* Philadelphia, 1992, Hanley & Belfus, p 69.

21. Humayan MS, Presky SK, LaFrance ND, et al: Local cerebral glucose abnormalities in the mild closed head injured patients with cognitive impairments, *Nucl Med Commun* 10:335-344, 1989.

22. Jane JA, Steward O, Gennarelli T: Axonal degeneration induced by experimental noninvasive minor head injury, *J Neurosurg* 62:96-100, 1985.

23. Kay T: The unseen injury: minor head trauma, Framingham, Mass, 1986, National Head Injury Foundation.

24. Kay T: Neuropsychological diagnosis: disentangling the multiple determinants of functional disability after mild traumatic brain injury. In Horn LJ, Zasler ND, editors: *Rehabilitation of post-concussive disorders,* Philadelphia, 1992, Hanley & Belfus, p 109.

25. Leininger BE, Kreutzer JS: Neuropsychological outcome of adults with mild traumatic brain injury: implications for clinical practice and research. In Horn LJ, Zasler ND, editors: *Rehabilitation of post-concussive disorders,* Philadelphia, 1992, Hanley & Belfus, p 169.

26. Lezak MD: Newer contributions to the neuropsychological assessment of executive functions, *J Head Trauma Rehabil* 8:1, 24-31, 1993.

27. Mateer CA: Systems of care for post-concussion syndrome. In Horn LJ, Zasler ND, editors: *Rehabilitation of post-concussive disorders,* Philadelphia, 1992, Hanley & Belfus, p 143.

28. Norre M: Rationale of rehabilitation treatment for vertigo, *Am J Otol* 8:31-35, 1987.

29. Oppenheimer DR: Microscopic lesion in the brain following head injury, *J Neurol Neurosurg Psychiatry* 31:299-306, 1968.

30. Povlishock J, Becker D, Cheng C, Vaughan G: Axonal change in minor head injury, *J Neuropathol Exp Neurol* 42:225-242, 1983.

31. Povlishock J: The morphopathologic responses to experimental head injuries of varying severity. In Becker D, Povlishock J, editors: *Central nervous system status report: 1985,* Richmond, Va, 1985, Byrd Press, p 443.

32. Reitan RM, Davison LA, editors: Clinical neuropsychology: current status and applications, Washington, DC, 1974, Winston & Sons.

33. Rimel RW, Giordani B, Barth JT et al: Disability caused by minor head injury, *J Neurosurg* 9:221-228, 1981.

34. Ruff R, Buchsbaum M, Troster A et al: Computerized tomography, neuropsychology, and positron emission tomography in the evaluation of head injury, *Neuropsychiatry, Neuropsychology, and Behavioral Neurology* 2(2):103-123, 1989.

35. Schoenhuber R, Gentllini M: Neurophysiological assessment of mild head injury. In Levin HS, Eisenberg HM, Benton AL, editors: Mild head injury, New York, 1989, Oxford University Press, p 142.

36. Strich SJ: Shearing of nerve fibers as a cause of brain damage due to head injury, *Lancet* 2:443-448, 1961.

37. Thatcher RW, Walker RA, Gerson I, Geisler FH: EEG discriminant analysis of mild head trauma, *Electroencephalogr Clin Neurophysiol* 73:94-106, 1989.

38. Therapeutics and Technology Assessment Subcommittee, American Academy of Neurology: Assessment: EEG brain mapping. In American Academy of Neurology Position Statement, 1989.

39. Van Zomeren AH: Reaction time and attention after closed head injury, Lisse, 1981, Swets & Zeitlinger.

40. Wilson JT, Wiedmann KD, Hadley DM, Brooks DN: The relationship between visual memory function and lesions detected by magnetic resonance imaging after closed head injury, *Neuropsychiatry, Neuropsychology, and Behavioral Neurology* 3:255-265, 1989.

41. Wilson JT, Wyper D: Neuroimaging and neuropsychological functioning following closed head injury: CT, MRI, and SPECT, J Head Trauma Rehabil 7(2):29-39, 1992.

42. Wrightson P, Gronwall D: Time off work and symptoms after minor head injury, *Injury* 12:445-454, 1981.

43. Yokota H, Kurokawa A, Otsuka T et al: Significance of magnetic resonance imaging in acute head injury, *J Trauma* 31:351-357, 1991.

44. Zasler N: Neuromedical diagnosis and management of post-concussive disorders. In Horn LJ, Zasler ND, editors: *Rehabilitation of post-concussive disorders,* Philadelphia, 1992, Hanley & Belfus, p 33.

15 Eye Injuries

Eye injuries in the workplace are distressingly common and often result in considerable loss of vision. Even more distressing is the fact that most of these injuries are preventable. Occupational eye injuries account for approximately 22% of all eye injuries. Recent studies have highlighted the high rate of acute eye injuries and the significant toll they take on the vision of American workers. Approximately 1000 American workers injure their eyes in work-related accidents each day,[3] and about two thirds of those who are injured were not using protective eyewear.[3] The latter statistic is significant because, in one study, workers using protective eyewear that met American National Standards Institute (ANSI) code Z87.1 of 1979 had no severe injuries.[3]

Eye injuries cost more than $133 million a year in lost production, medical expenses, and workers' compensation payments. This, of course, does not factor in the personal suffering and anguish caused by such injuries.

A study by the National Eye Trauma System Registry[1] showed that men accounted for 97% of all injuries in the workplace and 75% of eye injuries in workers under 40 years of age. Projectiles caused about 60% of eye injuries, and most projectile injuries resulted in vision worse than 20/200.

Construction work and automobile repair carry a high risk of eye injury.[2] Metal work, agriculture, the military, and fishing also have a larger than usual share of ocular injuries.

The occupational health team bears a significant responsibility for preventing these injuries. Careful attention to reducing risks where possible and to insisting on the use of protective eyewear in high-risk work sites certainly will reduce the human and financial costs of these problems.

ANATOMY

Management of eye injuries has improved markedly, partly because we are more knowledgeable about the detailed anatomy of the eye. Ophthalmologists historically have used magnified imaging of the eye to better detect and more effectively treat ocular disease. Today, even for practitioners who are not ophthalmologists, a careful examination of the eye requires some magnification. More and more emergency rooms and occupational health clinics have a slitlamp biomicroscope, and we recommend that all medical personnel use it whenever possible. It may make a critical difference in the treatment of ocular injuries, whether sorting out the different causes of red eye and ocular pain or managing trauma such as foreign bodies or perforating injuries.

The most important components of ocular anatomy are illustrated in Fig. 15-1, which shows the internal and external ocular structures on a quarter cutaway section view. We have limited our descriptions to the structures commonly injured in the workplace.

Eyelid

Both upper and lower eyelids contain eyelashes (cilia) and a cartilaginous plate (tarsal plate), which protect the eye itself. The upper and lower lid margins join at the medial and lateral canthus. A lacrimal drainage apparatus, located medially, includes the punctum (the opening in the lid) and a canaliculus (duct), which runs beneath the skin to the lacrimal sac.

Sclera

The sclera is the thick outer coat of the eye. It normally is white and opaque and approximately 1 mm thick. Blunt ocular trauma may rupture the sclera at its thinnest point, behind the insertion of the extraocular muscles.

Limbus

The limbus is the junction of the cornea and sclera and a common landmark in describing ocular injuries.

Iris

The iris screens out light by means of the dark-pigmented epithelial layer on its posterior surface. With blunt trauma the blood vessels serving the iris may be torn, causing hyphema (hemorrhage within the anterior chamber of the eye), or the root of the iris may be torn away from the sclera, causing iridodialysis (separation or loosening of the iris).

Ophthalmology: Study Guide, American Academy of Ophthalmology, San Francisco, Calif, 1987, used with permission.

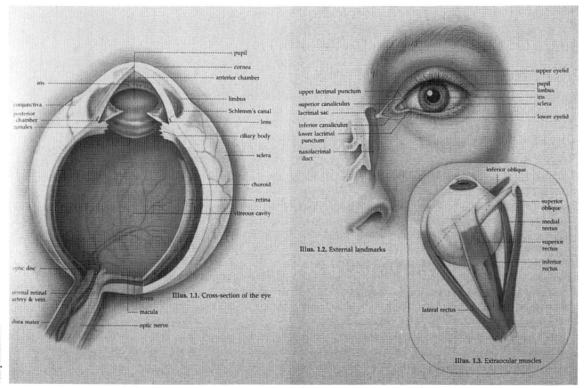

Fig. 15-1 Highlights of ocular anatomy.

Conjunctiva

The conjunctiva is a thin, vascular, mucous membrane lining the surface of the sclera (bulbar conjunctiva) and the inner surface of the lids (palpebral conjunctiva). It produces some of the components of tears and reacts in characteristic ways in viral, bacterial, and allergic conjunctivitis.

Cornea

The cornea serves as the major refractive surface of the eye. Abrasions of the surface layer usually are painful. Most foreign bodies penetrate no deeper than the superficial layer; however, some may perforate or lacerate it.

Anterior chamber

The anterior chamber is a space formed by the cornea anteriorly and the iris posteriorly. Perforating corneal injuries may cause it to collapse.

Lens

The lens is a transparent structure lying behind the iris that adds to the eye's refracting system. It may become opaque (cataract) after ocular trauma.

Retina

The retina is the neural tissue that contains the rods and cones, which together with the ganglions,

nerve fiber layer, optic nerve, and optic tract are responsible for transmitting visual input to the brain. Blunt trauma may create a hole in the retina, with subsequent retinal detachment and loss of peripheral vision.

Macula

The macula, the central area of the retina, is responsible for fine central vision. Color vision and the most acute visual perception are located in the macula. Blunt ocular trauma may cause a hole or degeneration, resulting in loss of central vision.

Choroid

The choroid is a vascular, pigmented tissue layer between the sclera and retina. It provides nutrition to and removes waste from the retina.

MEDICAL HISTORY

Accurate and complete historical data are crucial for diagnosing and treating eye injuries. Questions that should be asked in all cases include:
1. What happened? When did it happen?
2. Are one or both eyes affected?
3. What is the current level of vision?
4. What was the prior level of vision?
5. How does the current level of vision compare to the previous level?

6. What are the symptoms?
7. Are symptoms other than decreased vision present?
8. How long have these symptoms lasted?
9. Are the symptoms worsening, abating, or stable?
10. Have there been any prior eye problems or surgery on the eye?
11. Were high-speed or rotary machines involved in the accident, or anything that might present the possibility of foreign bodies from metal-to-metal impact?
12. Was chemical exposure involved? Was any first aid given at the site of injury?

CLINICAL EXAMINATION

To detect all significant damage, an eye examination should include the following components:

1. Check of visual acuity
2. External examination of the lids and bones around the eye
3. Status of conjunctiva (redness or discharge)
4. Pupillary function (reaction to light and to near stimulus)
5. Examination of eye movement with comments

DIAGNOSTIC PEARLS

A topical anesthetic can be a useful adjunct in performing an ocular examination after trauma, especially if the patient has pain or when the lids are hard to open. This can be safely given if there is no evidence of rupture of the globe. Once a drop has been given, the patient may allow opening of the eyelids. There are a number of devices to pull the eyelids open which are commonly available in emergency rooms; however, a paper clip, shaped as in the illustration (Fig. 15-2), can be as useful as a preformed eyelid retractor. Upper eyelid eversion is another technique that is helpful to examine for occult foreign bodies (Fig. 15-3).

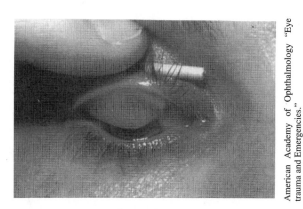

Dr. Otis Paul

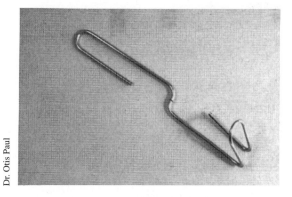

Fig. 15-2 Paper clip retractor.

American Academy of Ophthalmology "Eye trauma and Emergencies."

Fig. 15-3 Upper eyelid eversion.

on the completeness and symmetry of eye movements (nystagmus should be reported if present)
6. Examination of the anterior segment (conjunctiva, sclera, cornea, iris, lens)
7. Examination of the posterior segment (vitreous, retina, optic nerve)
8. Check of intraocular pressure (as indicated)
9. Confrontation visual fields (as indicated)

COMMON WORK-RELATED EYE INJURIES
Corneal abrasion

Abrasions of the corneal epithelium caused by minor injuries, flash burns, welder's keratitis, or contact lens overwear may be treated by the primary care physician. The corneal epithelium tends to regenerate rapidly and usually heals completely within 24 to 48 hours.

The symptoms of corneal abrasion are foreign body sensation, tearing, pain, photophobia, and possibly a red eye. Often the eye is squeezed shut, preventing appropriate examination.

Initially the foreign body sensation is the most prominent symptom. As time passes, a severe, aching pain may develop that worsens when the eye is exposed to light. This photophobia indicates that at least some iritis is present. The patient's vision is somewhat blurred and can be better evaluated after a topical anesthetic ophthalmic solution has been applied. Because fluorescein stains the denuded or damaged areas of the cornea, bright yellow-green fluorescence detected with a cobalt blue or Wood's light indicates damaged or absent corneal epithelium (Fig. 15-4).

Treatment is designed to promote rapid healing, restore comfort, and prevent secondary infection. It should include a medium-duration topical cycloplegic drop (such as cyclopentolate or homatropine) to relieve the pain caused by reflex spasm of the ciliary body muscles. Common cycloplegic drugs and their duration are shown in Table 15-1.

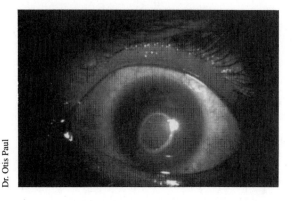

Dr. Otis Paul

Fig. 15-4 Corneal abrasion. Notice fluorescein staining.

DIAGNOSTIC PEARL

A slitlamp greatly facilitates diagnosis of a corneal abrasion and examination of the cornea for foreign bodies. If a slitlamp is not available, using fluorescein with magnification loupes and cobaltblue illumination is the best choice.

If the patient is in severe pain, oral analgesics with codeine should be prescribed. After the appropriate pain-relief agent has been administered, a topical ophthalmic antibiotic may be applied as well. The most important part of the treatment is a pressure patch, which is made by folding an eyepad in half and placing it gently against the closed eye, followed by an additional pad. The patient must keep both eyes closed while the pressure patch is taped firmly to the affected eye. The patch should remain on the eye for at least 24 hours, and follow-up evaluation by an ophthalmologist is indicated if the patient is not pain free in 24 to 48

Table 15-1 Common cyclolplegic drugs: this table is an approximate guide, as the times may vary by effectiveness of application, color of iris, and severity of ocular inflammation.

Drug	Duration
1% tropicamide (Mydriacyl, others)	1-2 hours
1% cyclopentolate (Cyclogyl, others)	3-4 hours
2% homatropine (Homatropine, others)	6-8 hours
1% scopolamine (Isopto-Hyoscine)	10-12 hours
1% atropine (Isopto Atropine, others)	4-7 days

hours or if his discomfort increases after pressure patching.

> **WARNING:** *Under no condition should topical anesthetic solutions be used to relieve pain because they have toxic effects on the corneal epithelium. The anesthetic damages the epithelium each time it is applied, resulting in greater pain when the anesthetic wears off; thus a vicious cycle is started that cannot readily be broken. A properly applied eye patch prevents this.*

> **WARNING:** *It should be noted that corneal abrasions caused by a fingernail or vegetable matter (such as a tree branch or sharp leaf of a plant) heal more slowly and warrant referral to an ophthalmologist; these abrasions tend to recur and pose the risk of an associated fungal keratitis. Steroid eye medications are strongly contraindicated because they may enhance fungal growth.*

Foreign bodies

A common cause of corneal foreign bodies is use of a grinding wheel without wearing safety goggles (Fig. 15-5). When foreign bodies of this type are superficial, they can be removed relatively easily with a moist, cotton-tipped applicator. When these particles are located deeper, an experienced clinician can remove them with a sharp-tipped instrument under magnification (preferably a slitlamp). The hub of a 23-gauge needle can be placed on a cotton-tipped swab for better control while removing corneal foreign bodies (Fig. 15-6). The approach is from below in case the patient rolls his eye upward during the procedure (Bell's reflex).

Using a hammer, with its tempered surface, against another hard-tempered steel object raises the risk of a more serious, perforating, intraocular foreign body because the tempered surfaces, when hitting one another, tend to fracture and break off, shooting small metallic shards. It is important to

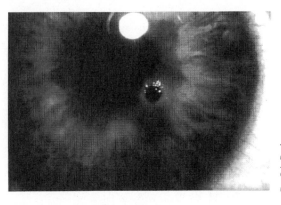

Dr. Otis Paul

Fig. 15-5 Corneal foreign body.

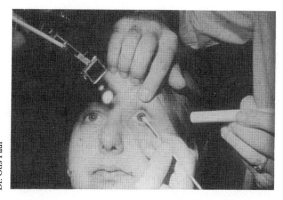

Fig. 15-6 Technique of removing corneal foreign body.

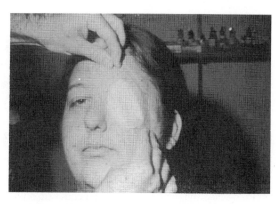

Fig. 15-7 Proper placement of simple eye patch.

examine the eyelids, iris, and lens in patients with corneal abrasions and foreign bodies for evidence of ocular perforation, particularly if an explosion or use of a hammer was involved in the accident. The examination should include careful inspection of the corneal wound for a perforation tract and viewing of the iris to check for perforation, bleeding on the surface of the iris, or adhesion of the iris to the peripheral cornea (Fig. 15-8). The sclera must be examined carefully for sites of perforation, particularly for any evidence of uveal protrusion through the sclera; this appears as a bluish or grayish discoloration beneath the conjunctiva associated with a spot of hemorrhage (Fig. 15-8). The eyelids also should be examined for perforation sites because such a site may be the beginning of a tract that perforates the sclera, risking damage to the retina or optic nerve.

Chemical burns

Chemical burns are a true ocular emergency; the injured person or coworkers must irrigate the eye immediately at the injury site. Serious vision loss is possible even if the injury initially does not seem severe.

TREATMENT PEARL

An ocular patch is made with sterile gauze. It is applied over the closed eyelids and held in place with layers of tape running from the center of the forehead to the cheek (Fig. 15-7). The patch is more effective when applied with pressure. The skin of the forehead is pulled down and the skin of the cheek is pulled upward to immobilize the lids. The lids should not be able to move beneath the patch. Applying a pressure patch in this way affords maximum comfort and healing. A loose patch may actually slow corneal healing and prolong the occupational disability.

Alkali burns generally are more damaging than acid burns, because they penetrate ocular tissues faster. Drain and chemical cleansers, detergents, fertilizers, and industrial solvents are the most common sources of alkali burns. The extent of ocular damage from these burns may not be apparent at first. Corneas that at first are relatively clear can become opaque and vascularized.

If a telephone call is received about a chemical eye burn, the caller should be instructed to start irrigation immediately with the nearest source of water. The eyelids should be held apart during irrigation at the injury site. The eye should be copiously irrigated at the site for about 5 minutes, and then the patient should be taken to the emergency room.

A patient with a chemical burn should receive immediate attention. Vision testing and paperwork should be postponed. Topical anesthetic drops should be placed in both eyes. The lids are gently retracted with a Desmarres retractor or the paper clip retractor described in Fig. 15-2. The eyelids and conjunctiva must be thoroughly searched for chemical residue or particulate matter from the acid or alkaline agents, and any residue or debris should be removed with cotton swabs or forceps. Everting the lids helps in detecting and removing

---

TREATMENT PEARL

It is of no value to delay treatment in search of a solution that might neutralize the type of chemical that originally was splashed into the eye. "Neutralizing" solutions also can cause significant chemical or thermal reactions that can increase the extent of injury. Immediate irrigation (within 1 minute) is the primary concern, and the volume of the solution irrigated should more than adequately neutralize any residual acidic or alkaline properties of the chemical.

particles lodged in the fornices. The eye should be continuously irrigated with a balanced salt solution, normal saline, or Ringer's solution for 10 minutes, regardless of any previous irrigation. A continuous, rapid-drip IV apparatus is effective for irrigation if the solution is directed across the everted eyelid, culs-de-sac, and cornea. If both eyes are involved, it is important to alternate irrigation frequently between them.

After the particulate matter has been removed and irrigation completed, a topical cylcoplegic drug should be instilled, such as 1% cyclopentolate drops. Topical antibiotic drops also are applied, and then a sterile patch is put in place. If the damage is anything more than minor, the patient should be referred promptly to an ophthalmologist. A mild chemical burn (conjunctival injection and no or mild corneal involvement) can be followed closely by the primary care physician. Short-term use of a steroid-antibiotic eyedrop can ease the pain and injection.

Ocular trauma

Examination. In cases of ocular trauma, both eyes and the surrounding structures should be examined completely and the results recorded. The inspection should cover visual acuity, the pupil and retina, external structures, and eye movement.

Visual acuity. Visual acuity must be recorded as specifically as possible. If a Snellen chart is not available, the examiner should determine the patient's ability to read printed material at hand. The type of print used and the distance at which it was read should be recorded.

It is important to know whether vision is equal in both eyes and whether it was equal before the injury. If the patient cannot read letters, the examiner should determine whether he can count fingers or perceive hand motions, or whether there is a response to light. If visual acuity is normal, the confrontation visual fields should be tested. Occasionally patients do not recognize loss of part of the visual fields as such, and later describe this condition as a general loss of vision.

Pupil and retina. The examiner also should note direct and consensual pupillary light reactions. In cases of monocular vision loss, the most useful objective test in ophthalmology is the afferent pupil test, or Marcus Gunn test (it also is known as the swinging flashlight test); an abnormal result indicates a relative afferent pupil defect (Marcus Gunn pupil).

The Marcus Gunn (or swinging flashlight) test is conducted by holding a flashlight in front of one eye for 3 seconds, then swinging it rapidly to the other eye for 3 seconds, and then back again. When the flashlight is shone into the abnormal eye, the pupil paradoxically dilates and then constricts when the light is swung in front of the normal eye. The test turns on the fact that light shown into one eye drives both pupils equally. If one neural pathway is not functioning as well as the other, light shown into the "weaker" eye does not cause pupillary constriction in *either* eye. This is manifest as a relative dilation of *both* pupils when the light is shown into the bad eye and constriction of *both* pupils when the light is shown into the normal eye.

Marcus Gunn pupil indicates a significant problem in the retina or in the neural pathways to the chiasm. Such conditions as a large retinal detachment or traumatic injury of the optic nerve can cause an afferent pupil defect. However, *whenever these conditions are bilateral, even if severe, Marcus Gunn pupil will not be present.* A previously undetected afferent pupil defect is always cause for concern. The box below lists conditions associated with Marcus Gunn pupil.

External structures. It is important to examine the external ocular structures by palpating the orbital rims and by looking for evidence of proptosis (protrusion of the eyeball). This generally is more readily detected if the examiner looks at the eye from above while the patient looks downward. A light should be used to examine the anterior chamber for signs of perforation; oblique illumination should be used to check the depth of the anterior chamber, which should be compared with that of the other eye.

CONDITIONS ASSOCIATED WITH MARCUS GUNN PUPIL (UNILATERAL OR ASYMMETRIC)

Large retinal detachment
Generalized retinal disease
Optic neuritis
Optic atrophy
Tumor of the optic nerve
Certain lesions of the chiasm

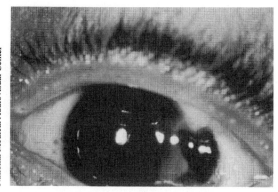

Fig. 15-8 Uveal prolapse and ruptured globe. Prolapse of dark iris and ciliary body is noted through scleral wound.

The sclera should be examined for evidence of uveal prolapse through the sclera, which may occur in addition to the more obvious prolapse of the iris through lacerations in the cornea. If a penetrating injury or a ruptured globe is suspected, the eyelids should not be manipulated. Retraction and eversion of the upper and lower lids facilitates inspection for a foreign body or for lesions near the equatorial region of the globe. Anesthetic eyedrops and fluorescein are useful for eliciting the patient's cooperation and detecting any epithelial damage. A topical anesthetic such as 0.5% proparacaine hydrochloride (Ophthaine, Alcaine) relieves pain almost instantly and allows a more deliberate and thus adequate evaluation.

Eye movement. Orbital hematoma may cause generalized restriction of eye movement. An orbital blowout fracture may result in upgaze restriction and diplopia (in these cases, the inferior tissues of the orbit are trapped in the fracture, preventing upward movement because of attachment to the inferior rectus muscle). When diffuse limitation of eye movement is accompanied by proptosis, the head and eye should be auscultated for a bruit; if present, this suggests a fistula of the carotid cavernous sinus.

If the *fundus* is visible, the examiner should look for edema or retinal hemorrhage or detachment. If perforation is suspected, an intraocular foreign body should be sought. If any of these findings are present or if the examiner suspects a penetrating injury or foreign body, the patient should be referred immediately to an ophthalmologist. Immediate referral is also warranted if the red reflex is absent, because the cause may be a condition such as hyphema, cataract, or vitreous hemorrhage.

X-ray films should be taken if there is a question of facial or orbital fracture or of an intraocular or orbital foreign body. The most efficient exami-

WARNING: *When treating a chemical burn caused by tear gas or an aerosol spray, the clinician should remember that these agents can injure the eye sufficiently to cause a ruptured globe or to push a foreign body into the eye.*

nation for an intraocular foreign body in the back of the eye is done with an instrument called the indirect ophthalmoscope, which allows a steroscopic view of the entire peripheral retina. However, most primary care physicians are not trained to use this instrument.

Common traumatic injuries

Ruptured globe. A ruptured globe must be identified early and managed appropriately to protect the eye from further damage. Good vision may be obtained, even with a full-thickness laceration of the sclera and cornea with prolapse of the iris and uveal tissue (see Fig. 15-8).

An ocular examination should be done before the patient is sent for x-ray films or laboratory procedures. If an ophthalmologist is not immediately available, the examining physician can use a slit-lamp, which usually is kept in or near the emergency room. Taking the time for a slitlamp examination often pays off with more diagnostic information than can be acquired with immediate x-ray films and laboratory testing. This initial examination is crucial when an intraocular foreign body or penetrating injury is suspected because, if such an injury is present, manipulation of the eye during the imaging process could aggravate the damage. Such cases should be referred immediately to an ophthalmologist, and the injured eye should be shielded before the patient is transported. A metal shield made specifically for this purpose may be used, or a shield can be fashioned from a paper cup, cardboard, or plastic (Fig. 15-9).

A ruptured globe should be suspected with any of the following:

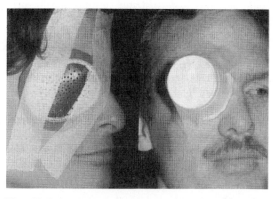

Fig. 15-9 Protective shield for ruptured globe. This shield may be a metal shield made specifically for this purpose, or a shield can be fashioned out of a paper cup, cardboard, or plastic.

1. A history of severe blunt trauma, projectile injury, contact with a sharp object, use of a grinding wheel, or trauma caused by hammering metal on metal
2. Subconjunctival hemorrhage
3. Conjunctival laceration
4. Uveal prolapse (indicated by dark tissue, either iris or ciliary body, on the surface of the globe)
5. Irregular or pear-shaped pupil (the peak of the pupil often points to the perforation site)
6. Hyphema (blood in the anterior chamber)
7. Lens opacity (cataract)

If a ruptured globe is suspected, the clinician should stop the examination immediately to avoid manipulating the eye, which could increase the amount of intraocular tissue that prolapses. The eye should not be patched because pressure from the patch may further extrude the contents of the globe. A protective shield, as previously described, should be placed over the eye to safeguard it from pressure.

WARNING: *Imaging studies to search for an intraocular foreign body should not be done until an ophthalmologist has performed an ocular examination.*

Hyphema. Serious eye damage can be caused by an injury that does not actually rupture the globe. Hyphema (blood in the anterior chamber) arises from a tear in peripheral iris vessels and usually is caused by blunt, nonpenetrating ocular trauma (Fig. 15-10). In most cases hyphema can be identified with a flashlight. A slitlamp greatly facilitates detection of blood in the anterior chamber. Patients with hyphema should be treated as though they have a ruptured globe and referred to an ophthalmologist as soon as possible. Treatment usually involves some combination of restricted activity, a protective eye shield, cycloplegia, topical steroids, and systemic aminocaproic acid (Amicar). Hyphema may be complicated by repeat bleeding into the anterior chamber, which typically may occur 5 days after injury. This condi-tion is associated with an increased risk of glaucoma. Blunt trauma may also lead to late development of glaucoma, cataract, and retinal detachment.

Orbital trauma. Fractures of the orbit are asso-

DIAGNOSTIC PEARL

One fourth of patients with hyphema have other, concomitant ocular injuries such as vitreous hemorrhage, subluxed lens, and retinal damage.

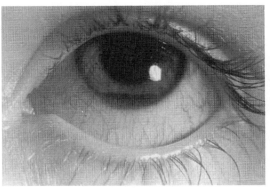

Self-Instructional Materials in Ophthalmology, National Medical Audiovisual Center

Fig. 15-10 Hyphema. Note blood level inferiorly.

ciated with swelling, ecchymosis, and hemorrhage into the orbital tissues. Signs may range from minor lid ecchymosis to major orbital hemorrhage with proptosis. Orbital trauma also may cause subconjunctival hemorrhage; however, most of the time an isolated subconjunctival hemorrhage is a benign finding.

Minor orbital trauma is treated with cold compresses and analgesics. Follow-up evaluation is advised to detect any worsening of the findings. Major orbital trauma with hemorrhage and edema may produce proptosis with secondary corneal exposure. If increased intraocular pressure poses a threat to vision, emergency surgical decompression of the orbit may be required.

Orbital fractures may be associated with these findings:

1. Diplopia
2. Epistaxis
3. Decreased sensation over the cheek and upper lip
4. A palpable disruption in continuity of the bone when the fracture involves the orbital rim
5. Point tenderness at the site of the fracture

If any of these findings is present, a skull x-ray film and/or detailed imaging studies, such as computed tomography (CT) or magnetic resonance imaging (MRI), is indicated. A blowout fracture does not warrant surgery in and of itself. Surgical repair, if warranted, often is delayed for at least several days and often several weeks, because the diplopia may be transient.

WARNING: *One fourth of patients with orbital floor fractures have associated occult ocular trauma. Referral to an ophthalmologist is strongly indicated.*

Lid lacerations. Lid lacerations can be caused by blunt trauma, direct injury with a sharp instrument, or a dog bite. The primary care physician should assume that lid lacerations are accompanied by globe lacerations until proven otherwise. Diagnosis and treatment of the more occult ocular problem often may take precedence over the more obvious lid laceration.

A lid laceration (Fig. 15-11) requires the attention of an ophthalmologist if one of these findings is present:

1. *Laceration involving the lid margin.* The lid margins must be repaired in layers to provide normal lid function and avoid long-term ocular complications such as corneal injury.
2. *Involvement of the canalicular system.* When the medial third of the upper or lower lid is lacerated, the tear drainage system commonly is lacerated as well. Effective repair includes reapproximation of the severed lacrimal drainage system.
3. *Deep lacerations of the upper lid.* The laceration may involve the levator muscle; if this is not repaired, permanent ptosis results.
4. *Fat prolapse.* Deep lacerations may be associated with fat prolapse; this also indicates a high risk of occult eye injury, intraocular foreign body, or impairment of lid function.
5. *Any significant loss of tissue.* These injuries may require skin grafting.

Superficial lid lacerations that do not involve the eyelid margin do not usually require the assistance of an ophthalmologist. Care must be taken to avoid retraction of the lid margin because this will impair lid function and preclude a good cosmetic result. Tetanus prophylaxis is recommended. Superficial foreign bodies in the wound should be removed to avoid skin irregularity and pigmentation changes. Again, the possibility of foreign body

Self-Instructional Materials in Ophthalmology, National Medical Audiovisual Center

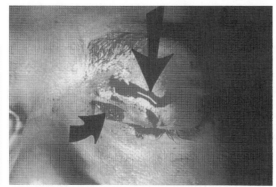

Fig. 15-11 Lid laceration. Large arrow points to simple laceration that can easily be repaired. Small arrow points to laceration through lid margin and possibly the lacrimal drainage system. This requires expert repair.

penetration of the eye must always be investigated with lid lacerations.

Further details on evaluation and treatment of ocular trauma are available in the American Academy of Ophthalmology's slide script program, "Eye Trauma and Emergencies." It can be obtained by writing the American Academy of Ophthalmology, 655 Beach Street, P.O. Box 7424, San Francisco CA 94120. The program also can be obtained by calling the AAO at 415-561-8540 and asking for customer service.

Eye pain

As in any organ system, eye pain may have many causes. Determining the timing of events and associated problems is important in distinguishing among such diverse conditions as sinus disorders, vascular disease, ocular inflammatory disorders, and ocular trauma. The patient may believe that his eye pain is due to a work injury or condition, such as "a lot of dust in the air at my job." Because defining the cause can be challenging, the clinician must consider the spectrum of differential diagnoses outlined below.

Associated sinus disease. With maxillary or frontal sinusitis, patients commonly complain of associated symptoms such as rhinorrhea (nasal discharge). An important sign is tenderness with pressure over the sinus.

Ocular inflammatory diseases. Ocular inflammatory diseases include uveitis, episcleritis, scleritis, and optic neuritis. They can be isolated to the eye or associated with systemic syndromes such as Reiter's disease or ulcerative colitis. Symptoms usually include a dull, aching pain and photophobia (sensitivity to light). The difference in light sensitivity between eyes often can be appreciated by passing a flashlight first from one eye to the other. Another possible finding is a perilimbal flush (a collection of dilated blood vessels adjacent to the limbus of the eye, with the remainder of the conjunctiva minimally involved). The pupil is somewhat smaller on the affected side, and a slitlamp examination will show the white blood cells in the anterior chamber.

Trauma. Trauma can result in hyphema, iritis, and retinal injury. If the anterior chamber is deep, it probably is safe to dilate the pupil. When iritis is the cause of pain, dilation will reduce the patient's discomfort and allow examination of the retina for possible retinal injury (see the previous discussion of ocular trauma).

Elderly patients often complain of a fleeting ocular pain that may have no detectable cause. Assuming the rest of the ocular examination is normal, the most likely cause of pain in these cases is ischemia.

COMMON EYE PROBLEMS

The following conditions are complaints commonly seen by practitioners in the primary care setting. Most of these problems become bothersome while the individual is at work, and they may impair safe job performance; however, although in some cases these problems may be exacerbated or aggravated by work activity, they usually are not caused by the job. They are included because they occur so often and because of the common misconception that they are solely job related.

Problems related to the video display terminal

Whether the patient is chained to a computer because of work demands or is a victim of "computer rapture syndrome," prolonged use of a video display terminal (VDT) is characterized by a number of symptoms. Ocular symptoms include tearing, blurred vision, or a burning sensation. Generalized symptoms are fatigue, headaches, musculoskeletal pain, and a cramping sensation associated with prolonged periods without an opportunity to stretch or shift positions. These symptoms can exacerbate underlying ocular problems that otherwise might not have been noticed.

A number of specific ocular conditions may become significant with prolonged use of a VDT. One such condition is uncorrected near vision. People who are hyperopic (farsighted) may have symptoms associated with near work at an earlier age than those who are myopic (nearsighted). The nearness of the VDT and the prolonged use associated with generalized fatigue may make reading-related symptoms prominent, which would not occur while reading a book with good illumination and posture. Ocular convergence problems also may emerge as a tendency for the eyes to lose binocular fixation, with associated symptoms of blurred vision and diplopia at near. Asymmetric refractions become more symptomatic when prolonged near-vision tasks are required, and a careful balancing of the reading prescription is necessary to minimize these symptoms.

Treating these problems requires careful assessment of the precipitating circumstances in an examination that includes refraction at distance as well as at near; assessment for strabismus at distance as well as at near; and careful attention to imbalance in the strength of the prescription for glasses. These conditions must be corrected first when evaluating patients with VDT-associated problems, and referral to an ophthalmologist or optometrist is warranted.

Some patients assume that the ocular problems are the cause of headaches, neck aches, and generalized discomfort. Therefore a comprehensive ocular examination is necessary to assess the role of the eyes in the entire symptom complex.

It also is important to reduce background glare from lights or a window. Dealing with this problem includes assessing the patient's posture, the position and angle of the monitor, and the relative position of the hands for keyboard tasks. (See Chapter 22 for further discussion of musculoskeletal problems associated with repetitive motion.) General ventilatory conditions in the area of the computer and monitor must be assessed for adequacy as well. What ultimately manifests as an ocular complaint may require comprehensive assessment sensitive to a number of postural and environmental conditions in the workplace.

Visual loss

It is critical to distinguish the acuteness of the visual loss and whether the patient had a preexisting decrease in vision or ocular problem. It is important to know (1) whether the visual loss is transient or persistent; (2) whether the visual loss is monocular or binocular; (3) the course of vision loss over time; (4) the patient's age and general medical health; and (5) any documentation of normal vision in the past.

Patients with gradually decreasing vision and blurred vision do not usually represent an emergency; however, it is important to establish the chronicity of the problem. One refractive problem that occasionally is seen in the emergency room is unrecognized loss of a contact lens. Because these patients usually are nearsighted, vision should be tested with a Snellen chart both at distance as well as at near; if vision is normal at near but blurred at distance, myopia (nearsightedness) is the most likely diagnosis. Another way to detect refractive error as a cause of blurred vision is to test the vision with a pinhole. If the vision becomes normal (at least 20/25) with a pinhole, the cause is most likely a refractive error. Occasionally patients with diabetic ketoacidosis may suffer a marked change in refractive error where the decrease in vision can be improved by having the patient look through a pinhole. Sulfa-related drugs can also enhance myopia.

It is important to test the pupillary reactions with the swinging flashlight test (Marcus Gunn test; see page 234).

Differential diagnosis
Opacity of the media
CORNEAL EDEMA. With corneal edema the normally crisp corneal light reflex may suddenly become dull, and the usually clear cornea takes on a ground glass appearance. Corneal edema can be caused by a rapid increase in intraocular pressure from angle-closure glaucoma or by an acute her-

pes simplex virus infection. Urgent referral to an ophthalmologist is warranted.

HYPHEMA. Blood in the anterior chamber (hyphema) after trauma may reduce vision. Blood cells layer at the inferior portion of the anterior chamber (Fig. 15-10) if the patient has been upright for a while; this is more easily detected with a bright light or slitlamp. Urgent referral is warranted for hyphema of any cause.

CATARACTS. Cataracts generally develop slowly; however, in rare cases they may occur suddenly after trauma. Routine referral is appropriate.

VITREOUS HEMORRHAGE. Vitreous hemorrhage may occur after trauma, but it also may accompany diabetes or retinal detachment. Urgent referral is warranted.

Retinal disease

RETINAL DETACHMENT. Acute vision loss is characteristic of retinal detachment. Patients often report flashing lights followed by a large number of floaters, then a shadow or "spider web" over the peripheral vision in one eye. Some may describe this as a curtain. An afferent pupil defect (Marcus Gunn pupil) may be present. Once the pupil is dilated, the retinal detachment is much easier to detect. Urgent referral is warranted.

MACULAR DISEASE. In a young person, edema in the center of the macula may cause a decrease in vision associated with a syndrome called central serous choroidopathy; this produces an elevation of the sensory retina in the region of the macula. In an older person, sudden loss from macula disease is most commonly associated with bleeding from a neovascular abnormality associated with macular degeneration. Urgent referral is warranted.

VASCULAR OCCLUSIONS. Retinal artery occlusions are a relatively common cause of sudden loss of vision. Central retinal artery occlusions may be preceded by transient periods of monocular vision loss called amaurosis fugax. An ipsilateral afferent pupil defect usually is present. Examination with an ophthalmoscope shows narrowed retinal arterioles and a pale optic nerve. If the retina is edematous throughout the posterior central region, the reddish foveal region may give the appearance of a "cherry red spot." Emergency treatment is directed to rapidly decreasing the intraocular pressure and dilating the blood vessels in an attempt to allow the obstructing embolus to pass into a less critical, smaller-caliber vessel. Treatment may include rebreathing carbon dioxide (10% Carbogen gas), intravenous acetazolamide (500 mg), digital massage of the globe through closed eyelids, or even paracentesis of the eye. Emergency referral and consultation can save vision.

Retinal vein occlusions also may cause sudden visual loss. They are characterized by multiple retinal hemorrhages and may require laser treatment.

TEMPORAL ARTERITIS. Temporal arteritis is a potentially blinding and fatal disorder. This condition should be considered an emergency because ocular involvement may occur within hours of onset. The disorder tends to occur in people over 65 years of age and often is accompanied by scalp tenderness, migrating myalgia, jaw claudication, loss of appetite, and generalized malaise.

Red eye

Most conditions that cause red eye are not dangerous. However, if red eye is associated with pain or reduced vision, the problem is likely to be more serious. Urgent referral is warranted if pain is present.

The differential diagnosis of nontraumatic red eye includes conjunctivitis, subconjunctival hemorrhage, iritis, corneal infection, and acute glaucoma. When inflamed, the conjunctival blood vessels dilate and are readily apparent against the white sclera. The cause usually can be determined through a clinical history and thorough examination. However, an ophthalmologist should be consulted if an infection is suspected and the vision is impaired or if the condition seems to be progressing despite conservative treatment.

Subconjunctival hemorrhage. Subconjunctival hemorrhage often is frightening to the patient, who notices the sudden appearance of a red or "blood" spot on the eye without any concomitant ocular symptoms (Fig. 15-12). Although these isolated broken capillaries sometimes may be associated with trauma, blood dyscrasias, or hypertension, most are of unknown etiology, benign, and self-limited, clearing within a few days. Subconjunctival hemorrhages are easily differentiated from

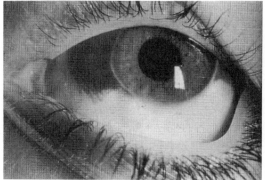

Self-Instructional Materials in Ophthalmology, National Medical Audiovisual Center

Fig. 15-12 Subconjunctival hemorrhage. Note clear areas.

other causes of red eye by their localization, the presence of normal conjunctiva around them, and the lack of symptoms. Patients with recurrent subconjunctival hemorrhages should be screened for hypertension, blood dyscrasias, or other ophthalmologic problems. Remember that a subconjunctival hemorrhage can mask a perforated globe, so ask about possible antecedent trauma.

Conjunctivitis

Viral conjunctivitis. Eye infections ordinarily are not considered work-related injuries unless they occur in the context of an "epidemic" among a group of workers or in special circumstances, such as direct transmission from patient to health care worker. Viral conjunctivitis is highly contagious and may be transmitted by fingers or contaminated towels. So many epidemics have been reported in the workplace that it is known as "shipyard conjunctivitis." Hand washing and separate towels are important to prevent the spread of this infection by both health workers and those infected. Because of the risk of large-scale contagion, a patient working in a factory, health care facility, or restaurant should be quarantined from fellow employees.

The most common cause of viral conjunctivitis is the adenovirus. The disease produces a discharge that usually is watery. The eyelids may stick together on awakening. A useful diagnostic check is that preauricular lymph nodes usually are present in severe adenovirus infections and may be an important sign in differentiating viral from bacterial conjunctivitis. The patient may have an associated upper respiratory infection, sore throat, fever, or generalized malaise, but this varies considerably. Viral conjunctivitis usually is self-limiting, and no specific treatment is indicated. An antibiotic is indicated if the conjunctivitis becomes purulent and a secondary bacterial infection appears. However, most infections clear without any specific treatment.

It is important to remember that (1) if the conjunctivitis persists longer than 10 days or (2) if pain, photophobia, or decreased vision is present, the patient should be referred to an ophthalmologist. Steroid-containing eyedrops should be avoided because they may activate a latent herpes virus infection, which can cause permanent corneal scarring and loss of vision.

Bacterial conjunctivitis. Bacterial conjunctivitis is rarely considered work related unless it occurs as a superinfection of work-related viral conjunctivitis or a work-related eye injury. All common bacterial pathogens may cause conjunctivitis. The most common offenders are *Staphylococcus, Streptococcus, Haemophilus,* and *Pseudomonas* species. If the patient has a mild, purulent dis-

---

DIAGNOSTIC PEARL

Culture and sensitivity testing should be done with any purulent, acute conjunctivitis, especially if gonococcal infection is suspected. A smear will show the intracytoplasmic inclusion gram-negative diplococci. If such an infection is suspected or is demonstrated by Gram's stain, the patient should be referred immediately to an ophthalmologist, because the cornea can be directly penetrated and infected by these organisms. Once in the cornea, these infections tend to spread rapidly and can cause permanent loss of vision and even loss of the eye.

---

charge and a clear cornea, the primary care physician may begin treatment. Warm compresses applied four times a day should be included in the treatment regimen. Topical ophthalmic antibiotic solutions (such as 10% sulfacetamide) applied four times daily should be prescribed for 5 to 7 days. A topical ophthalmic ointment, such as bacitracin, erythromycin, or gentamicin, may be added at bedtime for 7 to 10 days. The patient should be instructed to cleanse the eye of discharge and the lids of crusting. Referral is recommended in cases of persistent discharge or redness after 4 days.

With conjunctivitis, the pattern of redness tends to be more concentrated in the palpebral area, where the conjunctiva lines the lids, rather than near the cornea. If the discharge is copious and purulent, *Pseudomonas* or gonococcal infection should be considered.

Allergic conjunctivitis. Allergic conjunctivitis is characterized by lid or conjunctival edema often associated with a watery, white, stringy discharge. Itching is a hallmark symptom and often a useful way to distinguish this condition from viral conjunctivitis. Allergic conjunctivitis commonly is associated with hay fever, asthma, and eczema in patients with a history of these problems. Contact allergy is associated with drugs, chemicals, or cosmetics.

These conditions should be treated symptomatically with oral and topical antihistamines and by eliminating the offending allergen if possible. Vasoconstrictors containing naphazoline or phenylephrine are useful in mild cases. Although currently not commercially available, topical 4% chromolyn applied four times a day may prevent itching. If the condition does not respond to these local forms of treatment, the patient should be referred to an ophthalmologist.

Eye irritation. Bland ocular preparations are useful for mild eye irritation resulting from minor chemical or particulate exposure, such as smog or dust. Artificial tear preparations are useful; these also can be used when a chemical known to be only mildly irritating (petroleum products, mouthwash, mild detergents, weak acids) is splashed into the eye. However, if the chemical is unknown or toxic to ocular tissues (alkaline products), the eye must be irrigated immediately at the job site (see previous discussion) to save vision.

Two conditions that commonly cause symptoms of ocular irritation are pinguecula and pterygium, both of which may be associated with exposure to sun, wind, and dust. A pinguecula, which represents a degenerative process of the conjunctiva in the palpebral fissure, appears as a yellow-red discoloration (Fig. 15-13). A pterygium is an extension of this process onto the cornea and can be recognized by a gray-white growth onto the cornea (Fig. 15-14). Both of these conditions can be exacerbated by conjunctivitis of any cause and may become red when exposed to irritants in the air, such as smoke or smog.

Topical artificial tears can help relieve symptoms in these conditions. The patient also should be strongly urged to use ultraviolet protective lenses outdoors. Topical vasoconstrictors, which can be used four times a day, help reduce the redness. However, vasoconstrictors do not treat the underlying condition, and their effectiveness tends to diminish with time. Sometimes switching to a different preparation may work. If the symptoms are severe or the pterygium seems to be growing into the cornea, referral to an ophthalmologist is indicated.

DIAGNOSTIC PEARL

The presence of photophobia is a useful symptom in distinguishing iritis from allergic conjunctivitis and viral conjunctivitis.

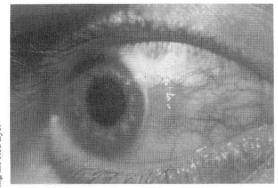

Fig. 15-13 Pinguecula.

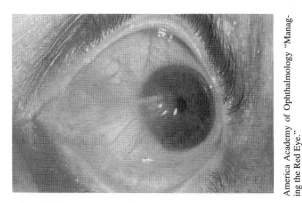

Fig. 15-14 Pterygium.

Iritis. A patient with iritis tends to have a characteristic circumcorneal redness, pain, photophobia, and decreased vision. The pupil on the affected side is smaller than the other. Iritis frequently accompanies other inflammatory conditions such as rheumatoid arthritis, sarcoidosis, urethritis, and bowel disorders. It also may be caused by blunt trauma to the eye. Early treatment of this condition is indicated, and prompt referral is the preferred method because untreated or improperly treated iritis can result in glaucoma and cataracts.

Corneal inflammation and infection. Acute corneal disorders typically are associated with pain, a small pupil, photophobia, and blurred vision. The primary care physician will note that corneal smoothness and clarity give way to an irregular corneal surface and opacification.

In addition to observing an irregular corneal reflection with a penlight or, preferably, a slitlamp, the clinician can use fluorescein dye to detect the loss of corneal epithelium, as seen in abrasions. When applied, the fluorescein spreads over the cornea, and the dye adheres where there is a defect in the surface, a loss or damage of epithelial cells. It is important to allow the tears to dilute the fluorescein or to rinse it out before examining the cornea. The affected cells are stained a bright green and can be seen most easily with a cobalt blue light (see Fig. 15-4).

In temperate climates, herpes keratitis is the most common cause of corneal opacification. Herpes simplex virus type I (HSV) is the more common cause of ocular infection, but infection with HSV II may occur as well. Corneal involvement with the herpes virus manifests as a red eye with a foreign body sensation. Fluorescein staining shows the characteristic dendritic lesion. The patient should be referred to an ophthalmologist immediately. HSV infection of the cornea can lead to corneal opacification, iritis, and loss of vision. Fortunately, if caught in time, modern treatment usually is effective in reducing or eliminating visual loss.

Bacterial keratitis (corneal ulcer) tends to appear as a red, painful eye with a purulent discharge. Bacterial keratitis may be a complication of extended-wear contact lenses. Examination with a light may show a discrete corneal opacity; this is commonly associated with decreased vision, and referral to an ophthalmologist for confirmation and treatment should be considered an emergency (Fig. 15-15).

Acute glaucoma. Rapid elevation of intraocular pressure occurs when outflow of the aqueous is suddenly blocked. This tends to occur in individuals with small eyes whose iris can bunch up and block the aqueous drainage system. An attack may occur after physiologic dilation of the pupil in dim light or after using eyedrops containing sympathomimetic or parasympatholytic agents such as topical vasoconstrictors or mydriatics.

Characteristically, a patient experiencing an acute attack of angle-closure glaucoma complains of ocular pain, frontal headache, blurred vision, and halos around lights. Nausea and vomiting also may be present if the attack lasts long enough. Angle-closure glaucoma is a rare problem. Depending on the presenting symptoms, other causes that should be considered are cerebral aneurysm (headache and a fixed, dilated pupil) or even abdominal disorders, including appendicitis (nausea, vomiting, and abdominal pain).

In a patient with acute glaucoma, the eye usually is red and the pupil is middilated and oval; the cornea is cloudy, and the intraocular pressure is markedly elevated. Generally the symptoms appear in one eye only, although both eyes are predisposed to this condition. If an ophthalmologist cannot treat the patient immediately, the primary care physician should initiate treatment. This should include topical 2% pilocarpine drops every 15 minutes and 500 mg of acetazolamide orally or parenterally. Oral glycerine or isosorbide (1 g/kg body weight) served over ice and drunk slowly by the patient will help stop the acute attack. The longer the intraocular pressure remains high, the greater the risk of permanent vision loss.

In summary, many conditions produce a red eye. Conjunctivitis usually is diagnosed easily and treated by the primary care physician. However, when decreased vision, ocular pain, photophobia, circumcorneal (limbal) redness, corneal edema, corneal ulcers, dendrites and abnormal pupil, and/or elevated intraocular pressure are noted, the patient should be referred to an ophthalmologist.

More detailed evaluation and advice on managing red eye can be found in the AAO's slide script, "Managing the Red Eye." It can be obtained by writing the American Academy of Ophthalmology, 655 Beach Street, P.O. Box 7424, San Francisco CA 94120. The script also may be obtained by calling the AAO at 415-561-8540 and asking for customer service.

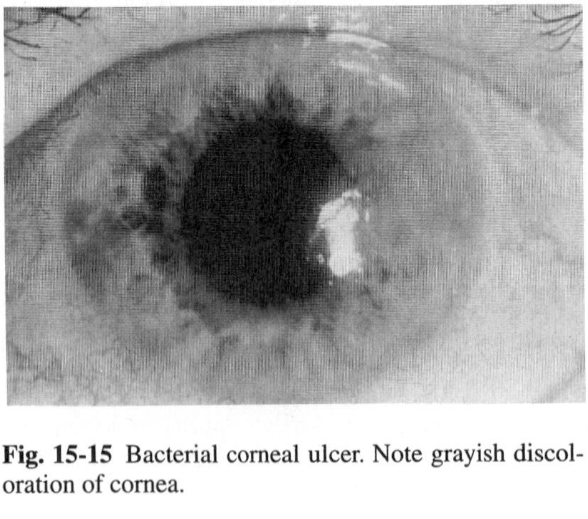

Stye

Patients commonly believe that occupational exposure to particulate matter in the air increases the risk of developing conjunctivitis, blepharitis, and styes. These conditions are not considered work-related injuries.

Stye/hordeolum. A stye is called a hordeolum when it is acute; it may look like a pimple near the skin surface adjacent to the lashes.

Stye/chalazion. The meibomian gland secretes the oily compound of the tears. Numerous meibomian glands arranged along the tarsal plate drain posteriorly to the eyelashes on the lid margin and, when obstructed, may produce a chronic swelling called a chalazion.

Treatment of a stye or chalazion is aimed at promoting drainage of the inflamed glands. Warm compresses applied for 15 to 20 minutes four times a day are highly effective for acute or subacute lesions. The compresses may have to be continued for weeks until drainage occurs. Topical sulfa or antistaphylococcal antibiotics may be of some value. Should the chalazion become chronic and nontender, drainage is best achieved by incision and curettage by an ophthalmologist. Systemic antibiotics are not indicated for this localized lid disorder unless it is accompanied by a diffuse cellulitis.

Blepharitis. Blepharitis is a chronic lid inflammation affecting the eyelashes and glands surrounding the eyelashes. The most common causes are staphylococcal infection and seborrhea. Typi-

Self-Instructional Materials in Ophthalmology. National Medical Audiovisual Center

Fig. 15-15 Bacterial corneal ulcer. Note grayish discoloration of cornea.

---

cally the patient complains of a foreign body sensation, burning, and discharge on the lashes. The eyelids tend to stick together on awakening. With chronic infection, some of the lashes may be lost.

Treatment is directed toward proper lid hygiene, using warm compresses to loosen the crusting, and mechanically cleansing the lashes with a nonirritating shampoo such as baby shampoo or one of the commercially available products designed for this purpose (such as Eye Scrub). An antibiotic ointment, such as erythromycin or bacitracin, should be applied at bedtime for 2 to 3 weeks to treat the lid margin infection. Topical antibiotic solutions such as gentamicin or 10% sulfacetamide should be added if an associated conjunctivitis is present. Oral antibiotics such as tetracycline or erythromycin are reserved for treating refractory cases.

Blepharitis is easily treated at the workplace in an occupational health clinic (although it is not considered a work-related injury). Referral to an ophthalmologist is needed only when the condition persists and does not respond to treatment for several weeks.

WARNING: *It is important to differentiate lid and anterior orbital cellulitis from styes.*

Cellulitis. Cellulitis of the eyelids manifests as a diffuse, erythematous edema. The lids often are tender to the touch, and they may be swollen shut. Visual acuity and eye movement are normal, and there is no proptosis. These cases should be treated with systemic antibiotics and warm compresses. Topical antibiotics are indicated if conjunctivitis is present. Referral to an ophthalmologist is warranted if the condition progresses or does not respond within 48 hours.

Orbital cellulitis. Cellulitis may extend posteriorly into the orbit, creating a true medical emergency. Because this development threatens vision and even the patient's life, the primary care physician should be aware of this and should be prepared to consult promptly with an ophthal-

---

---

mologist. The signs and symptoms include red, swollen lids and conjunctiva. Pain on eye movement and restriction of movement often is present; this characteristic distinguishes orbital from more anterior uveitis. The eye may protrude forward (proptosis) because of the posterior orbital inflammation. The optic nerve may be involved, which is signaled by decreased vision with an afferent pupil defect and edema of the optic disc. This condition warrants emergency ophthalmology referral.

Problems related to contact lens

Many employees wear contact lenses, and they often come initially to an occupational health clinic. Two typical contact lens problems are overwear and lens displacement.

Overwear. After wearing a contact lens for an excessive period of time, a patient will come in complaining of pain, blurred vision, and seeing halos around lights. With a hard contact lens, these symptoms generally are the result of corneal abrasion or, in more subtle cases, corneal edema secondary to hypoxia. Treatment includes removing the lens to check for a corneal infection. Cycloplegic and antibiotic drops, as well as a pressure patch, are applied.

Although the cornea epithelializes within 12 to 24 hours, the contact lens should not be worn until the cornea is well healed, which takes about 4 or 5 days. The patient should be advised to wear glasses during that period or to wear a lens on only one eye.

Soft contact lens also may produce these symptoms, but the condition usually takes much longer to develop. Some patients continuously wear their lenses for 2 to 4 weeks and then develop the symptoms of overwear described previously. For this reason, as well as to prevent corneal infections, ophthalmologists and optometrists now are recommending that more and more patients go to a daily-wear regimen and avoid wearing their lenses overnight.

Lens displacement. Lens displacement is more common with hard lenses, which can be realigned by using gentle pressure through the lids. The lens may be removed with a suction cup and then reapplied to give proper centration. The patient may continue to wear the lens if no corneal abrasion is involved.

Double vision

Head injuries in the workplace may produce associated diplopia even after seemingly minor trauma. It is important to take a careful neurologic history for a patient who complains of double vision. True diplopia, which means that two separate, equally bright images are visualized, with one of the images disappearing when one eye is closed, signifies a misalignment of the visual axes of the two eyes.

Sometimes patients state that they have double vision, when they mean they have blurred vision in one eye. This may be due to something as minor as a mucous strand in the tear film or inadequate refraction. To a careful observer who does not have adequate spectacle correction, uncorrected astigmatism typically appears as two discrete, slightly separated, blurred images. These problems typically cause *monocular* diplopia and persist when one eye is closed. It is important to note in the history whether the diplopia is transient or steady; sudden or gradual in onset; and horizontal, vertical, or diagonal.

Diplopia may be a presenting sign in neurologic disorders such as third, fourth, or sixth cranial nerve palsy. These conditions have characteristic patterns of diplopia and warrant urgent neurologic or ophthalmic referral, or both.

Because evaluating the causes of diplopia is difficult and the examination is complex, an urgent ophthalmology referral is indicated.

EYE SAFETY

Effective eye safety programs need to be emphasized in the workplace. From the smallest shop to large industrial concerns, ocular health and safety features are vitally important. This task is best undertaken by the occupational health team.

The occupational health team evaluates and preserves vision and eye health by assessing the workers' vision and the safety of various job tasks. This typically involves the services of a variety of professionals, including occupational and primary care physicians, ophthalmologists, nurses, optometrists, opticians, industrial hygienists, safety personnel, and others. Paramedics and a first aid team also may be involved.

Such a program has three basic components: (1) screening the vision of the worker; (2) determining the vision requirements and eye hazards at the job; and (3) requiring that all workers wear the appropriate protective and corrective eyewear (see Chapter 34, Personal Protective Equipment).

Vision screening

Vision screening provides the occupational health team with basic information about workers' vision that is necessary to place workers in the jobs they can perform safely and successfully. A variety of visual functions must be assessed, including visual acuity, visual fields, binocular function, oculomotor balance, and color vision. It also is important to examine for active eye disease. The visual acuity and binocular function should be screened during the preemployment physical examination and during periodical physicals thereafter. A corrected visual acuity of 20/40 or less warrants referral to an ophthalmologist or optometrist.

Screening also may be necessary when an employee returns to work after a layoff, illness, or prolonged vacation, or as part of an accident investigation. The frequency of vision screening depends partly on the particular vision requirements of the job and partly on the worker's age. Annual screening is advised for workers whose jobs demand excellent vision, such as crane and mobile equipment operators.

The screening examination should check the accuracy of distance vision, depth perception, and peripheral vision; these are essential to the safe and effective performance of most jobs. Binocular screening is most easily performed with a binocular testing instrument, which is a fast, accurate, standardized, and portable means of determining the distance and near vision of each eye separately and of both eyes together. It also tests muscle balance, screens for color vision, and measures depth perception. Using these machines, a trained technician can screen the average worker in less than 7 minutes.

Determining vision requirements and eye hazards

Two basic methods are used to determine a job's vision requirements. One method uses statistics to help define the association between successful job performance and the worker's visual skills. The second method is to observe a job on site to evaluate the visual demands involved. Both methods provide valuable information, although the observational method generally is preferred because it reflects the specific condition of the work area.

The statistical method uses the Purdue vision standards, which describe the visual skills associated with successful performance of various job tasks. For example, the Purdue vision standards indicate that a machine operator should have a distance and near acuity of 20/30 in each eye, in addition to normal depth perception and muscle balance. This means that individuals who have this level of visual acuity, depth perception, and muscle balance statistically are more likely to be productive machine operators than those who do not have these characteristics. It is important to note that the degree of the worker's vision skills is not in itself as critical as whether those skills and abilities meet the vision demands of the job. The Purdue vision standards can help make this determination and should be applied as basic guidelines, with modification as necessary, combined with information obtained by assessing the actual job site.

Because each individual is different and statistical evaluations can describe only the performance of groups, observing an actual job site provides the best information to help ensure that a particular worker's vision skills properly match the vision demands of the job. One way of using this information is to develop a general classification of jobs according to the degree of visual attention required: critical, moderate, or light. Once such a classification system is established, standards can be set for each level, with workers placed in those jobs for which they are best qualified. The best way to carry out an effective on-site observation is to perform a "vision job analysis." An in-plant vision job analysis involves the collaborative effort of an occupational health team, with the plant medical director or occupational nurse, eye consultant, safety engineer, and others all working together. A small plant may use the services of a medical eye consultant. Each job studied should be recorded by its title and code number, and a brief description should indicate the specific training or seniority required.

The following six points are important vision elements that the health team should assess at the job site:

1. The various environmental factors important to the vision performance of each job
2. The distances at which the worker must see and the size of the work area
3. The colors of the site and the degree of illumination
4. The quality of light, brightness ratios, shadows, and presence of glare (to obtain objective information about the amount of illumination present)
5. The type of visual attention required (concentrated, fixed and detailed; or casual, changing and gross)
6. The direction of gaze required (fixed or moving)

The health team then should assess eye hazards. Any conditions that might threaten the safety of workers or others in the area should be noted, such as the impact of metal on metal, dust and flying particles, acids, caustics or solvents under pressure, molten metal, and intense heat or radiation (such as ultraviolet, visible, or infrared rays). The health team should gather information about eye injuries reported earlier at each work site. Basic safety eyewear should be worn at all times, even by visitors, in areas containing hazards to the eye.

Finally, it must be stressed that responsibility for a successful program does not stop with the occupational health team. Management must provide services and ensure careful, overall planning. Day-to-day enforcement of the safety rules is imperative, and appropriate disciplinary measures must be carried out when necessary. A continuing education program is needed to enlist the active support of labor, so that workers, union leaders, and supervisors recognize the benefits of an eye care program. Too many injuries occur when, "I had just finished the job, took off my goggles, and had just one more thing to do. . . ."

Promotional activities are also important. Newsletters, posters, safety films, lectures, and rallies are effective ways to spread the word about the importance of eye safety in the workplace. Safety incentive awards, such as the Wise Owl Club, sponsored by the National Society to Prevent Blindness, can be useful in this effort.

The importance of eye safety for workers cannot be overemphasized. As many as 90% of all job-related eye injuries can be prevented by proper implementation of an effective eye care program. By providing vital services for eye health and safety in the workplace, the occupational health team can help preserve the precious gift of vision.

REFERENCES

1. Dannenberg AL, Parver LM, Brechner RJ, Khoo L: Penetrating eye injuries in the workplace: the National Eye Trauma System Registry, *Arch Ophthalmol* 110:843-848, 1992.
2. Karlson TA, Klein BE: The incidence of acute hospital-treated eye injuries, *Arch Ophthalmol* 104:1473-1476, 1986.
3. Schein OD, Hibberd PL, Shingleton BJ et al: The spectrum and burden of ocular injury, *Ophthalmology* 95:300-305, 1988.

SUGGESTED READINGS

American Academy of Ophthalmology: Eye trauma and emergencies.
American Academy of Ophthalmology: Managing the red eye.
American Academy of Ophthalmology: Ophthalmology study guide.
American Academy of Ophthalmology: The worker's eye.
Catalano RA, editor: *Ocular emergencies,* Philadelphia, 1992, WB Saunders.
Duane's *Clinical ophthalmology,* vol 5, chapter 47, 1991.
Newell F, editor: *Ophthalmology: principles and concepts,* ed 6, St Louis, 1986, Mosby.

16 Injuries to the Skin

Skin disorders are one of the most common on-the-job concerns, and they may not be reported to medical personnel if the skin condition has an insidious onset, is chronic, or is considered "part of the job." If a chronic or subacute skin disease worsens with workplace exposures or eventually leaves the employee unable to complete a job task, the person may seek medical advice. If an acute skin eruption or chemical burn occurs, the employee may be more likely to visit the medical office. Chemical burns, chemical exposure, and penetrating skin trauma are discussed in other chapters. This chapter focuses on other skin diseases that may occur or may be exacerbated in the workplace, particularly contact dermatitis, which accounts for more than 90% of cases of occupational skin disease.

ANATOMY

The microanatomy of the skin correlates with major skin functions, as outlined in Table 16-1.

The skin's major function, relevant to occupational diseases, is its role as a physical barrier to exogenous insults, either chemical (water, irritants, solvents) or physical (including ultraviolet radiation or mechanical friction).

The stratum corneum of the outer epidermis is the most important component of the physical barrier. It may be disrupted by mechanical injury (fissuring), excessive hydration and maceration, or dermatoses. Wet work leads to hydration of the stratum corneum, which enhances skin penetration of some substances that can trigger skin damage.

There are regional differences in the stratum corneum. It is thickest on the soles and palms. Thus exogenous substances penetrate less well at these sites, and substances moderately irritating to the hand may lead to inflammation more on the sides and dorsal aspects of the fingers and hands. The stratum corneum is thinnest on the eyelids and in the genital area; therefore substances inadvertently transferred from the hands (where there may be no dermatitis) may penetrate and cause an inflammatory reaction at these seemingly "unexposed" sites.

The major dermatosis associated with abnormal barrier function and skin reactivity is atopic dermatitis (atopic eczema). Individuals with atopy (crudely defined as having a personal or family history of childhood asthma, hay fever, and/or flexural eczema) may be more prone to the development of symptomatic skin inflammation with repeated contact with water, chemicals (even those listed as "safe" substances on the material data safety sheets [MSDS]), or airborne particulate material. This scenario emphasizes the importance of appropriate protective equipment for the job task.

Mechanical injury to the skin, especially frictional shearing of the surface, may acutely disrupt epidermis from dermis, leading to friction blisters. Repetitive frictional motion stimulates thickening of the stratum corneum, which clinically may lead to hyperkeratosis ("callus" formation). This rapidly thickened outer layer is a protective response, but flexion or extention of the hyperkeratotic sites (as on the palmar surface) may lead to fissures that disrupt the stratum corneum barrier and may subsequently allow penetration of irritants or become secondarily infected.

The skin is also immunologically active, and epidermal Langerhans' cells may become primed to recognize external substances (such as poison oak or poison ivy, metals such as nickel, additives in rubber gloves) and trigger an inflammatory reaction that is seen clinically as allergic contact dermatitis. The epidermis is also the site of melanocytes, which are responsible for pigment production and distribution, which are important to ultraviolet protection. Caucasian individuals, in particular, need additional sun protection if they are to be working outdoors. Melanocytes are sensitive to skin injury and inflammation, and any skin injury may cause temporary or permanent discoloration.

The dermis is the site of blood vessels, nerve endings, collagen support, and the skin appendage structures (hair follicles, sweat and oil glands). Sites with increased vasculature and innervation, such as the face, upper chest, volar forearms, and fingertips, may be more prone to redness and to symptoms of burning, itching, or stinging with physical insults such as heat, cold, or irritants. Injuries that penetrate the dermis lead to scarring because the connective tissue support and the appendages are disrupted.

Table 16-1 Skin structure and function and disease correlates

Structure	Function	Disease examples
Epidermis		
Stratum corneum	• Physical/chemical barrier	Desquamation/chapping Callus
Viable epidermal cells	• Stratum corneum synthesis • Metabolism of some topical agents • Inflammatory recruitment when perturbed	Contact dermatitis Superficial infections Hyperkeratosis
Melanocytes	• Melanin pigment production (ultraviolet protection, skin color)	Postinflammatory pigment change Chemical-induced leukoderma
Langerhans' cells	• Immune recognition • Inflammatory recruitment	Allergic contact dermatitis
Dermis		
Blood vessels	• Nutrition • Thermoregulation • Participants in inflammatory reactions	Flushing Urticaria Vibration-induced Raynaud's syndrome
Tissue mast cells	• Inflammatory mediator release	Contact urticaria
Nerves	• Tactile, itch, pain perception	Neuropathy
Connective tissue	• Mechanical support • Wound repair	Scar
Hair follicles	• Production of hair	Folliculitis
Sebaceous glands	• Sebum production	Oil acne
Eccrine sweat glands	• Thermoregulation	"Prickly heat" (miliaria)
Subcutaneous fat	• Thermoinsulation • Mechanical protection	
Hair	• Social	Alopecia
Nails	• Tactile manipulation	Paronychia Traumatic dystrophy

The subcutaneous tissue consists of fat and neurovascular bundles. The subcutaneous fat is important for thermal insulation and mechanical cushioning. Areas with minimal subcutaneous fat (nose, ears, bony prominences) are more susceptible to cold injury or to mechanical trauma to underlying structures.

KEYS TO THE MEDICAL HISTORY

The history of the dermatitis can yield important information that helps determine contributing factors (see Fig. 16-1, Evaluation of skin disease). A description of the patient's job tasks and exposures, hobbies or second job exposures, and use of topical products should be noted. The personal history, particularly of prior atopic eczema or psoriasis, also can provide clues about skin conditions that may be exacerbated by some workplace exposures. The following points are the key elements in the history when evaluating work-related dermatitis:

• *Is the dermatitis in a site that would relate to workplace exposures? What are the exposures?*

Hands are the site of most occupational dermatitis. Forearm, upper chest, and facial sites may also be involved, particularly with airborne exposures. With some exposures or dermatitis, covered or distant sites can become involved, which may lead the clinician away from the likelihood of a work-related origin. It is important to determine where on the skin the lesions first developed.

• *Are there exposures to potential irritants or allergens in the workplace* (see Fig. 16-2, Potential cutaneous irritants or allergens in the workplace).

The MSDS may not give clues; "safe" substances, such as water, can be very irritating to the skin with *frequent, repetitive,* or *cumulative* exposure or if the patient has a skin injury (even "trivial" ones such as paper cuts or abrasions).

Allergens need be present in only small amounts to trigger dermatitis when in contact with the skin of a susceptible individual. MSDS lists only ingredients present in more than 1% of the final product, and it may not list, for example, the

EVALUATION OF SKIN DISEASE

Keys to the medical history

- Date of onset
- Body site at onset
- Patient's description of symptoms and signs
- Subsequent spread to other sites
- Effect of weekend, vacation, layoff, work procedure, treatment
- Job title and description of tasks
- Type and frequency of exposures
- Hand washing, protective equipment method and frequency
- Other workers affected
- Personal history
  Contact dermatitis
  Other skin disease
  Hobbies, other jobs
  Topical products used

Keys to the clinical examination

- Lesion type (eczematous, redness, vesicles, scale, crusts?)
- Distribution (consistent with exposures?)
- Signs of other skin disease
  Psoriasis
  Atopic dermatitis
  Dermatophyte infection

Fig. 16-1

biocides (preservatives) that may cause allergic contact dermatitis.

Ambient environment (hot, dusty, low humidity) can contribute to dermatitis, and personal protective equipment such as rubber gloves, face masks, or steel-toed work boots also may cause skin problems.

- *Is there a temporal relationship between workplace exposures and the onset of dermatitis?*

This point can be tricky because of the variables of cumulative effect, repetitive or frequent exposures, minor skin injuries, and ambient environment mentioned previously. *There does not have to be anything new or different in the workplace* for a dermatitis to occur in a long-term employee. Strong irritants may cause symptoms and dermatitis within minutes to hours of initial exposure. In these cases, multiple exposed employees may have skin involvement. Weak irritants may take weeks to years of exposure to cause dermatitis. Because contact allergy is an immunologic reaction that requires sensitization and this sensitization can occur at any time after exposures, there is no predictable time course between exposure and the onset of dermatitis.

POTENTIAL CUTANEOUS IRRITANTS OR ALLERGENS IN THE WORKPLACE

Irritants

Water (frequent or repetitive exposure)
Soaps and detergents
Petroleum distillates
Organic solvents
Acids/alcohols/alkalis
Cutting fluids
Plant/animal products
Mechanical friction/repetitive motion

Allergens

Acrylates
Biocides
Epoxy resin
Formaldehyde
Rubber additives
Poison ivy/oak
Nickel, cobalt, chromate
Neomycin

Fig. 16-2

- *Was there a skin injury requiring medical treatment?*

As mentioned previously, injuries to the skin can disrupt the barrier function and lead to increased penetration of irritants and allergens that may cause dermatitis, even if there was no problem with exposure to intact skin. Even when the injury is visibly healed, the barrier function of the skin may be weak. First-aid treatment of skin injuries may also be a source of contact dermatitis. For example, the benzocaine in soothing sprays, the neomycin in topical antibiotics or drops, the thimerosal used as a preservative in eye drops, or the adhesive in bandage material may cause dermatitis at the injury site.

- *Did the dermatitis improve with removal of the employee from the job site?*

Generally, contact dermatitis slowly improves if the triggering exposures are avoided and the damaged skin is protected from further insults. A weekend or week away from work may not be an adequate interval to see significant improvement, and sometimes improvement may occur over months, particularly at sites where subsequent irritant exposures are difficult to avoid, such as the hands.

If an employee is moved from one job task to another because of dermatitis, it is important to determine differences in the exposures between the work stations. If the employee continues to have dermatitis, what is the same: direct exposures, airborne exposures, hand soap, protective gear?

• *What are the exposures to the involved skin sites at home, with hobbies, or at a second job?*

Skin injuries and irritation also may occur away from the job site and may set the stage for or worsen job-triggered dermatitis. On the other hand, an employee may be convinced that a dermatitis is work related because the eruption occurs on a workday, when the history points to the cause being, say, poison ivy resulting from yard work several days earlier.

• *Does the patient have a history of atopic dermatitis ("eczema") or psoriasis?*

Such a history does not necessarily solve the question of "preexisting." Patients with skin disease may be considered as having work-related exacerbation if there are cutaneous irritant or allergic exposures and the dermatosis becomes significantly worse at an exposed site or develops at new sites compatible with workplace exposure.

CASE STUDIES
Case 1

A patient with scalp and elbow psoriasis who develops palmar involvement several months after beginning work packing boxes for a moving company may be considered to have a work-exacerbation of psoriasis stemming from the mechanical irritation of the skin on the hands.

Case 2

An employee with a history of atopic eczema and mild hand dermatitis controlled with over-the-counter corticosteroids begins work as a hair dresser. Exposures include water, hair, shampoo, permanent wave, and coloring products. The hand dermatitis gradually worsens to the point that the employee must miss work and needs potent prescription topical or oral corticosteroids to control the dermatitis. This condition also may be considered work related, because the contact dermatitis exacerbates the atopic dermatitis.

DIAGNOSTIC AND LABORATORY STUDIES

Contact dermatitis is primarily a clinical diagnosis based on eczematous appearance and distribution related to exogenous exposures. Irritant contact dermatitis (the most common occupational type) which involves nonimmunologic direct skin damage is entirely a clinical diagnosis; there is no confirmatory test.

Patch tests

The probable causative agent for *allergic* contact dermatitis may be identified through epicutaneous

patch tests. Patch tests are a diagnostic method that can reproduce an immunologic (allergic) reaction on the patient's skin. Only standardized substances should be used to avoid false-positive or irritant reactions. Commercially available test substances for important industrial allergens (metals, rubber, adhesives, acrylates, biocides, fragrance) are helpful in screening patients for a possible allergic component to their dermatitis. The suggested readings at the end of this chapter include useful resources dealing with the patch test method and occupational allergic contact dermatitis.

The diagnostic patch test technique requires physicians to have experience in patient selection, application, reading, and interpretation, as well as in the determination of relevance to the clinical situation and exposures. It generally is in the patient's best interest to have this evaluation done by a dermatologist or other physician experienced in the technique.

Biopsy

Skin biopsy generally is nonspecific for eczematous dermatoses, and it is not recommended as a primary diagnostic technique.

Microbiologic examination and cultures

For any vesicular or crusting lesion, secondary bacterial infection (especially with *Staphylococcus aureus* or a group A beta-hemolytic streptococcus) should be considered and can be confirmed by bacterial culture. With a scaling, thickened plaque, dermatophyte fungal infection should be ruled out by potassium hydroxide (KOH) testing of a skin scraping or by a fungus culture.

DIAGNOSIS AND MANAGEMENT OF CONTACT DERMATITIS
Differential diagnosis

Primary and secondary bacterial infections, such as impetigo, can have an eczematous appearance. Atopic dermatitis with secondary infection is common, and superimposed irritant contact dermatitis must be considered in this setting. For the dry, lichenified, and scaly skin of chronic contact dermatitis, the clinical appearance is nonspecific; psoriasis, dermatophyte fungus, neurodermatitis (lichen simplex chronicus), and noneczematous dermatoses should be ruled out. Occasionally contact dermatitis has an appearance that mimics primary dermatoses such as lichen planus or purpura.

Treatment
Acute contact dermatitis

1. *Exposures and other irritants* must be removed (both on the job and at home).

2. *Astringent dressings* with tap water compresses or Burow's solution should be used for 20 minutes twice daily.

3. *Topical corticosteroid ointments* may be applied once or twice daily. Mid- to high-potency strengths may be used for short periods.

4. If acute dermatitis is severe, *systemic corticosteroids* may be used; for example, prednisone, approximately 0.5 to 1 mg/kg/day in a single morning dose for 2 to 3 weeks, with optional tapering (shorter "dosage packs" may lead to rapid rebound of the dermatitis).

5. *Bacterial superinfection* is treated with oral antibiotics to cover *S. aureus* and group A beta-hemolytic streptococci.

6. No additional topical products should be used.

7. Follow-up should be done on the patient within 1 to 2 weeks, and possible triggering exposures should be reviewed before the patient is returned to the work site. Protective measures and further evaluation, such as referral to a dermatologist for consultation and patch testing, should be considered.

Chronic contact dermatitis

1. The dry, thickened skin of chronic dermatitis often responds to *hydration and lubrication.* Application of a bland emollient, such as white petrolatum or a corticosteroid ointment, is most helpful after the affected skin has been soaked in water.

2. Secondary fissuring may improve with lubrication and a reduction in mechanical forces. Oral antibiotic treatment may also aid healing.

Prevention

1. Barrier creams usually are of no benefit once dermatitis has developed.

2. Careful selection of protective equipment may be helpful. Rubber allergy should be ruled out as the cause of the dermatitis before rubber gloves are recommended. Before equipment can be chosen to protect the patient from the triggering exposures, those exposures must be accurately identified.

3. Workers and management must be educated about potential irritants and allergens in the workplace. The clinician should be alert to clusters of dermatitis complaints, which may indicate irritant contact exposures.

CASE STUDIES
Case 1

A 28-year-old man had a traumatic injury to his left middle finger on the job. The injury required surgical repair, and the wound healed well, but a persistent, vesicular, pruritic eruption developed at the site. Therapy was changed from a neomycin-bacitracin-polymyxin triple antibiotic to bacitracin ointment. The problem persisted. Treatment with an oral antibiotic did not help. Patch tests confirmed a contact allergy to neomycin and bacitracin. Avoiding these agents and use of a topical corticosteroid ointment led to resolution.

Diagnosis: *Post-traumatic allergic contact dermatitis.*

Comment: *Approximately 3% to 5% of exposed individuals may become allergic to neomycin. Patients allergic to neomycin can co-react to bacitracin. The work-related injury was the precipitating event.*

Case 2

A 43-year-old operating room nurse complained of progressive worsening of "chapped hands." She had always noted some dryness and itching in winter months, but now the itching had increased to the point of interfering with sleep. She had changed to "hypoallergenic," powder-free rubber gloves without improvement. She did not describe hives or itching that increased with glove use.

Initial impression: *Irritant contact dermatitis caused by frequent hand washing and surgical scrubs. Contact allergy to gloves, detergent, and lotion ingredients must be ruled out.*

Workup: *Midpotency topical corticosteroid ointment helped, as did 1 week away from work. Patch tests showed a contact allergy to thiuram mix, rubber accelerators found in the gloves the nurse had been wearing.*

Diagnosis: *Occupational irritant contact dermatitis and allergic contact dermatitis to rubber ingredient, relevant to glove use in the workplace.*

Comment: *Appropriate glove selection improved (but did not cure) the condition and allowed the nurse to return to work with "baseline" episodes of irritant dermatitis. "Mixed" pictures of an irritant combined with allergic contact dermatitis are common. Product substitution can be misleading, because there is no consensus on the definition of "hypoallergic."*

Case 3

A 24-year-old hairdresser complained of hand eczema that began within the first month of full-time employment. When she was in cosmetology school and subsequently working part-time, she did not have much of a problem with her hands. History showed childhood asthma, which she outgrew, but no eczema. A weekend off work made no difference, but a 5-day vacation helped.

Initial impression: *Irritant contact dermatitis to water, friction (hair handling), and cosmetic ingredients. The patient has a history of atopy but no dermatitis prior to a threshold quantity of workplace irritant exposures.*

Workup: *Because of exposures to potential allergens, patch tests were done; the results were negative.*

Diagnosis: *See previous case.*

Comment: *The nature, frequency, and duration of irritant exposures can be important factors. For this patient, reducing such exposures by rotating job responsibilities away from irritants or using protective gloves for some exposures may help. Hairdressers and others with "wet work" exposures are prone to work-related irritant contact dermatitis. It is important to rule out an allergic component.*

Case 4

A 38-year-old machinist had a 4-month history of hand dermatitis that started as itchy water blisters and became painful, thick, cracked skin on both palms. No other sites were involved. Nothing changed at work, and he was in the same department for 15 years. He had "no time" for hobbies.

Initial impression: Irritant contact dermatitis—exposures include mechanical injury to skin caused by repetitive motion, machinery coolants, metal parts, and waterless hand cleaner. Because of the change, and particularly the history of vesicles at onset, allergic contact dermatitis should be ruled out.

Workup: Patch tests were done and showed a positive reaction to benzocaine and to methylchloroisothiazolinone/methylisothiazolinone. The latter is a biocide found in the water-based oil used at work.

Diagnosis: Irritant and allergic contact dermatitis. The diagnosis of irritant dermatitis is based on exposure history, and allergic contact dermatitis was confirmed by patch tests. Change to another type of coolant led to slow improvement. In this setting, with ongoing irritation, the improvement may be in terms of months, and intermittent flares are possible despite strict allergen avoidance. Because there was no history of the patient using a benzocaine-containing product, the positive result on the patch test for benzocaine was determined not to be relevant to the patient's current dermatitis. Patient education is important to teach the patient about other potential sources of his allergens, to help avoid future outbreaks.

Case 5

A 53-year-old car salesman had a 4-week history of severe itching and vesicular dermatitis involving his face, neck, and arms below his shirtsleeves. He had the worst outbreak each Monday morning when he came to work. He was not using any aftershave or skin lotions, did not work outside or in the bodyshop/maintenance area, and did not take any medicines.

Initial impression: Because of the distribution and appearance, airborne or photo-contact dermatitis must be ruled out. Further history showed that each weekend he had been remodeling and painting his home.

Workup: Patch tests were done to rule out an allergic contact dermatitis. There was a positive patch test to epoxy resin, relevant to the epoxy-based paint and two-part adhesive used in the remodeling work. Epoxy resin was used in the body shop area, but the patient did not work in that building, which reduced the likelihood of airborne exposure to epoxy in the workplace.

Diagnosis: Airborne allergic contact dermatitis to epoxy, not work related.

OTHER OCCUPATIONAL SKIN DISEASES

Contact dermatitis far outweighs other dermatoses in terms of occupational occurrence. However, a few other skin diseases may be associated with workplace exposures.

Acne

Acne may develop or worsen, particularly in hot, oily environments. Skin contact with aerosols of tars, oils, or petroleum distillates may aggravate acne, and mechanical factors such as friction from face masks or clothing may contribute to localization of acne lesions.

Sun exposure and skin cancer

Outdoor occupations put workers at risk for acute effects (sunburn) and chronic cumulative effects of ultraviolet exposure. The chronic effects include photoaging (thickened, wrinkled skin, and actinic keratoses) and the potential for developing nonmelanoma skin cancers, especially basal cell and squamous cell carcinomas. Protective clothing (hat, long sleeves) and daily use of sunscreen can reduce these sun effects. All workers with outdoor exposure should be educated about this protection.

Paronychia

Acute, tender swelling of the nail fold areas may occur with minor trauma to the skin. Treatment with antistaphylococcal antibiotics and incision and drainage are helpful. Chronic, less symptomatic paronychia is more likely to be seen in employees with frequent water exposure and is often due to *Candida* organisms. Treatment with topical antifungal lotion and protection of the skin to promote dryness can be helpful.

Calluses

Thickened skin at sites of mechanical friction is well known as an adaptive protection measure of skin. Some individuals may develop calluses that are "too thick" and that may crack and limit motion. Reviewing the ergonomics of the job task

---

DIAGNOSTIC PEARLS

1. Suspect irritant and/or allergic contact dermatitis as factors in any worker with hand dermatitis or other eczematous dermatoses.

2. Detail exposures. Do not rely too heavily on material safety data sheets (MSDS).

3. Slow or minimal improvement away from work does not exclude the job as a potential source.

4. There does not have to be something "new" in the workplace for contact dermatitis to occur.

5. Clinical history alone is not reliable for establishing the cause of *allergic* contact dermatitis. Referral for patch test evaluation is indicated.

6. Be cautious about predicting rapid recovery or advising a job change.

may be helpful. Judgement should be used in trimming or reducing callus.

Contact urticaria

Immediate, hivelike reactions at the site of skin contact with substances such as latex or animal proteins (as in fish and meat handlers) have been reported. It is important to recognize and document these cases because some types of contact urticaria may be associated with respiratory symptoms and anaphylaxis.

SUGGESTED READINGS
General

Adams RM, editor: *Occupational skin disease,* ed 2, Philadelphia, 1990, WB Saunders.

Fisher AA, editor: *Contact dermatitis,* ed 3, Philadelphia, 1986, Lea & Febiger.

Rycroft RJG et al, editors: *Textbook of contact dermatitis,* New York, 1992, Springer-Verlag.

Patch test method

Adams RM: Panels of allergens for specific occupations, *J Am Acad Dermatol* 21:869-874, 1989.

Marks JG Jr, DeLeo VA: *Contact and occupational dermatology,* St Louis, 1992, Mosby.

Occupational causation and impairment

Doege TC, editor: American Medical Association: *Guides to the evaluation of permanent impairment,* ed 4, Chicago 1993, AMA.

Mathias CGT: Contact dermatitis and worker's compensation: criteria for establishing occupational causation and aggravation, *J Am Acad Dermatol* 20:842-848, 1989.

Prognosis and outcome

Birmingham DJ: Prolonged and recurrent occupational dermatitis: some whys and wherefores. In Adams RM, editor: *Occ Med State Art Rev* 1:349-356, 1986.

Hogan DF, Dannaker CJ, Maibach HI: The prognosis of contact dermatitis, *J Am Acad Dermatol* 23:300-307, 1990.

Pryce DW et al: Soluble oil dermatitis: a follow-up study, *Contact Dermatitis* 21:28-35, 1989.

17 Burns

Through the centuries, humans have faced the devastating effects of burn injuries. Although the exact figure is not known, it is estimated that in the United States, more than 500,000 burn patients are seen annually in the emergency room, and burn patients account for approximately 100,000 hospital admissions each year.[1] Approximately 12,000 patients die as a result of their injury. Half of all major burns occur in patients under 20 years of age, and 30% occur in children under the age of 1 year.[2] Over the years the progress in burn treatment has paralleled the advances in acute trauma care, pioneering in particular shock resuscitation, nutritional support, wound management, and infection control. The complexity and diversity of the physiologic changes that occur over a prolonged period with a burn injury require an organized team approach. The final success or failure of treatment of a burn patient is measured not only by the patient's survival but also by his functional and social rehabilitation.

ANATOMY

The skin is a highly specialized structure composed essentially of two layers: the epidermis (outer layer) and the dermis (inner layer) (Fig. 17-1).

The skin varies in thickness from 0.5 to 6 mm. The epidermis contains (1) an outer layer, the stratum corneum, which is composed of nonviable, keratinized cells that have a protective function, and (2) an inner layer of nucleated cells, the stratum germinativum (basal layer), which contains melanocyte- and keratin-producing cells. Melanocytes, which are derived from neural crest cells, provide melanin, which absorbs and scatters ultraviolet radiation. Between the stratum corneum and the stratum germinativam are the stratum spinosum and stratum granulosum, which essentially consist of keratinocytes in various stages of differentiation. The impermeable stratum corneum acts as a barrier, preventing fluid loss and penetration of bacteria and foreign bodies.

The dermis, which is 20 to 30 times thicker than the epidermis, contains a supportive matrix composed of collagen and elastin in which vascular, lymphatic, and nervous structures are located. Epidermal appendages such as hair follicles and sweat glands are also present in close contact with the stratum germinativum. If this layer is destroyed by a burn, the skin's capacity to regenerate (reepithelialization) is lost, and a skin graft may well be necessary.

The skin also has antibacterial properties, specifically in the sebum, that destroy bacteria such as *Staphylococcus* and *Streptococcus* organisms. Sebum also helps lubricate the skin's surface. Regulation of body temperature is another important function of the skin. Adipose tissue is a good insulator and does not conduct heat.

PATHOPHYSIOLOGY

Despite continuing, intense research, the immediate changes in tissues after a thermal insult are still poorly understood. The skin, the largest organ in the body, has three main functions: (1) to prevent water loss by maintaining a constant temperature, (2) to act as a barrier against microbial invasion, and (3) to house nerve endings. The devastating effects of a burn injury are the result of changes in or loss of these functions.

The human body can tolerate temperatures up to 40° C; at higher temperatures protein denaturation occurs and exceeds the capacity of cellular repair. Jackson and Mac described the three classic zones of injury: (1) a central zone of coagulation with irreversible cell death, (2) a zone of stasis where cell survival is questionable, and (3) the periphery, consisting of a zone of hyperemia where the tissue usually is viable and the damage reversible (cells in this zone usually recover in 7 to 10 days).[6]

After a burn, there is a transient phase of vasoconstriction followed by opening of precapillary sphincters, which results in increased transcapillary filtration, vasodilation, and edema formation, which reaches its maximum at 18 to 24 hours after injury. It probably is caused by the severe hypoproteinic state of the burned patient.

Human skin is damaged by an immediate heat injury and by a delayed injury that occurs secondary to progressive dermal ischemia.[7] The damage is mediated by the release of many potent vasoactive and inflammatory mediators, including prostaglandins, kinins, oxygen radicals, serotonin, histamines, and complement. The activities of

255

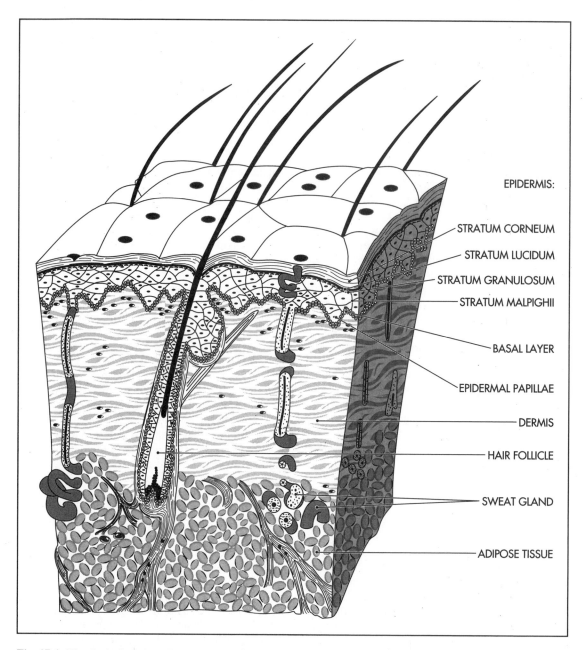

Fig. 17-1 Histological section of the skin.

these products are complex and still poorly understood.

Many other physiologic changes also occur. With major burns, a 10% reduction in red cell mass occurs in the first 24 hours after injury, along with production and release of a circulating factor that causes transient depression of myocardial activity and shuts down production of bone marrow. The degree of change in the normal functioning of all the physiologic systems is directly proportional to the severity of the burn injury, which makes a serious burn such a potentially devastating illness.

ETIOLOGY

It is important to determine the causative agent in the burn injury, because in most cases this determines the depth and extent of the burn. Most superficial burns are caused by scalding liquids and steam, whereas a flame injury will most likely cause a full-thickness burn. A flash explosion, electricity, or chemicals can cause significant burns, and each may need a different approach.

It also is important to ascertain the specific circumstances of the injury by carefully questioning the patient or co-workers, supervisors, firefighters, or police officers. A flame injury sustained in a closed place may be accompanied by respiratory problems.

EXTENT OF BURN

Evaluating the extent of the body surface involved and the depth of the burn are necessary to determine the proper treatment. A rough estimate of the extent of the burn in an adult can be made by using the "rule of nine." With this system, the body is divided into 11 units that are multiples of nine (Fig. 17-2). The head and neck together equal 9%; each upper extremity, 9%; the anterior trunk, 18%; the posterior trunk, 18%; each lower extremity, 18%; and the perineum and genitalia, 1%. By determining the portion of each unit involved, the burn area can be quickly estimated.

With smaller burns, the "rule of palms" also can be applied, which assumes that the palm of the patient's hand is equivalent to 1% of the total body surface area. In children, the hand represents a larger proportion of the total body surface area, and a different and more accurate method is needed. The Lund and Browder chart (Fig. 17-3) is recommended for estimating the extent of burns in children.

DEPTH OF BURN

The patient's age determines the natural thickness of the skin and also the amount of stress the person can withstand.[2] Along with the extent of the burn and the patient's age, the depth of the burn is a primary determinant of mortality with thermal injury (Table 17-1).

The depth of the burn is difficult to estimate correctly with current methods of evaluation. Furthermore, the fact that the depth is not uniform throughout and may be progressive with time complicates the picture. Evaluation by an experienced surgeon has an accuracy rate of about 50%:[5] tossing a coin is about as useful a technique. Knowledge of the cause is helpful; scald burns are more superficial than flame burns, and chemical and electrical burns tend to be deeper than they first appear. Burns are classified and recorded as first, second, or third degree (Fig. 17-4).

First-degree burns

Sunburns and scald burns are examples of first-degree burns. Histologically, the injury is limited to epidermal layers, with local erythema and pain being the classic symptoms. Healing usually occurs in 1 week without scarring. Symptomatic relief can be accomplished with moisturizing lotion, even though no specific therapy is necessary. The use of topical antimicrobial agents is controversial. They probably are unnecessary if the burn is indeed minor and does not include areas of deep partial-thickness injury. First-degree burns are not included when calculating the total body surface area burned to estimate fluid requirements.

Second-degree burns

The designation second-degree (or partial-thickness) burn implies destruction of the epidermal layer and the dermis, but sparing of the *deep* epidermal structures (hair follicles and sweat glands). The wound generally appears moist and pink, with blisters and bullae (Fig. 17-5). Whitish areas, paleness, and absence of blanching on pressure indicate a deeper burn.

An important concept is that partial-thickness injury may progress in depth over time because of ischemia or infection. Hydrating and protecting the wound may protect the tissue and prevent conversion to a full-thickness injury. Healing of a second-degree burn may result in wound contractures or hypertrophic scarring, with both cosmetic and functional impairment. Healing generally occurs in 2 to 3 weeks.

Third-degree burns

Third-degree (or full-thickness) burns are histologically characterized by destruction of the epidermis and the deep dermis. These wounds have a firm, leathery texture and a degree of charring on the surface. Etiologic factors usually include electrical, scalding, flames, or chemical causes. Thrombosed vessels can be seen, and unless the wound is small (less than 2 cm), a full-thickness burn invariably requires grafting. Pressure sensation may be present in full-thickness burns because these receptors are beneath the dermis, and pin-prick sensation may be absent in partial-thickness burns. Therefore, sensation is not as helpful for differentiating burn depth as was once believed (Fig. 17-6).

INHALATION INJURY

Pulmonary complications are the most common cause of death in patients with major burns, and they are the single most important factor that affects survival. Particular attention to the airway should always be paramount in a patient injured by flames in a closed space. Inhalation injury can be categorized into three stages: (1) acute pulmonary insufficiency, (2) pulmonary edema, and (3) bronchopneumonia.

The term "inhalation injury" refers to damage to the respiratory tract. Typically, suggestive symptoms are hoarseness, stridor, wheezing, coughing, and carbonaceous sputum. Because the airway dissipates inhaled heated air, inhalation injury is more

AREA	(AGE-YEARS)					% 2nd DEGREE	% 3rd DEGREE	% TOTAL
	0-1	1-4	5-9	10-15	ADULT			
HEAD	19	17	13	10	7			
NECK	2	2	2	2	2			
ANT. TRUNK	13	17	13	13	13			
POST. TRUNK	13	13	13	13	13			
R. BUTTOCK	2½	2½	2½	2½	2½			
L. BUTTOCK	2¾	2½	2½	2½	2½			
GENITALIA	1	1	1	1	1			
R. U. ARM	4	4	4	4	4			
L. U. ARM	4	4	4	4	4			
R. L. ARM	3	3	3	3	3			
L. L. ARM	3	3	3	3	3			
R. HAND	2½	2½	2½	2½	2½			
L. HAND	2½	2½	2½	2½	2½			
R. THIGH	5½	6½	8½	8½	9½			
L. THIGH	5½	6½	8½	8½	9½			
R. LEG	5	5	5½	6	7			
L. LEG	5	5	5½	6	7			
R. FOOT	3½	3½	3½	3½	3½			
L. FOOT	3½	3½	3½	3½	3½			
				TOTAL				

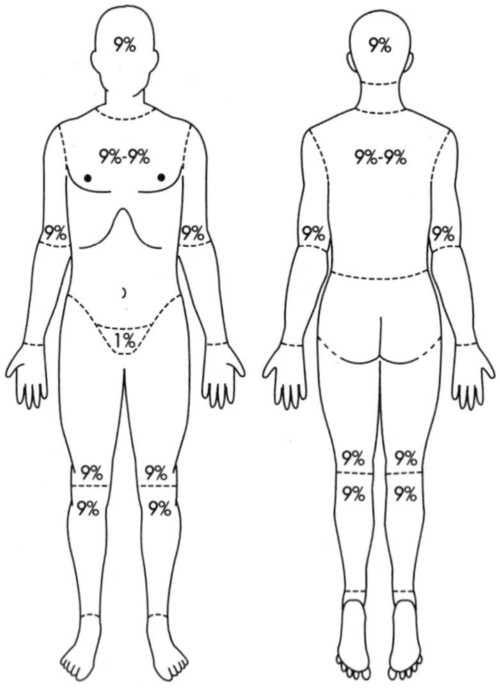

Fig. 17-2 Lund and Browder chart *(top);* rule of nines *(bottom).*

AREA	(AGE-YEARS)					% 2nd DEGREE	% 3rd DEGREE	% TOTAL
	0-1	1-4	5-9	10-15	ADULT			
HEAD	19	17	13	10	7			
NECK	2	2	2	2	2			
ANT. TRUNK	13	13	13	13	13			
POST. TRUNK	13	13	13	13	13			
R. BUTTOCK	2½	2½	2½	2½	2½			
L. BUTTOCK	2½	2½	2½	2½	2½			
GENITALIA	1	1	1	1	1			
R. U. ARM	4	4	4	4	4			
L. U. ARM	4	4	4	4	4			
R. L. ARM	3	3	3	3	3			
L. L. ARM	3	3	3	3	3			
R. HAND	2½	2½	2½	2½	2½			
L. HAND	2½	2½	2½	2½	2½			
R. THIGH	5½	6½	8½	8½	9½			
L. THIGH	5½	6½	8½	8½	9½			
R. LEG	5	5	5½	6	7			
L. LEG	5	5	5½	6	7			
R. FOOT	3½	3½	3½	3½	3½			
L. FOOT	3½	3½	3½	3½	3½			

BURN EVALUATION TOTAL

SEVERITY OF BURN

1st DEGREE =

2nd DEGREE =

3rd DEGREE =

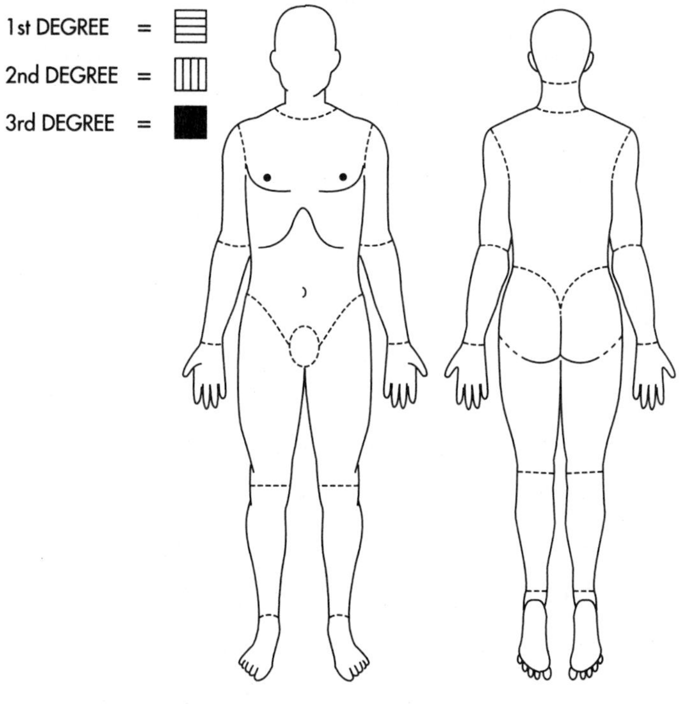

Fig. 17-3 Lund and Browder chart.

Table 17-1 Characteristics of burn depth

Degree	Depth	Pain	Characteristics
First	Epidermal layers only	Painful	Red, dry skin. May peel later
Second (Partial thickness)	Superficial to deep. Extends from epidermis to superficial to deep dermis	Moderate to very painful	Moist skin, intact or ruptured vesicles; skin color mottled white to pink or red
Third (Full thickness)	Down to and including subcutaneous tissue or fascia	Minimal pain	Skin is pearly white to dark or charred; loss of all epidermal appendages

a chemical injury produced by components of smoke than an injury caused directly by heat. Toxic material such as ammonia or sulfur dioxide are released in gases during fire. Some of these materials react with mucous membranes to form strong acid and alkali. Other, lipid-soluble material can cause direct tissue damage, including decreased ciliary function, thereby impeding the clearance of bacteria. Symptoms may be delayed 24 to 48 hours as the edema and inflammation progress, with the potential for late airway obstruction.

Many of the clinical signs suggestive of inhalation injury (facial burns, singed nasal vibrissa, carbonaceous sputum, hoarseness) are inaccurate, having a high incidence of false positives. Seventy percent of patients with inhalation injury have facial burns, but 70% of patients with facial burns do not have inhalation injury. The initial chest x-ray film usually is normal. Direct laryngoscopy may show inflamed, edematous vocal cords, but fiberoptic bronchoscopy remains the most accurate method for evaluating inhalation injury. Pulmonary injury also may be assessed by a xenon ventilation-perfusion scan.

Treatment of suspected inhalation injury should begin in the field, and oxygen must be given even if the patient is asymptomatic. Arterial blood gas values and the carboxyhemoglobin level should be determined while the patient is in the emergency room; if there is any sign of airway obstruction, an endotracheal tube should be placed. Bronchodilator therapy should be used to prevent bronchospasm. Prophylactic use of antibiotics or corticosteroids does not offer any benefit.[4] It is important to remember that the resuscitative fluid requirement is greatly increased in cases of inhalation injury.

Carbon monoxide intoxication should always be considered in patients who are involved in a fire-related accident. This gas is colorless and odorless and has an affinity with hemoglobin 200 times greater than oxygen. The diagnosis is made by measuring the carboxyhemoglobin concentration

in the blood. Symptoms of intoxication include headache, nausea, and weakness. If intoxication is more severe, neurologic signs and coma may occur. Treatment consists of administering 100% inspired oxygen and, in severe cases, intubation. Hyperbaric oxygen therapy should be considered in these cases, if available. (See Chapter 18 for further discussion of respiratory injuries.)

EVALUATION IN THE FIELD

Treatment of a severe burn begins at the scene of the accident, where the patient's clothing must be removed. The patient must be placed supine under a clean, dry sheet to minimize contamination. A clean cloth soaked in tepid water should be used to cool the injury. Placing ice or home remedies, such as ointment or butter, over the burned areas should be discouraged. Immediate attention to the airway, breathing, and circulation (ABCs of resuscitation) is essential. Ventilation should be established, and if the patient is unconscious, an oral airway or an endotracheal tube should be placed. If a transport time longer than 30 minutes is anticipated, a large-bore intravenous line should be started and Ringer's lactate solution administered.

Frequent evaluations are mandatory, and cardiac monitoring is advisable, especially in cases involving electrical injury or underlying cardiac problems. Concomitant traumatic injury, such as a cervical spine injury, should be addressed, and if carbon monoxide injury is suspected, the patient should be given oxygen. With chemical burns, copious irrigation with water often minimizes the extent of injury.

FLUID REQUIREMENTS

Patients with partial- or full-thickness burns that involve more than 20% of the total body surface area (TBSA) require fluid replacement (Table 17-2). Children may require fluid replacement with smaller burns because of inadequate oral intake.

The fluid resuscitation is calculated from the actual time of injury, not from the time the patient

BURN FORM

NAME__________________________

AGE_____ NUMBER____________________

BURN RECORD. AGES 7 TO ADULT.

DATE OF OBSERVATION______________

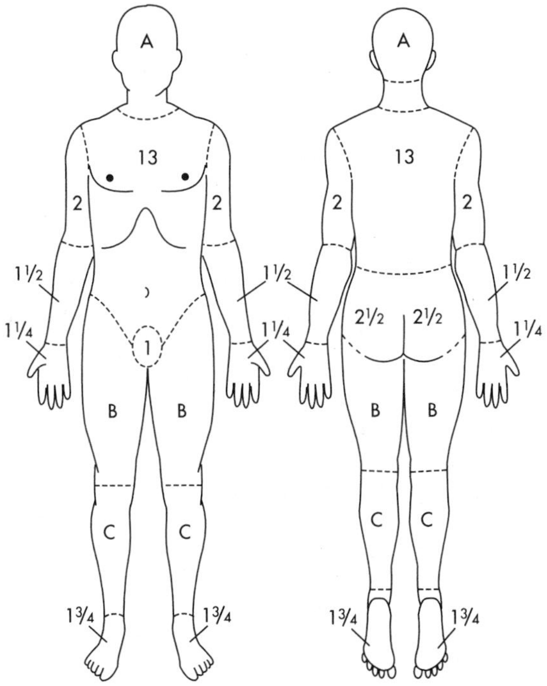

1st DEGREE

2nd DEGREE

3rd DEGREE

RELATIVE PERCENTAGES OF AREA AFFECTED BY GROWTH

AREA	AGE 10	15	ADULT
A ½ OF HEAD	5½	4½	3½
B ½ OF ONE THIGH	4¼	4½	4¾
C ½ OF ONE LEG	3	3¼	3½

% BURN BY AREAS

PROBABLE 3RD° BURN: HEAD___ NECK___ BODY___ UP ARM___ FOREARM___ HANDS___ GENITALS___ BUTTOCKS___ THIGHS___ LEGS___ FEET___

TOTAL BURN: HEAD___ NECK___ BODY___ UP ARM___ FOREARM___ HANDS___ GENITALS___ BUTTOCKS___ THIGHS___ LEGS___ FEET___

BURN FORM

NAME__________________________

AGE_____ NUMBER____________________

BURN RECORD. AGES BIRTH 7½

DATE OF OBSERVATION______________

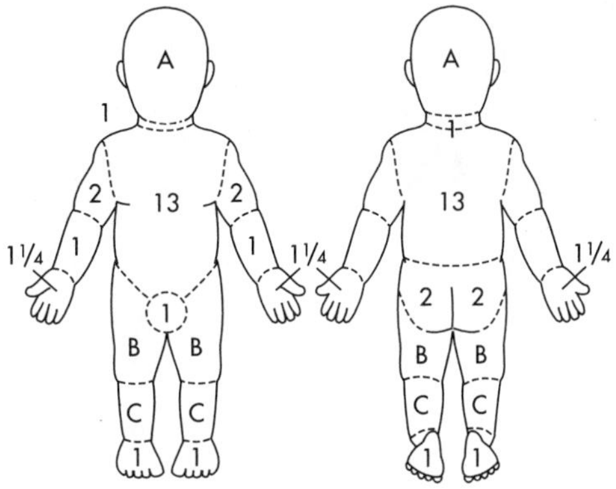

1st DEGREE

2nd DEGREE

3rd DEGREE

RELATIVE PERCENTAGES OF AREA AFFECTED BY GROWTH

AREA	AGE 0	1	5
A ½ OF HEAD	9½	8½	6½
B ½ OF ONE THIGH	2¾	3¼	4
C ½ OF ONE LEG	2½	2½	2¾

% BURN BY AREAS

PROBABLE 3RD° BURN: HEAD___ NECK___ BODY___ UP ARM___ FOREARM___ HANDS___ GENITALS___ BUTTOCKS___ THIGHS___ LEGS___ FEET___

TOTAL BURN: HEAD___ NECK___ BODY___ UP ARM___ FOREARM___ HANDS___ GENITALS___ BUTTOCKS___ THIGHS___ LEGS___ FEET___

SUM OF ALL AREAS_____ PROBABLY 3RD°_____ TOTAL BURN_____

Fig. 17-4 A sample form for recording burn location and severity.

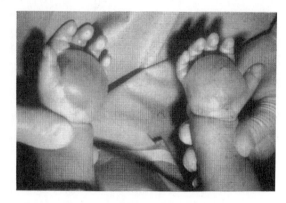

Fig. 17-5 An example of second degree burns.

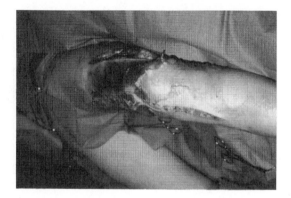

Fig. 17-6 An example of third degree burns.

gets to the hospital. Most methods are based on the patient's body weight and the percentage of the body surface area burned. The most commonly used formulas to calculate the fluid resuscitation requirement are the Brooke, Evans, and Baxter formulas. The best initial fluid to use is Ringer's lactate. In adults, the replacement recommenda-

tion is 2 to 4 ml of Ringer's lactate, multiplied by the patient's weight (in kilograms), multiplied by the percentage of body surface area burned. In children, the figure is 3 to 4 ml. The formula calculates the fluid requirement for the first 24 hours. Half of it is given in the first 8 hours (Baxter formula). Changes in the fluid administration rate should be based on urine output of 0.5 ml/kg/hour in adults and 1 ml/kg/hour in children. A pulse rate below 110 beats per minute usually is a good indicator of adequate resuscitation. Blood pressure is not a reliable indicator of resuscitation because of the release of catecholamines.

The urine should also be checked for hemochromogens. Electrical and deep burns may damage red blood cells (with the release of hemoglobin) and muscles (with the release of myoglobin). In such cases, alkalinization of the urine should be accomplished with 40 to 50 mEq of sodium bicarbonate in a liter of intravenous fluid to improve solubility in the renal tubules. An osmotic diuretic, such as mannitol, should be used, given as a 12.5 g bolus and 125 g in each liter of intravenous fluid.[3]

As emphasized, the formula chosen should be used to estimate the fluid requirement and modulated by the individual clinical response. Patients with inhalation and electrical injuries require more fluid, whereas older patients with cardiopulmonary disease may be more sensitive and require close monitoring.

TREATMENT
Burn wound care

The following criteria are guidelines for admitting a burn patient to the hospital:

- *Adult:* >15% TBSA partial-thickness burn
- *Child:* >10% TBSA partial-thickness burn

Table 17-2 Fluid replacement formulas for first 24 hours

Source	Colloid	Electrolyte solution	Water	Rate
			ml	
Brooke*	0.5 ml/kg/% BSA burned	1.5 ml/kg/% BSA burned	2000	½ first 8 hr ¼ second 8 hr ¼ third 8 hr
Evans*	1 ml/kg/% BSA burned	1 ml/kg/% BSA burned	2000	½ first 8 hr ¼ second 8 hr ¼ third 8 hr
Baxter†		4 ml/kg/% BSA burned		½ first 8 hr ¼ second 8 hr ¼ third 8 hr

BSA = body surface area.
* Approximately one-half the amount estimated for the first 24 hours is given the second 24 hours.
† Only maintenance fluids are given the second 24 hours; colloid is given as necessary.

- >2% full-thickness burn
- Smoke inhalation injury
- Partial- or full-thickness burns on hands, feet, genitalia, perineum, face
- Associated injury or illness (diabetes, coronary artery disease, patient taking steroids or immunosuppressive drugs)
- Some electrical burns
- Some chemical injuries
- Child abuse

Sterile precautions, including gowns, gloves, and mask, should be observed to avoid contamination. The burned area should be gently cleansed with a diluted soap and water mixture to remove the necrotic tissue. Blisters contain inflammatory mediators (thromboxane) that are known to be detrimental to the microcirculation; therefore, blisters should be aspirated, leaving the epithelium intact because it serves as a barrier against bacterial contamination.

First-degree burns

Excessive exposure to ultraviolet rays or scald injury usually is responsible for first-degree burns. Intravenous fluids normally are not necessary. Topical and oral analgesics may be used. With extensive sunburn, symptoms such as nausea and malaise sometimes may develop, but they seldom are severe enough to justify admission to the hospital.

Use of a topical antimicrobial agent is controversial. It usually is unnecessary for a truly shallow burn unless it covers a large surface of the body. The ideal antibacterial cream should be relatively painless and nonallergenic, have a bacterial spectrum target for the ecology of the wound, and should not inhibit epithelialization.[7] A nonstick, porous gauze saturated with a non-petroleum-based lubricant should be used as initial dressing, along with a bulky layer of gauze. The dressing should be changed twice a day. Tetanus prophylaxis is important, and follow-up is essential in 24 hours. Alternatively, the wound may be treated with Polysporin or Bacitracin and a nonstick porous gauze. It is important to instruct the patient to minimize edema through elevation, when possible, and to perform range-of-motion exercises during the healing period.

Second-degree burns

Partial-thickness burns usually are caused by a scald injury. Immediate immersion in cold water helps limit the depth of the injury but is not effective after the first 30 minutes except to relieve pain. Blister fluid contains inflammatory mediators that are detrimental to the microcirculation. Furthermore, it has been shown that wound desiccation converts the zone of stasis and deepens the burn. Therefore, aspiration of the blisters, leaving the epithelium intact, is physiologically sound. If the blisters are totally debrided, it is important to prevent desiccation with an appropriate moist dressing.

After cleansing and debridement, the burn should be temporarily covered with a dressing that does not impede epithelialization. A biosynthetic dressing such as Biobrane (knitted nylon fabric bonded to a silicone membrane coated with collagen peptides) can be applied to shallow wounds, covered by a compressive dressing to ensure adherence, and left in place. The external dressing can be removed once the Biobrane is adherent and the patient has been discharged. If Biobrane does not adhere, the wound is deeper and probably requires skin grafting. A shallow wound alternatively can be treated with an antimicrobial cream (Silvadene) and a dressing to prevent desiccation (Table 17-3).

An elevated temperature, purulent discharge, or other signs of infection should alert the physician to take the dressing down. If the burn involves an extremity, the limb should be kept elevated. If the hand is burned, it should be splinted with the interphalangeal joints extended, metacarpal joints flexed, and wrist extended (the position of function). Active and passive range of motion should be instituted at each dressing change. Face and neck burns should be treated with an open technique and antibiotic ointment.

Partial-thickness burns should be healed in 3 to 4 weeks.

Third-degree burns

Flame burns, electrical burns, or immersion in hot liquid may be responsible for third-degree, or full-thickness, burns. Circumferential full-thickness burns that involve the extremities may compromise circulation by acting as a tourniquet, resulting in pain, cyanosis, loss of distal pulses, and ischemia. In these cases, escharotomy should be considered in the emergency room. In the area of the full-thickness burn, an opening is made with a scalpel through the eschar down to subcutaneous tissue along the lateral and medial aspects of the extremity, across the joints, and to the dorsum of the hand or foot (Fig. 17-5). If the chest is involved, with impending respiratory insufficiency, longitudinal incisions are made along the midclavicular lines. Topical agents, such as Sulfamylon, that reduce bacterial proliferation and prevent septic complications are routinely used. Early primary wound excision and grafting is the treatment of choice in third-degree burns.

Table 17-3 Comparison of available topical agents for burn management

Agent	Technique of application	Advantages	Disadvantages
0.5% silver nitrate solution	2.5 cm thick coarse-mesh gauze dressing soaked every 2 hrs with solution; dressing changed every 12 hrs	Only minimal pain with application; occlusive dressing comfortable; decreased evaporative losses; easily used in grafted and ungrafted areas	Delays eschar separation; electrolyte abnormalities— hyponatremia, hypokalemia, hypocalcemia; discolors everything; does not penetrate eschar
10% mafenide acetate cream (Sulfamylon)	Apply every 24 hrs and replenish as needed; dressing usually not used	Penetrates eschar; easy to apply; nonstaining	Acidosis; burning pain with application; delays eschar separation; sensitivity reactions (10% to 15%); inhibits epithelialization
1% silver sulfadiazine cream	Apply every 24 hrs and replenish as needed	Easy to apply; nonstaining; minimal pain; no electrolyte or acid-base problems	Does not penetrate eschar well; delays eschar separation

CHEMICAL BURNS

Chemical burns are uncommon, accounting for only 3% of all burn injuries; however, they are responsible for more than 30% of burn deaths. Thus they require special consideration.

Chemical burns are caused by injuries from acids, alkalis, and organic compounds. The appearance of the wound may vary greatly. The injury primarily is due to the action of the chemical on the tissues and only secondarily to the heat liberated by the exothermic reaction.

Alkalis are present in various products, including industrial cleansers, cement, fertilizers, oven cleaners, and dry cleaning fluids. Acid is found in a wide range of products such as rust removers, acidifiers for swimming pools, and bathroom cleaners. Alkalis usually cause more tissue damage than acids. The reason for this is that acids tend to cause coagulation necrosis with precipitation of proteins, whereas alkalis tend to cause liquefaction necrosis, allowing more diffusion of the alkali deeper into the tissue. Phenol and petroleum products are common organic substances found in home products.

If the chemical remains on the skin, the wound will deepen. Therefore the areas involved must be flushed with large amounts of water. Irrigation should be continued for at least 30 minutes. Neutralization of the chemical is not indicated, because the heat released from the neutralization reaction may further deepen the injury. (See Chapter 25 for further discussion of chemical injuries.)

If the eyes are involved, copious irrigation with several liters of saline is required, and immediate ophthalmologic consultation is critical. It is also important to instruct first aid personnel to begin immediate irrigation with water. (See Chapter 15 for further discussion of eye injuries.)

Diesel and gasoline fuels (petroleum compounds) usually cause a partial-thickness burn secondary to prolonged skin contact. Absorption can cause systemic symptoms manifested by renal, hepatic, and pulmonary insufficiency.

Hydrofluoric acid is used by glass workers in rust removal and in the semiconductor industry. The chemical can penetrate deeply, causing ulceration and necrosis. Neutralization is achieved through copious irrigation, and many practitioners treat the area with calcium gluconate, which, by combining with fluoride ions, may prevent further tissue damage. A 2% calcium gluconate topical gel can be applied four to six times a day for 5 to 6 days. The gel is applied to all burned areas and massaged in by personnel wearing rubber gloves to prevent personal contamination. If a deep wound is present, subcutaneous infiltration with 5% calcium gluconate solution may be required. If the area involved is larger than 100 cm^2, the patient should be hospitalized and monitored in the intensive care unit for hypocalcemia; usually, 20 ml of a 10% calcium gluconate solution is added to the first liter of resuscitation fluid to prevent this condition.

Phenol injury is characterized by coagulation necrosis. Because it acts as a local anesthetic, phenol may cause damage before the patient experiences pain. It also can cause systemic toxicity. It is removed by using polyethylene glycol (PEG 300-400).

TAR BURNS

A tar burn is a thermal burn resulting from the heat content of the material. There is no chemical component to the injury. The tar should cool before it is removed. A petroleum-based solvent, such as Neosporin ointment or A&D ointment, may be used to remove the tar after it has cooled and solidified. Usually the top layer of the epidermis peels away with the tar or asphalt. The use of kerosene, gasoline, or acetone to remove tar should be discouraged because these agents may exacerbate the injury. In the first few days after injury, a decision should be made between excising and grafting of the wound versus waiting for healing. A burn specialist should be consulted if there is any question about proper management.

ELECTRICAL BURNS

Electrical burns are caused by the conversion of electrical energy to thermal energy. As the current courses through the body, heat is liberated in proportion to the resistance of the various tissues. The entry and exit sites of the current usually are self-demarcated, but the small size of the wound can be surprisingly out of proportion to the extent of the underlying damage. Frequently there is an associated flame burn from the heat of the electrical arc igniting clothing or causing a flash or flame. In high-voltage electrical burns, the extent of external damage may be impressive, resembling a blast injury. Attention should be given to the presence of underlying muscle damage, secondary edema, and progressive swelling that can lead to compartment syndrome.

In some cases an electrical current may also cause a progressive vascular injury, with vascular thrombosis and delayed tissue damage. Exploration, fasciotomy, and debridement of necrotic tissue constitute the treatment of choice. Myocardial damage, with ventricular fibrillation or infarction, may occur as a result of the current passing through the chest. Orthopedic injuries may be sustained after falls or from the violent muscle contractions caused by the current. Fluid resuscitation should be based on urine output (50 to 100 ml/hour) because it is impossible to accurately es-

timate the amount of fluid sequestered in the underlying tissues. Sodium bicarbonate and mannitol should be used to alkalize the urine and minimize the precipitation of pigments in the renal tubules and subsequent renal failure.

All patients suffering from high-voltage electrical injury should be admitted to the hospital because the symptoms and signs of internal damage may not become apparent until 24 to 48 hours after the injury. (See Chapter 31 for further discussion of electrical injuries.)

A topical bactericidal agent, mafenide acetate, is the agent of choice because of its high tissue penetration. The side effects of the drug (skin allergy, inhibition of carbonic anhydrase, and discomfort after application) should be monitored.

CONCLUSION

Most first- and second-degree burns can be handled by the occupational medicine physician. However, severe or extensive second-degree burns and most third-degree burns should be referred to a burn specialist.

Chemical burns require careful monitering but often can be managed by the primary care physician. Electrical burns require careful evaluation for underlying damage and late systemic complications.

REFERENCES

1. American Burn Association: Guidelines for service standards and severity classification in the treatment of burn injury, *Am Coll Sur* (Bull) 69:24, 1984.
2. Bolcker TG: Burns. In Converse JM, editor: *Reconstructive plastic surgery,* Philadelphia, 1964, WB Saunders.
3. Dimick AR, Wagner RG: Burns in emergency management of trauma.
4. Herndon P et al: Diagnosis, pathophysiology and treatment of inhalation injury. In Boswick JA, editor: *The art and science of burn care,* Rockville, MD, 1987, Aspen.
5. Hlava P, Moserova J, Konigova R: Validity of clinical assessment of the depth of a thermal injury, *Acta Chir Plast* 25:202, 1983.
6. Jackson D, Mac G: The diagnosis of the depth of burning, *Br J Surg* 40:588, 1953.
7. Robson MC, Smith DJ: Thermal injuries. In Jurkiewicz JM et al: *Plastic surgery: principles and* practice, St Louis, 1990, Mosby.

18 Respiratory Injuries

The respiratory tract is a common site of injury from occupational exposures. The widespread and increasing use of potentially toxic materials in the environment poses an ever expanding threat to both the upper and lower airways. Injuries caused by inhalational exposure can range from mild respiratory impairment to death. Early recognition and appropriate treatment by the physician of first contact can significantly reduce both morbidity and mortality and greatly affect the outcome for the patient. This chapter focuses on how to diagnose and manage common respiratory injuries.

ANATOMY

The respiratory tract is anatomically divided into three parts: the upper airways, the lower airways, and the lung parenchyma (Fig. 18-1). The upper airways are composed of the oronasal passages and the larynx, and the lower airways are composed of the tracheobronchial airways. The pulmonary parenchyma is primarily made up of terminal respiratory units, which contain the alveoli and supporting interstitium. This anatomic division of the respiratory tract has more than academic consequences because the structural differences serve important protective functions. Despite the greater effort required, humans tend to favor nasal breathing. Inspired air passes two acute bends before it reaches the relatively straight pharyngolaryngeal path. The anatomic arrangement of the nasal passages with the turbinates provides a large mucosal surface area that allows warming and humidification of inspired air.

The trachea begins at the lower border of the cricoid cartilage, distal to the vocal cords. The trachea, bronchi, and larger bronchioles form the conducting portion of the lower respiratory tract. The gas-exchanging portion, or terminal respiratory units, are composed of respiratory bronchioles, alveolar ducts, and alveoli. The airway lining as far as the terminal bronchiole consists of epithelial cells of the pseudostratified, columnar, and ciliated type. Interspersed with these are the mucus-secreting goblet cells. The terminal respiratory unit, in contrast, is composed of a number of different cell types, including type 1 and type 2 epithelial cells, alveolar macrophages, capillary endothelial cells, fibroblasts, and lymphocytes in the intraalveolar septa.

The site of deposition of inhaled materials depends on water solubility for gases and particle size for solids (Table 18-1). Water-soluble gases and particles larger than 10 μm in diameter tend to get deposited in the upper airways, whereas those without these properties gain access to the lower airways. Subsequent respiratory injury depends on both this property (site of toxin deposition) and on the type of cell/structure damaged.

EVALUATION OF RESPIRATORY INJURIES

A detailed evaluation of the individual can successfully identify and diagnose respiratory injury in most cases. The following four areas of approach are recommended: (1) detailed history, including occupational and environmental exposures; (2) thorough physical examination; (3) use of appropriate imaging studies; and (4) pulmonary function testing.

History

A thorough history of both the patient's complaints and her environmental and occupational exposures is essential. Work practices should be extensively explored, with attention given to types and duration of exposures, whether appropriate environmental controls are present, and whether respiratory protective gear is used. Material Safety Data Sheets (MSDS) should be sought, if available. These documents profile the important health, safety, and toxicologic properties of the product or mixture ingredients, and under federal law the employer must give them to the worker or her health care provider on request. When possible, actual industrial hygiene data on the level of exposure and the agent to which the patient was exposed should be obtained. The history should probe into the patient's home living conditions, hobbies, and social habits, because these may contribute to or cause the lung injury.

Physical examination

The physical examination may be helpful if abnormal, but it generally is insensitive for detecting

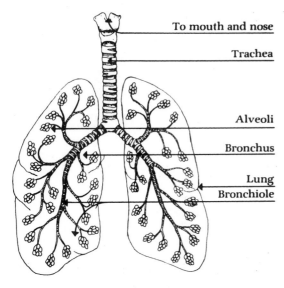

To mouth and nose

Trachea

Alveoli

Bronchus

Lung
Bronchiole

Fig. 18-1 Anatomy of the respiratory tract.

mild respiratory tract injuries. The vital signs and the level of respiratory distress, if any, should be initially assessed. The examiner should check for cyanosis and finger clubbing. Examination of the skin and eyes may reveal signs of irritation and inflammation. Oropharyngeal and nasal areas should be inspected for signs of ulceration and irritation. Of course, wheezing, rhonchi, crackles, or pleural rubs on chest auscultation suggest respiratory disease. When crackles are heard, it is important to examine the cardiovascular system for evidence of left ventricular failure. Isolated right ventricular failure suggests the possibility of cor pulmonale, resulting from chronic, severe lung disease with hypoxemia.

Imaging studies

A chest x-ray film should be part of the work-up when lung injury is suspected. However, normal x-ray findings do not exclude significant damage to the lung. In the period immediately after an in-

halational injury, the chest film often is normal. In contrast, dramatically abnormal chest films can be seen in individuals without significant lung injury who are exposed chronically to iron oxide or tin oxide. With individuals exposed to dust, chest films should be interpreted according to the International Labor Office (ILO) classification for pneumoconiosis in addition to the standard interpretation. Abnormalities on the chest film do not necessarily correlate with the degree of pulmonary impairment or disability. These are better assessed by pulmonary function testing and arterial blood gas (ABG) determination.

Computed tomography (CT). Computed tomography (CT) is a radiologic technique involving scans of axial cross-sections of the thorax; this produces tomographic slices, which are more defined than those of standard radiography. CT is better able to detect abnormalities of the lung parenchyma and the mediastinal structures than conventional radiography, in large part because it is more sensitive to differences in density. When done after an intravenous contrast medium has been administered, CT scanning is considered the imaging study of choice for evaluating the pulmonary hila.

High-resolution CT scanning (HRCT) incorporates thin collimation (1 to 2 mm, rather than the 10 mm used in conventional CT scanning) with high spatial-frequency reconstruction algorithms that sharpen interfaces between adjacent structures. Studies suggest that HRCT is more accurate than conventional CT or chest x-ray films in assessing for the presence, character, and severity of a number of diffuse lung processes, such as interstitial lung disease. These studies are especially useful in the evaluation of asbestos-related pulmonary parenchymal and pleural diseases.

Pulmonary function tests

Pulmonary function testing is used to detect and quantitate abnormal lung function. Spirometry can

Table 18-1 Determinants of site of deposition in the respiratory tract

Water solubility		
Degree of solubility	*Examples*	*Site of deposition*
High	Ammonia, formaldehyde	Upper airway
Moderate	Chlorine, sulfur dioxide	Upper and lower airways
Low	Nitrogen oxides, phosgene	Small airways and alveoli
Particle size		
Diameter		
>10 μm		Upper airway (nose, oropharynx, larynx)
>2-5 μm		Lower airways
<3 μm		Alveoli

and should be done in most evaluating centers; however, a well-equipped pulmonary function laboratory is needed for measuring lung volume and diffusing capacity, and for gas exchange analysis and exercise testing.

The most valuable parameters of pulmonary function are the forced expiratory volume in 1 second (FEV_1), the forced vital capacity (FVC), and the FEV_1/FVC ratio. These parameters constitute (1) the best method of detecting airway obstruction and judging its severity, and (2) the most reliable assessment of overall respiratory impairment. A simple portable spirometer can be used to obtain the necessary measurements. The results can be compared with predicted values from reference populations (adjusted for age, height, and sex) and expressed as a percentage of the predicted value. Because the commonly used reference populations consist entirely of Caucasians, problems may arise in using predicted values to evaluate nonCaucasian patients. Typically, the predicted value is reduced by 10% to 15% to correct for the generally smaller lungs of nonCaucasians.

Another commonly used single-breath test that reflects the degree of airway obstruction is the peak expiratory flow rate (PEFR) test. Portable instruments such as the mini-Wright peak flow meter or peak flow gauge can be used for this test (Fig. 18-2). The major limitation of the PEFR test is that the patient usually records the readings herself, and thus there is a potential for malingering. Despite this limitation, the test is useful for detecting changes in airway obstruction in the same person over a period of time. Serial peak flow measurements are especially valuable in the diagnosis of occupational asthma to document delayed responses after the work shift is over.

Bronchoprovocation tests

Pulmonary function responses to inhaled histamine and methacholine are relatively easy to measure and indicate the presence and degree of non-

specific hyperresponsiveness of the airways. Non-specific provocation tests are especially useful in diagnosing asthma. A measure of airway obstruction (such as FEV_1, airway conductance, or airway resistance) is obtained repeatedly after progressively increasing the dose of histamine or methacholine to generate a dose-response curve. The test usually is terminated after a 20% fall in FEV_1 (or a 100% increase in airway resistance). Patients with asthma typically respond with such a change in lung function after a relatively low cumulative dose of methacholine.

COMMON INJURIES
Inhalation of noxious gases, fumes, and mists

Short-term exposure to high concentrations of noxious gases, fumes, or mists generally results from industrial or transportation accidents or fires. Inhalational injury from high-intensity exposure can cause severe respiratory impairment or death.

Inhaled materials can produce toxic effects by the following mechanisms (see also Table 18-2):

- *Simple asphyxiation* resulting from replacement of atmospheric oxygen by other gases such as methane or nitrogen;
- *Tissue asphyxia* resulting from pulmonary absorption of agents capable of interfering with oxygen transport or poisoning cellular respiratory enzymes (such as carbon monoxide, cyanide, and hydrogen sulfide);
- *Nonrespiratory effects* resulting from pulmonary absorption of agents such as lead or hydrocarbon solvents;
- *Excessive stimulation of physiologic responses* (bronchorrhea and/or reflex bronchoconstriction); for example, inhalation of sulfur dioxide in concentrations too low to cause morphologic evidence of injury; and
- *Direct cellular injury* by agents such as ammonia, chlorine, nitrogen oxides, and phosgene.

Only the last two processes have direct pulmonary effects. The site of injury depends on the physical and chemical properties of the inhaled agent. As discussed earlier, the site of deposition is determined primarily by water solubility. Other important factors are the duration of exposure and the minute ventilation of the victim. The concentration of an inhaled water-soluble gas such as formaldehyde is greatly reduced by the time it reaches the trachea because of the efficient scrubbing mechanisms of the moist surfaces of the nose and throat. In contrast, a relatively water-insoluble gas, such as phosgene, is not well absorbed by the upper airways and thus may penetrate to the alveoli. The effects of inhalational exposure to such

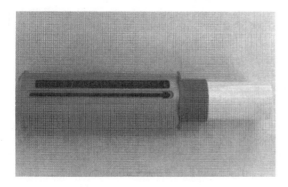

Fig. 18-2 Mini-Wright peak flow meter.

Table 18-2 Toxicity from inhaled materials

Mechanism	Toxins
Simple asphyxia	Nitrogen, methane (replacement of atmospheric oxygen)
Tissue asphyxia	Carbon monoxide, cyanide, hydrogen sulfide
Nonrespiratory effects resulting from pulmonary absorption	Hydrocarbon solvents (benzene), lead
Exaggeration of normal physiologic response	Formaldehyde, sulfur dioxide
Direct mucosal cell injury	Ammonia, chlorine, nitrogen dioxide, phosgene

toxic materials can range from transient, mild irritation of the mucous membranes of the upper airways to fatal adult respiratory distress syndrome (ARDS) (Table 18-3).

Specific agents

Ammonia. Ammonia (NH_3) is a colorless, strongly alkaline, highly water-soluble gas that has a characteristic pungent odor. It has a wide variety of uses: as a domestic cleaning agent, as a refrigerant, and as a raw material in the manufacture of plastics, cyanide, synthetic fibers, and petroleum products. Ammonia has an odor threshold between 40 and 50 ppm, and its distinctive odor usually provides adequate warning of exposure. The lethal concentration is about 500 ppm.

Adverse pulmonary effects depend on the concentration inhaled. Low-dose exposure usually produces local irritation of conjunctival membranes and the upper airway. Moderate exposure can result in hoarseness, coughing, bronchospasm, nausea, and vomiting. Acute high-level exposure can cause hemoptysis and ARDS. Long-term sequelae from exposure can range from bronchiectasis to reactive airway dysfunction syndrome (RADS). This recently described syndrome, an asthmalike illness characterized by nonspecific airway hyperresponsiveness and no preexisting history of respiratory disease, increasingly is being recognized as a sequel to exposure to high doses of respiratory irritants.

EVALUATION. In most cases details about the exposure should establish ammonia as the causative chemical. The more serious exposures generally occur after major spills caused by industrial or transportation accidents. The early effects depend on the level of exposure; they may range from mild conjunctival and irritation of the upper respiratory membrane (low-dose exposure) to life-threatening laryngeal edema (high-dose exposure).

The initial focus of the physical examination is the airway. If the nose and throat are badly burned or if the patient has hoarseness or stridor, chemical laryngitis should be suspected. Early wheezing suggests that the exposure was relatively heavy.

The chest x-ray film usually is normal immediately after exposure. Chemical pneumonitis and pulmonary edema (ARDS) may develop within 4 to 6 hours of heavy exposure. ABG measurements may show hypoxemia before radiographic evidence of parenchymal injury emerges.

MANAGEMENT. Treatment of ammonia-induced injuries should include immediate decontamination of exposed cutaneous and conjunctival areas by irrigation with water. If facial cutaneous burns are noted, intubation should be considered and, in the process, the larynx should be directly viewed to determine the extent of injury. Supplemental oxygen should be administered if there is any sign of respiratory distress. Wheezing should be treated with an inhaled bronchodilator.

Patients who develop pulmonary edema/ARDS require treatment in the intensive care unit, including mechanical ventilatory assistance. However, if these patients can be supported through the acute phase of the disease process, they may recover with no significant loss of lung function. Permanent respiratory impairment after chemical bronchitis from ammonia inhalation has been reported

Table 18-3 Effects of inhalation of irritant gases

Injury site	Effects
Eye, nose, and oropharynx	Erythema, mucosal membrane edema, ulceration, burns
Upper airways	Laryngeal ulceration and edema, mucosal inflammation and/or burns
Lower airways	Tracheobronchitis, interference with mucociliary clearance, bronchorrhea, airway edema, atelectasis
Pulmonary parenchyma	Pulmonary edema/ARDS, bacterial pneumonia stemming from impaired clearance

as a result of persistant asthma (RADS) or bronchiectasis.

Chlorine. Chlorine (Cl), a green-yellow gas, is a potent oxidizing agent that forms hydrochloric acid (HCl) in the presence of water. It is less water soluble than ammonia. Chlorine has a distinctive odor, and the odor threshold is approximately 3 ppm. Levels above 25 ppm are considered highly threatening to life. Chlorine is a commonly used gas in the chemical industry. Exposure can result from transportation accidents, in the paper and pulp manufacturing industry, from swimming pool decontamination efforts, and in the home when bleach (which contains sodium hypochlorate) is mixed with acid cleaners.

Exposure concentrations determine the degree of pulmonary injury. Low-level exposure leads to irritative symptoms of the conjuctivae and upper respiratory tract, whereas higher concentrations can cause chemical bronchitis and pneumonitis/pulmonary edema. Severe chest discomfort, coughing, vomiting, and headache can occur with high-level exposure.

EVALUATION. Evaluation of a patient after chlorine inhalation differs somewhat from that after ammonia inhalation because chlorine is less likely to cause laryngeal edema and more likely to penetrate to the lower respiratory tract. Spirometry may show airway obstruction relatively early after exposure. The x-ray film usually is normal immediately after inhalation, but changes consistent with pneumonitis or pulmonary edema may develop 4 to 6 hours after severe exposure. In heavily exposed patients, ABG measurements may show significant hypoxemia.

MANAGEMENT. Treatment consists of removing the patient from exposure and supportive care. Inhaled beta$_2$-agonists and supplemental oxygen may be required immediately after inhalation of chlorine. If chemical pneumonitis and pulmonary edema develop, mechanical ventilatory assistance and support in the intensive care unit (ICU) may be needed. Although inhaling chlorine gas clearly can cause acute respiratory tract injury, controversy exists about the potential for long-term pulmonary sequelae. There are well-documented reports of persisting airflow obstruction, nonspecific airway hyperresponsiveness, and sequential reduction in residual volume after acute exposure to chlorine gas. Until this controversy is resolved, it would seem prudent to follow exposed individuals with periodic clinical examinations and frequent pulmonary function testing, monitoring for the development of any persistent respiratory impairment.

Sulfur dioxide. Sulfur dioxide (SO$_2$) is a highly irritating, colorless, water-soluble gas that is ap-

proximately twice as dense as air. Its odor threshold is approximately 0.5 ppm, and exposure to concentrations in the range of 6 to 10 ppm causes immediate irritation of the respiratory tract. On contact with the respiratory mucous membranes, the gas is rapidly hydrated and oxidized to form sulfurous acid. Occupational sources of sulfur dioxide include industries that produce paper, refrigeration plants, fruit processing, and petroleum refining. It may also be produced by a variety of industrial processes, including smelting of sulfide-containing ores (lead, copper, zinc), and paper processing. The National Institute for Occupational Safety and Health (NIOSH) has estimated that more than half a million workers may have had sulfur dioxide exposure. Because of the high water solubility of sulfur dioxide, the nasopharynx and upper respiratory mucosa are the tissues most vulnerable to injury.

EVALUATION. At relatively low concentrations (1 to 50 ppm), most of the gas is deposited in the upper respiratory tract, mainly in the nasopharynx and hypopharynx. Higher levels of exposure exceed the capacity of these structures to absorb the gas, and penetration may occur to the level of the larynx, trachea, distal airways, and alveoli. The symptoms and signs depend on the level of exposure. Immediately after exposure, the patient may develop burning of the eyes, nose, and throat, with episodes of coughing, chest discomfort, and dyspnea. Physical examination may show signs of conjunctivitis with corneal burns, erythematous pharyngitis, and signs of pulmonary edema. Extremely high exposure to sulfur dioxide can cause pulmonary edema, through its mechanisms of direct cellular toxicity.

MANAGEMENT. Treatment of a sulfur dioxide inhalational injury is identical to that described above for a chlorine-induced injury. Survival after the acute exposure can be complicated within 2 to 3 weeks by the recurrence of respiratory symptoms. There are some reports in the literature of episodes of pathologically diagnosed bronchiolitis obliterans in patients who initially survived the acute exposure. There is also evidence of persistent airflow obstruction that lasts for as long as 4 years after exposure. Because of the potential for bronchiolitis obliterans, a therapeutic trial of corticosteroids may be warranted in patients who develop persistent symptoms of respiratory disease after acute exposure.

Phosgene. Phosgene, or carbonyl chloride (COCl$_2$), is a colorless gas that is almost $3\frac{1}{2}$ times denser than air, poorly water soluble, and highly lethal. It has a relatively low odor threshold (1 to 1.5 ppm), and its smell has been described as similar to that of freshly mown hay or green corn. Because the range between odor threshold and toxicity is narrow, odor is not an adequate warning of exposure. Commercially phosgene is used primarily as an intermediate in the manufacture of isocyanates. It also is used in the manufacture of pesticides, pharmaceuticals, and dyes.

Phosgene can be produced by pyrolysis of chlorinated hydrocarbons, a common method of exposure arising from arc welding of metal surfaces that were previously cleaned with chlorinated hydrocarbon solvents. Workers at risk of phosgene exposure are the 10,000 or more involved in its manufacture, as well as firefighters, fire victims, welders, and paint strippers. Because of its poor water solubility, phosgene is only mildly irritating to the upper respiratory tract. Once inhaled and deposited in the lower lung, it slowly hydrolyzes to hydrochloric acid and carbon dioxide over a period of 24 hours. The generation of hydrochloric acid is highly irritating to the pulmonary parenchyma, where it causes necrosis and sloughing of tissue.

EVALUATION. The initial focus after phosgene inhalation is the lung parenchyma. Exposed individuals may complain of mild eye and throat irritation. Up to 8 hours later, dyspnea, chest tightness, and cough may develop. Symptoms may progress to herald the onset of chemical pneumonitis and pulmonary edema. The chest x-ray film generally shows changes consistent with parenchymal injury, and ABG measurements show hypoxemia.

MANAGEMENT. The individual should be removed from the exposure, and supplemental oxygen should be administered. Chemical pneumonitis and pulmonary edema/ARDS should be treated with appropriate supportive measures. Because of the delayed reaction to inhaled phosgene, patients exposed to significant concentrations should be observed for a minimum of 24 hours. Serial periodic clinical examinations, chest x-ray films, and ABG determinations are useful in monitoring the progression of disease. There is no evidence to support the use of prophylactic antibiotics or corticosteroids, nor is there literature describing the long-term sequelae of exposure.

Nitrogen oxides. More than 1 million people in the United States are potentially exposed to nitrogen oxides (NO, NO_2, N_2O_4). Workers known to be at risk are silo fillers exposed to fresh silage, chemical workers exposed to by-product gases from the manufacture of dyes and lacquers, coal miners following shot firing, welders using acetylene welding equipment, and workers involved in the handling of nitric acid. The nitrogen oxides (of which nitrogen dioxide is the most important in terms of exposure) are poorly water soluble and therefore penetrate to the small airways and alveoli.

EVALUATION. Individuals exposed for brief periods to nitrogen dioxide in concentrations above 50 ppm are at risk of developing acute respiratory problems. Nitrogen oxides react with water to form nitric acid, which can induce direct tissue inflammation and destruction in the lower airways. Symptoms often are not noted until significant oropharyngeal mucosal injury has occurred. Depending on the level and duration of exposure, the patient may experience varying degrees of breathlessness, a persistent cough that often produces blood-streaked sputum, and a sensation of choking. Physical examination may reveal a fever, cyanosis, and signs of respiratory insufficiency. Crackles may be auscultated over the lung fields. A granulocytic leukocytosis and chest x-ray signs of pulmonary edema are commonly seen with significant exposure.

MANAGEMENT. Treatment for the acute phase is symptomatic, with oxygen therapy, assisted ventilation if necessary, and hemodynamic monitoring. If the patient recovers from acute exposure, a relapse may develop within 3 to 6 weeks of the initial exposure. This is characterized by fevers, chills, varying degrees of dyspnea, and a persistent cough. On physical examination, the patient may be cyanotic, have bibasilar crackles, and diffuse expiratory wheezing on chest auscultation. The chest x-ray film may show discrete, small, nodular densities with focal infiltrates. This presentation is consistent with the diagnosis of bronchiolitis obliterans, which histologically is characterized by inflammation and fibrosis in and around small bronchi and bronchioles. The small airways often are occluded with cellular and exudative material and fibrin. Treatment of this complication is controversial; some reports support the use of corticosteroids to reduce the respiratory bronchiolar inflammation.

The risk of developing permanent respiratory impairment after acute symptomatic exposure to nitrogen oxides has not been well defined. A few reports in the literature have documented the persistence of respiratory impairment, primarily chronic bronchitis and an obstructive pulmonary impairment, but these reports are by no means conclusive.

Fire smoke. Smoke from fires is a complex mixture of gases and aerosolized particles. With a smoke inhalational injury, the physician must consider the various agents that may be present in the smoke, including (1) toxic gases irritating to the airways and pulmonary parenchyma; (2) chemical asphyxiants, such as carbon monoxide and cyanide; and (3) steam heat and hot particulate matter, which may cause edema of the upper airways and vocal cords. Thus there is potential both for injury to the entire respiratory tract and for systemic toxicity.

Thermal burns usually are confined to the supraglottic region. Dry inhaled smoke is commonly in the temperature range of 260° to 280° C (500° to 536° F) and has a low heat capacity. The upper airways, primarily the nasopharynx and hypopharynx, are effective in cooling the hot, dry smoke, so that by the time it reaches the subglottic regions, it has cooled to about 50° C (122° F). In contrast, inhaled smoke with a high water content has a much greater heat capacity, which may exceed the protective mechanism of the upper airway. This is especially true in individuals who have inhaled steam, which has a heat capacity almost 4000 times that of dry smoke. In such cases, the lower airways can suffer significant thermal injury.

In addition to the dangers of thermal burns, inhaling toxic gases can complicate the respiratory injury of fire victims. Gases liberated from the combustion or pyrolysis of a wide range of organic and synthetic materials are toxic to the respiratory tract. Furthermore, the specific chemical composition of fire smoke can differ greatly among fires. The evolved gases can be considered under the two broad categories of irritants and chemical asphyxiants. The major irritants are ammonia, chlorine, hydrogen chloride, nitrogen dioxide, phosgene, acrolein, and sulfur dioxide. The major asphyxiants are carbon monoxide and cyanide, which can significantly affect tissue oxygen delivery and cellular respiration. These effects can be compounded by a relative absence of oxygen resulting from consumption by the fire. In addition to gases, acid aerosols can cause the pH of the smoke to be as low as 1 and can contribute significantly to injury of both the upper and lower respiratory tracts.

EVALUATION.   Certain clinical findings suggest significant inhalational injury resulting from a fire. Facial burns, inflamed nares, and early sputum production and wheezing are such findings. The level of consciousness at the scene of the fire often correlates with the degree of inhalational injury. Any victim with altered consciousness should be suspected of having carbon monoxide intoxication. As with other types of toxic inhalational injury, the chest x-ray film may be normal in the early stage of the disease process. ABGs and oxyhemoglobin saturation should be measured. A low oxyhemoglobin saturation with a normal arterial oxygen pressure (Pao_2) should alert the physician to the possibility of carbon monoxide intoxication. If possible, carboxyhemoglobin should be mea-

sured. Significant metabolic acidosis should alert the clinician to the possibility of cyanide or hydrogen sulfide intoxication.

Direct laryngoscopy or fiberoptic bronchoscopy is recommended by some to assess for laryngeal edema. If it is present, endotracheal intubation should be considered. However, it is by no means clear as to who will develop life-threatening upper airway obstruction. A conservative approach of careful clinical monitoring of the victim in an intensive care unit may be appropriate. If bronchoscopy is performed, evidence of significant inhalation injury includes erythema, edema, ulceration, and/or hemorrhage of the airway mucosa. If particulate material was inhaled, it may be visualized on the airway mucosa. Simple spirometry or PEFR measurements to detect early airway obstruction often are useful. Flow-volume loops have been used both to diagnose upper airway obstruction and as a more sensitive detector of early lower airway obstruction than simple spirometry or PEFR. Measurement of diffusing capacity has been suggested as a sensitive indicator of pulmonary parenchymal injury, but it is difficult for severely ill patients to perform.

MANAGEMENT.   At the scene of the fire, high-flow oxygen via face mask should be administered to most victims (Table 18-4). Victims over 40 years of age and those with frequent extrasystoles or tachycardia should be monitored via telemetry en route to the hospital. A mental status examination should be performed even in fully ambulatory victims because of the potential for central nervous system (CNS) effects. Hospitalization for a minimum of 24 hours should be considered for all victims with mental status abnormalities and for asymptomatic fire victims with a high probability of smoke inhalational injury (those with facial, nasal, or oral burns; those with significant elevated carboxyhemoglobin levels; and those with exposure to toxic fumes in confined spaces). Because respiratory tract injury may progress after admission, serial evaluations of the patient's status must be performed. These evaluations should include vital signs, including respiratory rate, CNS status, degree of airway obstruction (serial spirometry or PEFR measurements are more reliable than chest auscultation), ABG determinations, and chest x-ray films. Electrocardiograms and cardiac monitoring should be done in patients over 40 years of age, with chest pain, or with irregular heart rates because of the possibility of carbon monoxide–induced myocardial ischemia. Supportive care of patients known to have had smoke inhalation at the time of admission should include (1) maintenance of an adequate airway; (2) removal of mucus and debris from the tracheobronchial tree; (3) reversal

Table 18-4 Management of toxic inhalation injury

Indications for medical assessment

Exposed in a poorly ventilated, enclosed space
Altered mental status
Age over 60 years
Facial burns
Chest pains, shortness of breath
Known combustion of synthetic material

Indications for hospital admission

Abnormal results on mental status examination
Significant respiratory tract symptoms (shortness of breath, cough, chest tightness, wheezing, hoarseness)
History of chronic obstructive pulmonary disease (COPD) or ischemic heart disease
Elevated carboxyhemoglobin level (>20%)

Indications for admission to intensive care unit

Altered level of consciousness
Abnormal ABG measurements (hypoxia, hypercapnia, acidosis)
Upper respiratory tract symptoms of hoarseness, wheezing
Abnormal spirometry (obstruction, decreased diffusing capacity)
Facial burns

Indications for intubation

Respiratory distress
Severe laryngeal obstruction
Depressed level of consciousness

---

of airflow obstruction; and (4) correction of hypoxemia. Victims with stridor, hoarseness, or severe facial, nasal, or oral injuries should be closely monitored with serial ABG measurements for respiratory insufficiency and intubated if necessary.

Vigorous bronchial hygiene measures are required in patients who develop severe tracheobronchitis. Drainage of mucus plugs and respiratory secretions should be encouraged by postural drainage, chest physical therapy, deep inspiratory maneuvers, and adequate hydration. If the patient is intubated, the airways should be suctioned frequently to remove any adherent soot that may contain irritant and corrosive chemicals. Some authors recommend fiberoptic bronchoscopy to lavage off this adherent material.

Bronchospasm should be treated with inhaled beta$_2$-agonists and anticholinergic agents. Corticosteroids should be used only in patients with bronchospasm who are unresponsive to bronchodilators.

Hypoxemia can be corrected by the previously mentioned measures plus supplemental oxygen.

Refractory hypoxemia despite a vigorous treatment plan suggests severe pulmonary parenchymal injury.

Lung injury may develop into ARDS with significant inhalational exposure. Mechanical ventilation with positive end-expiratory pressure (PEEP) often is required to correct the hypoxemia associated with this complication. Hemodynamic monitoring and strict fluid management are the keys to a successful outcome.

The role of prophylactic administration of corticosteroids in the treatment of toxic inhalation injury remains controversial. The proposed advantages of reducing parenchymal inflammation and subsequent fibrosis need to be weighed against the patient's increased susceptibility to a nosocomial pneumonia. At this stage, routine use of corticosteroids cannot be recommended.

The prognosis from smoke inhalational injury is related to the degree of concomitant burns. Mortality rates in individuals with no associated burns are in the range of 5% to 10%. However, in those with severe cutaneous burns, the mortality rate is 50% to 80%. Facial burns, even without significant body involvement, and an elevated carboxyhemoglobin level (over 15%) are predictors of a high rate of inhalational injury and mortality. Little data are available on long-term morbidity from smoke inhalation. Anecdotal evidence shows an increased incidence of airway hyperresponsiveness and an asthmalike syndrome in victims of smoke inhalation. Some evidence suggests that firefighters, who are repeatedly exposed to smoke inhalation, have an increased prevalence of airway hyperresponsiveness. However, it is difficult to extrapolate findings from repeated occupational exposure to a single massive exposure.

Occupational asthma

Asthma is a clinical condition characterized by intermittent respiratory symptoms (dyspnea, chest tightness, wheezing, and cough), airway hyperresponsiveness to a variety of nonspecific stimuli, and reversible or variable airway obstruction. Occupational asthma can be defined as variable airway obstruction related to exposure in the workplace to airborne dusts, gases, mists, or fumes. Occupational asthma can be caused by either exacerbation of preexisting asthma or new onset of disease. Work-related variable airway obstruction can be caused by classic type 1 hypersensitivity reactions, pharmacologic effects, inflammatory processes, and direct airway irritation. More than 200 etiologic agents have been implicated for occupational asthma, and it is becoming increasingly more prevalent in the occupational setting. The prevalence of occupational asthma appears to be increasing, and it is estimated to constitute up to 15% of all asthma cases.

Sensitizer-induced occupational asthma results from "allergic sensitization" to a substance or material in the work site. Sensitizing agents known to cause occupational asthma can be divided into high-molecular-weight (>1000 daltons) and low-molecular-weight compounds (Table 18-5). High-molecular-weight compounds tend to cause occupational asthma by means of type 1, IgE-mediated reactions, whereas the mechanism or mechanisms of low-molecular-weight compounds currently are unknown. Sensitizer-induced asthma is characterized by a period of clinical latency after exposure begins, nonspecific airway hyperresponsiveness, and specific responsiveness to the etiologic agent. The mechanism of irritant-induced asthma also is unknown, but there is no clinical evidence of sensitization. Irritant-induced asthma may develop abruptly and involves persistent, nonspecific airway hyperresponsiveness but not specific responsiveness to the etiologic agent. Irritant-induced asthma often follows a single intense exposure (RADS), but it appears that lower level exposure of longer duration (months to years) also can cause the disease.

Evaluation. The diagnosis of occupational asthma is made by confirming the diagnosis of asthma and by establishing a relationship between asthma and the work environment. The diagnosis of asthma should be made only when both intermittent respiratory symptoms and physiologic evidence of reversible or variable airway obstruction are present. The relationship between the asthma and workplace exposure may fall into any of the following symptom patterns: (1) symptoms occur only at work; (2) symptoms improve on weekends or vacations; (3) symptoms occur regularly after the work shift; (4) symptoms progressively increase over the course of the work week; and (5) symptoms improve after a change in the work environment.

Clinical history. At least one of the cardinal symptoms of wheezing, shortness of breath, coughing, and chest tightness should be elicited while the patient is at the workplace, or within several hours of leaving it. Often the patient's symptoms improve during days off or while she is away from her usual job. With persistent exposure, the symptoms may become chronic and lose their temporal relationship to the workplace. Concomitant symptoms of an upper respiratory tract irritant and conjunctivitis may also be noted. The physician also should suspect occupational asthma if an otherwise healthy individual has a history of recurrent episodes of work-related "bronchitis" characterized by coughing and sputum production in an otherwise healthy individual. High-molecular-weight sensitizers typically cause immediate or dual responses, but low-molecular-weight sensitizers tend to induce isolated, late-phase responses that may occur many hours after the work shift is over.

Work environment. Appropriate evaluation for possible occupational asthma requires a detailed history of the work environment. Attention should be given to the agents to which the patient is exposed, the type of ventilation in the workplace, whether respiratory protective equipment is used and, if possible, the level of exposure (whether it is high or low, or if accidental exposure through spills ever occurs). A helpful clue to a significant problem in a workplace is the presence of other workers with episodic respiratory symptoms. Obtaining Material Safety Data Sheets for all materials in the workplace to which the patient states she is exposed can be helpful. Finally, if any uncer-

Table 18-5 Common causes of occupational asthma

Mechanism	Example
Without "sensitization"	
Endotoxin effects	Cotton dust (textile workers)
Anticholinesterase effect	Organophosphate pesticides (agricultural workers)
Inflammatory response	Ammonia, chlorine (custodial workers, paper manufacturing)
Irritant response	Dusts, fumes, vapors, cold (construction workers, chemical workers)
With "sensitization"	
High-molecular-weight compounds	Animal proteins (laboratory workers, shellfish handlers)
IgE mediated (complete allergens)	Plant proteins (coffee workers)
	Enzymes (food processors, detergent manufacturing)
Low-molecular-weight compounds	
IgE mediated (haptens)	Antibiotics (pharmaceutical workers)
Unclear mechanism of action	Acid anhydrides (plastics industry, epoxy painters)
	Diisocyanates (polyurethane foam producers, painters)

tainty exists, a visit by a qualified industrial hygienist to the workplace is invaluable.

Physical examination. The detection of wheezing on chest auscultation is helpful, but the physical examination often is normal in asthmatic patients who are not currently suffering from an exacerbation.

Imaging studies. Chest x-ray films are normal in most individuals with asthma because the disease involves the airways rather than the lung parenchyma. Hyperinflation and flattening of the diaphragms, indicating air trapping, may be seen in some. Fleeting infiltrates, which indicates mucus plugging, and bronchial wall thickening, which reflects chronic inflammation, may also be noted.

Pulmonary function tests. As noted previously, spirometry for measuring FEV_1 and FVC is the most reliable method for assessing airflow obstruction. However, because asthmatic patients typically have reversible airflow obstruction, they may have normal lung function during intervals between acute attacks. The response to inhaled bronchodilator administration has been used as a measure of airway hyperresponsiveness. A 15% improvement in FEV_1 after bronchodilator inhalation often is considered a significant improvement, indicating hyperresponsive airways. Cross-workshift spirometry, when available, can provide objective evidence of occupational asthma. A fall in FEV_1 of more than 10% across a workshift suggests an asthmatic response.

Serial recording of patient measurements of PEFR over a period of weeks to months often is the best way to document the work-related aspect of asthma. The patient records her PEFR every 2 to 4 hours while awake, as well as respiratory symptoms and medication use. When interpreting the log, attention should be given to any work-related pattern of change. A 20% or greater diurnal variability in PEFR has been considered evidence of an asthmatic response (Fig. 18-3). The major advantage of serial PEFR measurement over spirometry is the ability to detect late-phase responses that occur after work hours.

Bronchoprovocation tests. Methacholine or histamine challenge is believed to be the most sensitive test for nonspecific airway hyperresponsiveness. Such testing can be particularly valuable if it demonstrates an increase in airway responsiveness when the patient returns to work and a decrease when she is away from work. Specific inhalational challenge testing (challenging the patient with the specific agent at levels and under conditions that mimic workplace conditions) can be done for medicolegal purposes or to determine the precise agent in a complex situation. However, specific challenge testing is time-consuming, potentially dangerous, and usually should be reserved for evaluating patients for whom there is diagnostic uncertainty.

Skin tests and serologic studies. Allergy skin tests with common inhalant and food allergens can be used to establish whether the patient is atopic. When high-molecular-weight compounds are responsible for occupational asthma, skin tests with the appropriate extracts may help identify the etiologic agent. Extracts of materials such as flour, animal protein, and coffee yield positive skin test results in specifically sensitized individuals. Skin testing may also be helpful for a few low-molecular-weight compounds such as platinum salts.

IgE antibodies assayed by the radioallergosorbent test (RAST) or by enzyme-linked immunosorbent assay (ELISA) may confirm exposure to allergens such as flour, animal proteins, acid anhydrides, plicatic acid, or isocyanates. However, positive skin reactions and/or the presence of specific antibodies do not always diagnose or predict the development of clinically manifested occupational asthma.

Management

Acute asthma exacerbations. Acute asthma attacks requiring treatment in the Emergency Room should be treated with supplemental oxygen, $beta_2$-agonists, corticosteroids and, if infection is suspected, antibiotics. Hospitalization should be considered in more severe cases because a late-phase inflammatory response may occur some hours after initial evaluation.

Long-term management. Once the diagnosis of occupational asthma has been made, the proper treatment is to remove the worker from further exposure to the offending agent. This may be achieved through modifications in the workplace. It may be possible to substitute the offending agent with a safer one. Improved local exhaust ventilation and enclosure of specific processes may also be helpful. With irritant-induced asthma, the use of personal protective equipment may lower exposure to levels that do not induce bronchospasm. Chronic long-term treatment with inhaled $beta_2$-agonists and inhaled steroids allow the patient with irritant-induced asthma to remain in the workplace. Workers who are allowed to continue in the job should have regular follow-up visits, including monitoring of lung function and nonspecific airway responsiveness.

With sensitizer-induced asthma, however, it may be necessary to remove the worker completely from the workplace, because exposure to even minute quantities of the offending agent may induce bronchospasm. The patient should be considered 100% impaired on a permanent basis for

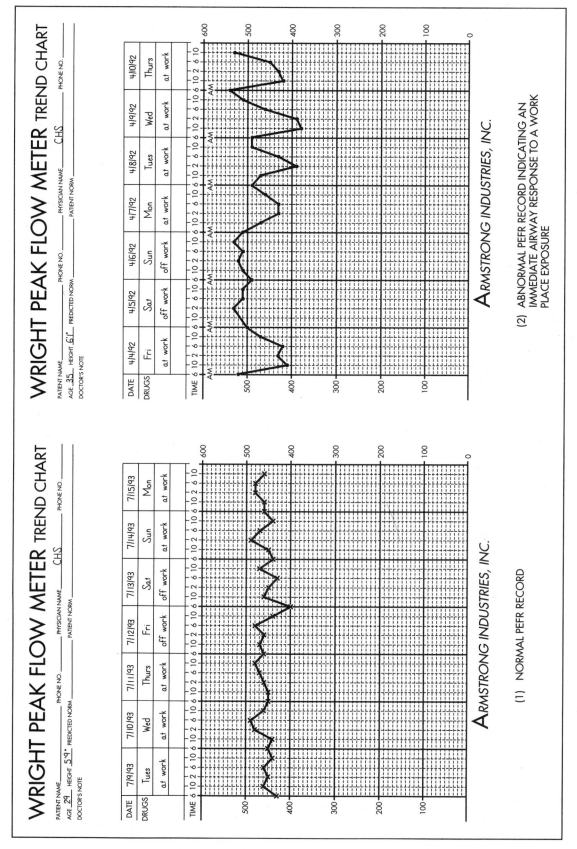

Fig. 18-3 (1) Normal PEFR record. (2) Abnormal PEFR record indicating an immediate airway response to a work place exposure.

the job that caused the illness and for other jobs with exposure to the same causative agent.

General measures. In addition to avoiding specific agents at work, the patient should be encouraged to avoid exposure to other irritants that may exacerbate asthma, such as welding fumes, dusts, and tobacco smoke. Minimizing exposure to household dust and avoiding exposure to household pets also may help.

Prevention. Prevention of further occupational asthma should be considered in all workplaces where cases are diagnosed. This can be achieved primarily through environmental control of processes known to involve exposure to potential sensitizers and irritants. Protecting workers by using appropriate ventilation systems or respiratory protective equipment should be recommended. Avoiding high exposure from leaks and spills that may initiate the development of occupational asthma is essential. Educating the work force in proper handling procedures also can contribute to reducing the incidence and prevalence of the condition.

Severity of disease. Once occupational asthma has been diagnosed, an attempt should be made to classify the degree of impairment or disability. An approach to evaluating impairment in patients with asthma was recently promulgated by the American Thoracic Society. A key issue is that asthma is a dynamic disease that does not generally result in a static level of impairment. The criteria used for impairment rating are (1) the degree of baseline airway obstruction by spirometry, (2) measurement of airway responsiveness, and (3) medication requirements. Assessment for impairment or disability should be reported after optimization of therapy and whenever the patient's condition changes substantially, whether for better or worse.

Natural history. Several follow-up studies of patients with occupational asthma caused by such agents as diisocyanates, flour, antibiotics, and Western red cedar showed persistence of symptoms and nonspecific airway hyperresponsiveness for periods up to 11 years after removal from the offending agent. Factors that affect the long-term prognosis of the patient with occupational asthma are the duration of symptoms before diagnosis, the lung function test values, and the degree of nonspecific airway hyperresponsiveness. Those who do poorly have a delayed diagnosis, lower lung function values, and a greater nonspecific airway hyperresponsiveness; hence the importance of early diagnosis and early removal from further exposure to the causative agent.

Examples of occupational asthma

Asthma caused by diisocyanates. Chemicals of the diisocyanate group are widely used in indus-tries manufacturing surface coatings such as polyurethane, insulation materials, car upholstery, and furniture. The most commonly used diisocyanate is toluene diisocyanate (TDI) in the form of the 2,4 and 2,6 isomers. Because of its high vapor pressure, the less volatile agent methylene diphenyl diisocyanate (MDI) is used in some production processes. Other diisocyanates, such as hexamethylene diisocyanate (HDI), naphthylene diisocyanate (NDI), and isophorone diisocyanate (IPDI) also have commercial uses. These chemicals are all highly reactive because of the $-N = C = O$ groups, which easily react with biologic molecules and thus are potent respiratory tract irritants. Inflammation of the upper respiratory tract occurs in almost everyone exposed to TDI levels of 0.5 ppm or more.

Five major patterns of airway response to TDI have been described in humans: (1) occupational asthma of the sensitizer type, which occurs in 5% to 10% of workers weeks to months after the onset of exposure; (2) chemical bronchitis; (3) acute but asymptomatic deterioration of respiratory function during a work shift; (4) chronic deterioration of respiratory function associated with chronic exposure to low doses; and (5) persistent asthma or RADS after exposure to high doses.

Asthma caused by exposure to dusts of cotton, flax, hemp, or jute. Asthma caused by exposure to cotton dust (byssinosis) occurs in certain workers in the cotton textile industry. The characteristic symptoms are chest tightness, coughing, and labored breathing 1 to 2 hours after the patient returns to work after several days off. The symptoms usually resolve overnight and on subsequent days become milder until by the end of the work week the worker may become asymptomatic. The prevalence of byssinosis is higher in individuals with a longer exposure history and with higher respirable dust exposure (such as during opening and carding) and lowest in those with a shorter exposure history and lesser dust exposure (such as during slashing or weaving).

The pathogenic mechanism underlying the disease remains unclear. Several immunologic and nonimmunologic mechanisms have been postulated. Dust extracts can cause direct release of histamine and contain bacteria that can induce a number of inflammatory responses.

Asthma caused by metal salts. Complex salts of platinum, used in electroplating, platinum refinery operations, manufacture of fluorescent screens, and jewelry making, are known to give rise to occupational asthma. Specific IgE antibodies to platinum salts conjugated to human serum albumin have been found in sensitized workers by RAST. Rhinitis and urticaria frequently accompany the asthma, and this triad sometimes is called "platinosis." Nickel, vanadium, chromium, and cobalt are among other metals known to cause occupational asthma.

Asthma caused by anhydrides. Epoxy resins often contain acid anhydrides as curing or hardening agents. Phytalic anhydride, trimellitic anhydride (TMA), and tetrachlorophthalic anhydride (TCPA) are several of the more commonly used acid anhydrides. Occupational asthma occurs in a small percentage of exposed workers. The serum of affected workers typically contains specific IgE antibodies against acid anhydride–protein conjugates.

Trimellitic anhydride exposure can give rise to four clinical syndromes: (1) symptoms of immediate airway irritation; (2) immediate rhinitis and asthma; (3) late asthma with systemic symptoms of fever and malaise; and (4) infiltrative lung disease (hemorrhagic alveolitis) with hemoptysis and anemia.

Asthma caused by wood dusts. A wide variety of wood dusts are known to cause rhinitis and asthma. Western red cedar is the best described. This wood contains plicatic acid and a number of volatile compounds such as tropolones, which are believed to be responsible for causing asthma through a combination of immunologic and non-immunologic mechanisms. There often is a long period between onset of exposure and onset of symptoms, and asthma develops in only a small proportion of those exposed. A small dose of plicatic acid can induce a severe asthmatic attack in a sensitized individual.

Hypersensitivity pneumonitis

Hypersensitivity pneumonitis, also known as extrinsic allergic alveolitis, refers to an immunologically mediated inflammatory disease of the lung parenchyma that is induced by inhalation of a variety of organic dusts. Although there are many different types of hypersensitivity pneumonitis, the basic clinical and pathologic findings are similar regardless of the nature of the inhaled dust. The mechanism or mechanisms by which inhaled dusts induce hypersensitivity pneumonitis are not fully understood; however, it is clear that the disease process depends on a complex interaction between environmental, genetic, and other host-related factors. Although specific IgG antibodies to the offending agent appear necessary, they are not sufficient, because only a minority of exposed workers with such antibodies actually develop the disease.

Numerous agents are known to cause hypersensitivity pneumonitis (Table 18-6). Occupational exposure in farmers, mushroom workers, sugar refining workers, grain workers, and wood workers have all been associated with hypersensitivity pneumonitis. In addition, exposure to hypersensitivity pneumonitis–inducing agents may occur from contaminated central heating and humidification units. Potential causative agents of hypersensitivity pneumonitis include animal and plant products, low-molecular-weight chemicals (TDI, MDI), and microorganisms (actinomycetes, bacteria, fungi, amoebas). One of the better known exposure settings is pigeon breeding, where avian proteins are the offending antigens.

Evaluation. Exposure to an appropriate antigen in a sensitized individual may result in either an acute or chronic syndrome.

Acute form. The acute and more common form of hypersensitivity pneumonitis usually occurs within 4 to 6 hours after intense exposure to the offending antigen. Symptoms of chills, fever, malaise, myalgia, coughing, headache, and dyspnea are commonly noted. Physical examination may reveal an ill, cyanotic patient with bibasilar inspiratory crackles on chest auscultation. Acute hypersensitivity pneumonitis often is misdiagnosed as an acute viral syndrome or pneumonia, because it tends to closely mimic these conditions. Laboratory findings may show a leukocytosis with

Table 18-6 Examples of hypersensitivity pneumonitis

Disease	Source of antigen	Antigen
Farmer's lung disease	Moldy hay	Thermophilic actinomycetes
Bagassosis	Moldy pressed sugar cane	Thermophilic actinomycetes
Mushroom worker's disease	Moldy compost	Thermophilic actinomycetes
Humidifier lung	Contaminated humidifiers	Thermophilic actinomycetes
Maple bark disease	Contaminated maple logs	*Cryptostroma corticale*
Sauna taker's disease	Sauna water	*Pullularia* spp.
Miller's lung	Wheat weevils	*Sitophilus granarius*
Pigeon breeder's disease	Pigeon droppings	Altered pigeon serum (IgA?)
Malt worker's lung	Malt dust	*Aspergillus clavatus*
Sequoiosis	Contaminated wood dust	*Graphium* spp., *Pullularia* spp.
Detergent worker's disease	Detergent	*Bacillus subtilis*

a left shift and eosinophilia in some patients, and elevation of acute phase–reactant serum proteins. ABG values may show hypoxemià, which worsens with exercise.

Chest x-ray findings may be completely normal even in symptomatic individuals. Typically, however, the acute phase is associated with a reticulonodular pattern or general coarsening of bronchovascular markings. Often, ill-defined, patchy densities that tend to coalesce may be seen. These infiltrates usually are bilaterally distributed but can be focal and frequently spare the apices.

Pulmonary function testing may show a decrease in the FEV_1 and FVC with an unchanged ratio consistent with a restrictive impairment. A decrease in pulmonary diffusing capacity reflecting impaired gas exchange also is typical of the acute presentation. In rare cases a patient may develop a late-phase reaction. The acute form generally progresses for up to 18 to 24 hours and then begins to resolve. The syndrome may subsequently recur with reexposure to the antigen.

Chronic form. Recurrent low-level exposure to an antigen that causes hypersensitivity pneumonitis may result in the insidious onset of chronic, irreversible interstitial lung disease. Progressive respiratory impairment with the symptoms of coughing, dyspnea, weakness, and weight loss may develop without acute episodes. Physical examination may show central cyanosis, digit clubbing, and auscultatory signs of advanced pulmonary fibrosis. Chest x-ray findings include diffuse interstitial fibrosis and progressive loss of lung volume. Pulmonary function testing shows a restrictive pulmonary impairment with a decreased diffusing capacity.

The diagnosis of hypersensitivity pneumonitis should be suspected in patients with episodic respiratory symptoms and signs of restrictive disease. A careful history can elicit the onset of respiratory symptoms with exposure to the offending antigen. The temporal relationship of symptom development after exposure is crucial to the diagnosis. Additional supporting evidence is provided by the remission of symptoms after extended absence from the source of the antigen and the reappearance of symptoms on resumption of exposure.

Serologic studies demonstrating specific IgG precipitating antibodies by gel diffusing techniques are positive in most patients with hypersensitivity pneumonitis, although such antibodies may also be detected in healthy exposed individuals. False-negative results are frequently due to the wrong choice of antigens.

Skin tests have not been particularly helpful in the diagnosis of hypersensitivity pneumonitis, because many of the preparations are nonspecifically irritating, and as many as 50% of healthy exposed individuals have positive responses.

Inhalational challenge studies with the suspected antigen may assist in the diagnosis of hypersensitivity pneumonitis. Antigen extracts may be administered in an aerosolized form and followed by frequent pulmonary function testing. Specific challenge testing should be conducted only by a laboratory experienced in the technique. Although such challenges provide the "gold standard" for confirming a direct relationship between a suspected offending antigen and the disease process, workplace studies involving the actual conditions of patient exposure are safer and usually easier to conduct.

Analysis of bronchoalveolar lavage fluid obtained by fiberoptic bronchoscopy in patients with hypersensitivity pneumonitis often demonstrates an increased number of cells with a significant elevation in the percentage of T lymphocytes. In contrast to sarcoidosis, where the T lymphocyte elevation is primarily CD4+ helper cells, in hypersensitivity pneumonitis, the elevation is composed of CD8+ suppressor cells.

In difficult cases, lung biopsy may be necessary to confirm the diagnosis. Open lung biopsy is preferred because transbronchial biopsy may not provide adequate tissue for pathologic inspection.

Management. The key to successful treatment of hypersensitivity pneumonitis is avoiding the antigen. This may be achieved through engineering controls or improved workplace ventilation, or both. Respiratory protective equipment may also help reduce the patient's exposure. If the symptoms persist despite these measures, the patient must be removed from the job causing the exposure.

Pharmacologic agents are required only in the treatment of moderate to severe episodes of acute hypersensitivity pneumonitis. Corticosteroids remain the mainstay of treatment; tapering doses of prednisone, beginning with 60 mg/day, often are required over 2 to 3 weeks. Therapy should be continued until there is significant clinical and radiographic improvement. If bronchospasm is present, $beta_2$-agonists and oxygen should be administered. Intensive care unit support may be needed in particularly severe cases.

Patients with a diagnosis of hypersensitivity pneumonitis should have frequent follow-up, especially if continued exposure to antigen is possible. Significant pulmonary morbidity may occur if persistent exposure is allowed.

Inhalational fevers

The term "inhalational fevers" refers to a variety of syndromes that involve short-term but debilitating flulike symptoms (Table 18-7). They occur after inhalation of relatively high concentrations of metal fumes, combustion products of fluorinated resins, endotoxin-contaminated dust, and dust from moldy silage, grain, or compost. Unlike occupational asthma and hypersensitivity pneumonitis, which require either susceptibility or sensitization, the attack rate for the inhalational fevers is high; most people experience symptoms as a result of high-level exposure to the etiologic agents. This section does not attempt to deal with all the known syndromes; rather, it describes two representative entities: metal fume fever and polymer fume fever.

Metal fume fever. When certain metals are heated to their melting point, metal oxide fumes are generated. The particle size of the generated fumes ranges from 0.1 μm to 1 μm in diameter, although aggregation, with the formation of larger particles, readily occurs. Inhaling freshly formed fumes can cause metal fume fever, an acute, self-limiting, flulike illness. The most common cause of this syndrome is inhalation of zinc oxide, which is generated from molten bronze or from welding galvanized steel. Less commonly implicated are oxides of other metals, including cadmium, copper, and magnesium. The underlying pathogenesis of metal fume fever is poorly understood. One hypothesis is that fume inhalation causes fever by stimulating an inflammatory response in the lungs, with an associated release of cytokines that cause systemic symptoms.

Evaluation. It is estimated that more than 700,000 workers in the United States are involved in welding operations; thus the potential for inhalational exposure and metal fume fever is great. The clinical syndrome begins 3 to 10 hours after exposure to metal oxides. Typically the patient notices a metallic taste associated with throat irritation, followed within several hours by the onset of a nonproductive cough and dyspnea. Fever, chills,

and malaise are common. Occasionally nausea, vomiting, headache, and myalgia are noted. Physical examination during the episode may show a febrile patient with crackles and wheezing on pulmonary auscultation. Laboratory evaluation frequently reveals a leukocytosis with a left shift and an elevated serum lactate dehydrogenase. The chest x-ray film often is normal but may show an increase in the bronchovascular markings. Pulmonary function tests often show a transient decrease in vital capacity and pulmonary diffusing capacity. ABG measurements may show hypoxemia in severe cases. Symptoms generally peak at 18 hours and resolve spontaneously, with complete resolution of abnormalities within 1 to 2 days.

Management. Treatment of metal fume fever is directed toward alleviating symptoms. Controlling the elevated body temperature with antipyretics and oxygen therapy for hypoxemia remain the mainstays of therapy. There is no evidence that steroid therapy has any benefit. Prevention relies on appropriate environmental controls. There are no good data on the long-term sequelae of repeated exposure.

Polymer fume fever. A syndrome similar to metal fume fever may occur after inhalation of combustion products of polytetrafluorethylene resins (Teflon) and polyvinyl fluoride. The properties of Teflon — strength, thermal stability, and chemical inertness — make it a widely used product in the manufacture of nonstick cooking utensils, radios, and other electrical appliances, and as an insulating material. Once Teflon is heated to temperatures above 300° C (572° F), numerous degradation products are formed which, when inhaled, cause the syndrome. Potential for exposure arises during welding of metal coated with Teflon, during the operation of molding machines, and while smoking cigarettes contaminated with the

Table 18-7 Examples of inhalational fevers

Illness	Inhalation exposure
Humidifier fever	*Micropolyspora faeni* – contaminated aerosols from forced air conditioning and humidification system
Pontiac fever	Aerosols of *Legionella pneumophilia* – contaminated water
Metal fume fever	Inhalation of freshly formed metal oxides or respirable metal dust
Polymer fume fever	Inhalation of the pyrolysis products of tetrafluorethylene resins (polytetrafluroethylene and polyvinyl fluoride)
Mill fever	Inhalation of dusts containing cotton, flax, soft hemp, or kapok (possible role for gram-negative bacterial endotoxin contamination of these dusts)
Organic dust toxic syndrome (ODTS)	Inhalation of organic dust from hay, moldy silage or other organic dusts (these mixtures contain bacteria, bacterial products, fungal spores, hyphae, feed grain silage, animal danders, pollens, and insect parts)

polymer. The pathogenesis of polymer fume fever is unknown.

Evaluation. Exposure to a high concentration of polymer fumes causes a fever to develop within several hours. Often this occurs toward the end of the work shift or in the evening after work. Chest pain or tightness associated with dyspnea and sometimes coughing are followed by malaise, myalgia, fever, and chills. Physical examination reveals a febrile patient with tachycardia and, in the vast majority of cases, a normal pulmonary examination. Leukocytosis with a left shift occasionally is seen. The chest x-ray film usually is normal, as are pulmonary function tests. The symptoms are self-limiting and resolve within 12 to 48 hours. Exposure to high concentrations of polymer fumes may lead to the development of severe pulmonary edema in some individuals. In such cases the symptoms, signs, and radiographic features are similar to those for pulmonary edema from other causes.

Management. Although recurrent attacks are a source of discomfort to the patient, there is no scientific literature demonstrating long-term, adverse health sequelae from recurrent episodes of polymer fume fever. Despite this, a conservative approach to management includes periodic follow-up of those who have experienced recurrent episodes. Finally, as with most types of occupational respiratory disease, the condition can be prevented through the use of appropriate environmental controls to reduce exposure.

Hard-metal disease

Hard metal is a cemented alloy of tungsten carbide with cobalt, although other metals such as titanium, tantalum, chromium, molybdenum, or nickel may also be added. These cemented carbides have found wide industrial use because of their properties of extreme hardness, strength, and heat resistance. They are primarily used in the manufacture of cutting tools and drill tips.

Workers exposed to hard metal are at risk of developing interstitial lung disease, the so-called hard-metal disease, and occupational asthma. The putative cause of both these diseases is the cobalt constituent of hard metal. Some workers may have features of hard-metal–induced airway and parenchymal diseases. Individuals at risk for these diseases are those that work in the manufacture of the alloy, grinders and sharpeners of tungsten carbide tools, diamond polishers and others who use disks containing cobalt, and metal coaters who use powdered hard metal.

Evaluation. Occupational asthma caused by cobalt in hard-metal workers is similar to that caused by other low-molecular-weight sensitizers.

Thus the remainder of this section focuses on hard-metal–induced interstitial lung disease. Patients may complain of symptoms of dyspnea on exertion, coughing, sputum production, chest tightness, and fatigue. Physical examination may show evidence of respiratory compromise with accessory respiratory muscle use and, in advanced cases, evidence of cyanosis. Digital clubbing and pulmonary crackles on chest auscultation may also be observed.

Chest x-ray abnormalities include both rounded and irregular opacities that are bilateral and that can occur in any lung zone. There are no associated plain film abnormalities of the pleura or lymph nodes to aid in the differential diagnosis.

Pulmonary function testing in patients with hard-metal disease may show evidence of both a restrictive ventilatory impairment and decreased diffusing capacity. These abnormalities may be present even if the chest x-ray film is normal.

Management. The primary treatment of hard-metal disease is removing the patient from further exposure, and the response may range from complete recovery to continued progression of the disease. Because the disease tends to progress, aggressive therapy with prolonged courses of steroids or immunosuppressives (e.g., azathioprine or cyclophosphamide), or both, have been tried. However, the disease may progress despite prolonged therapy. A conservative approach of complete removal from cobalt exposure may be wise for patients with interstitial lung disease because at least one case report exists of a worker who developed rapidly fatal lung disease with continued exposure to cobalt.

The following features of hard-metal–induced interstitial lung disease should be kept in mind: (1) a long history of exposure is not necessary; (2) relatively rapid progression to impairment is common; (3) the diagnosis often is made on the basis of pathologic examination of lung tissue rather than by clinical evaluation; (4) the disease may not resolve after exposure ceases; and (5) cytotoxic therapy may play a role in treatment.

Pneumoconioses

The pneumoconioses are a group of lung conditions caused by deposition of mineral dust in the lung and the subsequent reaction of lung tissue to this dust. The major diseases in this group are silicosis, asbestosis, and coal worker's pneumoconiosis.

Silicosis. Silicosis is a parenchymal lung disease caused by inhalation of silicon dioxide, or silica, in crystalline form. Silica is a major component of rock and sand. Workers who may be exposed include miners, sandblasters, foundry workers, glassblowers, quarry workers, ceramic workers, and tunnelers (Table 18-8).

Exposure to silica can lead to one of three disease patterns: (1) chronic simple silicosis, which usually follows many decades of exposure to respirable dust with less than 30% quartz; (2) subacute/accelerated silicosis, which generally follows shorter, heavier exposures (4 to 8 years); and (3) acute silicosis, which often is seen following intense exposure over several months to fine dust with a high silica content.

Chronic silicosis is characterized by the formation of silicotic nodules in the pulmonary parenchyma and hilar lymph nodes. The lesions in the hilar lymph nodes tend to calcify and eventually may impinge on or erode into airways. Although calcification of the hilar lymph nodes in an "eggshell" pattern is not always seen, its presence with diffuse, nodular lung disease indicates silicosis. Lung parenchymal involvement tends to have a predilection for the upper lobes. Progressive massive fibrosis (PMF) can complicate a minority of cases; this is caused by the coalescence of small lesions into larger fibrotic masses, often with obliteration of blood vessels and bronchioles. Progressive massive fibrosis tends to occur in the upper lung fields, and the lesions may cavitate secondary to ischemic necrosis.

Accelerated silicosis is similar to chronic silicosis except that the time span is shorter and the complication of PMF is more common.

Acute silicosis is a rare condition seen in individuals who are exposed to high concentrations of free silica dust with particles ranging from 0.5 to 3 μm in diameter. Such exposure often occurs in the absence of adequate respiratory protection. The characteristic findings differ from chronic silicosis in that the lungs show consolidation without silicotic nodules, and the alveolar spaces are filled with fluid similar to that found in pulmonary alveolar proteinosis.

The pathogenesis of silicosis is believed to involve cytotoxicity secondary to the chemical properties of crystalline silica. The inhaled silica particles are deposited in the distal airways and then phagocytosed by alveolar macrophages. The phagocytosed particles cause direct chemical damage to lysosomal membranes, leakage of proteolytic enzymes, and subsequent cell death. This cytotoxic effect is believed to be the first step in the subsequent development of fibrosis.

Evaluation. Chronic simple silicosis has few symptoms and signs. With complicated silicosis involving progressive fibrosis, increasing dyspnea is noted, initially with exertion and progressing to dyspnea at rest. Physical examination often is normal. Chest pain and digital clubbing are not features of the condition, and other diagnoses should be sought if these are present.

Chest x-ray films usually reveal small, round opacities in both lungs, with a predilection for the upper lung zones. If an adequate occupational history is obtained from the patient, along with a thorough review of the chest x-ray film, the diagnosis of silicosis should not present any great difficulty. Pulmonary function testing in patients with simple silicosis usually is normal but occasionally may demonstrate evidence of a mild restrictive ventilatory defect and decreased lung compliance. In addition, a mild obstructive impairment occasionally is found in patients with simple silicosis, often as a result of chronic bronchitis caused by nonspecific dust effects or smoking, or both. Complicated chronic silicosis is associated with greater reductions in lung volume, decreased diffusing capacity, and hypoxemia with exercise.

The incidence of mycobacterial disease, both typical and atypical, is higher in silicosis. Fungal diseases (especially cryptococcosis, blastomycosis, and coccidioidomycosis) are also seen with greater frequency. Impaired macrophage function caused by silica-induced cytotoxicity may be responsible for the increased incidence of mycobacterial and fungal infections. Certain connective tissue disorders, such as scleroderma, also are noted more often in patients with silicosis.

Management. There is no known treatment for silicosis, therefore management is directed toward preventing progression and complications. Continued exposure should be avoided, either through

Table 18-8 Occupations at risk for silicosis

Industry	Occupation
Ceramics: manufacture of pottery and stoneware	Workers at any of the dry stages of the process
Foundries: ferrous metals, nonferrous metals	Molder, knockout man, fettlers, coremakers, casters
Quarrying: granite, sandstone, slate, and sand	Drillers, hammerers, diggers
Mining: underground and surface	Miners, drillers, tunnelers, developers, stoppers
Abrasives	Sandblasters, abrasive manufacturing workers
Miscellaneous	Dental technicians, glass makers

environmental controls or by removing the patient from the source of exposure. Increased surveillance for tuberculosis should be instituted. If a patient with silicosis has a positive result on the tuberculin skin test, isoniazid (300 mg/day) should be prescribed for 1 year. With acute silicosis there may be a role for whole-lung lavage, because progression to severe respiratory insufficiency and death is common with this disorder.

The prognosis for patients with chronic silicosis is good, especially if they are removed from exposure. The major complications are mycobacterial or fungal infections and PMF. Mortality remains high in those who develop the latter complication.

Asbestosis. Asbestos is the name for the fibrous forms of a group of mineral silicates. The most common types of asbestos are chrysotile, amosite, crocidolite, and anthophyllite. The properties of durability, heat resistance, and ability to be woven into textiles have made asbestos a popular material for a wide variety of industrial applications. Common occupational exposure involves asbestos mining and milling, the manufacture or installation of insulation for ships or buildings, asbestos cement manufacturing, and asbestos textile manufacturing. Many insulators, sheet metal workers, pipe fitters, boilermakers, and welders are known to have been subjected to significant exposure.

Asbestosis refers to the diffuse interstitial pulmonary fibrosis caused by inhalation of asbestos fibers. The inhaled fibers are deposited in the alveolar ducts and terminal respiratory bronchioles, where they are phagocytosed by macrophages. Type 1 alveolar epithelial cells are injured by the transepithelial migration of asbestos fibers from the air space to the interstitium and by mediators released by alveolar macrophages as they phagocytose free fibers reaching the alveolar air sacs. A peribronchiolar inflammatory response ensues, involving fibroblast stimulation and eventual fibrosis. Many factors are thought to play a role in the initiation and progression of the disease, including the type and size of fiber, the intensity and duration of exposure, the patient's age, a history of cigarette smoking, and individual host responses. A dose-response relationship exists, such that pulmonary asbestosis is more common in individuals with a higher exposure level. Once pulmonary asbestosis has begun, it may progress even if the patient is removed from continued exposure. Finally, there is a considerable latency period (approximately 20 years) between exposure and development of the disease.

Evaluation. The clinical diagnosis of pulmonary asbestosis is made by a thorough exposure history, clinical examination, pertinent imaging studies, and pulmonary function testing. The clinical symptoms are indistinguishable from those of any other gradually progressive, interstitial pulmonary fibrosing disorder. Progressive dyspnea and nonproductive cough are the most prominent symptoms. Bibasilar crackles with a "Velcro" quality can be auscultated over the posterolateral chest in the mid to late phase of inspiration. The crackles of asbestosis are unaffected by coughing.

Imaging studies that are helpful are the chest x-ray film and CT scanning of the chest. The posteroanterior chest x-ray film shows characteristic irregular or linear opacities distributed throughout the lung fields but more prominent in the lower zones. There is loss of definition of the heart border. Possibly the most useful finding is a pleural thickening, which does not commonly occur with other diseases causing interstitial pulmonary fibrosis. Diaphragmatic or pericardial calcification is almost a pathognomonic sign of asbestos exposure. ILO classification of chest x-ray films by a NIOSH-certified "B reader" can further assist in the diagnosis of less obvious cases of pulmonary asbestosis. Conventional chest CT scanning is more sensitive than chest x-ray films for detecting pleural disease but not for parenchymal disease. High-resolution CT scanning is the most sensitive imaging method for detecting early asbestosis.

Depending on the disease's severity, pulmonary function testing shows varying degrees of restrictive impairment (decreased FVC and total lung capacity), decreased diffusing capacity, and reduced pulmonary compliance. Because asbestosis begins as a peribronchiolar process, reduced flow rates at low lung volumes, indicating small airway obstruction, may be seen.

Management. There is no known treatment for pulmonary asbestosis. Fortunately, only a minority of those exposed are likely to develop radiographically evident disease, and, of those who do, only a small percentage develop any significant pulmonary symptoms or pulmonary impairment. The worker with asbestosis should be removed from further asbestos exposure because the risk that parenchymal scarring will progress appears to increase with cumulative asbestos exposure. Any other factors that may contribute to respiratory disease should be reduced or eliminated. This is especially important in the case of cigarette smoking because some evidence indicates that this habit may contribute to the initiation and progression of disease.

Preventing asbestos-related lung injury involves strict control of the workplace environment to reduce exposure. In addition, OSHA requires medical surveillance of all currently exposed workers.

Coal worker's pneumoconiosis. Two different respiratory injury syndromes may result from inhalation of excessive amounts of coal dust: chronic bronchitis and coal worker's pneumoconiosis (CWP). This section deals with the latter syndrome. Miners who work at the coal face in underground mining and in transportation of coal within the mine are at a high risk of contracting this disease. It is more commonly seen with the mining of anthracite than bituminous coal. A heavy coal dust burden is required to induce significant disease, and the condition is rarely seen in those who have spent less than 20 years underground. Other occupations at risk for CWP are those involved in the mining and milling of graphite in carbon plants and in the manufacture of carbon electrodes.

The coal macule is the primary lesion in CWP. It is formed when the inhaled dust burden exceeds the mucociliary clearance mechanism of the lung. This leads to retention of coal dust in the terminal respiratory units. Prolonged retention causes lung fibroblasts to secrete a limiting layer of reticulin around the dust collection. This in turn leads to the formation of the coal nodule, and, with progressive enlargement of these lesions, the bronchiole wall weakens and the bronchiole dilates to create a focal area of centrilobular emphysema. Initially there is a predilection for the upper lung lobes, but, as the disease progresses, the lower lobes become involved. A small proportion of miners (fewer than 5%) develop complicated disease. Progressive massive fibrosis (PMF), similar to that described for silicosis, can occur even if there is no further exposure to coal dust. Progressive massive fibrosis is characterized by the development of bulky, irregular masses in the posterior segments of the upper lobes and apical segment of the lower lobes. As in silicosis, PMF can lead to respiratory insufficiency. Finally, Caplan's syndrome may occur in coal miners with rheumatoid arthritis; this disorder is characterized by the appearance of rapidly evolving, rounded densities on chest x-ray films. These densities have a propensity to cavitate and histologically are composed of layers of necrotic collagen and coal dust. The pulmonary disease may precede or coincide with the onset of the arthritis.

Evaluation. Coughing and sputum production are common symptoms among coal miners and often are the result of chronic bronchitis from dust inhalation. In complicated CWP, the patient complains of increasing dyspnea, initially with exertion, later at rest. In rare cases the patient reports a cough that produces small amounts of black sputum, which comes from rupture of a cavitating PMF lesion. The physical signs of emphysema (hyperinflated chest, resonant percussion note, distant breath sounds) may be elicited. Severe PMF may be associated with the symptoms and signs of pulmonary hypertension.

In simple CWP the chest x-ray film shows small, rounded opacities in the lung parenchyma. First seen in the upper zones, they may involve the lower zones in the later stage of the disease. In contrast to silicosis, "eggshell" calcification of the hilar lymph nodes is unusual. Complicated CWP/PMF is diagnosed when the parenchymal opacities exceed 1 cm in diameter.

Pulmonary function testing varies, depending on the stage of the disease. In simple CWP, no significant pulmonary function abnormalities are seen. In complicated disease, a mixed restrictive and obstructive picture is seen, with decreased diffusing capacity and abnormal arterial blood gases. Interpretation of any pulmonary function tests in a coal miner should be undertaken with the knowledge that she can develop both chronic bronchitis and CWP.

Management. In simple CWP, the patient is almost always asymptomatic and the disease follows a benign course. In complicated disease, the patient can have mild to severe respiratory symptoms and significant pulmonary impairment. In such cases, depending on the degree of impairment, the worker should be removed from continued exposure to dust. Unlike with silicosis, no increase is seen in either pulmonary tuberculosis or fungal infections of the lung. In all cases dust exposure should be minimized through strict environmental controls and worker respiratory protection.

Other pneumoconioses. Other mineral dusts capable of causing pulmonary parenchymal fibrosis include graphite (which causes a disease similar to CWP), kaolin and calcined diatomaceous earth (which cause a silicosis-like disease), and talc (which causes a disease that has features of both silicosis and asbestosis). Aluminum metal dust also can cause pneumoconiosis.

Beryllium disease

Beryllium is a light-weight, tensile metal with a high melting point and good alloying properties. It has a wide range of applications in modern industrial processes. Although beryllium is no longer used in the manufacture of fluorescent light tubes, it is commonly used in the ceramics, electronics, aerospace, nuclear weapons, and power industries. Workers at risk are those involved in processes that generate airborne beryllium, including melting, casting, grinding, drilling, extracting, and smelting of beryllium.

Two major syndromes result from beryllium exposure: acute and chronic beryllium disease.

Acute beryllium disease. The acute form of beryllium disease is a toxic dose–related lung injury characterized by acute irritation damage to the upper airways, bronchiolitis, chemical pneumonitis, and pulmonary edema. The intensity of exposure determines the clinical presentation with either an acute fulminating variety or an insidious variety. Clinically the condition is similar to toxic pneumonitis from other causes, and its management is not significantly different.

Chronic beryllium disease (CBD). The chronic variety is a multisystem disorder in which granulomas develop throughout the body but especially in the lung. Chronic beryllium disease is similar to sarcoidosis, and it occurs in only a small fraction of exposed individuals. There is no clear dose-response relationship, and the cause of the disease appears to involve specifically sensitized T-lymphocytes.

Evaluation. Patients with chronic beryllium disease generally have more than 2 years of beryllium exposure, and in some cases the disease develops insidiously after a latency period lasting up to 15 years. The type of exposure usually is one that generates either beryllium dust or fumes, such as welding, burning, or casting. Often a meticulously obtained occupational history is required to establish beryllium as the causative agent.

Common symptoms are dyspnea, chest pain, weight loss, fatigue, and arthralgia. Physical examination may show digital clubbing in as many as 30% of cases, cyanosis, and inspiratory crackles in the later stages of the disease. Renal calculi and palpable hepatosplenomegaly may develop in a small proportion of patients. In advanced disease, pulmonary hypertension and cor pulmonale may develop.

Hyperuricemia, hypercalciuria, and hypergammaglobulinemia occasionally are noted on laboratory testing.

Chest x-ray findings include ill-defined nodular or irregular opacities, and mild hilar adenopathy in as many as 40% of patients. Calcification of the nodules sometimes occurs. In those with relatively minor beryllium exposure, the pattern is that of a diffuse, finely granular haziness with relative sparing of the lung apices and bases.

The results of pulmonary function tests may be normal with mild disease, but often there is some degree of restrictive impairment and reduction in diffusing capacity. Resting arterial hypoxemia and further desaturation with exercise are common with moderate and severe disease.

The classic histopathologic findings on examination of lung tissue are noncaseating granulomas, which eventually lead to interstitial fibrosis. Multinucleated giant cells are seen in most cases.

Because of the similarity between CBD and sarcoidosis, several tests have evolved to help determine if beryllium exposure has occurred. The beryllium patch test gives a positive result in many patients with CBD, but unfortunately its use can no longer be advocated because it can actually cause sensitization to beryllium and exacerbations of disease in those already sensitized. The urine beryllium concentration can establish recent exposure but is unrelated to disease status. Lung tissue and lymph nodes can be analyzed for beryllium content but, as with urine testing, tissue beryllium levels merely establish exposure and do not confirm disease status. A relatively specific blood lymphocyte transformation test (LTT) is invaluable in the diagnosis of CBD. The sensitivity of LTT can be increased if lung lymphocytes obtained from bronchoalveolar lavage are used.

A new classification system has been proposed for the diagnosis of beryllium lung disease (Table 18-9). This classification relies on the LTT to confirm sensitization to beryllium and transbronchial biopsy of lung tissue to confirm the presence of disease, in addition to the usual tools of chest x-ray films and pulmonary function testing.

Management. Because of the probable hypersensitivity pathogenesis of the disease, a patient with CBD should be completely removed from further beryllium exposure. A trial of corticosteroids is warranted in symptomatic patients with documented pulmonary physiologic abnormalities, because this may induce a remission in some. If steroid therapy is initiated, objective parameters of response such as chest x-ray films and pulmonary function test results should be serially monitored to adjust appropriately the dose and duration of treatment. Because the disease has the propensity

Table 18-9 Diagnostic criteria* for beryllium lung disease

---

1. History of exposure to beryllium
2. Beryllium-specific immune response
   Positive peripheral blood LTT test
   Positive bronchoalveolar lavage LTT
3. Histopathology on lung biopsy compatible with beryllium disease
   Noncaseating granulomas, or
   Mononuclear cell infiltrates
4. Constellation of clinical findings that may include any of the following:
   Respiratory symptoms or signs;
   Reticulonodular infiltrates on chest x-ray film or other imaging technique;
   Altered pulmonary physiology with restrictive and/or obstructive physiology, decreased diffusing capacity for carbon monoxide.

---

* All four conditions must be present.

to develop into chronic irreversible pulmonary fibrosis, careful monitoring of the patient is necessary. The possibility that beryllium may be a lung carcinogen increases the importance of having the patient stop smoking.

Chronic bronchitis

Chronic bronchitis is a condition characterized by inflammation of the bronchial tree. It is manifested by a persistent cough that produces sputum on most days for at least 3 months of the year for at least 2 successive years. Inhalation of irritant dusts, fumes, and gases can cause chronic simple bronchitis, (i.e., persistent sputum production without airflow obstruction) (Table 18-10). Whether workers with chronic simple bronchitis are at risk of developing chronic airflow obstruction and permanent respiratory impairment has yet to be completely resolved. The development of permanent respiratory impairment may depend on a variety of host factors such as preexisting, nonspecific airway hyperresponsiveness, protease-antiprotease activity, and whether the worker is a cigarette smoker.

Evaluation. Once chronic bronchitis has been diagnosed, establishing a causal role for an occupational exposure often is difficult; it is based on the history obtained from the worker because no specific diagnostic tests are available. The symptoms of cough and sputum production that are temporally associated with workplace exposure should be elicited. Workers who smoke are at greater risk of developing respiratory symptoms, and a work-related contribution to their symptoms should be considered. Concomitant upper respiratory tract inflammatory symptoms, eye irritation, and an increased incidence of symptoms among coworkers are all features that suggest a work-related problem. Physical examination often is totally normal, with no evidence of pulmonary abnormality. Spirometry and expiratory flow-volume curves may or may not show evidence of obstructive airway disease. A nonsmoking worker exposed to high concentrations of an irritant at the workplace who has evidence of airflow obstruction should be suspected of having occupationally induced chronic bronchitis.

Management. Because chronic bronchitis often has a multifactorial cause, a multifocal approach to management should be taken. If the worker smokes, she should be encouraged to stop. Work exposure to the suspected agent should be reduced or eliminated. Pharmacologic agents of benefit are the beta$_2$-agonists, inhaled steroids, and inhaled anticholinergic agents. Frequent follow-up of the patient should be undertaken, with particular attention to symptoms and worsening airflow obstruction on serial spirometry.

The prognosis of patients exposed to irritants in the workplace has not been well described. However, some data suggest that accelerated loss of ventilatory function can occur. In light of this, it may be prudent to assume that all workers with chronic work-related bronchitis are at risk of developing permanent respiratory impairment. Those with worsening symptoms or lung function abnormalities should be considered for removal from further exposure.

Pleural disorders

The pleura is the serous membrane that lines the lung parenchyma, the mediastium, the diaphragm, and the rib cage. It is divided into the *visceral pleura,* which lines the lung surface, and the *parietal pleura,* which lines the remaining structures. The primary cause of occupationally induced pleural disease is asbestos dust, although talc and mica can cause benign pleural disease and zeolite can cause mesothelioma.

Benign pleural effusions. Pleural effusions resulting from asbestos exposure may occur in up to 3% of exposed individuals. The risk of developing an effusion is greater in those with heavy exposure to asbestos, and, if it does develop, it does so within 5 to 20 years of the initial exposure. A pleural effusion can be attributed to asbestos if (1) the patient has a significant history of occupational exposure, with an appropriate latent period since onset of exposure; (2) other known causes of pleural effusion can be excluded; and (3) a repeat evaluation of the effusion within a minimum of 2 years confirms that it is benign.

Table 18-10 Known or suspected causes of chronic bronchitis

Minerals	Coal
	Silica
	Silicates
	Metals (dusts and fumes)
	Oil mists
	Fiberglass
Organic substances	Cotton
	Grain
	Wood
Inorganic gases	Sulfur dioxide
	Chlorine
	Nitrogen oxides
Plastic constituents	Diisocyanates (polyurethane)
	Epichlorhydrin (epoxy)
	Acid anhydrides (epoxy)
	Phenolics
	Formaldehyde

Evaluation. Most patients who develop pleural effusions from asbestos exposure have no symptoms. Physical examination in those with large effusions may show diminished rib cage expansion, dullness to percussion, and absent air entry on the side of the effusion. Chest x-ray films typically show small to moderately large, unilateral pleural effusions. Bilateral involvement occurs in about 10% of cases. Pleural thickening may be noted, although often an effusion antedates diffuse pleural thickening. The pleural liquid is a sterile exudate with a predominance of polymorphonuclear leukocytes or mononuclear cells.

Management. As stated previously, it is essential to exclude other, more serious causes of pleural effusion. Regular follow-up and pleural fluid reevaluation are essential; there is no known treatment for the condition. The natural history is one of frequent recurrences, and in 20% of cases, extensive fibrosis of the parietal pleura develops. In most cases, however, the effusion clears spontaneously within a year without leaving any residual pleural disease. There is no evidence that a benign effusion predisposes to future development of mesothelioma.

Pleural plaques. Pleural plaques are circumscribed areas of pleural thickening that are the most common x-ray findings with chronic asbestos exposure. Plaques usually involve the parietal pleural surface and tend to occur over the central portions of the hemidiaphragm, especially at the cardiophrenic angle, and along the inferior posterolateral aspect of the lower ribs. The proportion of individuals with pleural plaques who have concomitant pulmonary asbestosis may be as high as 50%; consequently, the physician should have a high degree of suspicion for the existence or future development of pulmonary asbestosis.

Evaluation. Bilateral pleural plaques are almost invariably the result of past asbestos exposure, and their prevalence is related to the intensity of exposure and the duration since onset of exposure. Individuals with a greater exposure have a greater chance of developing plaques. In patients without pulmonary parenchymal disease, plaques rarely cause signs and symptoms. The diagnosis often is made from a routine chest x-ray film in which uncalcified plaques appear as ill-defined, misty opacifications of the middle or lower zones of the lung fields when lying at right angles to the x-ray beam. When plaques lie parallel to the beam, they appear as slightly to moderately protuberant linear or ovoid opacities along the costal or diaphragmatic margins. If calcified, they have an irregular, unevenly dense appearance. Although oblique x-ray views are recommended by some, chest CT scanning provides the most sensitive and specific technique for confirming the presence of plaques. Pathologically, the plaques are composed mainly of collagen, with little accompanying inflammation. If viewed through an electron microscope, asbestos fibers can be found in the lesions.

Management. A patient with a past history of asbestos exposure and pleural plaques on a chest x-ray film should be assessed for pulmonary asbestosis (this condition is discussed earlier in the chapter). Even if no evidence of parenchymal disease is found, the patient should be monitored yearly or every 2 years for possible development of this complication. Previously it was thought that individuals with pleural plaques and no parenchymal disease did not suffer from respiratory impairment. However, there is evidence that heavily exposed workers with radiographic evidence of plaques but no asbestosis tend to have decreased lung function in comparison to workers with similar exposure histories whose chest x-ray films are normal.

Because of the risk of bronchogenic carcinoma, cigarette smoking should be discouraged. The increased risk of lung cancer is not due to the plaques but to the cumulative dose of asbestos exposure; the plaques merely act as a marker of exposure.

Diffuse pleural thickening involving both visceral and parietal pleura also can result from past asbestos exposure. Such thickening occasionally is associated with a restrictive-type respiratory impairment, even in the absence of parenchymal asbestosis.

Mesothelioma

Malignant mesotheliomas are rare pleural tumors. As many as 80% occur in individuals exposed to asbestos. The exposure dose of asbestos may be extremely small, and the latency period between exposure and onset of disease ranges from 30 to 40 years. Crocidolite and amosite appear to be the types of asbestos fiber with the highest potential for inducing mesotheliomas. Other risk factors for developing pleural mesotheliomas are exposure to the mineral zeolite and thoracic irradiation.

Evaluation. Mesotheliomas generally manifest with the symptoms of chest pain and dyspnea. The chest pain usually is nonpleuritic and often is referred to the upper abdomen or the shoulder with diaphragmatic involvement. Other common symptoms are fever and weight loss. The clinical findings are influenced by the histologic type of the tumor. Epithelial and mixed mesotheliomas are more commonly associated with large pleural effusions, whereas mesenchymal tumors rarely have an associated effusion. Patients with the epithelial type are more likely to have supraclavicular or axillary lymph node involvement and extention to the pericardium. Those with the mesenchymal type have a higher incidence of extrapulmonary metastases.

Chest x-ray findings suggest a pleural effusion, but without either a meniscus or a contralateral shift of the mediastinal structures. In advanced cases, tumor is noted to encase the lung, the mediastinum is shifted toward the side of the tumor, and the involved hemithorax is contracted. Chest CT scans are especially helpful in the diagnosis of mesothelioma and often show a thickened pleura with a distinctive irregular or nodular internal margin.

Pleural fluid analysis shows a serosanguineous exudate that often is quite viscid. The cellular content is a mixture of mesothelial cells, differentiated and undifferentiated malignant mesothelial cells, and varying numbers of lymphocytes and polymorphonuclear leukocytes. Cytologic examination of the fluid may suggest malignant mesothelioma, but it is rarely diagnostic. An open thoracotomy or thoracoscopy with multiple biopsies usually is required to confirm the diagnosis.

Management. The treatment of malignant mesothelioma rests primarily on palliation of symptoms. Radiotherapy, chemotherapy, and surgical treatments have been attempted, but there are no good data to show that these prolong life.

Carcinoma of the respiratory tract

A number of agents found in the workplace have been implicated in the cause of carcinoma of the respiratory tract (Table 18-11). Therefore a detailed occupational exposure history should be obtained from any patient with a case of newly diagnosed carcinoma of the nasal sinuses, larynx, or lung. It is beyond the scope of this chapter to deal with these diseases, and we recommend that the reader consult a relevant textbook.

CASE STUDIES
Case 1: Occupational asthma

A 56-year-old maintenance mechanic at a rifle manufacturing plant has a history of recurrent episodes of coughing that produce yellowish sputum, and increasing exercise intolerance for the past 4 months. He has been diagnosed by his personal physician as having bronchitis and has been treated with several courses of antibiotics during this period. He is an exsmoker (30 pack-years but quit 5 years ago) who experienced no respiratory symptoms before the onset of these episodes of "bronchitis." Yesterday he developed a mildly productive cough, chest tightness, and dyspnea approximately 4 hours after cleaning the ventilation ducts of a spray booth used to coat rifle stocks with varnish. He originally thought he was "catching the flu" but came to the emergency room because of progressive dyspnea. He has waited several hours to be seen, however, and now feels better.

Physical examination reveals the patient to be somewhat anxious but in no acute respiratory dis-

Table 18-11 Occupational causes of respiratory tract cancer

Carcinoma of the nasal sinuses	
Substance	*Exposure Setting*
Nickel	Nickel refinery workers
Chromium	
Wood dusts	Carpenters
Oil mists	Lathe operators
Carcinoma of the larynx	
Substance	*Exposure Setting*
Asbestos fibers	Insulators and friction product manufacturing workers
Sulfuric acid	Sulfuric acid mist during pickling operations in the steel industry
Bronchogenic carcinoma	
Substance	*Exposure Setting*
Asbestos	Insulation workers
Arsenic	Smelting of copper, zinc, and lead; pesticide production
Bix (chloromethyl) ether	Production workers
Chromium (hexavalent)	Pigment manufacturing, leather manufacturing, chromium ore processing, electroplating
Polycyclic aromatic hydrocarbons	Coke oven workers, rubber workers, aluminum reduction workers, roofers
Mustard gas	Production workers, soldiers
Nickel	Nickel refining
Radiation	Uranium mining, hard rock mining

tress. His vital signs are: blood pressure (BP), 160/94 mm Hg; pulse, 100; respiratory rate, 24; afebrile. The remainder of the examination is within normal limits, except that he coughs repeatedly with forced exhalations and has a somewhat prolonged expiratory phase on chest auscultation. The chest x-ray film and complete blood count (CBC) are normal.

Additional questioning shows that the patient worked for 15 years as a plumber and pipe fitter in another section of the rifle plant. As a result of layoffs, he was transferred to the finishing area a little less than a year ago. About 6 months ago, during a temporary shutdown, he spent 1 solid week cleaning varnish spray booths without experiencing any respiratory symptoms. He wears a throw-away dust mask when cleaning the spray booths. He has no history of allergies or asthma. No coworkers are ill.

A phone call to the occupational health nurse at the rifle plant reveals that the varnish used in the spray booth is a two-part polyurethane compound that contains toluene diisocyanate (TDI). Spirometry in the emergency room is difficult for the patient to perform because of the coughing spasms but shows a slightly decreased FEV_1/FVC ratio (0.68) consistent with a mild obstructive defect.

The patient's history of episodic respiratory symptoms coupled with mild airway obstruction suggests the diagnosis of asthma. Because of his history of intermittent exposure to TDI, it is likely that he has occupational asthma. The work-related nature of the asthma can be confirmed by cross-shift spirometry on a day when there is TDI exposure or with serial peak flow measurements over several weeks during which such exposure occurs. The patient should not be exposed further to TDI.

Case 2: Toxic inhalational injury

A 32-year-old meat cutter at a local packing company is taken by ambulance to the emergency room after an explosion at the plant. He was in good health before the explosion. He was trapped in a relatively enclosed area of the plant for approximately 10 minutes after the explosion. He was exposed to a cloud of gas that burned his eyes, nose, and throat and caused him to feel nauseated and to vomit. His eyes, nose, and throat are still "burning," and he developed a headache approximately 20 minutes after being rescued. His vision is slightly blurred. Several coworkers who were also taken to the emergency room have similar but somewhat less intense symptoms.

Additional questioning reveals that he has worked at the packing plant for the past 10 years without health problems except for carpal tunnel syndrome of his right wrist, which required surgical release approximately 3 years ago. He has no allergies and no history of asthma. He has smoked a pack of cigarettes a day since age 18.

Physical examination shows the patient to be in considerable distress, primarily because of eye irritation. His vital signs are: BP, 150/92; pulse, 90; respiratory rate, 22; afebrile. His conjunctivae are inflamed, and his corneas are somewhat clouded. There is excessive tearing, and the nasal and pharyngeal mucosa are inflamed. Auscultation of the chest reveals inspiratory stridor and expiratory wheezing. The remainder of the examination is normal. The chest x-ray film is normal, as are routine blood tests.

Several firefighters who helped evacuate the workers from the plant after the incident think that a tank of ammonia used as a refrigerant exploded. The patient's arterial blood gases on room air are: pH, 7.45; carbon dioxide pressure (PCO_2), 32 mm Hg; oxygen pressure (PO_2), 75 mm Hg. The peak expiratory flow rate (PEFR), using a portable meter in the emergency room, is 250 L/minute (approximately 50% of the predicted value).

Ammonia is so irritating to the eyes and upper respiratory tract that exposed individuals tend to flee before sufficient inhalation to cause deep lung injury occurs. Unfortunately, this patient was unable to flee. The inspiratory stridor means that laryngeal edema is already present, and life-threatening upper airway obstruction is likely. The decreased PEFR indicates that significant bronchial exposure has occurred as well. Finally, the hypoxemia indicates that chemical pneumonitis is also developing despite the early normal chest x-ray film. This severely ill patient requires intensive care, and prophylactic intubation should be considered.

Case 3: Pulmonary asbestosis

A 77-year-old retired merchant seaman has had progressively increasing dyspnea for many years. He remembers dyspnea especially when climbing ladders onboard ship before his retirement in 1974 because of a bad back. His exercise tolerance currently is limited to walking 2 blocks on level ground (at a pace somewhat slower than his friends of the same age) or climbing one flight of stairs. He has a chronic cough that usually is nonproductive. He denies having any chest pain, wheezing, or hemopysis.

His occupational history begins in 1926, when he began working on farms in Texas as a casual laborer. From 1929 to 1942, he worked as a seaman in the Merchant Marines, primarily performing janitorial duties. He intermittently was required to clean up after other seamen had done "tear out" of asbestos pipe lagging. From 1942 to 1974, he worked as a laborer in local shipyards. He remembers hauling torn-out pieces of asbestos lagging out of the ships being repaired; he also remembers sweeping up dust from the decks of ships after laggers had completed their work. He states that his work clothes would get so dusty that he would look like a "snowman."

He denies ever smoking cigarettes, although he did chew tobacco in the past. He denies ever having pneumonia, tuberculosis, asthma, allergies, or chest surgery. He has a history of hypertension for which he currently is taking hydrochlorothiazide.

Physical examination shows a blood pressure of 140/90, a respiratory rate of 22, and a pulse of 108. He is afebrile. Abnormal clinical findings are primarily confined to the chest, with bilateral inspiratory crackles, especially at the bases, that do not clear with coughing. The heart examination and extremity examination are normal.

A chest x-ray film shows loss of definition of the heart and diaphragmatic borders and linear opacities distributed throughout both lungs, with a predominance in the lower zones. Calcified subdiaphragmatic pleural plaques are noted bilaterally. Pulmonary function tests reveals the following: FVC, 2.7 L (67% of predicted); FEV_1, 2.3 L (72% of predicted); FEV_1/FVC ratio, 0.85; total lung capacity (TLC), 3.8 L (68% of predicted); carbon monoxide diffusion (DLCO), 15 mm/min/Hg (56% of predicted).

Pulmonary asbestosis is the most likely diagnosis to account for the above clinical presentation. The patient has a history of significant occupational exposure to asbestos and an appropriate latency since the onset of exposure (longer than 20 years). His chest x-ray film shows findings consistent with interstitial fibrosis and calcified pleural plaques. The restricted lung volumes and diminished DLCO in the absence of any history of cigarette smoking or obstructive lung disease further support this diagnosis.

Case 4: Hypersensitivity pneumonitis

A 33-year-old white man has had a history of episodic fevers and chills associated with "weakness and lightheadedness" for several months. He also has a dry cough that appeared 1 month ago. After he began to experience exertional dyspnea, he went to his local emergency room, where a chest x-ray film was taken. He was told that it showed "pneumonia." He was treated with a 14-day course of erythromycin and advised to rest. He improved on this regimen, but soon after returning to work, his symptoms recurred. He returned to the emergency room, where he was prescribed a 14-day course of doxycycline and again encouraged to take time off work and rest. Despite initial improvement after closely following this treatment plan, his symptoms recurred within 5 days of returning to work. After a particularly bad morning of suffering from severe respiratory symptoms and generalized fatigue, he again went to the emergency room.

His occupational history revealed that he works as a computer programmer for a local software manufacturer. He works in a well-ventilated, modern building. None of his coworkers is ill. He mentions a part-time job as a magician. On further questioning, he discloses that he uses several pigeons in one of his tricks. He keeps these birds in a loft in the backyard of a friend's house. Because of his busy schedule, he tends to feed the birds and clean the cages in the early morning before going to his primary job. His friend took care of the birds during the periods the patient was advised to stay home and rest.

Physical examination shows a mildly distressed individual with the following vital signs: BP, 112/78; respiratory rate, 24; pulse, 114; temperature, 38° C (100.4° F). Bibasilar inspiratory crackles are auscultated on chest examination. Extremity examination reveals no evidence of cyanosis or digital clubbing.

A CBC reveals the following: normal hemoglobin (Hgb) and hematocrit (Hct), and leukocytosis of 13,400, with a differential of 78% polymorphonuclear cells, 14% lymphocytes, 3% monocytes, and 5% eosinophils. ABG determinations show a pH of 7.42, a Po_2 of 68 mm Hg, and a Pco_2 of 35 mm Hg. A chest x-ray film shows a diffuse, bilateral, reticulonodular infiltrate with normal heart size. The patient was referred to a pulmonolgist, who obtained the following studies: purified protein derivative (PPD) and cocci skin tests, both of which are negative (with a positive mumps test); pulmonary function tests, which reveal a mild restrictive defect with a normal FEV_1/FVC ratio and a normal DLCO; *Chlamydia psittaci* titers, which are negative for acute infection; and a hypersensitivity pneumonitis–precipitating antibody panel, which is positive for antibodies against pigeon serum.

The correct diagnosis is hypersensitivity pneumonitis caused by exposure to aerosolized pigeon droppings. The key to the diagnosis in this case is the episodic course of the illness coupled with evidence of interstitial lung disease. In more difficult cases, it may be necessary to extend the work-up to include specific inhalational challenge studies at the workplace or in the laboratory, fiberoptic bronchoscopy with bronchoalveolar lavage analysis and, in some instances, open lung biopsy. The patient should be advised to eliminate pigeons from his magic act and to give the birds away.

Case 5: Chronic bronchitis

A 34-year-old man seeks treatment for a chronic cough that produces small amounts of clear sputum. He first noted the symptoms more than 5 years ago, but the cough and sputum production have become worse over the previous 2 years. The cough is more prominent in the morning and occasionally produces discolored sputum. He denies having any shortness of breath, chest pains, or wheezing. He is otherwise well.

An occupational history reveals that the patient works as a grain handler at a local grain storage terminal. He has held this job since leaving high school at *age 17. He is exposed to large amounts of dust during the unloading of grain. He does not like to wear the standard dust masks that his employer supplies, because he finds them uncomfortable. By the end of the workday, he is covered in a fine dust. Lately he has noted that his cough is somewhat better during his days off. He has no hobbies, drinks alcohol occasionally, and has a 15 pack-year history of cigarette smoking.*

Physical examination is essentially normal. Spirometry shows a mild obstructive ventilatory defect. Lung volumes and DLCO are normal. A chest x-ray film is read as normal.

On the basis of the patient's history of chronic productive cough, he can be considered to have chronic bronchitis. Both occupational grain dust exposure and tobacco smoking are likely to be contributing to this problem. The patient should be advised to discontinue smoking and to wear a mask that filters respirable dust while at work. Annual medical surveillance with repeat symptom assessment and spirometry is indicated.

Case 6: Hard-metal lung disease

A 28-year-old Hispanic immigrant is referred from a local urgent care clinic because of bilateral upper lobe infiltrates noted on her chest x-ray film. The referring physician suspects tuberculosis. The patient has a nonproductive cough, weight loss, fatigue, and loss of appetite. She denies doing any recent traveling or having fevers or HIV risk factors.

Her occupational history indicates she has worked in a "tool and die" shop. Her chief duty for the past 2 years has been wet-grinding drill bits made of tungsten carbide. She does not wear any protective respiratory gear.

Physical examination reveals a thin, ill-appearing woman in no obvious distress. There are bilateral inspiratory crackles over both midlung zones that do not clear with coughing, and digital clubbing is present.

A repeat chest x-ray film confirms the presence of bilateral upper lobe linear infiltrates, which appear to have progressed when compared with the previous film. A CBC shows normal values. The PPD test result is negative, with a positive mumps control. Pulmonary function testing shows both a severe restrictive ventilatory defect and a severely decreased DLCO. Although resting arterial blood gases are normal, there is arterial oxygen desaturation with exercise. Bronchoscopy is performed to rule out an infectious process. The bronchoalveolar lavage fluid contains multinucleated giant cells, and the histologic characteristics of the transbronchial biopsy specimen are consistent with giant cell pneumonitis.

Tungsten carbide, or "hard metal," contains significant amounts of cobalt, which can cause an interstitial lung disease (hard-metal disease). This disease has a characteristic histology of giant cell pneumonitis. Because of the patient's relatively severe respiratory symptoms and pulmonary function abnormalities, she should be removed from further exposure and treated with high-dose oral prednisone.

CONCLUSION

Industrial and environmental toxins are ubiquitous; both workers and individuals face an ever-present risk of exposure to toxic levels of these agents. Because the percentage of the population that works outside the home is increasing, the potential for workplace exposure—and subsequent injury—is rising. The role of the primary caregiver is to recognize these injuries, treat them appropriately, and assist in preventing future injuries.

This chapter has dealt with the diagnosis and treatment of the commonly encountered respiratory injuries. Although most such injuries can be treated by the primary caregiver, it sometimes is necessary to refer more complicated or diagnostically difficult cases to a physician trained in occupational medicine. Always, the role of the physician is to help reduce impairment and disability and return the patient to a safe workplace.

SUGGESTED READINGS

Imaging studies

Aberle DR, Balmes JR: Computed tomography of asbestos-related pulmonary parenchymal and pleural diseases, *Clin Chest Med* 12:115-131, 1991.

Pulmonary function testing

Hankinson JL: Instrumentation for spirometry, *Occupational Medicine: State of the Art Reviews* 8(2):397-407, 1993.

Bronchoprovocation testing

Cartier A et al: Guidelines for bronchoprovocation in the investigation of occupational asthma, *J Allergy Clin Immunol* 84:823-829, 1989.

Inhalation of noxious gases, fumes, and mists

Brooks SM, Weiss MA, Bernstein IL: Reactive airways dysfunction syndrome (RADS): persistent asthma syndrome after high-level irritant exposure, *Chest* 88:376-385, 1987.

Harkonen H et al: Long-term effects of exposure to sulfur dioxide, *Am Rev Respir Dis* 128:890-893, 1983.

Kern DG: Outbreak of the reactive airways dysfunction syndrome after a spill of glacial acetic acid, *Am Rev Respir Dis* 144:1058-1064, 1991.

Schwartz DA, Smith DD, Lakshminarayan S: The pulmonary sequelae associated with accidental inhalation of chlorine gas, *Chest* 97:820-825, 1990.

Occupational asthma

ATS Statement: Guidelines for the evaluation of impairment/disability in patients with asthma, *Am Rev Respir Dis* 147:1056-1061, 1993.

Burge PS: Use of serial measurements of peak flow in the diagnosis of occupational asthma, *Occupational Medicine: State of the Art Reviews* 8(2):279-294, 1993.

Chan-Yeung M: Occupational asthma, *Chest* 98(5):148S-161S, 1990.

Hudson P et al: Follow-up of occupational asthma caused by crab and various agents, *J Allergy Clin Immunol* 76(5):682-688, 1985.

Hypersensitivity pneumonitis

Richardson HB et al: Guidelines for the clinical evaluation of hypersensitivity pneumonitis. II, *J Allergy Clin Immunol* 84(5):839-844, 1989.

Inhalational fevers

Rom WM, editor: *Environmental and occupational medicine,* ed 2, Boston, 1992, Little, Brown.

Hard-metal disease

Balmes JR: Respiratory effects of hard-metal dust exposure, *Occupational Medicine: State of the Art Reviews* 2(2):327-344, 1987.

Pneumoconioses

Rom WM, editor: *Environmental and occupational medicine,* ed 2, Boston, 1992, Little, Brown.

ATS Statement: The diagnosis of nonmalignant diseases related to asbestos, *Am Rev Respir Dis* 134:363-368, 1986.

Chronic bronchitis

Becklake MR: Occupational exposures: evidence for a causal association with chronic obstructive pulmonary disease, *Am Rev Respir Dis* 140:S85-91, 1989.

Granulomatous disease

Kriebel D, Brain JD, Sprince NL, Kazemi H: The pulmonary toxicity of beryllium, *Am Rev Respir Dis* 137:464-473, 1988.

Pleural disease

Rosenstock L, Hudson LD: The pleural manifestations of asbestos exposure, *Occupational Medicine: State of the Art Reviews* 2(2):383-407, 1987.

19 Chest and Abdominal Pain

CHEST PAIN

In the grand scheme of occupational injury and disease, the incidence of chest pain is minor compared with such common maladies as "low back pain" or extremity injuries. In our own experience, the chief complaint of (anterior) chest pain accounts for fewer than 5% of patient visits. Although this presenting symptom is relatively uncommon, the potential significance of underlying disease underscores the need to take the complaint seriously (Fig. 19-1). In the emergency medicine setting, where chest pain also accounts for only a fraction of admitting complaints, failure to diagnose un-derlying disease accurately (such as myocardial disease) accounts for the greatest number of malpractice dollars spent. Timely and accurate diagnoses are essential for this group of disorders, in which morbidity and mortality are so common and often tragic.

The key to avoiding missed diagnoses of serious, potentially life-threatening disorders is stratification of patients and their complaints into high and low risk. The algorithm in Fig. 19-2 represents such a system.

SYNDROMES OF ACUTE CHEST WALL PAIN
Costochondritis

Costochondritis has been well described. Unlike the nonspecific, broad-banded chest pain that occasionally is attributed to this disorder, costochondritis describes a localized inflammation of the second, third, fourth, or fifth costochondral joints. Most often the pain is unilateral and confined to a single joint space along the sternal margin. The onset of pain varies, and the pain has been described as abrupt and spontaneous or as an indolent discomfort that advances slowly over many days. Although costochondritis has been described in association with other systemic disorders, including Reiter's syndrome, gonorrhea, rheumatoid arthritis, and multiple myeloma, the disorder more commonly appears as an isolated inflammation.

The physical examination is crucial to the diagnosis of this condition. A universal finding and criterion of costochondritis is localized tenderness over one or more costochondral joints. There may or may not be attendant induration and frank erythema overlying the affected cartilage and soft tissue (Tietze's syndrome). The affected joint is almost always tender (often exquisitely) to palpation by the examiner. Also, pain often is elicited by a positional change of the torso, coughing, the Valsalva maneuver, and movement of the upper extremities through their various planes of motion.

The examiner must remain vigilant regarding true visceral disease in patients with chest pain. The patient may well be thoroughly convinced that he is having a heart attack when in fact a less ominous diagnosis better fits the picture. Under such circumstances, patients are apt to be in a panic, sometimes hyperventilating and diaphoretic. Given the mixed clinical picture, determining the correct diagnosis from all the signs and symptoms requires considerable skill on the part of the examiner.

The cause of costochondritis remains elusive in most patients. Unfortunately, a directed, effective therapy also is lacking. Most physicians treat this disorder with nonsteroidal antiinflamatory drugs (NSAIDs), but data on the efficacy of this treatment are unavailable, and reports of successful treatment remain anecdotal. Other treatment modalities include application of warm, moist compresses and modest exercise regimens. In anxious individuals, reassurance probably is the single most important intervention.

Intercostal muscle sprain

The thorax is composed of bony skeletal ribbing bound by a multitude of soft tissues, including the parietal pleura and the transversus thoracis, internal and external intercostal, serratus anterior, and pectoralis minor and major muscles. As with other mechanical and kinetic stressors, when exceptional forces are directed against these tissues, as in trauma (such as a fall from a ladder), or when situations require exceptional movement and strength of the thorax (an attempt to "catch" the falling ladder), the soft tissue may be injured. Muscles of the thorax may be crushed or torn, or

Musculoskeletal	Cardiac	Pulmonary
Costochondritis	Coronary artery disease	Pneumonia
Intercostal sprain	Mitral valve prolapse	Bronchitis
Pectoral myositis	Aortic dissection	Pulmonary embolism
Chest stitch syndrome	Aortic aneurysm	Pleurisy
Trauma	Pericarditis	Pneumothorax
Contusion	Myocarditis	Mediastinitis
Rib fracture		
Pneumothorax		

Gastrointestinal	Other
Gastritis	Panic attacks
Esophagitis	Hyperventilation
Esophageal spasm	Herpes zoster
Peptic ulcer disease	
Pancreatitis	
Esophageal rupture	

Fig. 19-1 Differential diagnosis of chest pain.

both, in varying degrees. When the degree to which these tissues are injured is relatively minor, they typically are described as "sprained." As such, the cluster of injuries we describe as an intercostal (chest wall) sprain really does not constitute a single, specific pathologic condition; rather, it is a loose, generic grouping of ill-defined chest wall pain, the common denominators being pain and a history consistent with injury or exertion.

In high-risk individuals, it is critical to maintain a high level of suspicion for cardiac and pulmonary disease. Patients with true intercostal sprains generally respond well to reassurance, local compresses (often warm and cold in alternating fashion), and controlled exercise after a period of convalescence (generally 3 days to 2 weeks, depending on the severity of injury). Nonsteroidal agents generally are used for these conditions. At the least, they appear to confer some analgesia and are therefore justified.

Pectoral myositis

The syndrome pectoral myositis is an inflammation specific to the pectoralis group and particular to the pectoralis major. The pain most often is described as a dull, persistent aching that is exacerbated by use of the ipsilateral shoulder and upper extremity. As with other myositides, a diffuse tenderness is present on palpation. When it affects the left side of the chest, pectoral myositis may well be indistinguishable from ischemic cardiac pain, and therefore such cases should be evaluated at an appropriate facility.

Chest stitch (precordial catch syndrome)

A chest stitch is a spontaneous, acute pain that is sharp and knifelike. The pain usually is unilateral,

often lateral along the thorax, or may begin medially and then radiate laterally to the axillary axis. Generally the pain, or "stitch" as it sometimes is called, begins with a simple movement of the torso, such as getting dressed or tying shoelaces. The sharp bolt of pain may last several seconds or longer and is followed by a residual aching —a reminder, so to speak, against any similar movement in the future. The physical examination is unremarkable, as are the electrocardiogram, chest x-ray film, and pulse oximetry. Because this condition usually is fairly brief, lasting hours to days, generally only reassurance is required.

Fractured ribs

Simple rib fractures caused by moderate blunt trauma are a commonplace occupational injury. Although the vast majority of these injuries can be treated easily and heal uneventfully, even "simple" rib fractures may generate significant morbidity or even mortality under special circumstances. Appropriate evaluation and management, therefore, are essential to minimizing discomfort and excessive morbidity.

The diagnosis of a simple rib fracture often will be self-evident to the examiner (as it usually is to the patient). A history of blunt trauma to the thorax that is followed by acute, well-localized pain—often positional and pleuritic—is characteristic of such fractures. The physical examination reveals localized tenderness on palpation and often a palpable step off at the site of fracture. Pain that is referred to the suspected fracture with anteroposterior compression is good confirmatory evidence of a fracture. Also, local crepitus with respiration is a marker for rib fracture (as it may be for pneumo-

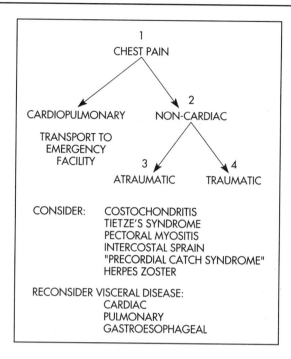

1
CHEST PAIN

CARDIOPULMONARY   2
NON-CARDIAC
TRANSPORT TO
EMERGENCY
FACILITY   3   4
ATRAUMATIC   TRAUMATIC

CONSIDER: COSTOCHONDRITIS
TIETZE'S SYNDROME
PECTORAL MYOSITIS
INTERCOSTAL SPRAIN
"PRECORDIAL CATCH SYNDROME"
HERPES ZOSTER

RECONSIDER VISCERAL DISEASE:
CARDIAC
PULMONARY
GASTROESOPHAGEAL

1. In evaluating the adult with chest pain, consideration of predisposing factors for cardiopulmonary disease is essential. In particular, risk factors such as age over 30 years, male sex, history of hypertension, hypercholesterolemia, diabetes mellitus, smoking, illicit drug use (e.g., cocaine and amphetamine), or family history of premature heart disease will heighten the suggestion of cardiac disease. Similarly, a history of smoking, asthma, and pneumothorax increases the likelihood of a primary pulmonary process.

Initial diagnostic tests that are useful for such patients include electrocardiography, chest radiography, and pulse oximetry.

Although the purpose of these tests is to **exclude** such nonoccupational etiologies, it is safe to assume that anyone presenting with a history or with a physical examination suggestive of cardiopulmonary disease should be referred to an appropriate emergency facility without further diagnostic studies at the workplace or at the occupational medicine clinic.

2. After acute cardiac and pulmonary disease has been excluded in the patient complaining of chest pain, the practitioner should further characterize the pain as either traumatic or atraumatic in etiology. For the patient who has experienced no injury by violence or extrinsic agent, the differential diagnoses should include those listed above (see 3).

3. The individual under the heading **atraumatic chest pain** may derive little benefit from further diagnostic studies. The diagnoses will be characterized by the history and physical examination alone.

If, on completion of a detailed H&P, the examiner is not confident of the diagnosis, a pathology of a deeper viscera should be reconsidered.

4. Chest pain that follows moderate or, on occasion, minimal trauma, should have the diagnostic benefit of chest radiography. Rib fractures and pneumothoracies will require this degree of diagnostic evaluation.

Possibilities including pulmonary injury might further require pulse oximetry or arterial blood gas analysis. Patients who show any hemodynamic instability (hypotension, weakness, pallor) for days or weeks following a history of modest trauma will require complete blood counts, chemistries, and further diagnostic imaging.

Fig. 19-2 Algorithm for diagnosing etiology of chest pain.

thorax). The patient generally complains of severe, unilateral chest pain that worsens with inspiration. He splints the chest and avoids deep inspiration or coughing because these tend to exacerbate the pain.

Patients with simple rib fractures are not significantly tachypneic or dyspneic. The appearance of real dyspnea, tachypnea, cyanosis, or accessory muscle retractions should alert the examiner to the likelihood of significant underlying respiratory distress. This may be secondary to an evolving pneumothorax, hemothorax, or significant visceral injury. Similarly, patients with underlying cardiovascular disease are less tolerant of even "simple" rib fractures than are healthy individuals.

Although often not essential for the diagnosis or treatment of rib fractures, our practice has been to investigate significant blunt trauma to the chest with x-ray studies. A standard PA and lateral view of the chest probably is inadequate for most of these patients. It has been well documented that these standard views fail to demonstrate as many of 50% of rib fractures, depending on the location of the injury. The correct approach, therefore, is to obtain an appropriate rib series if the history and examination warrant x-ray films at all. In patients with suspected respiratory compromise, pulse oximetry or blood gas analysis, or both, may offer further useful information.

The management of rib fractures involves analgesia, rest, and reasonable follow-up. These fractures often are terribly painful and lead to voluntary splinting of the thorax. Left untreated, some degree of atelectasis is likely to develop, increasing the likelihood of secondary infection and prolonged convalescence. Exterior supports, such as rib belts, may be comforting but may worsen the tendency to atelectasis. Adequate analgesia is essential. Depending on the severity of the pain, NSAIDs or narcotic analgesics may be used in the first week of injury. Acutely, some authors have advocated the use of intercostal nerve block with long-acting anesthetics. Depending on the anesthetic used, analgesia may last from 12 to 24 hours. In any event, such patients are routinely seen in follow-up in 1 or 2 days.

The nerve block procedure involves injecting 3 to 5 ml of anesthetic (such as Marcaine 0.25%) into the intercostal spaces, one space inferior and one superior, either just posterior to the site of the fracture or directly into the suspected fracture site. With a half-inch, 30-gauge needle, the physician injects subcutaneously to the flat of the rib; then, using a 22-gauge needle and aspirating, the physician advances 0.5 cm over the inferior margin of the rib, with the syringe and needle directed inferi-

orly, and (assuming no blood or air is withdrawn) deposits the anesthetic (Fig. 19-3).

Often multiple rib fractures may be treated conservatively in a manner similar to that outlined above. Presuming that the bellow's mechanism of the thorax remains intact and that no free-floating (flail) chest is present, multiple rib fractures may simply represent a "more of the same" musculoskeletal injury. However, the incidence of pneumothorax and underlying pulmonary contusion increases dramatically when increasing traumatic forces are applied to the thorax and result in multiple fractures. Therefore, the clinician must ensure that no pneumothorax, pulmonary, or cardiac contusion is present.

Various complications have been reported in association with first and second rib fractures. Principally, these have been tension pneumothorax and severe vascular injuries, including subclavian artery interruption and aortic injuries. Fractures of the first and second ribs are distinctly uncommon. Because these ribs are situated under the clavicle and scapula, forces usually required to fracture these elements must be especially severe. Careful attention must be given to examination of the lungs and the neurovascular integrity of the upper extremities with such injuries.

The ninth and tenth ribs overlie both a portion of the thorax and the abdominal viscera. Fractures of these bones not infrequently lacerate the underlying spleen and liver. Subsequent hemorrhage from these organs may be brisk and catastrophic, or it may be delayed by virtue of their mantlelike capsules. Delayed splenic rupture is an increasingly noted disorder that manifests with mild upper abdominal pain, weakness, and often orthostatic hypotension secondary to persistent, slow splenic hemorrhage. When the possibility of this

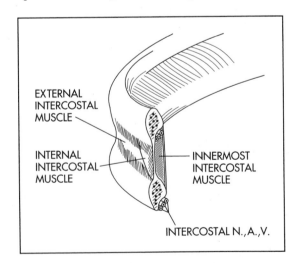

Fig. 19-3 Anatomy for nerve block of acute rib fracture.

condition exists, the diagnosis most often is made by abdominal computed tomography (CT) scan, although other diagnostic modalities, including ultrasonography and diagnostic peritoneal lavage, also have been used.

CASE STUDIES
Case 1

A 41-year-old pipe fitter comes to the clinic with a weeklong history of chest wall pain. He describes the discomfort as "central," or sternal, associated with movement and exertion, and improved with rest. He says he has no radiating pain or associated symptoms such as nausea, emesis, fatigue, pleuritic pain, or shortness of breath. Coincidentally, he has taken on a major contract within the past 2 weeks and admits to working "double time" in accordance with the needs of the plumbers and other subcontractors. He is a generally healthy person with no significant medical history or known coronary artery disease. However, he is a one-pack-per-day smoker.

The physical examination shows a healthy, robust man who is quite comfortable. The examination is remarkable only for mild, palpable tenderness over the left, second, and third costal cartilages. No erythema or induration is present. The patient notes a remarkable similarity between his exertional pain and the tenderness elicited with sternal massage.

Where does the examiner go from here? Further testing to rule out the possibility of underlying ischemic cardiac disease? Or treat this as a simple chest wall discomfort? How much importance may we place in the finding of reproducible chest wall tenderness? Clearly, the extent of evaluation depends in some measure on the resources available to the clinician and on the nuances of the physician/patient relationship. The larger answer, however, is not clear cut and depends on the circumstances and perspectives of those involved, as influenced by the clinical picture.

In this instance, a 41-year-old male smoker has new-onset chest pain. An electrocardiogram (ECG), at the very least, is in order. Chest wall tenderness, although perhaps comforting to the clinician and patient, is present in as many as 10% of patients who have an acute myocardial infarction. Evaluation beyond a normal ECG would be at the discretion of the examiner, according to the related history. If the examiner is not well convinced of the musculoskeletal cause of the patient's discomfort, the patient should be triaged at this point to a facility where further workup is possible. Stated in other terms, the primary responsibility of the occupational medicine physician generally is to identify and minister to a precise diagnosis. Where underlying, life-threatening disease may be involved, the primary responsibility is to confidently rule out such conditions before proceeding.

ABDOMINAL PAIN

Just as other broad and general categories of illness such as chest pain and headache have managed to find their place in consideration of the multitude of occupational-related disease, so, too, must we concern ourselves with the vast subject of abdominal pain; that is, patients who see the occupational medicine physician with complaints of abdominal, pelvic, or groin discomfort. The differential diagnoses entertained under such a heading are numerous, and our effort here shall be to help organize this large collection of conditions in a way more useful to the practitioner.

In the management of abdominal injuries, the occupational medicine physician is responsible for rapidly diagnosing and directing triage when necessary. Indeed, many of the diagnoses we will consider require investigation and/or therapy that is likely to be beyond the capacity of even the best-equipped industrial clinic. Figure 19-4 presents an algorithm for delineating the etiology of abdominal pain.

An employee who complains of belly pain may or may not have a work-related condition. Perhaps nowhere in occupational medicine is it more important to free the mind of this association. The physician must maintain a clear and unbiased mindset when approaching a patient with abdominal pain. The discomfort may truly originate from occupational hazards, as in blunt abdominal trauma or carbon tetrachloride liver disease, or it may be etiologically unrelated to the job, even though it may manifest, as in acute appendicitis, while the person is at work. As clinicians, our first and foremost responsibility is to understand the nature of the immediate illness, not the exact etiologic roots from which it developed. In fact, with a few notable exceptions, abdominal pain often is not a symptom of illness conceived *because* of work, but rather is symptomatic of an illness conceived *while* at work. As such, abdominal pain presents a challenging and frightening array of possibilities to negotiate and treat.

The epidemiology of "work-related" abdominal disorders is poorly understood. Some data exist for isolated conditions, such as the varieties of inguinal and abdominal hernias (discussed later in this chapter), but overall the issues of abdominal pain in occupational medicine remain unaddressed in the literature of this field. Whereas the percentage of cases involving abdominal pain seen in emergency and primary care facilities is significant (accounting in some studies for 15% to 20% of presenting complaints), the incidence of such chief complaints to our own occupational clinic is well below 5%. As with chest pain, however, the

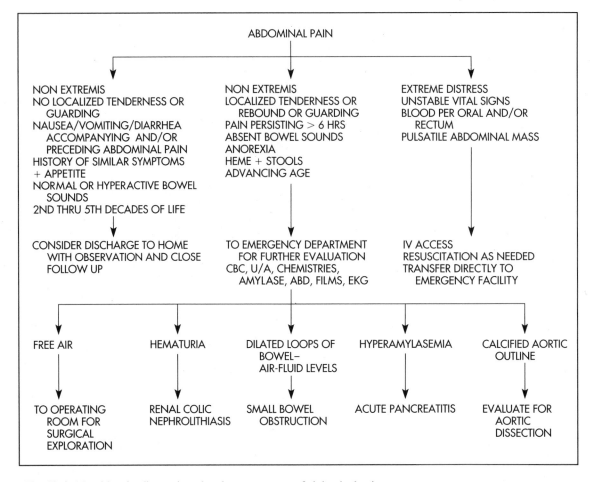

ABDOMINAL PAIN

NON EXTREMIS
NO LOCALIZED TENDERNESS OR
GUARDING
NAUSEA/VOMITING/DIARRHEA
ACCOMPANYING AND/OR
PRECEDING ABDOMINAL PAIN
HISTORY OF SIMILAR SYMPTOMS
+ APPETITE
NORMAL OR HYPERACTIVE BOWEL
SOUNDS
2ND THRU 5TH DECADES OF LIFE

NON EXTREMIS
LOCALIZED TENDERNESS OR
REBOUND OR GUARDING
PAIN PERSISTING > 6 HRS
ABSENT BOWEL SOUNDS
ANOREXIA
HEME + STOOLS
ADVANCING AGE

EXTREME DISTRESS
UNSTABLE VITAL SIGNS
BLOOD PER ORAL AND/OR
RECTUM
PULSATILE ABDOMINAL MASS

CONSIDER DISCHARGE TO HOME
WITH OBSERVATION AND CLOSE
FOLLOW UP

TO EMERGENCY DEPARTMENT
FOR FURTHER EVALUATION
CBC, U/A, CHEMISTRIES,
AMYLASE, ABD, FILMS, EKG

IV ACCESS
RESUSCITATION AS NEEDED
TRANSFER DIRECTLY TO
EMERGENCY FACILITY

FREE AIR

HEMATURIA

DILATED LOOPS OF
BOWEL–
AIR-FLUID LEVELS

HYPERAMYLASEMIA

CALCIFIED AORTIC
OUTLINE

TO OPERATING
ROOM FOR
SURGICAL
EXPLORATION

RENAL COLIC
NEPHROLITHIASIS

SMALL BOWEL
OBSTRUCTION

ACUTE PANCREATITIS

EVALUATE FOR
AORTIC
DISSECTION

Fig. 19-4 Algorithm for diagnosis and early management of abdominal pain.

simple numerical incidence belies the severity of the illness.

General approach

Before discussing the qualities of specific pain patterns, it would be useful to first separate abdominal pain into two distinct etiologic entities, traumatic and nontraumatic abdominal illness.

Case 2

A 27-year-old shipyard worker went to the occupational health clinic with diffuse abdominal discomfort and weakness, which he had suffered for 2 days. One week before the onset of these symptoms, the patient recalled slipping on the icy dock, landing painfully on his left chest and flank. He said the fall, "really knocked the wind out of me." He noted subsequent pain over the left hypochondrium but continued working until the present time. The review of systems was otherwise unremarkable.

The physical examination was notable for a young man in no acute distress. He was orthostatic both by blood pressure and pulse. The lungs were clear. The resting cardiac examination was normal. The abdomen was notable for mild palpable tenderness over the left hypochondrium. There was no splenomegaly. The bony

thorax was nontender and had no ecchymoses or rib deformity. The abdomen was otherwise nontender and had no masses, and normal periodic bowel sounds were heard.

A spun hematocrit from the clinic showed a value of 28. The patient was transferred to the referral hospital emergency department for further evaluation.

This case illustrates two points. The first is that the cause of abdominal pain may be obvious or, as in the previous example, it may be hidden in some past event or activity. Often the details are so obscured as to be completely mystifying. The second point is that from the perspective of patient care, it does not much matter. The clinician in the above case recognized the triad of abdominal pain, unstable vital signs, and anemia. Regardless of the cause, whether the young man had suffered a penetrating gastric ulcer, a traumatic diaphragmatic hernia, or a subacute splenic injury, the need for further emergency evaluation and treatment was clear.

The algorithm for blunt abdominal trauma (Fig. 19-5) may be useful, bearing in mind, of course, that obvious, severe blunt injuries are triaged immediately to a trauma care facility.

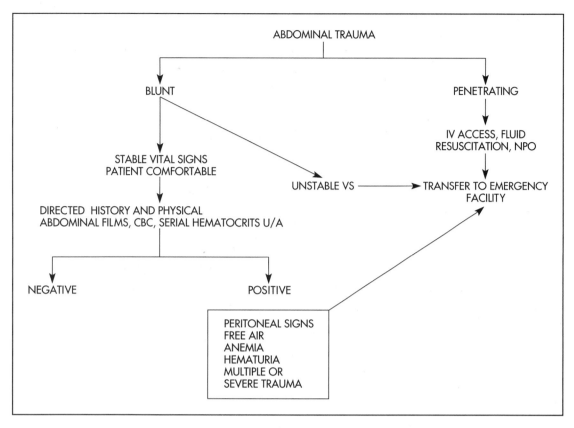

Fig. 19-5 Algorithm for abdominal trauma.

In short, individuals suffering blunt or penetrating abdominal trauma are likely to require further evaluation unless one can demonstrate that the injuries are minor. If the physician can perform limited radiologic and laboratory studies, so much the better. With a benign abdominal examination, normal vital signs, and a normal blood count and urinalysis, it may be appropriate to discharge a patient home after a period of observation. Serial hematocrits have been used to monitor blood volume, although we appreciate that a falling hematocrit valve may lag hours before reflecting significant blood loss. This is an inefficient and crude system at best. If there is sufficient trauma to warrant this degree of concern, the patient probably is best brought to the nearest emergency facility for appropriate diagnostics and care. Although it may be tempting to render complete care for the patient, the clinician should bear in mind that the consequences of *unrecognized* abdominal or thoracoabdominal injuries are likely to be devastating and irremediable.

Acute spontaneous abdominal pain

As in most of medicine, there is still no substitute for a careful, detailed history and physical examination. Often, as the patient chronicles his symptoms, the familiar pattern of some disease process begins to take shape. Less often, the clues buried in the narrative and examination are mystifying, and then, in the words of William Carlos Williams, "The hunt is on." The "hunt," as it were, begins with a careful history, with great attention paid to the onset, progression, and quality of pain.

Case 3

A 33-year-old woman employed in accounting seeks treatment for right lower abdominal pain, which has been increasing since she arrived at work about 4 hours ago. The pain has slowly progressed, and she notes that it is worse with positional movement, walking, and lifting. She was rearranging furniture in her office this morning and believes this may have contributed to her present situation. She is in excellent health generally and offers no other acute complaints.

Before moving on to the physical examination, what can we say about the history, which is sparse at best? What about the *onset* of her pain? Was it present on awakening? On retiring the night before? Was it gradual or abrupt? Sharp or diffuse, when first noted? What about the *chronicity* of the pain? How long has the pain endured? Has she experienced similar discomfort before? If this is the presentation of an acute appendicitis, it is unlikely she has experienced these symptoms before, whereas if she is familiar with this pattern of

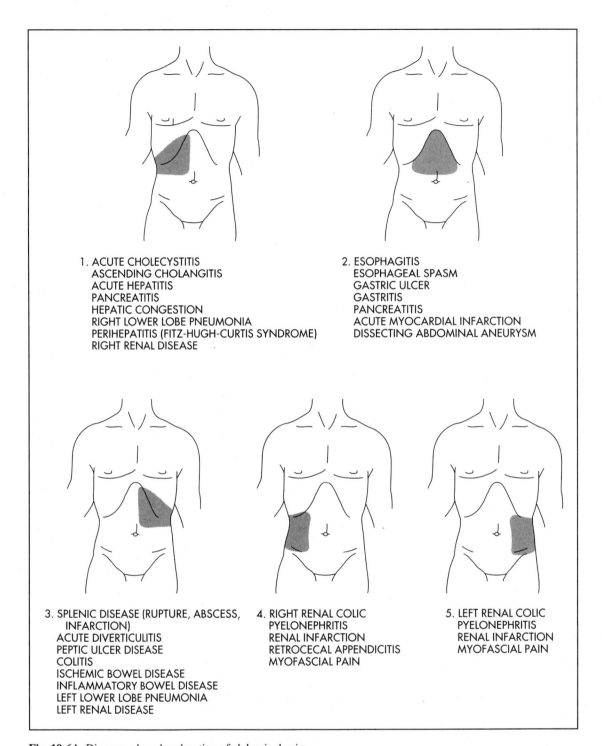

1. ACUTE CHOLECYSTITIS
   ASCENDING CHOLANGITIS
   ACUTE HEPATITIS
   PANCREATITIS
   HEPATIC CONGESTION
   RIGHT LOWER LOBE PNEUMONIA
   PERIHEPATITIS (FITZ-HUGH-CURTIS SYNDROME)
   RIGHT RENAL DISEASE

2. ESOPHAGITIS
   ESOPHAGEAL SPASM
   GASTRIC ULCER
   GASTRITIS
   PANCREATITIS
   ACUTE MYOCARDIAL INFARCTION
   DISSECTING ABDOMINAL ANEURYSM

3. SPLENIC DISEASE (RUPTURE, ABSCESS,
      INFARCTION)
   ACUTE DIVERTICULITIS
   PEPTIC ULCER DISEASE
   COLITIS
   ISCHEMIC BOWEL DISEASE
   INFLAMMATORY BOWEL DISEASE
   LEFT LOWER LOBE PNEUMONIA
   LEFT RENAL DISEASE

4. RIGHT RENAL COLIC
   PYELONEPHRITIS
   RENAL INFARCTION
   RETROCECAL APPENDICITIS
   MYOFASCIAL PAIN

5. LEFT RENAL COLIC
   PYELONEPHRITIS
   RENAL INFARCTION
   MYOFASCIAL PAIN

Fig. 19-6A Diagnoses based on location of abdominal pain.

symptoms, their onset will be familiar and thereby will help to distinguish them. Whereas, chronic pain typically begins as a dull, vague aching sensation, acute appendicitis frequently manifests abruptly and often is described as a sharp, searing pain.

What of the *severity* of the pain and the precipitating and/or alleviating factors? Were this renal colic, the pain might be expected to be intermittently breathtakingly severe, punctuated by periods of relative calm. There is little in the way of positioning, eating, or walking that significantly

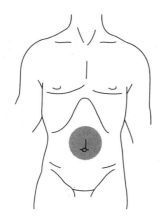

6. EARLY APPENDICITIS
   INTESTINAL OBSTRUCTION
   DIVERTICULITIS
   GASTROENTERITIS
   DISSECTING OR RUPTURED ABDOMINAL
      AORTIC ANEURYSM
   ISCHEMIC BOWEL DISEASE
   INCARCERATED OR STRANGULATED
      UMBILICAL HERNIA

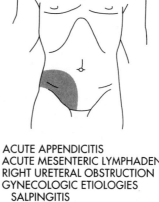

7. ACUTE APPENDICITIS
   ACUTE MESENTERIC LYMPHADENITIS
   RIGHT URETERAL OBSTRUCTION
   GYNECOLOGIC ETIOLOGIES
      SALPINGITIS
      TUBO-OVARIAN CYST
      RUPTURED OVARIAN CYST
      ECTOPIC PREGNANCY
      MITTELSCHMERZ
      ENDOMETRIOSIS

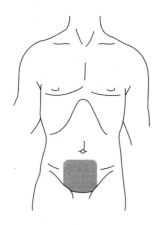

8. ACUTE CYSTITIS
   ACUTE PROSTATITIS
   URINARY RETENTION
   GYNECOLOGIC ETIOLOGIES
   INCARCERATED OR STRANGULATED
      INGUINAL/FEMORAL HERNIA
   PELVIC APPENDICITIS

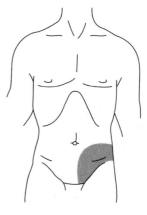

9. SIGMOID DIVERTICULITIS
   LEFT URETERAL OBSTRUCTION
   GYNECOLOGIC ETIOLOGIES
   ULCERATIVE COLITIS
   PSOAS ABCESS
   SIGMOID VOLVULUS

Fig. 19-6B Diagnoses based on location of abdominal pain.

affects the course of the impacted stone and its consequent pain. An ovarian cyst, on the other hand, often "quiets down" when the patient is supine. Alternatively, the pain may well be exacerbated by increasing lower abdominal pressure or Valsalva maneuvers. Pain during or just after

coitus is notorious for the presentation of ruptured ovarian cyst.

It may be useful to bear in mind the nature of visceral and somatic abdominal pain. Visceral (hollow gut) organs are principally innervated by the tiny, unmyelinated C-fiber nerves. These rather primitive sensors respond primarily to severe distention and forceful contractions of the gut. Consequently, "visceral" pain tends to be a diffuse, dull, poorly localized, and often persistent sensory experience. "Somatic" pain, conversely, is transmitted via larger, myelinated nerves that are found mainly within the parietal peritoneum. Painful stimulation of these nerves is characterized by sharp, knifelike pain that may localize with extreme precision. Thus early in the course of appendicitis, one experiences the visceral discomfort of a distended, engorged cecum appendix. The pain typically is diffuse, constant, periumbilical discomfort. Only much later, when a full-thickness inflammation of the appendiceal wall is achieved, with involvement of the surrounding peritoneum, do patients describe a well-localized pain over McBurney's point.

Physical examination

A thorough physical examination often is exceedingly useful in the rapid, accurate diagnosis of abdominal pain. It begins with an overall assessment. Attention to vital signs, state of hydration, and level of distress are all integral to the assessment. Not infrequently, the diagnosis is already revealed as the patient splints to one side or the other while stumbling toward the examination room. Once there, he refuses to undress or lay supine until the "wave of pain" has passed. Unless the patient is a woman and appears to be in her third trimester, the likelihood of renal colic is high. Similarly, if the patient is jaundiced and splints the right upper quadrant rather than the flank, an obstructive cholangitic process is likely at work. In the case of peritonitis, the patient typically lies deathly still because any movement is likely to stir the inflamed peritoneum. This is in stark contrast to renal colic, which prompts the sufferer to squirm throughout the painful seizure.

Palpation. Examination of the abdomen itself is the key, of course, to the physical diagnosis. This begins with a visual inspection. The clinician should observe for distention, as in obstruction of the bowel from adhesions or a sigmoid volvulus. Abdominal scars suggest the possibility of adhesions or prior abdominal illness, such as inflammatory bowel disease. Focal masses are uncommon findings but may signal an abdominal aneurysm, intussusception, or herniation of the abdominal viscera.

Visual inspection is followed by gentle palpation of the entire abdomen for masses and tenderness. Rebound tenderness is a useful sign for inflammation of the anterior peritoneum. These patients are also likely to show rigid abdomens

with involuntary spasm of the rectus abdominus sheaths. Visceral perforations occurring in the lesser peritoneal cavity (hemorrhagic pancreatitis) or the pelvis (acute salpingitis), or in the presence of obesity (fatty omentum) may not manifest early in their course with a rigid, boardlike abdomen as, for example, in a young asthenic individual with a ruptured appendicitis. Rigidity and rebound are primarily a function of *anterior* peritoneal irritation.

Percussion may also be useful to demonstrate rebound tenderness, or hyperresonance, in the case of abdominal distention. I have not found percussion very useful in delineating masses in an acutely painful abdomen. In patients experiencing great discomfort from abdominal pain, it is at once compassionate and informative to administer analgesics and then repeat the abdominal examination. Providing some analgesia for excruciating abdominal pain more commonly improves rather than obscures the essential features of the examination.

Auscultation. Bowel sounds generally conform to one of the following three familiar pathologic patterns.

1. *Loud, continuous borborygmi throughout the belly.* This may vary somewhat in intensity but remains fairly constant. Such bowel sounds are typical of hyperactive bowel, as seen in acute gastroenteritis (Norwalk or Rotavirus, Giardia infection, "food poisoning," and the like).

2. *High-pitched, crescendo-decrescendo tinkles with silences interposed between them.* These peculiar borborygmi often occur rhythmically and concurrently with abdominal spasms (peristalsis) and occur generally with mechanical intestinal obstruction.

3. *Absence of bowel sounds.* A silent bowel has several explanations, among the most worrisome of which is peritonitis. With an acute surgical condition, the belly rapidly loses normal peristalsis. Ileus is such a reliable finding that normal or hyperactive bowel sounds should lead the examiner to reconsider the diagnosis of peritonitis.

Location. The location of the abdominal pain and concurrent knowledge of abdominal anatomy are indispensable in the accurate diagnosis of abdominal illness. Location is arguably the best organizer in beginning the pursuit of a diagnosis (Fig. 19-6A and B, pp. 302-303). The clinician must pay attention to both the immediate location and the distribution of pain as it evolved from the onset. Left-sided inguinal pain in a young woman, for example, conjures a host of diagnoses. But inguinal pain that began as flank and back discomfort effectively limits the range of likely diagnoses.

Fig. 19-7 Differentiation between these hernias is not always clinically possible. Understanding their features, however, improves diagnostic accuracy.

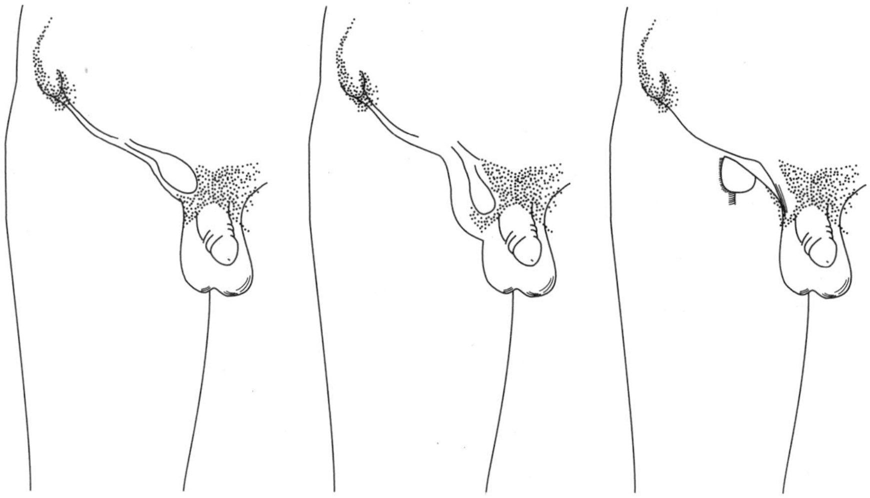

Features	Inguinal		Femoral
	Indirect	**Direct**	
Frequency	Most common, all ages, both sexes	Less common	Least common
Age and sex	Often in children, may be in adults	Usually men over 40, rare in women	More common in women than in men
Point of origin	Above inguinal ligament, near its midpoint (the internal inguinal ring)	Above inguinal ligament, close to the pubic tubercle (near the external inguinal ring)	Below the inguinal ligament, appears more lateral than an inguinal hernia and maybe hard to differentiate from lymph nodes
Course (With the examining finger in the inguinal canal during straining or cough)	Often into the scrotum. Hernia comes down the inguinal canal and touches the fingertip.	Rarely into the scrotum. Hernia bulges anteriorly and pushes the side of the finger forward	Never into the scrotum. The inguinal canal is empty.

Inguinal hernias

Case 4

A 27-year-old waiter seeks treatment for acute right-groin pain, which he noted 30 minutes before presenting to the occupational clinic. He was lifting a heavy tray overhead when he felt a sudden "pop" over the right inguinal region. He immediately felt a tender mass over this region of acute sharp pain. He said he had no nausea, vomiting, diarrhea, fever, chills, or other complaints.

The examination showed a healthy, anxious-appearing young man in moderate discomfort. The abdomen was remarkable for a 6 × 4 cm mass over the right groin. The mass was tender to palpation. Bowel sounds were appreciated over this nonreducible (incarcerated) tissue. The abdominal examination was otherwise be-

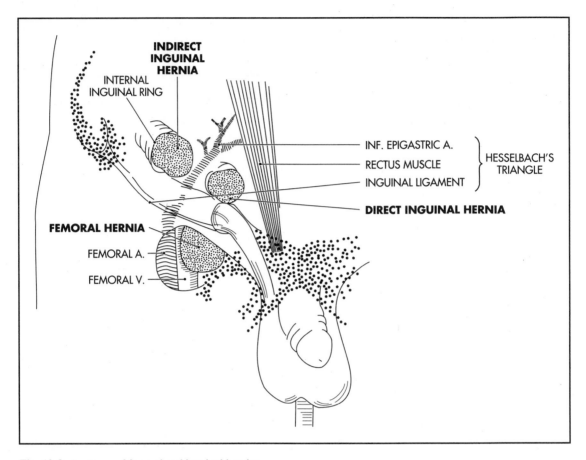

Fig. 19-8 Anatomy of femoral and inguinal hernias.

nign. The rectal examination was nontender, and the stool was heme negative.

Hernias may be organized into three principal types: inguinal, femoral, and ventral abdominal defects of the anterior/inferior abdominal cavity (Fig. 19-7, p. 305). Inguinal hernias are far and away the most common of these abdominal wall defects, as illustrated in the previous example. They account for 75% of all such hernias, the vast majority of these occurring in men. It is estimated that roughly 5% of all men develop an inguinal hernia at some time in their lives. Groin hernias manifest as both inguinal and femoral hernias. Inguinal hernias are further differentiated as either indirect or direct. These two varieties of inguinal hernias account for 85% of all such symptomatic patients (Fig. 19-8).

The patient mentioned previously most likely suffered an acute herniation of the indirect type. This defect is a common congenital anomaly in which the embryonic tissue known as the processus vaginalis remains patent. This is a tract of peri-

toneal tissue that stretches into the scrotum and closes during normal fetal life. Often these hernias are present at birth. There is a high likelihood of contralateral weakness once an indirect hernia has been discovered. The custom, therefore, is to correct both sites whether symptomatic or not when discovered in infancy.

In the case of the waiter, he, too, was born with a propensity for indirect herniation, but it was not until his twenty-fourth year that he became symptomatic. Other types of abdominal hernia, including direct inguinal hernias and ventral abdominal hernias, do not arise from congenital anomalies, but instead reflect simple structural failures of the wall containing and restraining the abdominal viscera. As might be predicted, therefore, these clinical presentations often are precipitated by environmental factors that tend to increase intraabdominal pressure, such as obesity, straining, lifting, prolonged and or strenuous labor, chronic obstructive pulmonary disorder, and advancing age. Although these hernias may be annoying and disfiguring, they rarely incarcerate or strangulate.

The existence of a patent processus vaginalis alone is not adequate grounds for defining a hernia. There should be some invagination of this potential channel for proper application of the term. The extention of tissue may be omentum, intestine, or simply fluid alone, as in hernias associated with ascites. Surgical statistics suggest that incarceration of intestinal tissue (an inability to reduce) occurs most often in indirect hernias. This figure generally is placed at around 10%. Once incarcerated, the protruding tissue may continue to swell, with resulting constriction of the vascular supply and strangulation of the tissue from its narrow passageway arising from the abdomen.

In the example of the waiter, the physical examination showed unequivocal evidence of a mass. The mass itself, along with the location, history, and auscultatory findings, was pathognomonic for an incarcerated hernia, which in this instance was of indirect origin. Identification is not always as simple as this. If the hernia has spontaneously reduced, proper identification depends on the examiner.

To examine for a hernia, the clinician should place the index finger over the scrotum, invaginating the redundant scrotal tissue, and palpate over the external inguinal ring. As this is done, the patient performs the Valsalva maneuver or coughs. If a hernia is present, the examiner will palpate tissue descending through the ring during these maneuvers, confirming a weakened abdominal wall. Identifying an incarcerated hernia that is strangulating is less challenging. Typically the incarcerated mass is exquisitely tender and nonreducible, and depending on the period of intestinal insult, the patient may already appear systemically ill. An elevated temperature, leukocytosis, and peritoneal signs may all be present.

The responsibility of the occupational physician is to diagnose and appropriately triage these patients. In the absence of incarcerated intestine, arrangements for urgent surgical repair (usually within 1 to 2 weeks) can be safely undertaken. If there is incarcerated tissue, the patient requires further emergency care. Generally this involves administration of narcotics and gentle reduction over 30 minutes to an hour. If systemic illness is also a factor, the patient should be surgically evaluated and explored without delay.

Femoral hernias

Femoral hernias are invaginations of abdominal contents through the femoral ring, through which passes the neurovascular bundle. Enlargement of the ring is thought to occur with advancing age and intra-abdominal pressures, as might be seen during pregnancy or obesity. These hernias are notoriously silent until incarceration occurs. Furthermore, when incarcerated, they do not readily reduce. Rather, if left unattended, they typically proceed to strangulate the affected portion of bowel.

Women are predisposed to these hernias. In this population, femoral hernias constitute one third of all groin hernias, whereas in the male subset, these hernias account for fewer than 2% groin hernias. Treatment is similar to that for other hernias. Incarcerated bowel still requires emergency attention, whereas asymptomatic, nonincarcerated hernias may be attended to urgently. As with other abdominal wall defects, extrinsic constraining devices work poorly and generally should be avoided.

SUGGESTED READINGS

Dunphy JE, Botsford TW: *Physical examination of the surgical patient,* ed 4, Philadelphia, 1975, WB Saunders.

Gushee DE, Holroyd BR: Chest pain. In Callaham M, editor: *Current practice of emergency medicine,* ed 2, Philadelphia, 1991, BC Decker.

Silen W, editor: *Cope's early diagnosis of the acute abdomen,* ed 17, New York, 1987, Oxford University Press.

Snell RS, Smith MS: *Clinical anatomy for emergency medicine,* St Louis, 1993, Mosby.

Wiener SL: *Differential diagnosis of acute pain by body region,* New York, 1993, McGraw Hill.

SECTION III
SPECIAL ISSUES

20 The Challenge of Patient Management

"Doctor, why do I still hurt? I've done everything you told me to, and I'm really no better. I want to work, but I just have too much pain. I can't work like this. What are you going to do?"

These and similar statements reflect the frustration too often felt by patient and practitioner during the course of treatment after an injury at work. When a patient's progress is slow and knotted with impediments, new complaints, and multiplying problem lists, we may, in mind or attitude, label the patient as difficult. We may consciously or unconsciously withdraw regard, attention, or treatment. The relationship changes from a healing partnership to a dispassionate, alienated, or even hostile association. Ultimately, the patient may find another health care provider.

This outcome hardly represents a satisfactory resolution, although both patient and practitioner may feel happily relieved of the frustration of dealing with each other. Although this abandonment may seem to free the practitioner from a problem patient, the real problem is not addressed, the case remains open, the patient continues to suffer impairment, and direction may be lost. Responsibility for case management is taken by no one or, less desirably, by the patient or others, often nonmedical personnel, whose primary goal centers on manipulating the case to an end point that may or may not be consonant with optimal medical care. A sense of despair, distrust, hopelessness, anger, or depression may exacerbate the patient's underlying problem and further distance the goal of full function, productivity, and a sense of well-being. The purpose of this chapter is to examine some of these impediments to healing and to suggest some approaches aimed at problem resolution.

WHAT ARE THE DIFFICULTIES?
Occupational medicine: a unique context

Throughout our medical training, we focus on the science of medicine. We study pathology, organ systems, and disease processes and apply this knowledge as our patients come in with various complaints or symptoms. We obtain a medical history, examine the patient, and order appropriate laboratory tests as we formulate a differential diagnosis and treatment plan. Often this formula works effectively, and the patient improves.

In this approach, the practice of occupational medicine does not differ significantly from that of any other field of medicine. In the practice of occupational medicine, we make diagnoses and initiate treatment plans. We suture wounds and treat ankle sprains just as our surgical and orthopedic colleagues would. We provide the same medical treatment for a cut or sprain that occurs at work as for one that occurs at home.

Yet there are particular aspects of an occupational medicine practice that can dramatically affect patient outcome and that reflect much of what makes occupational medicine unique as a practice specialty. One can practice medicine brilliantly, diagnose and treat incisively, and still mismanage a case from a workers' compensation standpoint. This failure to solve a patient's problem, despite practicing our best scientific medicine, prompts an examination of potential impediments in the course of patient care.

Medical care in a legal context. In traditional medical practice, the patient comes to the physician with a medical problem that she wishes to define, solve, and heal. There is an underlying assumption of positive motivation. In the field of occupational medicine, the underlying assumption of positive motivation may be eroded or challenged by the fact that we practice medicine, we diagnose and treat, in the context of the workers' compensation system. This means that we practice medicine in the context of a legal system, which by definition means that we practice in the context of an adversarial system.

Often the patient is sent to us by the employer, insurance carrier, or case manager. We most likely are not the patient's personal physician and were not chosen by the patient. Patients may come to our office with real concern about whether they will receive appropriate and objective treatment because we are, after all, company doctors. As we enter the examination room, we may well face this preconceived notion of who we are and what we will do before we even introduce ourselves. Certainly such an atmosphere colors the usual doctor-patient relationship and affects the chances for successful treatment or resolution of the problem.

This adversarial context is highlighted by the frequent variation between how the injury is described by the employer or supervisor and by the patient. A company representative may inform the physician that the employee complained of low back pain after a minor event at work.

"I want you to know that this guy had just been disciplined for poor job performance and had requested 2 days off for a long weekend camping trip. We couldn't give him the time off, and after 10 minutes of work today, he said he hurt his back. Just go over him and send him back to work, Doc," the company representative might say.

The patient, meanwhile, tells you that his supervisor "has had it in for me ever since I made some recommendations about how to improve our department. Sure, I wanted to go camping with my family, but we had cancelled the trip already. I know it looks funny, but my back really hurts. I can't work like this."

The physician may become entangled in a web that is spun before the patient even arrives at the clinic.

This potentially adversarial context underscores the need for sensitivity to the patient's underlying fear or distrust. It is useful to assess the degree to which this influences the patient's history or description of pain, as well as the consistency between the history and clinical examination. We may too hastily conclude that a patient is malingering when, in fact, an exaggerated description or demonstration of pain might simply be an attempt to convince us that a real problem exists.

Expectations and responsibilities. In the workers' compensation system, the practitioner confronts expectations from the patient, the employer, and the insurance carrier. How the physician embraces these expectations flavors the interaction between doctor and patient.

Patient's expectations. In traditional medical practice, both patient and physician reasonably expect that the presenting complaint will be appropriately diagnosed and treated. Such agreement establishes the context of partnership in the process of healing. In the ambulatory care setting, the patient is treated while continuing relatively normal daily activity, assisted by the physician through advice and treatment.

In the workers' compensation setting, there may

be other expectations. As noted previously, the patient may anticipate unfair treatment from a bureaucratic system and may expect an adversarial relationship with the caregiver and the insurance adjustor. The patient may expect the injury to be cured in one or two visits without loss of work-time and income, or the patient may expect to be sent home for extended rest after a trivial work injury. We must be alert to these expectations so that we can address the patient's underlying concerns. Remember that our medical advice is delivered in the context of the patient's expectations and may not be heard or may not be followed if it is misunderstood.

Employer's expectations. The employer, who ultimately pays the medical costs, expects us to return a healthy, productive employee to the workplace as soon as possible. The employer may expect the employee to continue work in spite of pain, as in "Look, doc, I broke my arm and didn't miss a day of work the whole time, and you keep my employee off work for a little sprain." This expectation of rapid cure is particularly true for soft tissue injuries such as low back pain, in which the clinical examination is relatively unrevealing and the pathologic condition is not readily observable to others.

The employer may also try to use the work injury to discipline a problem employee. He may request that we keep the patient off work for an extended period so that the worker suffers a greater financial impact or loses sick days or vacation days.

Also, the employer may expect all medical information on the employee. We must be judicious with regard to such communication. (See Chapter 6, Legal Issues, for further discussion of what information may or may not be passed along to the employer, and to Chapter 4, Administrative Aspects, for information about the logistics of communication with the employer.) If the patient believes that we are a direct conduit to the boss, she may withhold useful information or may shade the information that is presented to us. The patient's confidence in us will be undermined if appropriate confidentiality cannot be maintained.

Finally, the employer may press for a return to work at each clinic visit, adding pressure to our interaction with the patient. The employer may threaten to use another clinic if we do not return injured employees to work fast enough.

Insurance carrier's expectations. The claims adjustor may not only expect excellent and inexpensive medical care but may expect to manage or micromanage the case. We may find ourselves asking a clerk for permission to do our job. Physical therapy may not be authorized. Bone scans or magnetic resonance imaging (MRI) studies may not be authorized, or authorization for further diagnostic testing or treatment may be delayed pending investigation of the claim. Meanwhile the patient faces us expectantly from the examination table, and the employer wants to know why the case is progressing so slowly.

In this time of medical cost containment, we must recognize more than ever our responsibility to weigh the need for diagnostic testing or expensive, prolonged therapy. Certainly, the insurance carriers expect physicians to be appropriate and judicious when ordering. Most workers' compensation carriers have established an array of systems to review billing and practice habits.

Physician's expectations. As physicians, we expect to do our jobs with minimal interference or resistance. We may expect to walk into a room, do our medical science, and exit with a plan that will be carried out by others such as laboratory technicians, nurses, physical therapists, x-ray technicians, and pharmacists. We expect the full cooperation and participation of the patient. We may not expect a patient to resist taking medicine because she prefers herbal therapy. We may not expect the insurance carrier to deny authorization for treatment that has been ordered. We may not expect the employer to question our decisions regarding the work status.

We also expect to be paid whatever we charge. Some states have fee schedules that limit reimbursement for services rendered under workers' compensation. Some insurance carriers routinely send bills to a review organization that may automatically or arbitrarily reduce the billing category or fee. Payment is frequently delayed, further frustrating the practitioner.

It is useful to be aware of your own expectations as a counter to the frustration that you experience when they are not met.

Determining whether the injury is work related. Another unique aspect of occupational medicine is the demand that is placed on the physician to determine whether the injury is work related. The answer is simple when the injury is the obvious result of a specific incident at work, such as a cut, burn, or fall. Unfortunately, this line is blurred by concepts of cumulative trauma, work-related stress, aggravation of an underlying medical problem by work, and pain that may slowly worsen over days to weeks after normal work activity (such as light lifting) that may or may not have caused the problem.

The decisions regarding the cause of a particular medical problem take on importance in a time when, because of soaring medical costs, many workers have no private medical insurance or have

had their private insurance cut or limited as the result of company cost-control measures. There may be subtle or overt pressure on the employee to make an injury work related so that insurance will cover the medical costs. We may face an employee who tells us that her back hurt a little at work but became worse after she and a neighbor moved a dresser at home. The employee tells us that she loves her job, needs work to buy food for her family, and has no private insurance because she has worked only 4 months or is a part-time employee. "Doc, I can't afford to pay any medical bills, and I can't be off work without some income for food. Please help me. My family relies on me."

This tendency may be countered by an employer or insurance carrier who will deny that the injury is work related or will put a case on hold pending investigation. Employers whose insurance premiums are experience rated are motivated to decrease the number of claims to lower the cost of their insurance. The adjustor may take weeks or months to investigate a claim, interview witnesses, or undertake surveillance of the allegedly injured employee.

It is also important for the employee that we determine, as soon as possible, whether an injury is work related. Significant medical expenses can mount as we order diagnostic tests and therapy. If the workers' compensation carrier, after some investigation, denies the injury as work related, the private insurance carrier may not automatically cover the costs if we are not a member of the appropriate medical plan or preferred provider network. Suddenly the patient becomes responsible for a huge medical bill, and both parties may be unhappy at the outcome.

Once again, the practitioner is placed in the line of fire. The important issue at hand is not how to diagnose or how to treat a medical problem (the usual domain of the physician's practice) but whether the injury is covered by workers' compensation insurance. Although at first glance this issue may seem peripheral to doctoring, it nonetheless may be central to successful diagnosis and treatment. Also, the answer may not be a simple yes or no. An injury may be apportioned so that a certain percentage is considered work related and the remaining percentage is not.

Finally, remember that many patients who are sent to our clinics may already have a personal physician. We are the interlopers. Our role is best carefully defined and strictly confined to appropriate treatment of the work-related injury. Ongoing medical care for underlying, pre-existing, or non-work-related medical problems must remain with the primary care physician. This fact underscores the need to define the work-related aspects of any medical problem so that appropriate care can be delivered by the appropriate route.

Work status. Among the challenges of treating injured workers is the decision regarding work status after an injury. In treating occupational injuries, it is not enough merely to make a diagnosis and formulate a treatment plan. We must determine work relatedness and then, worse, must determine whether the patient can return to work. This skill is not commonly taught in our medical training. Nowhere are there clear, written guidelines for work status.

Unfortunately, the answer often is not as simple as whether the patient can or cannot return to work. Sometimes the person can return to modified work with lifting restrictions or with shorter hours or with limitations on sitting or standing. Making these judgments spotlights the art of practicing occupational medicine. Sometimes we have the aid of another physician's opinion or of adjunctive tests that help answer the question. More often, we must rely on our own experience or best guess.

The factors discussed previously define the context in which we practice medicine. They color and flavor our interactions with the patient and affect the healing process. We therefore must be aware of the dynamics involved as we treat injured workers so that we can find satisfactory resolutions to the problems that arise. Having outlined this context, let us examine some specific problems in case management and discuss avenues of response.

CASE STUDIES
Case 1

Eve cut her left index finger (DIP) on a piece of broken glass at work. The wound is properly sutured, and a 10-day follow-up appointment is made for suture removal. Eve asks, "What about work, Doc?"

Of course, we inquire about Eve's occupation and learn that she is a dishwasher. We may pause because the laceration is across the DIP joint, and we do not want dirty dishwater to result in an infection that could potentially involve the joint. Further inquiry clarifies that Eve works in the kitchen of a large hotel, where dishes are washed automatically by a machine. Eve has to lift trays of dishes onto a conveyor but does not hand-wash dishes. We instruct Eve to wear a finger cot or plastic wrap as needed to keep the wound clean at work.

This case points to the importance of understanding not only our patient's occupation but also the exact nature of the work. Do not assume that you and the patient have the same understanding of actual work activity simply from a job title.

When making decisions about work status, we must weigh the functional aspects of the job against the pathology of the injury, both in terms of actual limitations in function and potential for exacerbation or damage from continued use or exposure of the injured area.

Understanding the relationship between work demands and injury limitations should point us to an appropriate answer about work status. Remember that we have the option of prescribing activity modification or limitations that the employer may or may not be able to accommodate. We should put any medical restrictions in writing and give a copy to the patient, the employer, and the insurance carrier. Remember that some managers do not have the luxury of replacing an injured worker so that the required work can be done by a different employee while the injured employee performs a light duty assignment. The status slip may be thrown into a drawer, and the patient may be ordered to return to the usual job. At recheck appointments we should inquire about the patient's adherence to the modified duty assignment, particularly if the healing process is slower than we would expect.

We must also be alert to negative pressure from coworkers who may be doing extra work because our patient is on light duty. At times the injured worker may express a wish to return to full work before she is actually ready to do so to alleviate harassment from peers. Of course, the converse may be true. Modified duty may be a welcome relief from a difficult, demanding job or from an irascible supervisor. The patient's reluctance to return to normal work may be reflected in continued or new complaints of pain and impairment. Successful modified duty programs require planning, management training, commitment, and communication.

We may also prescribe splints, guards, and medication that will protect the injury and allow the employee to return to work safely. If we cannot balance the functional restriction with the required demand by modifying the job or protecting the injured area, we must remove the patient from work.

Although this previously mentioned decision process may seem intuitive, life is often not so straightforward:

You tell Eve that she can return to work as long as she wears a finger cot as necessary to keep the wound clean. She becomes agitated and tells you that there is no way she can keep it clean at work. She knows it will get infected. After further discussion, she bursts into tears and says, "I have two stitches in my finger. I can't work. Owww, it hurts too much. I never miss work, but I can't, I just can't. It hurts! It really hurts!" You hand the patient a box of tissue and sit back to reassess.

This situation requires sensitivity to the individual sitting in front of us. It may be appropriate to inform the patient that in our expert opinion, she can work without problem. We made a decision, and the patient must live with it. On the other hand, not all people respond the same to any given injury. Although an overwhelming majority of patients with a similar laceration would return to work, occasionally a person will be devastated by the injury and truly unable to function. It does not seem appropriate to punish people for their personalities. Remember that the employer hired the person we are treating, hired the person's skills, talents, personality, motivation, ability to cope, response to stress, strengths, and weaknesses.

A further caution in this case is Eve's contention that she knows the wound will get infected if she uses the hand. Patients who tell us that a return to work will make them worse may consciously or unconsciously backslide and experience an increase in their symptoms if forced to do so. Because our responsibility is to facilitate healing, restore function, and find the fastest means to an end, we must attend to the dynamics that might prolong disability. We must judge carefully when to press our opinion and when to be flexible.

We learn quickly that the injury is not a static bit of pathology but a kinetic experience set in a personality, in a belief system, in a family or social context, and in a complex psychologic theater. In short, it is set in an individual whose responses vary with the ongoing dynamics of life that continually affect the experience of pain, disability, motivation, and well-being.

Case 2

Sandra, a produce worker at the local supermarket, complains of back pain after a 20-pound box of artichokes falls from a pallet and causes her to twist backward. You diagnose a lumbosacral sprain, send her home with medications (NSAIDs and a muscle relaxant), and arrange to see her next week after a course of physical therapy. At that visit she has not improved. Physical therapy, including hot packs, ultrasonography, and appropriate back exercises is continued for another week, then another, then a fourth week. At a recheck visit your physical examination shows no significant deficit or pathologic condition. The patient tearfully tells you that she wants to work but can't even sleep at night because of pain. "I just can't go back to work. I'm really no better at all." The employer tells you that her coworkers say she is "running around shopping."

Several weeks into the course of treatment for a soft tissue injury (sprain), we may face a patient who states that she still hurts or that she is no better. Worse, the patient may tell us at each visit that she is "a little better." We may be lulled into thinking that the patient is making progress when, in fact, she is saying only what she thinks we want to hear because she wants to be pleasant and cooperative and wants to continue therapy.

This case highlights the need to reassess diagnosis and treatment at every visit. In a common case of low back pain in which progress is slow, we must look for other causes of continued symptoms or delayed recovery. It would be reasonable, in this situation, to get lumbosacral spine x-ray films between 5 and 8 weeks and to consider bloodwork regarding an underlying rheumatologic problem. Certainly by 6 weeks, a sound workup should be completed or well underway. If the diagnostic workup is unrevealing and progress is slow, consider consultation with a specialist. A fresh look at the patient may suggest other diagnoses or avenues of treatment. Be certain to supply the consultant with all available information to date *and* be clear about what information is sought from the consultant. Ask specific questions.

You order lumbosacral spine x-ray films and set up consultation with an orthopedist. The x-ray films are normal. The consultant informs you that he finds nothing that requires orthopedic intervention and agrees with your approach. "It's just a sprain. I asked Sandra to continue her care through you." At her next appointment, Sandra tells you that she is "a little better" but still hurts whenever she bends or tries to lift anything. Because her job involves lifting, she knows she cannot do it yet.

The consultant may not have a simple, magic answer to the dilemma. Sometimes more time is required for healing, and over another 2 or 3 weeks, the patient will recover. Our initial diagnosis of an uncomplicated lumbosacral sprain has been reevaluated and confirmed. Avoid *indiscriminate* use of MRI or computed tomography (CT) scans. Although these tests buy time and are convincing to reluctant patients or their attorneys, they usually have little impact on the ultimate course. The benefit may not outweigh the cost of the test. We must use these tests judiciously and wisely, not routinely and not out of desperation because we do not know what else to do.

Sandra's progress has been slow. We have reviewed the history and proceeded through an appropriate medical workup. We must at the same time reassess the treatment plan at every visit.

You ask Sandra what she does in physical therapy and speak directly to the therapist. You learn that she lies on a table for 20 minutes with hotpacks on her back. Then she lies another 8 to 10 minutes while the therapist performs ultrasonography. Then the therapist guides her through some exercises which, you learn, consist of gentle stretches. She is given a sheet of exercises to take home but does them only sporadically.

This passive approach to therapy may be useful for some patients. However, most patients can benefit from much more aggressive, hands-on therapy that includes manual therapy, manipulation, aerobic exercise, and aggressive strengthening. "Modality" physical therapy, like acetaminophen, feels good for a few hours but too often does little to advance the patient. If we order physical therapy, we must monitor the progress carefully at each visit. If progress is slow, we must make changes. If the approach is too passive, the therapist should spend more time on exercise. If the therapy is too aggressive, the therapist should be sensitive to the patient's limits. It is useful to refer routinely to several different therapists or therapy groups so that we can match the aggressiveness of their style to our patient's needs. It is also useful to educate ourselves with regard to physical therapy so that we can provide guidance to the therapist, particularly with regard to specific exercise regimens.

If after 2 weeks of physical therapy progress is negligible, we should make specific changes in the treatment plan. If progress remains negligible after another 2 weeks, we must strongly consider stopping physical therapy. We may easily fall into the habit of ordering more and more and more therapy because we do not know what else to offer. More of what does not work is still unlikely to work. Remember that the goal of therapy is to make the patient independent of it. When we order therapy, we must be judicious and must think about end points. If it does not help, stop it.

In this case, information from the employer (that the patient is "running around shopping") suggests that Sandra may not be as impaired as she reports during her clinic visits. Given the lack of objective findings and the length of time since the injury in the face of ongoing treatment, we might conclude that Sandra is malingering, is taking advantage of the system, and is simply trying to get out of work.

Unfortunately, this conclusion too often does not solve the underlying problem, whether it be physical, motivational, or psychologic. We must not lightly abandon our role as caregiver to assume the role of detective, investigator, or judge. If we tell Sandra that she must return to work because we find nothing wrong with her, we are closing a door, suppressing communication, and terminating our relationship—with or without resolution of the problem. In fact, Sandra may then simply find a more sympathetic practitioner. Rather than solving the problem, we have prolonged it, lost control over it, and lost the ability to have a positive effect.

Therefore, whenever we decide that our patient is malingering, we should use the opportunity as a warning to reassess the situation. We may, in fact, conclude that Sandra does not have a medical work-injury problem that needs further medical care. If so, we can clearly state this opinion and our reasons for reaching it. However, we must be certain that we are not swayed by our frustration with the patient's personality, beliefs, or sense of values, or by outside, less-than-objective, influences. We must also be certain that we have properly done our job as a medical care provider.

Sandra is sent to a different physical therapist, who, at your request uses an aggressive approach of manual therapy with aerobic and resistive exercise. At a recheck visit after 2 weeks of this therapy, Sandra reports that she "hasn't felt this good in a long time." She still gets occasional pain but feels that she can return to work. She does so successfully while completing 2 more weeks of conditioning physical therapy. She thanks you, adding that, "I was beginning to think you didn't believe me."

It is premature to presume malingering without a complete workup to rule out other causes of the pain and without modifying our therapeutic approach in an attempt to alleviate the symptoms. If we have satisfied these two criteria, and the patient remains disabled without any substantive medical explanation, then we may refine our definition of the problem. We must ask specifically what underlies, explains, or feeds the lack of progress.

Case 3

Susan, an ICU nurse, "wrenched my shoulder" during an emergency when she lifted a patient. The diagnosis was "shoulder sprain," and although her entire workup (which ultimately included an arthrogram) was negative, her progress was slow despite treatment with NSAIDs, steroid injection, and physical therapy. After 5 weeks of therapy, her range of motion was full, and there was no real pain, although she said, "It just doesn't feel quite right." She returned to a trial of full work and before completing one shift burst tearfully into your office: "My shoulder is killing me. I'm worse than when I first came here. What are you going to do? Please help me!"

We know Susan to be a highly trained and motivated professional who loves her job. She worked hard in physical therapy and demonstrated excellent arm and upper body strength. Neither we nor our consultant found any significant pathologic condition of the shoulder after a thorough evaluation. We are convinced that our diagnosis is correct and that we have not missed any significant medical problem.

One option at this point would be to order more physical therapy. Perhaps Susan returned to work prematurely and a little more time off and a little more physical therapy might solve the problem.

Another option would be to inquire further about the specific problem that Susan encountered when she returned to work.

Susan tells you that she really felt great when she got up to go to work. "I always notice my shoulder a little, but it really didn't bother me. I was doing OK until I bent over to plug in an IVAC. Then I got this pain in my shoulder again. I freaked out. I was afraid that I wouldn't be able to function in an emergency, that I'd hurt my patient or myself further. Is my nursing career over?" You hand her a box of tissues and sit back to reassess.

Susan has suggested the solution to her problem. The activity that caused her pain was not heavy lifting. The patient does not lack strength or range of motion. Therefore more physical therapy might not be the best choice at this time. The issue seems to be one of function and confidence in her ability to perform. Susan was referred to an occupational therapist.

The occupational therapist first performed a job analysis to clarify the physical, environmental, and emotional demands of Susan's job. Susan noticed pain with activity in certain positions such as reaching up to adjust monitors or infusion pumps. She also feared moving her patients. The pain was not severe, but the fear and emotional impact were.

The therapist then designed a brief, six-session course of rehabilitation aimed at modifying the way in which Susan performed the tasks that bothered her. She was taught how to move and lift patients without hurting herself. She pushed a wheelchair loaded with a light weight, then with a small person, then with a heavy person, first on a flat surface, then on an incline. Within a short time Susan was able to perform the functions of her job without problem and with confidence.

Within 2 weeks, the therapist knew Susan was ready to return to work; Susan knew that she was ready; and you knew that she was ready. She returned to full work without problem and shared with her coworkers the proper techniques of lifting and reaching.

This case illustrates the value of listening to the patient, identifying the specific problem, and aiming the solution as specifically as possible at the problem. Physical therapy is a valuable tool for alleviating symptoms and increasing strength and range of motion. If function or how the task is performed is the issue, consider alternatives such as occupational therapy.

Case 4

Don, a hospice worker, pulled an AIDS patient in a wheelchair upstairs and noted sudden, sharp low back pain. You diagnose a lumbar sprain. Don volunteers that he is healthy, HIV positive, taking no drugs, and has no history of opportunistic infections or other problems. His pain appears significant, and hydrocodone is dispensed.

When seen again 4 days later, Don states that the pain is severe and requests more hydrocodone. His examination is remarkable for lumbar paraspinous tenderness and spasm. There are no radicular signs. L/S spine x-ray films are normal, and physical therapy is ordered. After one physical therapy visit, Don phones, fearful and crying, because the pain continues to bother him even at night. When seen 1 week later, he tells you that the pain is killing him and that he needs some stronger medicine.

This case underscores the importance of getting past medical records and the names of other physicians who are seeing or have seen the patient. Certainly this case suggests drug-seeking behavior. As always, however, the physician's responsibility is to define the problem.

Given the severity of the complaints and the physician's gut feeling that something was wrong, an MRI scan was obtained early in the course. Don was found to have lymphoma with spine involvement. This diagnosis stunned everyone, because there was no history of pain. His symptoms came on after a specific event at work and seemed clearly related to lifting the wheelchair. His pain was real, as was his fear. In retrospect, Don admitted to occasional back pain, but he thought nothing of it. We must not be mislead by precipitous judgments about a patient's true motivation. Our job is to be objective and compassionate.

Case 5

Chuck, a construction worker, fell from a roof 10 feet to the ground. He got up, bruised and embarrassed, and continued to work. The next day he came to the emergency room with upper, mid, and lower back pain. X-ray films were negative, and he was referred to your office. Chuck denied any previous back problems. He has been a construction worker for 15 years and has had only minor accidents throughout that time. You diagnose cervical and thoracolumbar sprains and send Chuck to physical therapy.

At each visit Chuck feels better, but you and he are reluctant about a return to full work that involves climbing, lifting, bending, stooping, carrying, and squatting. All these activities bother Chuck. Several weeks slip by, and slowly Chuck improves. At 6 weeks his upper back pain is mostly gone, but he continues to note lower back pain. His MRI scan shows only a minor central disk bulge at one level. Your favorite orthopedic consultant has little to offer. Now, 2 months after the injury, you learn that Chuck, long ago, lost his job. He tells you that the pain bothers him at night and that he doesn't eat well when it bothers him.

It is now 11 weeks since the fall. Diagnostic studies are negative. Chuck tells you that "The physical therapy really seems to help me. I do OK for a day or two, and then if I overdo, wham, I get this pain. All I can do is lie down. I think if I get some more therapy, I'll get better."

Where is the end point? At what point is Chuck "permanent and stationary" with regard to his fall? Chuck seems willing and able, but not quite. Somehow his case has slipped along for months.

If we truly believe that we have completed our evaluation and have no further therapeutic options for the patient, we should consider declaring that he has reached maximum medical improvement (permanent and stationary). The process of defining any residual impairment or permanent disability can then begin. The process of returning Chuck to a productive life that is not about his pain can also begin. However, declaring someone permanently disabled has potentially devastating lifelong effects on the individual. In many ways, it rivets the problem to the person forever. This decision is best made after exhausting all other options (see the discussion in Chapter 36, Vocational Rehabilitation).

This case was not tightly controlled. Chuck seemed to be improving. Each clinic visit ended with a little more time off, a little more therapy. Each of us hoped that next time Chuck would be well. Yet, he never was.

In retrospect, the problem subtly and quietly shifted from one of acute injury to one of chronic pain. Neither the doctor nor the patient was aware of what happened or when. Chuck might benefit from referral to a pain clinic, although earlier intervention might have averted the fall into chronic pain and permanent disability. (See Chapter 21 for further discussion of pain clinics and pain management.)

The lack of an objective pathologic condition to explain the degree of impairment, the sleep disturbance, the loss of appetite, and the loss of job all point to depression, somatization, or both. Early probing inquiry, early dialogue with Chuck, or early referral for psychologic evaluation with regard to somatization might have defined and highlighted the real problem behind the experience of pain, allowing for effective early intervention.

Referral to a psychologist or psychiatrist is likely to be resisted by the insurance adjustor, who sees the referral as the nightmare of *a new stress claim*. We must be clear with the patient and the adjustor that we seek a one-time consultation to help clarify issues around the symptom, around the experience of pain. The consultant's report should help define the cause of the pain experience. If the symptom is the result of somatization, some form of counseling or psychotherapy will likely be recommended. Ordinarily, therapy aimed at underlying conflicts is not covered under workers' compensation, and this therapy may have to be paid for privately.

Occasionally a patient who has marginal ability to cope with ordinary life problems will be overcome by a work injury. A defined number of psychotherapy or counseling therapy sessions (usually 6 to 10) may in some states be covered under workers' compensation as appropriate to resolve a specific and temporary aggravation of an underlying problem. However, an end point can and must be defined. These few sessions, which are explicitly directed at returning the patient to the baseline (still marginally functional) state, are much less expensive than ongoing physical therapy while the patient remains off work and fails to progress. Such therapy allows closure of the workers' compensation claim and provides the patient with correct treatment that is more likely to succeed. (See Chapter 32 for further discussion of psychiatric issues and somatization.)

This case underscores the need to reassess diagnosis, treatment, and progress *at every clinic visit*. The patient may tell us that she is improving, but if she is still off work, intervention is demanded. Actions must speak as loudly to us as words.

Case 6

Judy, a receptionist in a physician's office, wrenched her back while carrying a 10-pound box of files. You diagnose a lumbar sprain, but her pain continues despite 6 weeks of physical therapy and medication. The orthopedic consultant tells you that her MRI scan is completely normal and that he can find nothing wrong with her. He follows her for a time, but 3 months after the injury, Judy returns to you.

She is upset as she tells you that she still experiences daily pain. She has returned to work but frequently is forced by pain to stop her activity and to rest. She has used all her sick days and still leaves work early on bad days. She says that the specialist has not helped. She has been through physical therapy with two different therapists and got a new chair at work. "After sitting for 15 minutes, my back is killing me. So I try to walk around for a while, but the pain just stops me." She tearfully asks you, "Am I going to have this pain all my life?"

Issues raised in the discussion of Chuck's case (Case 5) certainly apply to Judy.

You review the evaluation by your consulting psychologist, who does not find a psychiatric diagnosis. He notes that she has a low level of pain tolerance but that she does not fit the profile of somatization.

In select cases we might consider other treatment options. Judy has been through the approach of traditional medicine without much benefit. We might consider alternatives such as acupuncture, biofeedback, chiropractic adjustments, yoga, or one of the somatic therapies such as rolfing, Alexander work, or Feldenkreis.

Many patients benefit greatly from these approaches. We can arrange a trial of 6 to 10 sessions with the particular practitioner of the chosen approach and reevaluate the patient at the end of that time. We must also contact the workers' compensation carrier for prior authorization, which may or may not be granted. Usually a limited, direct therapeutic trial that is carefully monitored will be of negligible cost compared with total medical expenditures to date.

In this case, Judy was sent to a rolfer and miraculously improved. She received 10 sessions and was able to be discharged from further care. She thanks you profusely and feels that "I have my life back."

MEETING THE CHALLENGE

How do we meet the challenges that face us as we treat injured workers? We have discussed some of the hazards and offered some navigational aids. The above cases present options to consider when approaching the management of difficult clinical situations. Awareness of the following points may ease the decision process:

1. Thoughtfully assess the diagnosis at every visit. Gear the extent of your workup to the complexity of the case and to the degree of agreement between the defined pathologic condition and the patient's complaints.

2. Weigh carefully at each visit the patient's response to therapy and make changes accordingly. Use the full range of your therapeutic armamentarium as necessary.

3. Fulfill your responsibilities to all parties involved in the case and understand your charge to find the most appropriate and expedient solution to the problem.

4. Define your role. Be clear about whose advocate you are as you make decisions. As a caregiver, your primary responsibility is to your patient, even though in the workers' compensation system you have an expanded set of responsibilities.

5. Understand the dynamics of the workplace and the particular job tasks required of your patient as you contemplate work status.

6. Solicit input from other health care professionals who have seen your patient, including physicians, consultants, physical and occupational therapists, and vocational rehabilitation counselors.

7. Be candid with your patients. If you detect underlying fear, anger, distrust or believe that the patient may be exaggerating a complaint, share your observation and be open to the response.

8. View the workers' compensation claims adjustor as a partner who may provide valuable input or guidance in difficult cases.

This summary points to some of the tools that we can use to direct the course of a difficult case toward resolution.

There is another important factor that must be considered: ourselves. As practitioners, we must be aware that we may be part of the difficulty in a difficult case. Sometimes we do not hear patients. We do not attend to the dynamics playing out in front of us. We are not sensitive to the fullness of the communication coming from the patient or the subtle solutions that the patient is suggesting. We burst into the examination room with our mind elsewhere, annoyed that we have to spend time on someone's trivial complaints after a minor injury at work. We tightly ask our medical questions about when, where, and how much, throw the pieces into our mental hopper, pull out a diagnosis and treatment plan, and move along to the next patient. We may not even perform a thorough examination. Too frequently, patients say that, "The specialist walked in, spent 3 minutes asking questions, asked me to move my arm, and then told me to get some tests and come back in 3 weeks." This interaction does little to satisfy either party and certainly does not promote a smooth working relationship.

We must not forget that many patients cannot distinguish serious from minor pain and may be genuinely worried about their condition. We must not forget that medical care should be about well-being, not merely about repair. We must not lose the opportunity to have a positive impact on the patient's life because we are piqued at wasting time on what we judge to be a trivial problem. We therefore must be as sensitive about what our actions communicate to the patient as we are about what the patient's words and actions communicate to us.

In addition to being aware of and responsible about what we communicate, we must be clear about our own motives, about the forces or influences behind the decisions we make. Sensitivity to the patient demands sensitivity to ourselves. We must understand what dynamics affect our decisions in order to remain objective. As we discussed in Case 1, factors to be weighed when determining work status are (1) diagnosis and pathologic findings, (2) degree of impairment, (3) job tasks, (4) mechanical protection of the injury, (5) modified duty, (6) work environment, and (7) patient motivation.

On the basis of these criteria, we usually can reach a reasonable decision on any given patient's work status. But what can color, influence, or even change this decision? Consider your reaction to the following two patients whose first words to you are as follows:

Paul: "Look, Doc, I know I hurt my back, but I really like my job and need to work. I just need something for the pain and send me back to work."

Larry: "Look, Doc, I'm in a hurry. I'm meeting with my attorney in half an hour. I don't care what you say, I'm not going back to work!"

Do you react the same to Larry as to Paul? Does one influence you to be more or less firm in your decision? Would you attend to one more than the other? Would you spend more time with one than the other?

We must examine our own emotional responses to patients not only in terms of how these reactions influence our decisions but also as a signal that the particular case or patient requires careful attention to potential troubles. If we find ourselves angry, hostile, upset, or bored with a patient, we should consider the emotion as an alert to examine the dynamics carefully. These cases might require more careful objective testing or might prompt us to quickly define exact medical pathologic conditions or to explore the patient's work, social, family, and psychologic environment.

At a practical level, awareness of the complexity of forces around a work injury will help define and limit the treatment course when the patient's complaints continue in the face of no significant medical condition. We can chase symptoms for months if we believe that their only source is from damage to the body and that we must address them with therapy as long as they continue. In his twenty-third lecture, "The Paths of Symptom Formation," Sigmund Freud discusses symptoms:

In the eyes of the general public, the symptoms are the essence of a disease, and to them a cure means the removal of the symptoms. In medicine, however, we find it important to differentiate between symptoms and disease, and state that the disappearance of the symptoms is by no means the same as the cure of the disease.[1]

The converse is also true. The persistence of symptoms is by no means the same as persistence of organic disease or physical injury. The symptoms may actually reflect underlying pain or conflict that is unrelated to the specific accident at work. Therefore, as we treat injured workers, we are challenged constantly to define the problem, to define the cause to apply the correct solution. This solution, in some cases, may be a recommendation for psychologic counseling on a non-work-related basis. Clearly, arriving at this conclusion implies that we have carefully examined and ruled out any physical condition requiring further medical treatment. It also implies a solid working relationship with the patient and assumes honest communication with the patient about our conclusions and the patient's reactions to and concerns about these recommendations.

Treating injured workers offers the opportunity to practice medicine in a context that can positively affect people's lives beyond merely suturing a wound, setting a fracture, or treating an infection. People spend the majority of their waking hours in the workplace and often define themselves by their jobs (as we often do). The workplace can become a stage where internal struggles, conflicts, or dramas are played out. Awareness of these internal influences on the course of an injury can lead to solutions that are closer to healing than repair.

CONCLUSION

The challenge of treating injured workers is a challenge to practice the art of medicine. We must recognize that around every difficult patient is a difficult system with difficult practitioners. It is our job to define the difficulties and to find the proper resolution.

Solutions to the difficult cases require an understanding of the medical condition, the patient, the workplace, the psychologic dynamics, the workers' compensation system, and most importantly, ourselves as practitioners. We must be aware of what motivates and affects our decision-making process so that we can remain objective.

The challenge of patient care in the workers' compensation system is the challenge to practice medicine with art, grace, intelligence, and compassion in the face of a system that does little to honor or support such practice. Therein lies the experience of satisfaction from our work. Therein lies the reason we went into medicine. Therein lies healing.

REFERENCE

1. Freud S: Lecture 23, "The Paths of Symptom-Formation." *A General Introduction to Psycho-Analysis.* A series of lectures delivered at the Vienna Psychiatrical Clinic in 1916-1917, first published in German in 1917.

21 Pain Management

LOCAL AND REGIONAL ANESTHESIA

The management of painful injuries and the use of local anesthetics are important aspects of everyday treatment of occupational injuries. In discussing local and regional anesthesia, this chapter explains the mechanism of action, the nuances of clinical use, and the recognition, prevention, and treatment of adverse reactions to commonly used anesthetics.

The first local anesthetic was cocaine, an alkaloid found in the leaves of the *Erythroxylon coco* shrub from the Andes Mountains. Local anesthesia was achieved by allowing coco-drenched saliva to drip from the surgeon's mouth into the wound. In 1884 Koller, a colleague of Freud, used cocaine in the eyes, and he is credited with introducing local anesthesia into clinical practice. In 1885 Halsted demonstrated that cocaine could block nerve transmission, laying the foundation for nerve block anesthesia. The search for alternatives led to the synthesis of the benzoic acid ester derivatives and the amide anesthetics.

Although local anesthetics have been used for more than half a century, it was not until the 1960s that physicians gained a specific understanding of the physiochemical properties, mechanism of action, pharmacokinetics, and toxicity of these agents.

Pharmacology and physiology

The commonly used local anesthetic agents share a basic chemical structure:

aromatic segment
intermediate chain
hydrophilic segment

Within the basic structure, each agent's specific chemical composition determines its main physiochemical properties. These in turn are the principal determinants of the agent's pharmacologic activity: onset of action, potency, and duration of action.

The two main classifications of local anesthetics are based on the intermediate-chain linkage between the aromatic and hydrophilic segments: either an amino-ester or an amino-amide. The ester-type drugs include procaine, chloroprocaine, cocaine, and tetracaine. The amide-types include lidocaine, bupivacaine, mepivacaine, prilocaine, and etidocaine. The main difference between esters and amides is their metabolic pathways. Esters are hydrolyzed by plasma pseudocholinesterase, whereas acids are metabolized in the liver to enzymatic degradation.

Chemically, local anesthetics are poorly soluble, weak bases that must be combined with hydrogen chloride to produce the salt of a weak acid. In the resulting acidic solution, salts exist both as uncharged molecules (nonionized) and as positively charged cations (ionized). The uncharged form is lipid soluble, enabling it to diffuse through tissues and across nerve membranes; the charged form cannot do this. The ratio of the uncharged to charged form depends on the pH of the medium (vial solution or tissue milieu) and the pK_a (pH at which the charged form equals the uncharged form) of the specific agent.[1] When the pH of the solution or tissue decreases, a given agent exists more in a charged form; conversely, when the pH increases, the agent exists more in its nonionized, uncharged form, which can diffuse through tissues and nerves. Manipulation of the solution's pH is a useful tool for the physician.[2]

Local anesthetics are available in plain solution and premixed with epinephrine, both in single-dose ampules and multidose vials. The antibacterial preservative in the multidose vials is methylparaben, which has been implicated in many allergic reactions. Agents premixed with epinephrine contain an antioxidant to prevent deactivation of the vasoconstrictor. These solutions must be more acidic (pH 3.5 to 4) to maintain stability of the epinephrine.

Nerve impulse and transmission

The resting potential of a nerve (-70 MV) is the net result of marked differences in ionic concentrations on each side of the axonal membrane and the forces that maintain that difference. There is a surplus of sodium extracellularly and of potassium intracellularly. When a nerve is excited, the sodium channel opens and a slow influx of sodium begins, followed by a more rapid movement once a critical threshold has been reached. The influx of sodium and efflux of potassium creates the process known as the action potential. Repetition of the action potential cycle facilitates propagation of the nerve impulse, which is essentially unidirectional.

Mechanism of action

Anesthetic solutions exist in charged and uncharged forms, with the concentration of the uncharged form increasing in more alkaline milieus. It is only the uncharged, lipid-soluble form that crosses tissues and membrane barriers. Once the agent has penetrated the barrier, the uncharged form reequilibrates into uncharged and charged forms. It is now believed that both the charged and uncharged forms are responsible for activity, with the charged form predominating for most anesthetic agents.[3]

The most attractive theory concerning these drugs' mode of action involves their binding to a receptor that is on the inner surface of the nerve cell membrane.[4] The broad consensus is that the physiologic basis for neuro-blockade is prevention of sodium influx across the nerve membrane. Local anesthetics reduce sodium influx, which decreases the slope and amplitude of depolarization, thereby preventing the action potential from forming. If there is no action potential, no impulse can be transmitted, and conduction blockade is achieved. The result is local anesthesia.

Adverse effects

The use of local anesthetics is not without risk of adverse events. These events may be categorized into systemic toxic reactions, allergic reactions, effects on wound healing and infection, and local injuries.

Systemic toxicity. Systemic toxic reactions are rare, occurring in fewer than 0.4% of administrations of local anesthetic. Yet they are the type of serious reaction most frequently encountered.

These reactions are caused by high blood levels of local anesthetic, which result when the drug is absorbed from the injection site into the systemic circulation. This most often occurs with inadvertent intravascular administration. Toxicity most commonly occurs with higher concentrations or doses, injections at vascular sites, a rapid rate of administration, and the absence of a vasoconstrictor.

The earliest manifestation of systemic toxicity is central nervous system (CNS) stimulation, which results from blockade of inhibitory synapses. CNS depression follows as a result of direct depression of the medulla. The increasing order of CNS toxicity with a representative lidocaine concentration is as follows: numbness of the

tongue, lightheadedness, and tinnitus (4 ng/ml); visual disturbances (6 ng/ml); muscle twitching (8 ng/ml); convulsions (10 ng/ml); coma (15 ng/ml); and apnea (20 ng/ml).[1] Drowsiness is common with lower doses of lidocaine but not with bupivacaine or etidocaine (Fig. 21-1).

Cardiovascular toxicity at moderate blood concentrations (lidocaine, 3 ng/ml) produces a slight increase in cardiac output, heart rate, and arterial pressure. At concentrations above the CNS toxicity levels, local anesthetics cause direct myocardial depression, manifested as hypertension and bradycardia. In severe cases this can lead to cardiovascular collapse.

Factors affecting toxicity. Anesthetics are used in equipotent doses (for example, 1 mg bupivacaine to 4 mg lidocaine) and therefore are approximately equitoxic. On a milligram-for-milligram basis, the more potent agents are more toxic. Among the amide anesthetic agents, those with high lipid solubility and protein binding (in increasing order: etidocaine, bupivacaine, lidocaine, and mepivacaine) are more likely to be sequestered in tissue, allowing for slower absorption and lower blood levels. Anesthetics with a greater volume of distribution or more rapid clearance also produce lower blood levels. These characteristics create margins of safety for each anesthetic, with etidocaine having the greatest safety margin, followed by bupivacaine and lidocaine.

Maximum safe dose. The dose that produces a blood level of the drug just below the toxic level is defined as the maximum safe dose. Unfortunately, the maximum safe dosage for each anesthetic cannot be based on the patient's weight because studies have shown the volume of drug distribution to

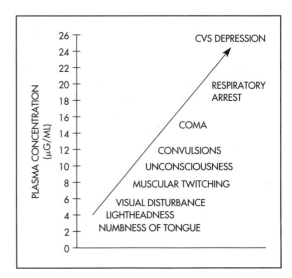

Fig. 21-1 Symptoms of systemic toxicity per lidocaine concentration.

be relatively constant. Maximum safe doses, as stated in the package inserts, should be taken only as guidelines. Most of them are based on animal experiments and use only absorption data. They vary with the site, the use of vasoconstrictors, and even the patient's condition. They often can be exceeded safely when administered accurately, yet they may be toxic even within the safe range if inadvertently injected intravenously (Fig. 21-2).

Allergic reactions. True allergic reactions are rare, accounting for only 1% to 2% of all adverse reactions. Esters, specifically the metabolite paraaminobenzoic acid (PABA), account for the great majority of these reactions. Amide solutions are rarely involved, and it is usually the preservative methylparaben (MPB), which is structurally similar to PABA, that is responsible. Hence, if multidose vials containing MPB are used, the response may appear as a cross-reaction to an ester allergy. Patients may also have an allergic response on contact with a local anesthetic as a result of previous sensitization to MPB, which is found in various creams, ointments, and cosmetics, or to PABA, an ingredient in many sunscreens.

Both delayed and immediate reactions can occur. Immediate hypersensitivity may produce a variety of signs and symptoms, from rhinitis and mild urticaria to bronchospasm, upper airway edema, and even full-blown anaphylactic shock. The onset may be immediate, occurring even during administration of the agent. These reactions should be treated with intramuscular diphenhydramine and subcutaneous epinephrine. In more serious reactions, intravenous epinephrine, diphenhydramine, and corticosteroids should be administered.

Physicians frequently face the problem of treating a patient who claims to have a history of local anesthetic allergy. Because true allergy is rarely

---

The drug concentration of an anesthetic solution or preparation is expressed as a percentage (bupivacaine 0.25%, lidocaine 1%).

A 1% solution contains 1 g/dl (10 mg/ml) of the anesthetic.

The strength of a solution or preparation can be calculated by moving the decimal point one place to the right:

0.25% = 2.5 mg/ml (e.g., bupivacaine)
0.5% = 5 mg/ml (e.g., tetracaine)
1% = 10 mg/ml (e.g., lidocaine)
2% = 20 mg/ml (e.g., viscous lidocaine)
4% = 40 mg/ml (e.g., cocaine)
5% = 50 mg/ml (e.g., lidocaine ointment)

Fig. 21-2 Calculating an anesthetic's strength.

the cause of previous adverse reactions, a careful history and use of prior medical records, if available, are crucial in evaluating these patients. The inquiry should attempt to uncover the cause of past reactions and the agent involved, the exact signs and symptoms, the amount of drug used, and the technique of administration. If an allergic reaction was present or cannot be excluded and the drug is known, an agent from the other class of anesthetics should be used.

If there is uncertainty about the specific agent involved, the physician should choose an alternative approach to management. This may range from general anesthesia if the wounds are extensive and the risks are acceptable to no anesthesia if minimal pain is expected and the procedure is short, such as one or two sutures in the scalp. Alternatives include parenteral narcotics, benzodiazepines, inhalation nitrous oxide, or a combination of these. Antihistamines such as diphenhydramine (Benadryl) have shown anesthetic properties when injected into wounds, although the mechanism of action is unknown. One recent study showed similar levels of early anesthesia with both 1% diphenhydramine and 1% lidocaine, although lidocaine had a significantly longer duration of action. The standard 5% parenteral form of diphenhydramine should be diluted to 1% for subcutaneous injection (1 ml diphenhydramine to 4 ml saline solution).[5]

Infiltration anesthesia

Injection of an anesthetic directly into the tissues to be surgically manipulated is called "infiltration anesthesia." It is indicated whenever good surgical conditions can be obtained with the use of this technique. It should apply to most minor surgical procedures. Field block anesthesia can be considered a form of infiltration anesthesia, because the agents, concentrations, and safe doses are the same. A field block involves a subcutaneous injection around the surgical site to create an anesthetic field.

The advantage of infiltration anesthesia over nerve block and general anesthesia is that it generally is quicker and safer. Local infiltration also can provide homeostasis, both by direct distention of tissue and by use of epinephrine. The major disadvantage, compared with nerve blocks, is that a relatively large dose of drug is required for a relatively small area.

Choosing an agent. The local anesthetics most commonly used for infiltration are 1% to 2% lidocaine, 0.5% to 1% procaine, and 0.25% to 0.5% bupivacaine (Table 21-1). Lidocaine has long been the agent most commonly used because of its excellent activity profile, low allergenicity, and low toxicity. Procaine is useful for patients who are al-

Table 21-1 Commonly used infiltration anesthetics

Drug	Plain solution		Epinephrine-containing solution		
	Concentration (%)	Max. dose (mg)	Duration (min/hr)	Max. dose (mg)	Duration (min/hr)
Short duration					
Procaine	0.5-1	500	15-45 min	600	30-120 min
Chloroprocaine	1-2	800	15-30 min	1000	30-90 min
Moderate duration					
Lidocaine	0.5-1	300	30-60 min	500	2-6 hr
Mepivacaine	0.5-1	300	45-90 min	500	2-6 hr
Prilocaine	0.5-1	500	30-90 min	600	2-6 hr
Long duration					
Bupivacaine	0.25-0.5	175	2-4 hr	225	3-7 hr
Etidocaine	0.5-1	300	2-3 hr	400	3-7 hr

lergic to amide anesthetics. Bupivacaine, with its prolonged duration, may be preferred if postoperative analgesia is desired.[6] Studies have shown that after laceration repair, patients treated with bupivacaine had less pain than those treated with lidocaine.

A longer-acting anesthetic may also be useful for prolonged procedures or for procedures that might be interrupted in a busy practice. The duration of anesthesia with lidocaine can be prolonged by adding epinephrine, sodium bicarbonate, or both. Epinephrine has the advantage of providing excellent hemostasis and slowing systemic absorption. Vasoconstrictors should never be injected into tissue that is supplied by end arteries. Use on fingers and toes, the nose, the pinna of the ear, and the penis may result in gangrene.

Proper technique. The proper technique of administration should be used to minimize pain, prevent bacterial spread, and avoid intravascular injection. For a given anesthetic, lowering the pH by adding epinephrine increases pain; raising the pH by adding sodium bicarbonate decreases pain. Numerous clinical studies have documented that alkalinizing the anesthetic reduces pain and stinging during injection.[7] This is true for both infiltration and digital block anesthesia.[8] The technique has improved patient satisfaction during minor surgical procedures involving skin infiltration.

To apply this technique with lidocaine, 1 ml of sodium bicarbonate (8.4%, 1 mEq/ml) is added to every 10 ml of anesthetic solution. Sodium bicarbonate probably works by increasing the ratio of nonionized to ionized molecules, rendering the pain receptors less sensitive, or by producing more rapid inhibition of pain transmission. The addition

of bicarbonate should not reduce the duration of action.

Local infiltration anesthesia should be administered before the wound is manipulated and cleaned to reduce the patient's discomfort. It is more comfortable for the patient, and equally as effective, if the anesthetic is injected subdermally rather than intradermally. Intradermal anesthesia, which raises a wheal, provides more rapid onset of anesthesia but is certainly more painful. Subdermal injection may take 5 to 10 minutes for onset of anesthesia. All injections should be made through the wound edge and not through a skin puncture, which is quite painful.[3] A slower infiltration rate is also more comfortable. Infiltrating as the needle is withdrawn after inserting the needle maximally allows space for the solution, which reduces the pain associated with tissue distention. The smallest needle possible should be used, such as a 27- or 30-gauge needle with a 10 ml syringe.

Nerve blocks

For most lacerations and injuries seen in the office or emergency department, infiltrative anesthesia is adequate and efficient. However, there are indications for peripheral nerve blockade. The general requirement is that the blockade provide anesthesia equal or superior to that offered by other techniques. Digital nerve blocks of the fingers and toes are commonly used and are indispensable to the practitioner. Nerve blocks would be preferred over infiltration when (1) tissue distension from local infiltration would hamper closure or compromise blood flow (fingertip); (2) anesthesia is required over a large area and multiple injections would be painful, or the amount of anesthetic needed for local infiltration exceeds the recommended dose; (3) a nerve block is the most efficacious form of treatment.

The factors influencing the choice of anesthetic for nerve block are similar to those for local infiltration. If analgesia is desirable after the procedure is completed, such as for repair of traumatic injuries, a long-acting anesthetic such as 0.25% bupivacaine would be appropriate; 1% lidocaine with epinephrine, where allowed, can be substituted. Care must be exercised not to exceed the recommended doses of anesthetic.

The procedure should be explained to the patient, including the pain of needle insertion, paresthesia that may be felt, and possible complications that may occur. Inserting the needle close to small nerves and "into" the nerve sheath of large nerves is the essential step in a successful block. The ease of locating the nerve varies with the anatomic relationship between the nerve and block site. Some sites have good structural landmarks immediately next to the nerve (e.g., prominent bones or tendons). For example, the digital nerves are reliably found at positions 2, 4, 8, and 10 o'clock around and just superficial to the proximal phalanx.

Digital nerve blocks. Blocking the digital nerves of fingers and toes is the most commonly used form of nerve blockade in the acute care setting. It is superior to local infiltration in most circumstances. Indications for chosing digital blockade include repair of finger lacerations and amputations, reduction of fractures and dislocations, drainage of infections, and removal of the nail.

Each finger is supplied by two sets of nerves, the dorsal and palmar digital nerves. The dorsal nerves run along the phalanx at the 2 and 10 o'clock positions, and the volar nerves are located at the 4 and 8 o'clock positions.

The palmar, or common, digital nerves are the principal nerves supplying the fingers. These nerves arise from the ulnar and median nerves at the wrist and supply sensation to the volar skin and interphalangeal joints of all five fingers. For the middle three fingers, it usually is necessary to block only the palmar digital nerves because they also supply the dorsal distal aspect of the finger, including the fingertip and nail bed.

The digital nerves can be blocked anywhere in their course, but the preferred site usually is the web space between the fingers because there is more tissue space here to accommodate the volume of anesthetic injected. After the skin has been prepared, anesthesia is deposited at the position of the four digital nerves (2, 4, 8, and 10 o'clock) using a 25- to 30-gauge needle. The needle is inserted on the dorsal surface just distal to the metacarpophalangeal (MCP) joint and along the lateral edge of the bone. The dorsal digital nerves are blocked first, and the needle is then passed lateral to the bone, toward the palmar surface, where more anesthetic is deposited after first aspirating. The procedure is then repeated on the opposite side of the finger. The total volume required is 4 to 8 ml. This technique produces a band of anesthesia at the base of the finger that can be massaged to promote diffusion of the anesthetic to the nerves. Epinephrine is contraindicated when blocking digital nerves because of possible vasospasm and ischemia. Nerve blocks are commonly used in toes, and the indications and techniques are similar.

SUMMARY

Appropriate, thoughtful use of local anesthetics is vital to the treatment of acute injuries and other painful conditions. Easing the patient's pain allows thorough assessment, supports directed, definitive treatment, and promotes patient compliance and satisfying outcomes.

MANAGEMENT OF CHRONIC PAIN
WILLIAM BAUMGARTL

Pain management has become a growing field in the 1990s. It is now not uncommon to find practitioners whose entire practice has developed around the management of chronic and acute pain. The field of medicine has responded to the new demand for pain management by developing fellowship training programs to promote a higher degree of treatment sophistication. 1993 became the first year that the American Board of Anesthesiology offered its first subspecialty board certification in pain management. Given this important trend, the purpose of this section is to review the concept of chronic pain management so that the occupational primary-care practitioner can know when to seek the unique services offered by a pain medicine specialist.

Effects of chronic pain

Chronic pain usually is defined as any pain syndrome that lasts longer than 3 months. However, the syndrome has much greater implications than duration of pain alone because the presentation and manifestations of chronic pain may take many different forms.

Almost anyone who has persistent pain for any extended period begins to manifest maladaptive functioning and behavior. Most patients develop at least some elements of depression and tend to withdraw from their work, friends, and family. This results in the loss of important emotional support structures at a time when the patient most needs them, increasing his stress and anxiety.

Unlike with acute pain, some patients with chronic pain may give no outward display of their pain, causing some people to doubt the degree of pain they feel. The patient's perception that other people cannot understand his level of pain leaves him angry and frustrated. Other patients with chronic pain may show extreme displays that are out of proportion to their level of pain in an attempt to seek help and understanding from caregivers. Over time the patient's response to the persistent pain becomes as debilitating as the pain itself, and the patient can devolve into a desperate, poorly coping, and incapacitated human being.

Pain management clinic

The treating physician must address all components of an injured worker's pain complaint to ensure optimal success. The primary goal, of course, is to resolve the painful condition that originally bothered the patient. However, it also is important to reverse the patient's depression, restore his social support structures and self-esteem, and renew his sense of well-being and physical functioning. The complex nature of this treatment requires support from several specialties, and the treatment often is best done with the assistance of a pain management clinic that packages these specialists and services together.

Pain clinics run by physicians usually take one of two forms: "block clinics," where the focus is limited to procedure-oriented diagnosis and treatment and "comprehensive clinics," which provide both diagnosis and long-term care and management. Either type may be multidisciplinary in scope, although this approach usually is characterisic of the "comprehensive clinic." As the specialty evolves, the trend is growing toward comprehensive clinics because of their versatility.

Referral to a pain clinic should be considered in any of the following conditions:

1. Any severe pain that the practitioner is unable to manage or uncomfortable in managing (cancer pain, postoperative pain, management of chronic use of narcotics).
2. Any pain condition at high risk of becoming chronic if not quickly resolved under the practitioner's care (sympathetically mediated pain, shingles, back pain).
3. Any patient with "red flags"—pain with a history of substance abuse, sexual abuse, physical abuse, depression, or secondary gain issues.
4. Chronic pain.
5. Specialized diagnostic assistance (selective nerve blocks, diagnostic sympathetic nerve blocks).
6. Specialized therapeutic assistance (epidural steroids, sympathetic nerve blocks, and implantable pain management devices, such as dorsal column stimulators, intrathecal pumps, indwelling catheters, and the like).

Process

The pain management process should begin with an attempt to get an accurate diagnosis of the patient's pain process and to identify all other related medical and psychosocial issues that may affect the problem.

Effective pain management cannot begin until the origin and pathway of the pain is identified. For example, the initial differential diagnosis for a patient with low back pain may include (1) pain originating from a muscular strain, (2) nerve root irritation or compression, (3) spinal stenosis, (4) vertebral compression fractures or instability, (5) referred pain from the facet joints or discs, (6) primary or metastatic bone disease, (7) Aortic aneurism, or (8) Renal disease.

Obviously, the treatment approach and the likelihood of success will differ, depending on which specific cause of pain is identified. A careful history and physical examination, along with diagnostic blocks, often are useful to help differentiate pain etiologies. In this example, half of the differential diagnoses may be ruled out by the history and physical examination alone. The remaining possibilities may be sorted by selectively blockading different structures in the back with precisely placed injections of a local anesthetic. These injections, often done with fluoroscopic assistance, can be useful in methodically "unplugging" different possible pain pathways and structures to identify the pain generator.

It is important to concurrently evaluate the patient's psychosocial structure. Does the patient give a history of physician shopping, multiple procedures, crying spells, marital and work discord, weight change, and sleep loss? All of these may be signs of depression or a marked loss of coping skills. A rough assessment of broad categories of psychologic functioning and well-being usually can be achieved by spending an additional few minutes during the examination specifically asking about depressive symptoms, family and job functional interactions, suicidal ideation, and a history of abuse. Patients who evidence problems in these areas probably warrant a full psychologic evaluation by a psychologist or other caregiver skilled in doing such assessments.

The value of this assessment should not be underestimated. It is often difficult to determine where emotional pain ends and physical pain begins; both may be present and real for the patient. Pain has two important components that create misery for a patient. Pain begins as a signal that is transmitted to the brain from some pain generator, and part of the patient's pain is certainly proportional to this signal. However, the other component of pain is how the brain processes and interprets the pain signal. This processing has tremendous impact on how the pain *affects* the patient. A soldier shot in the heat of battle may sometimes go hours before realizing that he has been wounded and before being aware of the pain of the wound. The same soldier may be crying in agony days later during a simple dressing change. Even with a circumscribed pain stimulus, such as an intramuscular injection, people exhibit varying pain tolerance. The resulting response to a given stimulus can range from no reaction to extreme crying and yelling. Patients with a history of abuse often attach traumatic associations to pain input, and, as a result, relatively minor pain becomes disabling for them. Cortical processing has a great deal to do with the resulting misery and impact of pain.

When a patient's pain has a strong emotional component, some of the distress can be reduced by behavioral modification and stress reduction. Depending on the chronicity and severity of the psychologic dysfunction, sometimes only a few sessions of psychotherapy and education are needed to restore a patient's sense of well-being. Patients with a history of abuse or who are psychologically defensive may require a more prolonged period of treatment. Patients with depression often do best with a combination of psychotherapy and antidepressant medication to restore their ability to function more quickly.

Attempting to treat a pain problem without addressing the psychologic components may seriously impair the success of the treatment. For example, severely depressed patients often claim to feel no improvement in pain despite all interventions. Concurrent treatment of their depression is imperative for any satisfactory outcome. Similarly, patients whose pain is mediated from secondary gain, such as a husband who is only treated sympathetically by his wife when he has back pain, may have trouble resolving their pain until the underlying issue (in this example, the marriage relationship) has improved. Psychologic "red flags" indicate the strongest imperative for multidisciplinary and multidimensional approaches, so that solutions to the pain problem can be effective.

Finally, it is important to stress that pain should be addressed as an urgent problem. Failure to treat acute pain aggressively not only prolongs the patient's suffering, it also often leads directly to the development of chronic pain patient, with all the complications described previously. The relief of

pain and suffering was the original goal of the physician in ancient Greece, and it should still be our goal today. When a patient has pain that is significant enough to affect his daily activities, a cause for the pain must always be sought. At the same time, the physician must be sure to follow-up immediately with a program for effective treatment. The best window of opportunity for treating pain occurs when the problem first arises. It can be hard to try to catch up months or even weeks later. The cost and failure rate of treatment escalates rapidly with time. If a practitioner feels uncomfortable managing a particular problem, the most effective time to seek consultation is early.

Procedures

Epidural steroids. Probably the best known service offered by most pain centers is injection of epidural steroids for back pain. A common cause of chronic back pain is herniation of a degenerated disc. This not only results in mechanical compression of neural tissue but also results in the release of the disc's contents. The disc contents are acidic and rich in phospholipase A_1, a strong inducer of arachidonic acid, as well as other inflammatory mediators, such as substance P.[9] Extrusion of this material is extremely irritating to neural tissue, particularly when this tissue is under compression. The rationale behind using steroids in the epidural space is that they can help block the inflammatory reaction caused by the chemical irritants, thereby speeding recovery.

By convention, steroids usually are given once a month for a total of three doses. This practice is supported by a study showing that 58% of 144 patients previously unresponsive to the first epidural steroid injection responded to a second or third epidural steroid injection.[10] Even when pain is reduced by the first injection, many practitioners believe that reapplication of steroids helps ensure the quiescent state of the back while the patient is recovering. Because insoluble steroid salts usually are used in the procedure, there is little reason to repeat doses of the steroid more often than every 3 to 4 weeks (the drug's duration of action). There have been no studies showing the optimal choice of steroids, dose-response relationships, or timing of steroids. Studies documenting their effectiveness have also been difficult to pursue because of the difficulty in controlling for the duration of symptoms and the exact nature of the pathologic condition of the back. However, the preponderance of data suggests that epidural steroids do reduce pain and restore activity,[11] with typical success rates ranging from 50% to 90%. The benefit of giving epidural steroids is highest when they are given early and when the duration of pain has been short.[11] One study reported a success rate of 69% in achieving satisfactory pain relief when steroids were given in the first year of symptoms.[10] This success rate decreased to 46% after 1 year.

At first glance, long-term follow-up studies show little apparent advantage to giving epidural steroids. More than 90% of patients with disc disease treated with or without epidural steroids recover without needing surgery.[12] The main value in giving epidural steroids lies in their short-term ability to speed recovery and get the patient back to work sooner. Epidural steroids have been associated with a higher incidence of return to work and higher rates of retention in work at 12 months.[13] Patients given these steroids also show less need for supplemental narcotic use and are better able to comply with physical therapy because of their increased comfort. It is my recommendation to consider epidural steroids early in the course of treatment for any patient with back pain caused by degenerative disc disease or nerve root compression that is unresponsive to noninvasive therapies. In well-selected patients, the speedier return to work will more than offset the cost of the procedures done early and will spare many patients needless misery while waiting to resolve their problems.

The most common complication associated with the use of epidural steroids is inadvertent puncture of the subarachnoid space, which has an incidence of less than 2%. This can result in a severe spinal headache for the patient and frequently necessitates an epidural blood patch to correct the problem. Bleeding, infection, and new nerve damage are exceedingly rare complications and are not normally of clinical concern.[11] Patients referred for epidural steroids should not be taking any aspirin products or other anticoagulant medications and should have no other active bacterial infections. Human immunodeficiency virus (HIV) disease does not contraindicate epidural injections as long as the patient has no platelet abnormalities and the usual sterile procedure precautions are observed. Because approximately 12.9% of epidural injections given "blindly" are misplaced,[14] many practitioners now routinely do these procedures under fluoroscopic guidance to verify correct placement. Fluoroscopy is also helpful when requesting blocks on patients who have undergone previous back surgery and who may have altered spinal anatomy.

Sympathetic nerve blocks. Reflex sympathetic dystrophy (RSD) is one name for a syndrome of sympathetic nerve dysfunction that sometimes occurs after even minor injuries. This syndrome, more correctly called sympathetically mediated pain (SMP), appears as a constellation of early skin

hypersensitivity, inflammation, and swelling after an injury. The original injury causes hyperstimulation of sympathetic nerve outflow. One of the sympathetic outflow functions is to innervate the sensory tissue and regulate the sensitivity and gain of the sensory nerve. When the sympathetic nerves are hyperstimulated, the sensory nerves become so hypersensitive that even cold air currents or light touch result in excessive sensory nerve discharge and intense pain. Patients keep the affected extremity protected close to their body, often covered with a warm material to protect it from cold cold drafts and chance contacts. When left untreated, the extremity later becomes cold and atrophic, leading to its classic name of reflex sympathetic dystrophy. At the advanced stage of the disease, the process becomes irreversible and usually results in permanent disability for the patient. (See Chapter 22, Cumulative Trauma/ Repetitive Motion Injuries for further discussion of RSD.)

The keys to resolving this syndrome are to recognize the process early and treat it aggressively. Mild cases may resolve spontaneously with a period of physical therapy, but it is important to proceed rapidly if the syndrome is severe or not resolving quickly. Referral for local anesthetic blockade of the sympathetic nerve supply to the affected area is necessary, both to confirm the diagnosis of the process and to initiate treatment. Fig. 21-3 shows the dramatic improvement in symptoms that usually results from sympathetic blockade. Repeated nerve blocks spaced closely enough together to provide prolonged pain relief usually allow the sympathetic nerves to "reset" and resume normal function. Blocks two or three times a week or more may be necessary until the process is controlled. The spacing of the blocks is then gradually increased to maintain quiescence of the sympathetic nerves. When SMP is treated early and aggressively, success in resolving the problem is high.

The sympathetic nerve supply to the head, neck, upper thorax, and hand passes through the stellate ganglion, which sits anterior to C7 in the neck.[15] Hence, sympathetic blockade to these areas is achieved with a stellate ganglion block. Sympathetic nerve supply to the lower extremities usually is disrupted at the lumbar sympathetic plexus chain, which lies anterior to the upper lumbar vertebrae.[16] Alternatively, Bier blocks, with the use of intravascular administration of local anesthetics and bretylium under a tourniquet, or epidural blockade of the affected area also effectively block sympathetic outflow to an extremity.[17]

Patients who achieve short-term pain relief with sympathetic nerve blockade but whose pain persistently returns may have some other pathologic

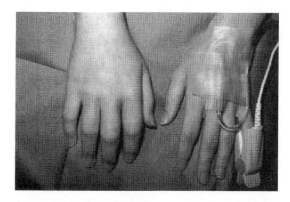

Fig. 21-3 A Young woman with an acute sympathetically mediated pain of her right hand. Note the marked edema. The patient was barely able to move her fingers and had severe pain to the slightest touch of her skin.

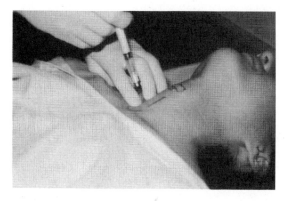

Fig. 21-3 B Same patient shown in Fig. 21 A receiving a stellate ganglion block.

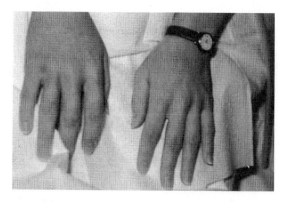

Fig. 21-3 C The same patient shown in Figs. 21 A and B two days after receiving a stellate ganglion block. Edema has been substantially reduced, and pain is nearly gone. The patient could now close her hands to make a fist.

condition that keeps stimulating the sympathetic nervous system. One common cause is coexisting injury of a nerve, causing neuralgia. A coexisting nerve injury with a sympathetically mediated pain is called a *causalgia*. Other causes of persistent pain include occult fractures, ligament disruption, or persistent tendonitis. Patients who do not demonstrate a progressive increase in the duration of pain-free intervals between blocks should be further evaluated for previously unrecognized disorders. If no underlying treatable problems are found, the patient can be treated with long-term disruption of the sympathetic nerves (a neurolytic block) or in extreme cases may require implantation of an electrical spinal cord stimulator.

Medical management with tricyclic antidepressants, NSAIDs, alpha-receptor drugs such as Minipress and clonidine, steroids, and sodium channel–blocking drugs such as mexiletine, often are appropriate adjuvant therapies to speed resolution of the process, but they are never acceptable substitutes for sympathetic nerve blocks in controlling the symptoms. Transcutaneous electrical nerve stimulation (TENS) units usually increase pain for these patients and rarely are helpful. Once the patient is made comfortable with blocks, it is important to proceed with a physical therapy program to restore function to the injured area. Physical therapy given without first addressing pain may actually aggravate the process in cases of severe SMP, by further increasing sympathetic outflow; and it is needlessly cruel to the patient.

CASE STUDIES

Case 1

A 56-year-old woman consulted a spinal surgeon about her low back pain, which radiated to her right buttock and leg and had lasted 6 months. The patient had an MRI scan, which showed evidence of a herniated L5 disc compressing the right L5 nerve root and marked facet hypertrophy. Nerve conduction studies had detected an S1 neuropathy. Her surgeon believed she might be a surgical candidate for decompressive laminectomy, but he was uncertain in proceeding because of the conflicting information from the studies. She was referred for a pain diagnostic consultation.

The patient's medical history was otherwise unremarkable. She appeared to have a good relationship with her husband and was still able to work part-time. She had no apparent secondary gain issues and reported only mild sleep disturbance. She was otherwise without evidence of depression. Her physical examination showed a pain distribution somewhat consistent with an L4 nerve root lesion, although she had a considerable amount of bilateral low back pain.

A series of diagnostic blocks were performed to help identify and localize her pain complaint. With the use of fluoroscopy, the L3, L4, L5, and S1 nerve roots were located, and electrical stimulating needles were placed in contact with the nerve roots. Each nerve root was individually stimulated, and it was determined that only stimulation of the L4 nerve root reproduced the distribution of pain in her leg. An injection of local anesthetic temporarily blocked the pain in her calf area, confirming part of the pathway of her pain transmission.

She persisted in having low back and buttock pain, not resolved even temporarily by injection of the L4 nerve root. Because her history and symptoms were consistent with a referred pain from her facet joints, the next step in diagnosis was to isolate the facets selectively. Again under fluoroscopic guidance, additional needles were placed to block the nerve supply to these joints. A series of injections enabled the specialist to isolate the low back pain to an origin from the lower lumbar facets. The blocks also showed that the pain was transmitted through the right and left L3, L4, and L5 facet nerves (the medial branch of the dorsal primary ramus nerve). Only when the facet nerves were blocked simultaneously with the right L4 nerve root was the patient's pain completely resolved.

On reviewing this information, the patient's surgeon believed she was no longer a candidate for any of the procedures he was considering. Although she had evidence of a pathologic condition at L5 and S1, these areas were actually not the source of her pain, and the blocks predicted that surgical interventions at these areas were not likely to relieve her pain. She was referred for a trial of additional therapeutic blocks to see if her pain could be managed nonsurgically. A repeat block of the L4 nerve root was performed with a long-acting steroid. The facet nerves were injected with small quantities of absolute alcohol to disrupt their function on a long-term basis. The patient had nearly complete resolution of her pain and returned to full work duties without further interventions.

Case 2

Originally, a 62-year-old woman consulted her general practitioner about new-onset groin and vaginal pain and burning 5 years ago. She believed that her pain began shortly after moving a box at work. A routine speculum and manual examination failed to show any abnormalities. The pain rapidly became more severe, and a repeat examination by a gynecologist was equally unrevealing. The woman was next sent to a urologist, who found no urologic abnormalities. Plain x-ray films of her pelvis were normal.

Her medical history was significant for chronic bouts of poorly managed depression throughout her life. She also had a history of sexual abuse as a child. She had remarried for a second time and had been in a stable marriage for more than 15 years. She worked as a housewife and had no lawsuits pending for her injuries.

Her pain persisted for a year without resolution. Because of the multiple red flags in her history, she was finally referred to a pain management clinic. Her initial medical screening was again benign, and note was made of the extensive psychosocial problems she had had throughout her life. Because she previously had been labeled as a sexually abused patient who had vaginal pain, the pain clinic practitioners thought the evidence for a psychologic basis to her pain was over-

whelming. It was decided to treat her with antidepressant medication, counseling, and biofeedback. The patient was extremely compliant with her treatment and underwent 3 years of counseling. Despite this, her pain persisted. Finally, in frustration, she sought new health care providers to treat her pain. A second gynecologist thought her pain may be referred from her uterus and proceeded to perform an abdominal hysterectomy. The patient developed pneumonia postoperatively and required a prolonged recovery in the ICU. Unfortunately, her pain persisted, unchanged by her surgery. She ultimately returned to the pain clinic for care, this time under a different provider.

Her presentation was quite compelling. She stated, with extreme frustration, "I have had this pain problem for 5 years now. I've done everything my doctors have recommended. I am no longer depressed, and I've become very well adjusted. I think I have resolved what happened to me as a child. I am not crazy, and I still hurt in my vagina!" In reviewing her records, the specialist believed that an accurate diagnosis of her pain problem had never been made. It was always presumed that her problem was attributed to her psychologic history, and an exhaustive workup of her problem had not been pursued. It was agreed that a thorough reevaluation with diagnostic blocks should be performed to try to localize her pain problem.

An epidural block done at the time of her hysterectomy had temporarily blocked her pain, suggesting that the pain originated at or below her lumbar area. To rule out referred visceral pain from any remaining pelvic tissue, a bilateral lumbar sympathetic block was performed, not to block the sympathetic nerves but to temporarily denervate the visceral afferents, which travel with the sympathetic nerve plexus at that location. This produced no pain relief for the patient (and would have predicted that the hysterectomy would have been ineffective in relieving her pain). The remaining likelihood of pain pathways suggested some process originating between the vagina and the sacrum. Serial blocks were planned, starting with the most distal portions of the nerve pathways. The first block attempted, a pudendal nerve block, produced complete pain relief for the patient. On careful reexamination of the area, the pain specialist detected a small lump in the deepest recess of the vaginal wall that previously had been missed. With the knowledge of the block results, a repeat gynecologic evaluation specifically addressing this area was requested. A subsequent surgical exploration revealed a benign tumor compressing the left pudendal nerve. Removal of this tumor relieved the woman's chronic pain.

Case 3

A 35-year-old woman had a history of severe right hand and wrist pain after receiving a new computer keyboard. After 2 months of protests, a different keyboard was finally provided, but her pain continued to worsen. Several physicians had been consulted in her care, and she had been treated with NSAIDs, splints, and physical therapy. Her pain rapidly escalated to the point that her hand had become tender to the slightest touch, and she constantly kept a mitten over it to protect it from drafts. Her ring had to be cut off her finger because of the marked swelling in her hand. Because of the extreme pain, she could no longer work. Her husband had also recently been laid off, and there was a great deal of stress at home, resulting in numerous fights. She was referred to a pain management clinic for evaluation.

The patient broke into tears frequently during her examination. She could hardly sleep at night because of the pain and rarely left the house. She was tired and frustrated. She had lost all desire for engaging in sex with her husband, much to his consternation, and this had been the cause of additional arguments.

Her past medical history was unremarkable. Her medications consisted of amitriptyline (25 mg) to help with sleep, ibuprofen (800 mg bid), and Vicodin (six tablets per day). She denied any lawsuits pending for her injuries.

Her physical examination showed a hand that had normal motor and sensory function. It was swollen and warm to the touch, with dramatic mottling of the skin. Even small motions of all joints were markedly painful. Light touch of the skin showed a stocking-type distribution of hypersensitivity extending up to the midforearm. Her neck and shoulder examination was normal save for diffuse muscular trigger points.

A presumptive diagnosis of sympathetically mediated pain was made on the basis of her physical examination. A subsequent stellate ganglion block showed complete pain relief in her upper extremity within 5 minutes of the block, and the hypersensitivity of her skin normalized. She was scheduled for a follow-up block 2 days later (Figs. 21-3 A, B, and C).

On her next visit, the edema in her hand had substantially resolved, and motion in all joints had improved. Her neck and shoulder stiffness had also improved. The patient stated she had $1\frac{1}{2}$ days pain relief from the first block, although she was now beginning to have some return of pain. A repeat stellate ganglion block was performed. Her medical management was also optimized by gradually increasing her dose of amitriptyline to a more therapeutic level of 100 mg/day and by increasing her ibuprofen to three times a day. After 3 more weeks of treatment, she had progressed only to getting a maximum of 3 days of pain relief from a block. Attempts were made to add alpha-active drugs, such as clonidine and Minipress, as well as physical therapy, but this additional intervention stretched the duration of action to only 4 days. The patient also was now noticing some tenderness in the radial portion of her wrist even after the stellate blocks.

Because of her failure to progress with repeated sympathetic blockade, she was referred to an orthopedic hand surgeon for evaluation. Further workup revealed a previously unrecognized carpal fracture with nonunion and ligament disruption from an old skiing injury. Wrist reconstruction was performed while the patient continued to receive intermittent sympathetic blocks. Her wrist pain finally resolved 8 weeks after surgery. During her period of recovery, she received six once-a-week, 1-hour counseling sessions focusing on the effect of pain on her behavior and began to address her marital problems. Her husband was invited to participate in the final two sessions. They were subsequently referred to a private marriage counselor. Her night sleep was finally restored after her dosage of amitriptyline was increased to 125 mg each night. Her mood also improved, and she began once again to go out with her old friends from work. She later was placed on light duty office work and returned to full-time work status.

In analyzing this patient's case, the repetitive-motion injuries from the new keyboard at her work probably resulted in a flare of the pain from her damaged wrist. This in turn led to an increase in sympathetic outflow, further increasing her pain and eventually establishing a cycle of sympathetically mediated pain. Sympathetic blocks confirmed a diagnosis of the sympathetically mediated pain but did not resolve the precipitating problem. Additional diagnostic work identified the remaining pathologic condition. The wrist reconstruction corrected the wrist problem, while ongoing sympathetic blockade prevented her sympathetic dysfunction from progressing and ultimately allowed function to return to normal. Counseling greatly reduced her stress level as she began to understand what had been happening to her and as she worked to restore her relationship with her husband. As her depression resolved, her motivation increased and she renewed her other support structures. Physical therapy restored mobility and strength to the damaged hand. The patient eventually retrained to a different office function. Although she had continued wrist stiffness after surgery, the severe, disabling pain never returned.

REFERENCES
Local and regional anesthesia

1. Vanstrum GS: *Anesthesia in emergency medicine,* Boston, 1989, Little, Brown.
2. Tetzlaff JE: Clinical effects of pH adjustment of local anesthetics, *Anesthetics Anesthesiology Review* 20(1):9-15, 1993.
3. Orlinsky M, Dean E: Anesthetic and analgesic technique in clinical procedures in emergency medicine. In Robert JR, Hedges JR, editors: *Clinical Procedures in Emergency Medicine,* Philadelphia, 1991, WB Saunders.
4. Savarese JJ, Covino BG: Basic and clinical pharmacology of local anesthetic drugs. In Miller RD, editor: *Anesthesia,* New York, 1986, Churchill Livingstone.
5. Dire DJ, Hogan DE: Double-blinded comparison of diphenhydramine versus lidocaine as a local anesthetic, *Ann Emerg Med* 22(9):66-69, 1993.
6. Hanke B: Advances in wound management in the emergency department, *Resident and Staff Physician* 39(1): 23-26, 1993.
7. McKay W, Morris R, Mushlin P: Sodium bicarbonate attenuates pain on skin infiltration with lidocaine with or without epinephrine, *Anesth Analg* 66:572, 1987.
8. Bartfield JM, Ford DT, Homer PJ: Buffered versus plain lidocaine for digital nerve blocks, *Ann Emerg Med* 22:216-219, 1993.

Management of chronic pain

9. Sella E: Noncompressive spinal radiculitis, *Orthop Rev* 21:827-832, 1992.

10. Warr AC, Wilkinson JA, Burn JMB, Langdon L: Chronic lumbosciatic syndrome treated by epidural injection and manipulation, *Practitioner* 209:53-59, 1972.

11. Benzon H: Epidural steroid injections for low back pain and lumbosacral radiculopathy, *Pain* 24:277-295, 1986.

12. Sheon R: Cost-effective care for low back pain, *Journal of Musculoskeletal Medicine* 8(1):57-81, 1991.

13. Dilke TFW, Burry HC, Grahame R: Extradural corticosteroid injection in management of lumbar nerve root compression, *Br Med J* 2:635-637, 1973.

14. Andrade S, Eckman E, Yates G: The value of preliminary interlaminar epidurography during the performance of interlaminar lumbar epidural injections, International Spinal Injection Society, vol 1, no 6, Sept 1993, pp 28-31.

15. Cousins MJ, Bridenbaugh PO: *Neural blockade in clinical anesthesia and management of pain,* ed 2, Philadelphia, 1988, JB Lippincott, pp 479-482.

16. Cousins MJ, Bridenbaugh Phillip PO: *Neural blockade in clinical anesthesia and management of pain,* ed 2, Philadelphia, 1988, JB Lippincott, pp 483-487.

17. Hord AH, Rooks MD, Stephens BO et al: Intravenous regional bretylium and lidocaine for treatment of reflex sympathetic dystrophy: a randomized, double-blind study, *Anesth Analg* 74:818-821, 1992.

22 Cumulative Trauma/Repetitive Motion Injuries

Cumulative trauma/repetitive motion injuries have been called the occupational epidemic of the 1990s. The Occupational Safety and Health Administration (OSHA) uses the term "cumulative trauma disorder" (CTD) to identify injuries that arise over time rather than as the result of a specific accident or incident. The U.S. press has promulgated the term "repetitive motion injury" (RMI) primarily referring to injuries stemming from the use of computers or video display terminals (VDTs). Another term, "repetitive strain injury" (RSI) was used widely in Australia during the 1980s epidemic in that country (NOHSC, 1986). In this chapter we use *repetitive motion injury,* and although we recognize that the disorder occurs in a variety of occupations, we have centered the discussion on keyboard use as the prototype for the ailment in this decade.

Historically, these are not new injuries. Bernardino Ramazzini (1633-1714) discusses diseases of weavers in the 1713 supplement to his 1700 treatise *De Morbis Artificum* (Diseases of Workers):

In the weaving-rooms where they are employed in making the cloth there are men who spend the whole day shearing the woven cloth with large heavy shears, a task which is naturally very fatiguing, above all for the arms and hands. . . . To relieve intense fatigue, gentle rubbing of the arms, thighs, and legs with oil of sweet almonds will be beneficial.

Ramazzini's description of diseases of scribes and notaries in 1713 translates easily to the afflictions of modern computer keyboard operators:

The maladies that afflict the clerks aforesaid arise from three causes: First, constant sitting; secondly, the incessant movement of the hand and always in the same direction, thirdly, the strain on the mind from the effort not to disfigure the books by errors or cause loss to their employers when they add, subtract, or do other sums in arithmetic. . . . In a word, they lack the benefits of moderate exercise, for even if they wanted to take exercise, they have no time for it; they are working for wages and must stick to their writing all day long. Furthermore, incessant driving of the pen over paper causes

intense fatigue of the hand and the whole arm because of the continuous and almost tonic strain on the muscles and tendons, which in the course of time results in failure of power in the right hand.

Ramazzini goes on to describe an acquaintance of his, "a notary by profession," whose history could easily be that of a modern office worker:

First, he began to complain of intense fatigue in the whole arm, but no remedy could relieve this, and finally the whole right arm became completely paralysed. In order to offset this infirmity, he began to train himself to write with the left hand, but it was not very long before it, too, was attacked by the same malady.

Heavy labor long has been associated with a variety of musculoskeletal problems that now would be classified as CTDs. However, our more recent problems have several causes. First, manufacturing of goods has changed from a craft-based process, whereby one or a few workers would produce a complete item, to assembly line production, initiated by Ford in 1905 and put into wide use over the next decades. As a result of this change, small muscle groups are being used hundreds or thousands of times per shift, performing the same small part of the production process. An automobile assembly worker may stand all day at a conveyor belt and turn screws on parts that flow past her 5000 times a day.

The widespread introduction of computers into information processing is a more recent change, one that certainly represents a significant change in work tasks. Computer technology has rapidly grown more powerful and smaller, and countless new applications are possible that previously were found only in the realm of science fiction. The focus has been on the VDT, but in fact this technology pervades all aspects of our lives, from grocery store scanners and library check-out lines to banking and clothing design (Bammer, 1987).

Additionally, a generalized speedup in the workplace has evolved, and fewer workers are asked to do more. This change was particularly evident in the economic recession of the late 1980s

333

and early 1990s. Layoffs have increased assignment workloads, and deadlines demand sacrificing coffee breaks, lunch, or brief rest and exercise breaks from keystroking. Journalists, for example, no longer stop to insert or remove a single sheet of paper from a typewriter; no longer stop to erase by hand; and no longer stop to write rough drafts by hand. Modern reporters do all text typing and editing on the keyboard, frequently take notes on the keyboard while interviewing by telephone, and even leave messages for colleagues on the computer E-mail system.

Ergonomic factors increase the risk of injury already posed by the escalation of repetitive motion tasks performed under increasing stress and time pressure. Until recently ergonomic considerations were not applied in the designing of work stations; work stations and tools were designed for the task, not the worker. Efficiency, cost, and aesthetics took precedence over fit and comfort for the worker. (See Chapter 35 for further material on workplace ergonomics.) (Drury, 1987; Feldman, 1983)

Psychosocial factors, such as job dissatisfaction and the stress caused when women, especially, hold down a full-time job and yet are still primarily responsible for the care of children and home, have also been implicated in studies searching for the etiologic factors in this epidemic of injuries (Linton, 1989).

Finally, the work force has become deconditioned. Modern patterns of living, which include (1) single adults and couples all working and frequently commuting long distances; (2) a lack of good physical education in schools and generally sedentary life-styles; and (3) the normal loss of muscle mass and strength that occurs with aging all combine to create a work force that often is deconditioned to the physical demands of repetitive work, leading to injury. An understanding of these factors is the key to successful diagnosis and treatment of these injuries.

ANATOMY

Cumulative trauma disorders can occur in any part of the body that is subject to the risk factors discussed here. This chapter focuses on upper extremity problems, but the clinician should recognize that low back injuries can very legitimately be considered CTDs in many settings, and although much rarer, lower extremity CTDs have been reported (Forst, 1988).

The anatomic structures most often affected, in order of frequency in our experience, are tendons and tendon sheaths, muscles, nerves, joints, and blood vessels.

Tendonitis and tenosynovitis are commonly found in the flexor and extensor tendons of the wrists and thumbs, the extensor tendons of the elbow, and the rotator cuff and biceps tendons of the shoulders. At the wrists the tendons are enclosed in sheaths, which supply lubrication for the finger movements. Risk factors include rapid, repetitive movements; pinching or grasping, particularly with force; awkward positions; nonneutral wrist position; and extended reaching at or above shoulder height (Luopajarvi, 1979; Reed, 1983).

Muscle spasm/pain syndrome, or "muscle strain," is the next most common injury seen in our clinics. An awkward, constrained posture is the most common cause, often deriving from lack of fit between the worker and work furniture. Common injury locations include the cervical paraspinous muscles, the trapezius and underlying muscles, and the forearm muscles (Maeda, 1986).

Nerve entrapment syndromes can occur anywhere from the cervical nerve roots distally through the shoulder and down the arm (Howard, 1986). Common locations include the cervical spine; the cubital tunnel at the elbow or Guyon's canal at the ulnar aspect of the wrist for ulnar nerve entrapment; the proximal forearm at the supinator muscle or the origin of the extensor digitorum communis for radial nerve entrapment; and under the pronator muscle or at the transverse carpal ligament for median nerve entrapment. The risk factors are similar to those for tendonitis but also include vibration exposure from hand-held power tools (Araki, 1988). (See Chapter 28 for further discussion of vibration-related injuries.)

Degenerative joint disease (DJD) occurs as a CTD in joints that are moving and loaded (i.e., weight bearing) in both animal models and epidemiologic studies (Acheson, 1970). Affected locations include the wrists, elbows, shoulders, knees, hips, and cervicolumbar spine.

It is important to note that osteoarthritis is not work related in office jobs or very light manufacturing. Significant weight stress (e.g., from commercial plumbing tools or foundry equipment) is necessary for upper extremity DJD to be considered occupational.

Thoracic outlet syndrome, or compression of the blood flow to the upper extremity, commonly occurs in jobs that require full arm extension, especially while holding weight. The anterior chest wall muscles can hypertrophy, which in deconditioned individuals is not balanced by enlargement of the back muscles, as it is in someone who exercises. Often the work requirements or body habitus also result in a head-forward posture. All these factors can cause compression of blood flow to the arms (resulting in numbness and tingling of the upper extremity, especially when the arm is elevated) that is relieved by lowering the extremity (Morse, 1992).

CLINICAL EVALUATION
Keys to the medical history

The medical history is critical not only to identify the correct diagnosis, but also to determine the work-relatedness of the medical problem. The history therefore begins with *standard questions* about symptom onset, duration, frequency, severity, and temporal associations, and very specific inquiry into what relieves or exacerbates the symptoms.

A detailed description of formal *treatment to date* is also needed. "Six weeks of physical therapy" could mean 6 weeks of hot packs and ultrasound or 6 weeks of intensive hand splinting, treatments, and exercises; each has a very different impact on the patient's course. Prescription and over-the-counter (OTC) drugs, as well as the patient's actual compliance, must be recorded. The clinician might also inquire about past chiropractic treatment and alternative therapies such as herbal remedies or acupuncture. How successfully these approaches alleviated the symptoms may help the physician better understand the severity of the complaint and its progression over time, and also may guide the therapeutic approach.

Occupational factors too often are insufficiently investigated when a history of cumulative injury is taken. The patient must be asked detailed questions about her workstation, tools, tasks, and practices. Workstation questions should seek a description of the type and height of the desk, bench, or worktable; the type, adjustability, and comfort level of the chair; the brand and model of computer; whether a mouse or trackball is used; and the location of these items on the work surface. Are "ergonomic aids" used, such as a wrist rest, footstool, and document holder? The use and type of other equipment, such as a telephone, calculator, keypunch, or stapler should be noted. Assembly line employees should provide a detailed description of the types of tools used (e.g., screwdriver, pliers), the handle material of the tools (hard plastic, metal, or rubber), and the location of all parts bins, including how far the worker has to reach to get frequently needed objects.

A useful approach to assessment of *work tasks* breaks down the day or week into the key tasks, such as 70% computer work, 15% telephone work, and tasks done occasionally or rarely, such as 5% mail sorting, 5% meetings, and 5% handwriting. The frequency and duration of exposure to risk factors are important issues in causality. Often two overlap. For example, many employees type on computer keyboards while processing telephone orders.

Obtaining a history of *work practices* involves assessing the patient's own approach to her job. Does she eat lunch away from or at her desk? Does she do overtime frequently or take work home? Does she get up and move around often, or does she remain working at her desk for hours? Does she "float" to different work stations? Does she get along well with her colleagues and supervisor? Does she enjoy her job and regularly do more than is required, or does she constantly feel that she is behind in her work? Is the work or office atmosphere stressful?

Perhaps the most important question to ask, in terms of causality, is *what changes were made* in the workplace during the several months before the onset of symptoms. Was the employee working on a big project with a deadline, working overtime, working faster because of a coworker's absence or layoff? Was the employee moved to a different work station, or did she get new tools (e.g., a new computer or a different one)? Did the employee just return from an extended vacation, illness, or pregnancy leave? Although these respites from work might seem beneficial, and sometimes are, they can predispose to deconditioning and thus increase the risk of injury.

A medical history of cumulative trauma must document *activities outside the usual job* that might cause or exacerbate the complaint. The frequency and duration of hobbies, "moonlighting" jobs, and exercise patterns should be explored. Playing tennis once a week is not likely to be an issue, whereas playing computer games for hours every night is significant.

The *past occupational history* should also be outlined; this can be done easily by having the patient fill out a form before the examination (Appendix A). The physician can then focus on previous jobs that might relate to the cumulative injury at hand. Past military service also should be explored in this light.

Finally, a careful, complete *standard medical history* should be reviewed. Again, a medical questionnaire should be completed before the examination and reviewed at the time of the examination; this ensures that nothing is missed and efficiently reduces the time spent on nonessential material. This medical history should include the past medical history, a review of systems, current medications, allergies, family and social histories, and use of alcohol, tobacco, or drugs. Specific medical conditions that might cause peripheral neuropathies or tenosynovitis, or both, must be explicitly ruled out. These include diabetes, hypothyroidism, lupus, rheumatoid arthritis, and other neuropathic or connective-tissue disorders.

Keys to the physical examination

The physical examination should begin with the patient undressed and gowned from the waist up. The physician should carefully *observe* affect (evidence of depression); upper extremity abnormalities (clubbing, cyanosis, erythema, or joint deformity); and body posture (especially "head forward" or "shoulder droop" position).

Neck and upper extremity *range of motion* (ROM) should be tested by having the patient follow the physician's movements. Any deviation should be checked against passive range of motion (AMA, 1988).

The examiner should *palpate* for tenderness along the cervical spinous processes and facet joints; for tenderness and spasm in the cervical paraspinous, trapezius, and other upper back muscles; for tenderness, swelling, or nodules along the rotator cuff and biceps tendons at the shoulder, the extensor tendons of the forearm, and the extensor/flexor tendons of the wrists and thumbs. Any trigger points should be specifically noted. The wrist and finger joints should be palpated for heat, bogginess, and effusion. The grind test for osteoarthritis in the thumb should be performed in anyone with thumb symptoms. The examiner should not overlook the presence of a ganglion, especially on the dorsum of the wrist or hand, although the finding may be incidental and unrelated to the symptoms. The temperature of the upper extremities should be noted, particularly any difference between the two hands.

Muscle *strength* is tested against the examiner, and the objective grip strength (as measured by Jaymar hand grip dynamometer) is recorded. "Objective" dynamometer measurements are useful to help track progress and document improvement.

A screening *sensory evaluation* is performed with a pinwheel, and *reflexes* at the biceps, triceps, and brachioradialis muscles are tested.

Provocative testing should be performed for the following clinical syndromes (see specific injuries below):

1. Lateral epicondylitis (resisted wrist extension)
2. Median nerve entrapment (resisted pronation; the wrist flexion test for 60 seconds [Phalen's test]; and Tinel's test, performed by tapping over the nerve)
3. Radial nerve entrapment (tenderness along the extensor muscle wad 4 to 5 cm distal to the lateral epicondyle; resisted middle finger extension)
4. Ulnar nerve entrapment (wrist extension/elbow flexion test for 60 seconds)
5. Thoracic outlet syndrome (evaluated by a modified Adson's test)

Imaging and laboratory studies

Evaluation of CTD/RMI rarely requires any additional testing. If additional studies are considered, the clinician should ask himself what effect the results will have on the patient's treatment or on the management of the workers' compensation claim. X-ray films may be useful if arthritis is suspected, and if these are ordered for the hands, the clinician should specify "high-resolution film"; the subtle changes of early hand-joint arthritis are difficult to detect on regular film because of the multiple tiny joints. Computed tomography (CT) or magnetic resonance imaging (MRI) scans are useful to confirm spine abnormalities, but disk problems in this area should be diagnosed clinically, and further imaging should be done only if the case does not progress well, if surgery is being considered, if malingering is suspected, or if an alternate diagnosis is being considered. Recently MRI has been promoted as a way to diagnose tendonitis and carpal tunnel syndrome. In fact these are clinical diagnoses, and MRI confirmation of either does not change the management at all. Thus it is warranted only in extremely rare situations.

If objective evaluation of nerve entrapment is needed, a nerve conduction/electromyography study (NCS/EMG) can be ordered (Corwin, 1989). Any patient being considered for surgery should have this study to confirm the presence and exact site of the entrapment. This is an expensive and unpleasant test, and likely may yield a negative result in early nerve entrapment. The clinician must remember that "early" in the course of nerve entrapment may mean 1 year or more, and that some patients with a real pathologic nerve condition that has been cured by surgery never have an abnormal NCS/EMG. NCS/EMG testing should not be ordered prematurely, because these diagnoses are best made by a good physical examination. A negative test result may send the wrong message to the patient, the employer and, importantly, to the insurance carrier, who may then deny benefits. On the other hand, the test can be very useful if entrapment at a higher site is suspected, or if double crush syndrome is in the differential diagnosis. In such cases the study should be done from the cervical paraspinous muscles distally, using the inching technique if warranted.

In some cases an appropriate alternative is to have an occupational therapist perform the Semmes-Weinstein monofilament test, which uses a series of pencil-sized wands, each with a single attached filament of sequentially heavier gauge, to test relative threshold levels of cutaneous pressure sensation. A decrement in light touch is the first manifestation of altered cutaneous sensation. This test costs far less, correlates very well with the NCS, and can easily be repeated to monitor clinical progress.

Hematologic tests are often ordered, but they are not warranted except in specific cases. If arthritis is suspected, it can be useful to obtain a complete blood count (CBC), erythrocyte sedimentation rate (ESR), antinuclear antibodies (ANA), and rheumatoid factor (RF), although these values often are normal in the early stages of disease. A chemistry panel (panel 20) may provide some evidence of metabolic abnormalities or alcoholism as a cause of polyneuropathy. Because diseases such as diabetes and hypothyroidism increase the risk of carpal tunnel syndrome, a fasting blood sugar, 2-hour postprandial blood sugar, or thyroid-stimulating hormone (TSH) test can screen for these diseases when the history or clinical examination warrants it.

Lyme disease is a new problem, with musculoskeletal and neurologic effects. It must be considered in outdoor workers or patients whose problems do not respond to treatment as expected, particularly if the patient has any history of outdoor activity in endemic areas. Practitioners, especially on the East and West coasts, must consider Lyme disease in the differential diagnosis.

TREATMENT

In developing an approach to treating CTD/RMI, the physician must weigh many factors, including the diagnosis; the duration of the symptoms; the intensity of the symptoms; the extent to which the symptoms disable the patient; the availability of alternate work; the patient's compliance with treatment; deleterious activities or hobbies outside the workplace; and other detrimental influences, such as stress, family or peer pressure, cultural bias, or psychologic factors (e.g., personality disorders, limited coping skills, and tendency to somatize). All these factors may well determine the success or failure of any therapeutic approach and therefore must be considered as the clinician determines a treatment plan.

The patient whose symptoms are long-standing, annoying, and even worsening, but not severe or disabling, will not likely require treatment with medication. We advise *ice* and a *home exercise program* in conjunction with the workplace modifications discussed below.

For more severe symptoms, *physical therapy, hand therapy,* or *occupational therapy* may be ordered. Generally we choose physical therapy for neck, upper back, and shoulder problems and hand and occupational therapy for more distal upper extremity complaints, particularly if the therapeutic goal centers on function or performance rather than on relieving symptoms. Acute problems respond to modalities such as ice and heat, contrast baths, hot paraffin, whirlpool, ultrasound, phonophoresis, iontophoresis, and electrogalvanic stimulation (EGS). Hands-on soft tissue work, deep cross-friction massage, stretching, and manipulation or mobilization may help greatly. We advocate early use of aerobic and strengthening exercises. However, if the symptoms are acute, exercise can worsen an already "overused" structure. When tolerated, an exercise regimen should start with isometric exercises and progress slowly with very light resistance (e.g., home exercises using a 6-ounce tomato paste can).

The physician might also wish to use a forearm, wrist, finger, or thumb *splint*. However, he should think carefully before splinting a joint that is designed to move. We ordinarily use splints to help control an acute inflammatory response or to alleviate troublesome symptoms. Used judiciously, splints promote healing, relieve pain, and allow the patient additional confidence and independence. Soft or elastic splints may provide some degree of support and certainly serve to remind the patient to protect the affected part from further stress. Splints should *never* simply be handed to the patient in a box; they should always be checked by a nurse or physician to ensure proper support and fit, and to ensure that there is no ulnar or superficial radial nerve compression by the splint (Rayan, 1983). For severe cases the splint should be custom-made for the patient by an occupational therapist. The patient should be encouraged to wear it only for times specified (i.e., in initial inflammatory periods, removing it for icing, contrast baths, and ROM exercises, and later only for decreasing periods during activities that hurt). Constant use of a splint within a few weeks causes significant disuse atrophy, which can leave the patient more susceptible to further injury later because of weakness.

The goal in applying a splint is to enable the patient to discontinue using it. The physician should be sensitive to a patient who "marries" the splint, because dependence may thwart the sense of responsibility, self-control, and functional autonomy that are the goals of successful therapy. Routine daily use of splints at work is discouraged in favor of a supportive workstation setup.

Medications

We generally try to avoid using pain medications. Not only do they treat nothing, but they may, by masking pain, allow the patient to do further damage through continued use of the injured area. If medicine is required, nonsteroidal antiinflammatory drugs (NSAIDs) are a good choice (assuming no contraindications, such as salicylate-sensitive asthma, acid-peptic disease, or renal insufficiency), because they tend to reduce acute inflammation and swelling and provide some analgesic effect. The physician must explain the desired purpose and the correct dosage interval of the medication to ensure the patient's compliance. Otherwise, the patient may take a pill only when she has severe pain, may never achieve steady-state therapeutic blood levels, and may report at follow-up visits that the medicine did not help at all.

Muscle relaxants have a limited role. We find them useful in the short term if a patient cannot sleep because of pain, or if marked, palpable spasm is present, as in cervical or upper back muscles. We do not recommend them for routine treatment of tendonitis or pathologic joint and nerve conditions.

Occasionally the physician might want to try other medicines (e.g., vitamin B_6 and diuretics in carpal tunnel syndrome, or amitriptyline in neuritic disorders). Use of these medications is not validated in the literature, but the physician may use them judiciously to prevent the patient from self-prescribing harmful doses.

We generally try to avoid steroid injections early in a treatment course, because the disease may well be marked by numerous acute symptom flares, and repeated steroid injections may have detrimental results, such as tendon thinning and rupture.

Surgery

In our experience surgery is very rarely needed and frequently is harmful. It should not be considered until *both* aggressive conservative therapy and workplace interventions have been tried (Harter, 1989). If surgery is elected, occupational or physical therapy should be strongly considered afterward. (See further discussion in the chapters on Hand Disorders and Shoulder and Elbow Disorders.)

Workplace intervention

Workplace interventions must occur as an integral part of medical management if treatment is to suc-

ceed. It accomplishes little to alleviate a patient's acute symptoms only to return her to the exact work condition that caused it. Problems with tasks, and practices, and the design of the workstation and tools must be corrected.

Workstation interventions in the typical office include raising or lowering work surfaces and providing lumbar support pillows, foot rests, document holders, adjustable keyboard trays, wrist rests, copy stands, mouse nests, electric staplers, and telephone headsets. Frequently used items should be moved close to the body to reduce reach. Tool handles should be covered with caulking material or thermophilic plastic to make them larger, softer, and rougher so as to reduce the force of grip and wrist deviation. A computer mouse or trackball can be modified with pieces of sponge applied with rubber cement to provide a custom grip and to reduce the finger flexion needed to depress buttons. Padded, contoured mouse nests may provide additional support for the hand and fingers, thereby reducing stress.

Work task intervention seeks to modify or eliminate deleterious activities. The physician should look first at deleting unnecessary elements of the job that increase exposure to high-risk actions or movements. In the electronics software industry, a certain amount of E-mail is personal trivia and can easily be reduced or eliminated. However, in some companies, E-mail may involve more than 200 pieces a day, requiring a significant amount of mouse and keyboard use just to review it, let alone to respond. Rotating tasks among workers or within the patient's own schedule helps reduce repetitive motion. Some industries with very high-risk tasks have a rigorous rotation schedule, so that an individual, for example, performs such a task for only 2 hours twice a week.

Work practice intervention should address individual work habits. The patient should be encouraged to slow her typing speed; to perform stand-and-stretch movements every 20 to 30 minutes (see Chapter 35); to eat lunch away from her desk; to take walks during the day; and to avoid overtime keyboard work unless it is absolutely necessary. We also ask the patient to practice keying with her forearms and wrists relaxed. Pianists who play more than a few bars of a Chopin etude with tense, tight forearms, wrists, and hands develop pain and cramping that stop the music. Just as a concert pianist learns to play relaxed, the worker too must learn to perform her repetitive fine-movement tasks with relaxed muscles. This skill, which is not fostered in a work environment that emphasizes deadlines and high-volume productivity, must be encouraged and consciously practiced. We also recommend regular relaxation activities, such as meditation, listening to music, jogging, swimming, or quiet time under a tree. Even 10 minutes 4 or 5 days a week helps counter workplace tension.

COMMON INJURIES

Further discussion of these injuries may be found in Chapter 8 (Hand and Wrist Disorders), Chapter 9 (Shoulder and Elbow Disorders), and Chapter 10 (Neck and Thoracic Spine Disorders).

Tendonitis

Wrist flexor or *extensor tendonitis* is characterized by a history of intermittent dull, aching pain progressing to persistent sharp, throbbing pain that may be punctuated by very sharp shooting sensations (Rowe, 1987). The pain is worse at the end of the day, worst at the end of the workweek and is relieved by rest, at least initially. Patients may have difficulty localizing the symptoms and often point to the entire wrist, hand, and distal forearm as sites of pain. The physician should be aware that patients may describe the pain as *weakness,* because the body, via neurologic feedback loops, tends to protectively splint injured areas, resulting in a subjective sensation of powerlessness. They may also experience the pain as *numbness,* particularly if swelling is present. Descriptions of pain as weakness or numbness should not mislead the clinician to a diagnosis of neuropathy if other findings in the history and the clinical examination point to tendonitis.

Tenderness to palpation over the tendons is the key physical finding. Erythema, swelling, crepitus, and heat may be present over affected structures. Sometimes ganglion cysts of the sheaths are present. If the above findings cannot be isolated to a specific tendon or tendons, the diagnosis of tendonitis should be reconsidered. Risk factors include rapid repetitive movements, awkward wrist positions, and forceful pinch or grip (Stern, 1990; Thorson, 1989). The differential diagnosis includes any of the inflammatory arthritides, such as lupus or rheumatoid arthritis, although these commonly involve significant synovitis, which is not usually found in CTD/RMI tendonitis.

Very early cases can be treated by aggressive workplace intervention, simple icing, and a soft splint. Cases that do not resolve rapidly (within 1 or 2 weeks), or that are older than 1 month should be referred for treatment to occupational and physical therapy. A nonsteroidal antiinflammatory medication may be used in acute cases (Janeci, 1980). (See Chapter 8, Hand and Wrist Disorders, subsection Cumulative Trauma Disorders, for further discussion of specific tendons that may be involved.)

De Quervain's tenosynovitis of the thumb is characterized by the same pain pattern described above, save that the patient usually points to the thumb and radial wrist when asked to locate the pain. Crepitus may be palpated along the radial forearm if significant fluid is present in the tendon sheath. A specific additional maneuver, Finkelstein's test, is performed by curling the thumb into the palm, wrapping the fingers around it, and supporting the forearm while applying gentle ulnar deviation to the wrist. Forceful deviation produces pain in many normal people. The treatment is the same as outlined above for tendonitis, but additional helpful measures include a custom-molded thumb splint and steroid injection. Wrist splints that leave the thumb free to wiggle are not effective. Differential diagnoses include osteoarthritis and intersection syndrome.

Lateral epicondylitis or *extensor tendonitis* at the elbow occurs in work that requires forceful gripping, especially with the wrists in extension, and work that involves rapid repetitive movements with the wrists extended (e.g., using a keyboard or calculator). Specific tests include resisted wrist extension, resisted third finger extension, and the magazine test. In the magazine test, the patient is asked to stand with her arm hanging at her side. She is handed three magazines, which she should hold in a pinch grip, and then is asked to flex her elbow, lifting the magazines. With a positive result, these maneuvers reproduce the patient's pain. The treatment is the same as for other types of tendonitis, although steroid injection may be tried twice. Physical therapy is helpful, including deep cross-friction massage, ice, iontophoresis, EGS, and graded wrist-extension exercises as tolerated. In our experience surgery has been a dreadful treatment choice that rarely produces happy results, although opinions differ regarding the success of surgical intervention (Powell, 1991). Patients uniformly report relief with a forearm band, which distributes the forces from the large extensor muscles over a wider area than the tendon insertion. In recalcitrant cases, a wrist splint (Collies splint) prevents forceful extension and may be used in conjunction with a tennis elbow strap.

Workplace interventions can include forearm supports, wrist rests, and devices such as rubber finger cots or gloves to make forceful grip and pinch easier. Lateral epicondylitis can have a prolonged and difficult course, particularly in the context of heavy work (e.g., warehouse work, plumbing, long hours of keyboard work). Cases often take over a year to improve, and the employee may well be left with residual pain.

Medical epicondylitis commonly results from

excessive keyboard use or from activity requiring repeated forceful wrist flexion, such as shoveling or applying and pressing price tags or decals. Cubital tunnel syndrome should be distinguished from medial epicondylitis. The examination and treatment are similar to those outlined above for lateral epicondylitis, translating for involvement of the flexor forearm muscles and tendons rather than the extensor group. Pain is reproduced with wrist flexion against resistance. However, a strong caution against steroid injection for medial epicondylitis differentiates the treatment somewhat from that recommended for lateral epicondylitis. Also, the ulnar nerve lies very close to the surface by the medial epicondyle area.

Rotator cuff tendonitis usually is seen in workers using their arms at shoulder height or above in extended positions. It also may occur with repeated shoulder flexion and extension, as in vacuuming (Bennahum, 1978). The patient complains of shoulder aching, which is often worse at night, and commonly cannot raise her arm or brush her hair. With anterior rotator cuff tendonitis, the pain may be referred to the deltoid area or the scapula. Palpation and testing range of motion against resistance usually allow the examiner to make the diagnosis. If impingement is suspected, the impingement test should be done, as described in Chapter 9. A plain x-ray film may show calcification of the tendon and will reveal the morphology of the acromion. An MRI scan is superb for identifying impingement, whereas diagnostic ultrasound is not generally helpful.

This problem may be very difficult to treat, and the employee must be removed from further work involving the aggravating activities. Physical therapy is useful in early cases, but, unfortunately, surgery is needed in a large number of impingement cases that do not respond to NSAIDs, physical therapy, steroid injections, and time.

Nerve entrapment syndromes

Ulnar nerve entrapment is common, with entrapment of the nerve occurring in the cubital tunnel at the elbow or in Guyon's canal at the wrist (Grundberg, 1989). Symptoms include numbness and tingling along the ring and little fingers and often along the forearm to the elbow. Risk factors include repeated wrist flexion and ulnar deviation, which compress the nerve in Guyon's canal, and repeated elbow flexion, which has been shown to stretch or compress the nerve in the cubital tunnel between the medial epicondyle and the olecranon. Treatment focuses on reducing or eliminating risk movements, and early cases may respond to simple ice, antiinflammatory medication, balm, and night splinting. In our experience occupational

therapy, physical therapy, and acupuncture also are useful (Adelaar, 1984).

Median nerve entrapment causes numbness and tingling in the thumb and first three digits. If the symptoms occur above the wrist, a higher lesion should be suspected, such as pronator teres syndrome from repeated pronation, thoracic outlet syndrome, double crush syndrome, or a non–work-related polyneuropathy (Adelman, 1982).

Carpal tunnel syndrome (CTS) is entrapment at the transverse carpal ligament of the wrist (Smith, 1977; Thurston, 1987). It is important to remember that many anatomic variants of median and ulnar nerve distribution are discussed in most anatomy texts, so the patient does not always have "classic" symptoms and signs. The wrist flexion (Phalen's) test is a key diagnostic test on physical examination. The patient holds the wrists in 90 degrees of flexion for 60 seconds and is asked to inform the examiner if numbness or tingling develops (DeKrom, 1990; Braun, 1989; Katz, 1990; Niosh, 1989). With wrist flexor tendonitis, this position is uncomfortable and may cause pain. However, such a report of pain does not constitute a positive test result; only the development of numbness or tingling is considered significant. Conversely, because of language differences, some patients may report pain when actually paresthesia is present; therefore the patient must be questioned carefully. Testing for Tinel's sign by tapping over the ligament with a reflex hammer or a finger may produce a shooting, tingling sensation, shocklike in character, with carpal tunnel syndrome and in some normal patients without CTS. However, in our experience the wrist flexion test is far more sensitive and specific.

Pinwheel testing for decreased sensation along the distribution of the median nerve is sometimes helpful, although patients can have hyperesthesia in very early stages of nerve irritation. Two-point discrimination testing has been advocated as a diagnostic tool, because it also is often abnormal in CTS. However, this test is not particularly helpful, because norms vary, and the diagnosis can be made without it.

Medical risk factors include hypothyroidism, diabetes, rheumatoid arthritis, joint-deforming osteoarthritis, and pregnancy. Workplace risk factors include rapid repetitive movements, deviated wrist positions, forceful pinch or grip, and vibration exposure (Cannon, 1981). Workplace interventions focus on these activities. Beyond identifying or treating any underlying medical condition, early management includes splinting, ice, and NSAIDs. If conservative treatment fails, steroid injections into the carpal tunnel have both diagnostic and therapeutic value. If the patient gets no relief, even temporarily, from a properly performed injection, the diagnosis should be reassessed. Temporary or permanent relief of symptoms from an injection not only treats the condition, it also confirms the diagnosis and suggests that a patient with recurrent flares might well respond to surgical release. Physical therapy or hand therapy may be of use in some cases, particularly if median nerve irritation results from swelling of surrounding tendons. If ordered, such therapy should be performed by an experienced therapist with established protocols specific to the particular stage or acuity of the disease. The clinician should not reflexively order standard physical therapy, because modalities alone and inappropriate use of exercise waste time and money; treat nothing; or, worse, may further exacerbate the condition. Occupational or hand therapy also has an important role in workstation evaluation or task retraining to minimize recurrent stress to the affected area. Carpal tunnel release is indicated for cases in which the symptoms have lasted longer than 9 to 12 months; in which abnormal NCS/EMG results indicate loss of motor function; and in which there is evidence of thenar atrophy on examination.

Muscle pain and spasm syndrome (muscle strain)

Muscle pain and spasm syndrome develops from a cyclic spasm and pain cycle. The initial injury, which usually results from awkward, constrained postures, produces isolated fiber spasm and consequent pain, which begets more spasm until significant fibers are recruited (Korinka, 1979; Sheehy, 1982). The resultant spasm is thought to constrict blood flow to the area. The subsequent decrease in the supply of nutrients and oxygen to tissues and the buildup of toxic metabolic waste products induce even more spasm and pain. In CTD/RMI cases, symptoms may be bilateral but often the unilateral, dominant side is affected most. The diagnosis is made by a history of intermittent stiffness progressing to pain, which can be quite sharp and significant. In some cases palpable knots of painful muscle spasm can be noted in the affected area, and pressure on these knots reproduces the pain. Treatment options include ice, balm, and physical therapy initially, and then stretching and strengthening exercises, aerobic exercise, "spray and stretch," and injection of specific trigger points when identifiable.

Degenerative joint disease

Degenerative joint disease (DJD) is seen in the context of moving "loaded" or weight-bearing joints and of vibration exposure from electrically powered hand tools. Typically, problems occur in the dominant hand, thumb, elbow, and/or shoulder of construction workers, who often have knee and lumbosacral spine findings as well. Absence of the problem in the nondominant upper extremity confirms the disorder's work-relatedness. DJD in the hands of typists and other computer workers is not work related according to our understanding of the pathophysiology, which requires significant weight to the joints.

Degenerative joint disease of the cervical and lumbosacral spine occurs with normal aging, but under some circumstances it may be considered a CTD. The relationship of lumbosacral spine DJD to heavy physical labor is obvious. Less obvious is the possible relationship between the disease and seated work, which has been shown to put more compressive force on the disks than standing. Typical office furniture, which is based on anthropomorphic measurements of white men in the U.S. Air Force, does not provide proper support for many women and workers from ethnic groups with smaller body sizes. These employees are forced to sit forward in the chair, because the seat pan is too long for their thigh length. As a result, they have no back support at all. Over the course of the workday, the spine may slump into an abnormal kyphosis, throwing the head forward and curving the spine into a C. Because the head and upper torso are heavy and the work requires head and torso movements, the setting is perfect for early development of DJD at both the cervical and lumbosacral spine. For the above reasons some suggest that select cases of cervical and lumbar DJD may in fact be related to these deleterious postures. Unfortunately, these postures also result from poorly designed car seats, overstuffed home furniture, and sagging beds, as well as from general public inattention to appropriate posture and exercise.

A history of morning stiffness and pain that worsens with activity, together with joint swelling and typical x-ray abnormalities, make the diagnosis. Evaluation of spine problems can be aided by an MRI scan for disk injuries and a CT scan for foraminal narrowing. Surgery is not indicated unless there is a history, confirmed by clinical findings, of progressive neurologic deficit or onset of intractable pain. Therefore treatment is conservative, focusing on self-managed joint protection techniques; exercise designed to strengthen other supporting tissues; and weight loss and aerobic exercise to decrease stressful loading, increase flexibility, and promote general well-being. If surgery is required, consideration should be given to newer techniques that hold promise of less reactive scarring, and to a postoperative course of physical therapy. Progression of the disease can be stopped or slowed only by preventing further repetition of the injurious movements and promoting exercise for postural retraining. For office work, proper seating is critical. Nonsteroidal antiinflammatory agents can be very useful in managing pain, but usage and side effects must be monitored. Some patients in whom NSAIDs are contraindicated or poorly tolerated (especially older workers with renal insufficiency or a high risk of ulcer disease) may be given acetaminophen and occasionally a mild narcotic.

Thoracic outlet syndrome

Thoracic outlet syndrome classically develops in a worker who performs repetitive tasks, frequently weight bearing, with her arms at shoulder height or above. The symptoms include numbness, tingling, and fatigue in the hands and arms, brought on quickly by raising the arms and relieved by lowering them. Patients with "head forward" posture and those who are significantly overweight may be at higher risk (see Chapter 8 on Hand and Wrist Disorders and Chapter 10 on Neck and Thoracic Spine Disorders).

Physical examination findings are limited, but obvious hand blanching may be seen on elevation. The modified Adson's test is performed by feeling for pulse amplitude and listening over the supraclavicular area for a bruit while the patient has her arms lowered. The patient then is asked to raise her arms, palms out, above her head and take a series of deep breaths over 1 to 2 minutes. Each breath is held as long as possible, then released and repeated. The examiner listens for development of a bruit and monitors pulse amplitude in the elevated wrist of the most affected side. The patient is asked to tell the examiner when symptoms develop. A clearly positive test result is one in which a bruit is heard in conjunction with symptoms. A change in pulse and hand blanching associated with symptoms are also positive findings, although symptoms alone can provide useful information. A very small percentage of patients have an extra congenital cervical rib, most often unilateral. A posteroanterior (PA) chest x-ray film can identify this condition, although requesting a prior film is sufficient, because the condition is present from birth.

Because thoracic outlet syndrome is not a disease but rather a structural abnormality (i.e., unbalanced muscle hypertrophy), treatment frequently only requires a series of exercises to stretch anterior muscles, to strengthen posterior chest and shoulder girdle muscles, and to move the head and neck into a more normal posture. A daily set of exercises that are reviewed once a week by a physical therapist usually corrects the problem in 6 weeks. For this reason, thoracic outlet syndrome can be a very satisfying diagnosis to make. Patients who fear that they have CTS and face surgery or long-term disability are very pleased with the results. Nocturnal numbness from sleeping with the neck flexed and arms curled tight is only partly corrected by the exercises. A change in sleep habits, including obtaining a lower pillow and sleeping on the back with arms out or wrapped loosely around another pillow, can help.

Once again, addressing work activity is critical. Moving objects closer and lower, standing to get something instead of reaching overhead, and providing forearm support for assembly work operations are all interventions that have been used successfully.

ASSOCIATED CONDITIONS
Depression

Depression may manifest with or develop during the course of CTD/RMI injuries. Patients often have been bounced around the system; have an employer who does not believe anything is wrong or who thinks the employee is malingering; have had several physician referrals with many diagnoses and therapeutic approaches; have become unable to perform routine activities of daily living; and have lost income and self-esteem.

Because the abnormal sleep patterns that result can heighten the pain and anxiety responses, it is important to ask the patient about emotional reactions to the injury, family and coworker attitudes, sleeping and eating patterns or disturbances, and so on. Intervention with antidepressants or limited behavioral or psychotherapy such as 10 sessions with a counselor, or both, may be tremendously helpful. The scope of any psychotherapy should be carefully defined and limited to the workers' compensation injury at hand, because other, non–work-related issues will certainly surface in the course of treatment for the work-related emotional reaction. We inform our patients, the adjustors, and the therapist directly that therapy is to be limited under workers' compensation and should be oriented toward resolving the issues raised by the injury. Any further treatment deemed necessary by the patient and therapist is the patient's own responsibility and must be billed to the patient's private insurance or paid for by the patient.

Reflex sympathetic dystrophy syndrome

Reflex sympathetic dystrophy syndrome (RSDS) is another associated condition that is rare, but it can be devastating (Patt, 1991). RSDS is a poorly understood neurovascular pain syndrome that occurs in the context of injury to a limb from acute or cumulative trauma. Because it is rare and because most case reports are end-stage descriptions, the early presentation is ill defined. There are many theories about the pathophysiology, but little is known except that an abnormal sympathetic reflex arc is set up between the central nervous system (CNS) and the injured limb. Early indicators in our clinical series include a change in the pain pattern and development of burning pain that worsens at night. CTDs usually are worse at the end of the workday and feel better with rest at night. Changes in hand temperature or color and the presence of edema are also warning signs, and the examiner sometimes can observe these changes directly. The affected hand may turn pale or purple and become swollen, in contrast to the opposite one. The physical examination reveals changes in range of motion as the joints stiffen, changes in temperature, and heightened sensitivity to light touch. The limb may be so sensitive that the patient holds it in what we call the "crystal arm" sign; namely, slightly flexed and extended away from the body to avoid touching anything. A previous case of tendonitis that often required significant palpation to elicit tenderness now will be impossible to touch at the site of injury, as are other parts of the arm.

We cannot overemphasize the importance of movement as part of treatment (Watson, 1987). We remove splints and have the patient begin to use the arm in the office. We order 2 weeks of daily physical therapy to urge range of motion and exercises such as scrubbing motions that further encourage upper extremity movement. Many patients require narcotics during this period, because the condition can be extremely painful. In addition, the patient is taught to carry an object in her hand at all times (e.g., a small rubber ball or toy) to roll around in the fingers, grasp, and squeeze. Abrupt muscle atrophy can develop when RSDS is not caught early. If the above techniques do not reverse the process within a few weeks, the patient should be referred to an experienced anesthesiologist or pain center for possible stellate ganglion block or other more sophisticated treatment (Duncan, 1988; Kettler, 1988; Linson, 1983). Failure to identify and reverse this process early can result in a frozen, atrophied, useless limb. See Chapter 21 on pain management.

CASE STUDIES
Case 1
A woman had worked in a secretarial pool for 12 years. Several years ago, her company purchased new computer equipment and redecorated the office. Several months ago, she noted the onset of extensor wrist aching and gradually developed shooting pain up the forearm. The physician diagnoses extensor tendonitis and treats the patient with ice and an NSAID.

She tells you that she saw a video on repetitive strain injury (RSI) during an office staff meeting and that she got a new wrist rest. She feels that her workstation is "just fine." However, her progress is slow despite the addition of a splint and physical therapy. Rather than wait week after week for the symptoms to improve, the physician requests a workstation evaluation by the occupational therapist who visits the woman at her job site. The therapist notes that the woman is forced to cock her wrists somewhat because the wrist rest is too wide and too low. The physician is amazed to note that the patient improves rapidly with a new, appropriate wrist rest.

Case 2
The assistant manager of a large chain supermarket seeks treatment for numbness, tingling, and pain, which he can localize only to the left wrist and hand. He notes occasional symptoms in his dominant right hand. The symptoms have been present for 8 months, but he has been "too busy" to seek care until now. Aspirin sometimes relieves the pain but lately does not help, because the symptoms seem to be worse. Several of his checkers have been diagnosed with carpal tunnel syndrome, and one told him that his symptoms were just like hers.

On examination, Tinel's and Phalen's tests yield positive results on the left and negative results on the right. The physician diagnoses left carpal tunnel syndrome. However, because the worse symptoms are in the nondominant hand, the clinician reviews the occupational and medical history. Because the patient is a manager, he does not check more than 3 to 4 hours a week and does little stocking. He does not regularly use a calculator or keyboard. A review of symptoms elicits a recent 20-pound weight gain, and the patient, responding to direct inquiry, recalls radiation therapy to his neck as a child. The clinician provides a splint, recommends ice and an NSAID, and orders a TSH test. At a follow-up visit, the patient notes the treatment has brought him some relief. The clinician informs him that his TSH value is markedly elevated and confirms the diagnosis of carpal tunnel syndrome. Because the patient's most significant risk factor is hypothyroidism because his symptoms are worse in the nondominant hand; and because he does no significant keying, checking, or repetitive wrist activity at work, he is instructed to follow up with his personal physician. The claim is determined to be unrelated to his work, and his future medical care is aimed at the underlying medical problem.

Case 3
A newspaper journalist complains of pain, some weakness, and occasional "funny feelings" in her left hand and wrist, particularly after rushing to complete a story to meet a deadline. Occasionally these symptoms move up the arm to the shoulder. She jogs, swims laps, and lifts weights 3 to 5 days a week to stay in shape. She

gardens, occasionally, enjoys mountain biking on weekends, has a new baby, and tries to maintain an active social life with her husband. The results of her examination are unremarkable, and the clinician recommends an assessment of her workstation. She is provided with an adjustable chair and a new wrist rest and instructed to take frequent small breaks from keying. Over the next few weeks the clinician sees her twice, with little change in her symptoms and examination results. X-ray films and laboratory studies are normal. The clinician reduces her keyboard time by 50% in an effort to provide symptomatic relief. Her complaints are unchanged, save that she hates the modified work schedule. She is referred to a hand specialist for further evaluation.

Five months later she returns to the clinician, stating that the hand specialist did more tests that were negative and put her on a vigorous exercise program in physical therapy to increase her endurance. She states that the exercise relieved her shoulder symptoms and that her neck felt looser, but that she dropped a coffee cup yesterday because her hand still feels weak. The hand specialist states that he could find no pathologic condition after several examinations and that he has nothing further to offer the patient. He recommends that, given the patient's fierce work schedule, she consider changing professions if she still has symptoms. The clinician's careful reexamination of the patient reveals nothing except some vague weakness in the left upper extremity. The clinician considers that months of examinations and laboratory and x-ray studies have been normal. The specialist, who has followed the patient for 5 months, finds nothing, and the clinician knows him to be a well-trained, thoughtful practitioner. The clinician is tempted to discharge the patient, but feels that something is just not right. He obtains authorization for a cervical MRI scan and is stunned to find a huge mass lesion at C2. The patient is referred immediately to a neurosurgeon, who removes a spinal cord ependymoma and tells the clinician that the patient is lucky she did not sever the remaining thread of cord during her vigorous exercise program.

Case 4

A 33-year-old kitchen worker comes to the clinic with a weeklong history of numbness and tingling in his dominant right fourth and fifth fingers and along the forearm to the elbow. He has been assigned to clean pots and wonders if he's gotten "carpal tunnel" from the job.

Because the clinician is very familiar with the patient's work, having treated a number of people from his department for various acute injuries, he suspects an alternate diagnosis and questions the worker about hobbies and other activities. He proudly announces that he was fishing the weekend before the symptoms developed, and in fact was successful in catching a 120-pound sturgeon, which took hours to reel in! He shows a picture, and at the clinician's request, duplicates his movements, which involve holding the rod with his left hand while winding the reel handle with his right, a movement that requires repetitive flexion and extension of his elbow.

His elbow flexion test is positive for increased numbness in the fourth and fifth fingers, and his sensation to pinprick by pinwheel is decreased there and along the forearm. The clinician diagnoses ulnar nerve entrap-

ment from nonoccupational reasons and sends him to his personal physician, who removes him from work on his own sick time.

Case 5

A 32-year-old warehouse worker is sent to the clinic for a second opinion. She has been off work for 8 months. She developed tendonitis in her right wrist after a particularly heavy inventory period, was initially treated with ice, NSAIDs, and a splint, and, when that failed, was pulled off work and has been off since. She was never sent to physical therapy but was seen by two orthopedic surgeons, one by referral for ongoing treatment at the request of her primary care physician after the first 2 months, the other for a recent second opinion.

She currently complains of burning pain along her whole forearm and hand, both sides, worse at night, and relieved only by not touching anything. In asking about her occupational history the clinician questions her about hobbies, and she responds with great fervor, "I can't even play my synthesizer any more!" Further questioning reveals that music is her avocation, and when she initially was removed from work, she purchased a music synthesizer and used it 7 to 8 hours a day for months. She did not make the connection between use of the instrument and worsening of her symptoms, because her actual job was such heavy work in comparison. She states that none of her other physicians asked her about hobbies.

On physical examination, she holds her hand and arm away from her body, immobile. She is very tender all over her forearm, and her hand is swollen and purple in color. She has decreased range of motion at the wrist and shoulder.

The clinician diagnoses reflex sympathetic dystrophy syndrome, and refers her immediately for therapy, urging her in the meantime to move her arm continuously. She improves somewhat, but 3 weeks later, the clinician notices early atrophy of her forearm extensor muscles. An immediate referral to a local anesthesia–based pain center confirms the clinician's diagnosis, and she receives the first of a number of stellate ganglion blocks and is given oral Tegretol. Her care is transferred to the pain center. Two years later, the clinician learns that she has undergone vocational rehabilitation and has just gotten a job as a receptionist in a medical office. She has required repeat blocks several times a year, including a month before beginning work.

DIAGNOSTIC PEARLS

- If it hurts worse in the morning and is stiff in the morning, it's not RMI, it's arthritis.
- A physician with a big practice is the first to make new diagnoses of such disorders as lupus and rheumatoid arthritis, so he must be alert to the signs.
- If the ESR is elevated, it's not RMI.
- Cervical radiculopathy must be considered in the differential diagnosis of forearm and wrist nerve entrapment syndromes.

- Tendonitis responds to icing in most cases, but if the patient has "poor circulation" or "cold hands," the physician should try heat, analgesic balm, and gloves with the fingers cut out.
- Alternative therapies should be considered for tough cases; acupuncture is very good for ulnar nerve irritation, Alexander massage/neuromuscular retraining can be beneficial in chronic, long-term, multiple-injury cases.
- Not all numbness and tingling in the hands is carpal tunnel syndrome. Ulnar nerve entrapment is more common, and thoracic outlet syndrome is often missed, especially because it frequently manifests with both nocturnal and daytime numbness.

CONCLUSION

Cumulative trauma disorders present a unique challenge to the practitioner, because there is little hard science behind much of the advice we provide. Ergonomic recommendations generally assume that a neutral position that minimizes stress and loading tends to alleviate the disorder. Until such time as controlled studies define the optimum chair or hand position, the least stressful type of keyboard, and the number of times a given activity or movement can be repeated without trauma, we are left to our experience, intuition, and observation in planning appropriate preventive measures. Nonetheless, the guidelines discussed above provide a useful approach to the problem of repetitive motion disorders. We anticipate further modification of work procedures, introduction of adjustable keyboards and other tools, redistribution of workloads, and refinement of ergonomic recommendations as reliable studies provide more data about the cause, pathophysiology, and treatment of CTD/RMI.

23 Building-related Disorders

Over the past two decades, health problems associated with newly constructed or remodeled buildings have become increasingly common, reflecting in part the increase in sealed or "tight" buildings with energy-efficient designs. Problematic design features include windows that do not open, with outside air provided only through a recirculating air-conditioning system, and modern building materials. The latter include compressed wood products, synthetic furnishings and floor coverings (carpet, vinyl), wall coverings (wallpaper, fabric), ceiling materials (acoustic tiles, "blown" gypsum), and insulation (fiberglass, rigid foam). As a result, the clinician must not only direct the diagnosis and treatment of the *patient* with building-associated health problems, she must also be familiar with the environmental factors within the *building* that can lead to illness, understand approaches to controlling these factors, and possibly be engaged in follow-up epidemiologic investigations to identify others who may be similarly affected. It is rarely possible to successfully treat a patient with building-associated health problems without addressing building-related environmental or related social factors, or both.

A number of terms have been used to describe building-associated health problems, including "sick building syndrome," "tight building syndrome," "indoor air pollution," "building-associated illness," and "building-related illness." These terms obviously are descriptive without ascribing a precise cause, but they generally imply sources of health problems relating to the indoor building environment. "Building-related illness" is probably the most inclusive of terms, connoting any health problem (regardless of precise cause) relative to the indoor environment. In this chapter the term "building-associated illness" is used in relation to *etiologic agents* known to be clinically or epidemiologically associated with building-related health problems, such as environmental tobacco smoke, carbon monoxide, allergic or infectious agents, chemical agents, and particulate matter. In contrast, the term "sick building syndrome"[43] is used to describe a situation in which a group of individuals develops excessive work-related symptoms such as headaches; eye, nose, and throat irri-

tation; fatigue; and dizziness without an identified cause, possibly related to other factors (fresh air, humidity, temperature and/or psychologic factors). In the diagnosis and treatment of building-related illness, the clinician should differentiate between "building-associated illness" and the "sick building syndrome": the former term implies a specific etiologic agent, whereas the latter term implies an environmental building problem related to the other factors mentioned.

This chapter is intended to provide the clinician with a brief overview of the epidemiology and causative factors associated with building-related illness. Several reviews of building-associated illness have been published that discuss these aspects in much greater detail.* These reviews provide useful information for the clinician interested in an overview of the epidemiology and environmental factors associated with building-related illness, but with few exceptions,[60] they provide little practical guidance for clinical management. Therefore this chapter focuses on the clinical diagnosis and treatment, and epidemiologic and physiologic evaluation of building-associated illness.

EPIDEMIOLOGY AND CAUSATIVE FACTORS
Building-associated illness

As mentioned previously, building-associated illnesses have a known etiology related to specific causative agents and sources (Table 23-1). Epidemiologic studies have documented an association between clinical signs and symptoms and indoor air exposure to these agents.

Environmental tobacco smoke. There is strong evidence of an association between environmental tobacco smoke (ETS) and acute symptoms of eye, nose, and throat irritation.[33,90] Occupant complaints of ETS smoke odor occur at lower concentrations than that associated with irritation from tobacco smoke pollutants,[126] and ETS exposure has been linked to building-associated illness in at least one study.[107] The National Institute of Occupational Safety and Health (NIOSH) has found

---

* References 23, 44, 50, 60, 80, 109, 110, 113, 114, and 119.

Table 23-1 Causes of building-associated illness

Etiologic agent	Source
Environmental tobacco smoke	Smoking coworkers
Combustion products	
Carbon monoxide	Vehicle exhaust, leaking combustion appliances
Nitrogen dioxide	Vehicle exhaust, leaking combustion appliances
Allergic agents	
Thermophilic actinomycetes	Air-conditioning systems, contaminated building materials
Mold, dust mites	and furnishings
Infectious agents	
Legionella pneumophilia	Water-cooled heat exchange equipment
Aspergillus flavus	Ventilation systems, contaminated water supplies
Mycobacterium tuberculosis	Aerosol from infected building occupants
Viral agents (measles, chickenpox)	Aerosol from infected building occupants
Chemical agents	
Formaldehyde	Building materials, furnishings
Volatile organic compounds	Building materials, furnishings, copy machines
Semivolatile organics	Pesticides
Respirable particulate	
Glass fiber	Ventilation systems

that a small fraction of investigations are related to ETS,[82] but no systematic studies have analyzed the proportion of building-related illness linked to this pollutant.[61] Nevertheless, it is clear that exposure to ETS may cause symptoms of respiratory irritation among building occupants.

Carbon monoxide. Carbon monoxide may become entrained into building ventilation systems through fresh-air intakes from parking garages, adjacent loading docks, or nearby commercial vehicles. Published documentation of carbon monoxide exposure in building-related illness is sparse,[46,129] but the physiologic effects of carbon monoxide on reducing tissue oxygen delivery are well known. Symptoms of headache, dizziness, light-headedness, nausea, and fatigue may occur with low-level exposure and resemble a flulike illness. Individuals with underlying atherosclerotic diseases may be more susceptible to myocardial ischemia with exposure to carbon monoxide.

Hypersensitivity diseases

Hypersensitivity pneumonitis. In hypersensitivity pneumonitis (extrinsic allergic alveolitis, HSP), sensitizing microorganisms (actinomycetes; *Cryptostroma, Aspergillus,* and *Penicillium, spp.;* and *amoebae*), animal and plant proteins (e.g., pigeon or parakeet antigens), rat urine, or low-molecular-weight compounds (e.g., detergent enzymes or iisocyanates) lead to acute recurrent pneumonitis or chronic interstitial lung disease.

HSP is an immunologically induced inflammatory disorder of the lung parenchyma that results from repeated inhalation of a variety of etiologic agents, including organic dusts and low-molecular-weight chemicals. The lungs typically show a granulomatous interstitial pneumonitis, with varying degrees of distal bronchiolitis obliterans. Initially, peribronchiolar granulomas tend to be prominent and fibrosis is minimal. However, HSP occasionally may progress to end-stage fibrosis.

HSP may arise in acute, subacute, or chronic forms, depending on the frequency, intensity, and duration of exposure. In acute cases, individuals may have onset within 6 to 24 hours of symptoms of fever, cough, shortness of breath, and chest tightness, with an x-ray film appearance of pulmonary infiltrates; symptoms abate hours to days after exposure ceases. In subacute cases, cough and dyspnea appear over days to weeks and may progress to respiratory insufficiency, leading to hospitalization for respiratory support. The chronic form manifests as an insidious onset of cough, exertional dyspnea, fatigue, and weight loss over a period of months (see Chapter 18, Respiratory Injuries).

One of the first reports of building-associated hypersensitivity pneumonitis occurred among four workers in an office building with a contaminated humidifier, among whom exposure to the thermophilic actinomycete of the *Micropolyspora* genus was associated with intermittent chills, fever, and work-related shortness of breath. Lung biopsy in one individual confirmed granulomatous interstitial pneumonitis.[10] Since then, numerous cases of building-associated hypersensitivity pneumonitis have been reported to be associated with contaminated humidifiers or air-handling units, or water-damaged materials such as carpets, furniture, or dividers.* In most systematic investigations of outbreaks, efforts have been made to correlate the presence of serum IgG precipitins with the presence of common saprophytic organisms or to an extract of building material, but the specific sensitizing antigen often cannot be identified.

Humidifier fever. Humidifier fever is an influenza-like illness characterized by fever, chills, myalgia, and malaise, which occur within 4 to 8 hours after exposure at work and resolve within 24 hours. Pulmonary symptoms and x-ray film appearance of infiltrates are rare. The syndrome was first reported in 12 employees in a carpentry workshop whose symptoms were correlated with exposure to a humidifier contaminated by mold.[99] Numerous additional reports have since been published.[4,42,48,98,100] Microbial agents that may contaminate humidifiers have been postulated as the cause of humidifier fever, including *Bacillus subtilis, Acanthamoeba polyphaga, Naegleria gruberi,* and endotoxins. It is not clear whether humidifier fever should be considered a distinct clinical syndrome or a milder form of humidifier-associated hypersensitivity pneumonitis because both disorders have been reported in association with exposure to similar antigenic agents.

Asthma. Occupational asthma may be caused or aggravated by workplace exposures and may be due to either sensitizing agents or irritants. In relation to building-associated illness, asthma was first documented by serial peak-flow measurements reported in two office workers with exposure to contaminated building humidifiers.[44] Work-related asthma subsequently has been reported in print works employees in a building with a humidifier contaminated by several microorganisms[26] and among employees of an office building[64] (see Chapter 18, Respiratory Injuries).

Allergic rhinitis. IgE-mediated symptoms of nasal congestion and discharge, itching, and sneezing may occur because of exposure to identified allergens (mites, dander, insect parts, fungi) in the indoor work environment. In contrast, nonallergic or vasomotor rhinitis may be due to occupational exposure to irritants or temperature or humidity extremes. Case reports or epidemiologic studies have not determined the prevalence of allergic rhinitis in building-associated illness, although it is acknowledged to be a common symptom.[72,131] Individual host factors, such as a history of atopy, age, upper respiratory infection, and a history of smoking are important risk factors in the

development of allergic sensitization.[66] It probably is not practical to distinguish between allergic and nonallergic rhinitis in building-related illness.[72]

Infectious agents. Infectious agents have been responsible for many outbreaks of building-related illness. In particular, *Legionella pneumophila* is a common bacterial contaminant of air-conditioning and potable water systems, and it is responsible for both legionnaires' disease and Pontiac fever. Legionnaires' disease, a bacterial pneumonia first described in 1976 among 182 members of the American Legion at a Philadelphia convention, has since been traced to aerosols from cooling towers, evaporative condensers, humidifiers, whirlpools, shower heads, and industrial cooling systems.[72] Hospitals and offices have been the sites of many outbreaks.[36,38,94,95] Most cases are associated with serotype I of the species *L. pneumophila.* Because the organism is ubiquitous in the environment, its presence in potable water and air conditioning components is common and does not necessarily imply the risk of clinical illness.[25] Pontiac fever, a self-limited illness characterized by fever, chills, headache, and myalgia, is also caused by a species of *Legionella* bacteria. First described in 1968 in Pontiac, Michigan,[49] it has since been reported to occur in buildings with contaminated air-conditioning systems, whirlpools, and industrial coolants.[135]

Other infectious diseases and agents, including measles,[18,104,105] the common cold,[24] *Aspergillus spp.*[1,6,111] and tuberculosis[30] may also be spread via ventilation systems. It is not clear to what extent sealed buildings may contribute to the spread of infectious diseases.[76]

Chemical agents. Among the chemical agents, *formaldehyde* has received the most attention as a cause of building-associated illness. The major sources of formaldehyde in modern buildings are urea-formaldehyde foam insulation, pressed wood products (particle board), floor coverings, carpet backings and glues, and new furniture and fabric finishes. Formaldehyde may cause eye and upper airway irritation in the 0.5 to 2 parts per million (ppm) range and has been reported to cause excessive complaints among occupants of mobile homes used as offices and among occupants of office buildings.[15,81] Formaldehyde at these levels probably cannot cause asthma.[50] In general, formaldehyde in the indoor building environment is detected at levels below that which would be expected to cause respiratory irritation and probably is not a common cause of building-related illness.

Volatile organic compounds (VOCs) make up a large and diverse group of organic substances that are frequently measured in the course of building-

---

* References 5, 17, 45, 56, 57, 59, 67, and 71.

related investigations. Sources of VOCs in the indoor building environment include paints, adhesives, furnishings, printed materials, photocopying machines, pesticides, floor adhesive, floor finishes, vinyl tiles, room freshener, and carpet shampoo.[118,124] Although VOCs generally are detected in indoor buildings at levels substantially lower than those permitted in the workplace, experimental studies have shown adverse upper respiratory and neuropsychologic effects (inability to concentrate, impaired memory) at levels below the presently accepted threshold for acute effects,[86,87] and VOCs have been reported to be associated with symptoms of upper respiratory irritation, headache, and fatigue in schools and office buildings.[62,92] However, a recent experimental study failed to find effects on neurobehavioral performance from exposure to low-level VOCs.[96]

Pesticides have also been reported to cause building-associated illness,[58,79] as have petrochemicals,[22,28,133] detergents,[29,70] and carbonless copy paper.[89] Fibrous glass may also become airborne from moisture or improper installation and produce symptoms of respiratory irritation or skin rash.

Sick building syndrome

Beginning in the 1970s, numerous complaints of symptoms relating to the office environment were reported to local, state, and federal agencies. Many of these episodes occurred in new or recently renovated office buildings where fabrics or furnishings were thought to be related to the occupants' complaints. Several hundred investigations have been conducted by NIOSH.[82] In only 19% of cases was contamination from an indoor source found; in 11%, an external factor was identified; and in 4%, building materials and fabrics were incriminated. In 50% of cases no source of contamination was determined; rather, the primary factor was found to be inadequate ventilation characterized by poor air distribution and mixing, temperature and/or humidity extremes, inadequate fresh air intake, and filtration problems.[130]

The prevalence of sick building syndrome is unknown, but it has been estimated that 20% of office workers report lost productivity as a result of inadequate air quality, with 30 million to 70 million exposed occupants.[137] It is estimated that at any one time, 10 million to 25 million workers in 800,000 to 1.2 million commercial buildings in the United States have symptoms typical of sick building syndrome.[137] Twenty-four percent of office workers who were surveyed reported poor air quality in their offices.[136] Several systematic epidemiologic studies have been conducted in several large offices. In one of the first, investigators found a higher prevalence of symptoms of mucous membrane irritation, headache, dry skin, and lethargy in occupants of six mechanically ventilated buildings compared with occupants of three naturally ventilated buildings.[44] The presence of a humidification system appeared to be associated with a higher rate of symptoms. An environmental assessment in one fully air-conditioned and one naturally ventilated office building found no significant differences in globe or dry bulb temperature, relative humidity, moisture content, air velocity, positive and negative ions, carbon monoxide, ozone, and formaldehyde concentrations.[106] In the so-called Danish town hall study, investigators found higher rates of mucous membrane irritation, fatigue, and malaise in mechanically ventilated versus naturally ventilated buildings, with higher rates among women, clerks, those using photocopiers, carbonless copy paper, or video display terminals, and among those occupants in buildings with a greater numbers of office workers.[115] Differences in symptom prevalence were related to organic floor dust, floor covering, number of workplaces in the office, building age, "fleece factor" (area of all textile floor coverings, curtains, and seats divided by room volume), "shelf factor" (length of all open, filled shelves and cupboards divided by room volume), and type of ventilation.[116] Eye symptoms (dryness, irritation, and inability to wear contact lenses) were related to specific ophthalmologic findings documented by slitlamp examination.[47] In a study of 42 different office buildings with 47 different ventilation conditions, buildings with local and central induction/fan coil units had the greatest mean number of symptoms per worker, followed by buildings with "all air" systems and buildings with mechanical or natural ventilation.[27] The most common symptoms were lethargy (57%), blocked nose (47%), dry throat (46%), and headache (46%), which were more than twice as common in buildings with local and centrally supplied induction/fan coil units compared with naturally ventilated buildings.

These three studies suggested that mechanical ventilation and the air change rate were less important than the type of air-conditioning and humidification system, work organization characteristics, gender, and job category. A reanalysis of data from six cross-sectional studies (including the three previously mentioned) that compared symptom prevalence in buildings with different ventilation types found consistently increased prevalence odds ratios for symptoms of headache, lethargy, and mucous membrane irritation in air-conditioned versus naturally ventilated buildings.[83] Humidification or mechanical ventilation without air-conditioning was not associated with a higher symptom prevalence, suggesting that symptom reporting was related to still-unidentified factors in sealed, air-conditioned buildings. In an analysis of factors related to reports of the sick building syndrome in 11 office buildings, total volatile hydrocarbon concentration and personal factors such as reported hyperreactive airways, sick leave as a result of airway disease, smoking, and psychosocial factors (work stress, work satisfaction, and climate of cooperation) were significantly associated with symptoms of eye, skin, and upper airway irritation, whereas atopic history, age, gender, or outdoor exposures were not.[91] These findings were also reported in occupants of primary schools.[92] A random population-based survey of symptoms of sick building syndrome found that symptoms were significantly related to both individual factors (atopy, nickel allergy, airways hyperreactivity) and environmental factors (urban residency, fresh paint, preschool children at home, work with video display terminals, work satisfaction, and climate of cooperation at work).[93] Using a linear-analog self-assessment scale to define symptoms at a specific point in time while simultaneously measuring environmental parameters in five building areas, symptoms of mucous membrane irritation and CNS symptoms were significantly related to volatile organic hydrocarbon concentrations, crowding, layers of clothing, and light intensity.[62] Another study in 15 office buildings found a significant relationship between symptom prevalence rates and levels of airborne viable bacteria and fungi, but not particulate matter,[55] whereas another study of a "sick building" found no relationship between reported symptoms and microbial contamination.[16]

Taken together, these studies indicate that several factors appear to be responsible for sick building syndrome, which may vary according to the building or population studied. Primary factors associated with the sick building syndrome are those related to fresh air, humidity, temperature, density of occupancy, building materials and work category. Many associated underlying causes may be responsible, such as inadequate design and maintenance of new and existing ventilations systems, lack of training of building operators, and poor employee morale (Table 23-2). Although it is clear that air-conditioned buildings are at risk of producing occupant complaints, it is not clear precisely what factors lead to an episode of building-related illness in any particular building. Investigations of "sick buildings" usually fail to show an association between measurable exposure factors and health effects. Additional studies are needed to assess the risk of sick building syndrome on the basis of analysis of exposures and ventilation characteristics, including additional stratified random samples of buildings and their occupants,[73,120] longitudinal studies,[117] field exposure studies using direct-reading or short-term sampling techniques,[63] and controlled laboratory experiments.[87]

Psychologic factors. Psychologic factors are important in the pathogenesis of sick building syndrome, particularly the social and organizational factors that may influence the development of symptoms among building occupants. "Mass psychogenic illness," which has been defined as a collective occurrence of a set of physical symptoms and related belief among two or more individuals in the absence of an identifiable pathogen,[31,] has been described in various occupational settings,[20,30,32,54] including office buildings, as an alternative explanation for a building-related problem.[39,52] Because many building-associated illness investigations fail to find a single identifiable cause of increased symptoms among the occupants, it is tempting to conclude that symptoms are a result of psychologic factors alone. A study of psychologic factors among building occupants with symptoms of sick building syndrome failed to find evidence of mass psychogenic illness when these occupants were compared with occupants of an unaffected building, but did find evidence that the occupants of the problem building had a significantly greater prevalence of psychologic symptoms derived from a standardized symptom checklist.[13] Scales from the Minnesota Multiphasic

Table 23-2 Factors associated with sick building syndrome

Factor	Associated causes
Insufficient fresh air	Building occupancy above design occupancy
	Low ventilation efficiency
	Renovation using strong contaminant sources
Extreme humidity	Condensation or leakage of water
Extreme temperature	Inadequate maintenance of heating, ventilation, and air-conditioning
	Inadequate training of operators of complex building system
Psychologic factors	Low employee morale, lack of recognition

Adapted from Stolwijk JA: Sick-building syndrome, *Environ Health Perspect* 95:99-100, 1991.

Personality Inventory indicated significantly greater defensiveness, resentment, distrust of authority, anxiety, and confusion among the "sick building" occupants, probably reflecting the effects of chronic stress as a result of uncertainty over the cause of their symptoms, unsatisfactory solutions to their problems, and management attitudes. These findings support the concept that psychologic, social, and organizational factors appear to be modifiers of individual and organizational responses to biologic, chemical, or physical perturbations of the office environment.[9] Aspects of the physical environment, job structure, work task, job control, management policies, and social support structures are important factors in outbreaks of sick building syndrome.[108] In contrast to episodes of mass psychogenic illness, symptoms among occupants of "sick buildings" typically develop over days to months, do not develop along visual sight lines, and cannot be explained by anxiety reactions with secondary hyperventilation.[9] Along with the evaluation of the environment, psychologic factors should be investigated as important effect modifiers in any episode of sick building syndrome, and underlying stressors and organizational characteristics should be treated with effective communication and social support.

Clinical evaluation

Case definitions. For building-related illness, case definitions for the various conditions depend on the history of work-related symptoms, physical examination findings, and appropriate diagnostic tests. In contrast, no uniform case definition exists for sick building syndrome (SBS). The World Health Organization first attempted to define this condition, which has been described as an unexplainable sensory irritation appearing in a large fraction of the occupants of the affected building[87] (Table 23-3). The term "SBS" generally is defined as occurring among a *population* of building occupants, but has also been applied to describe a single *individual* who manifests typical symptoms in the absence of an epidemiologic investigation.[131]

History of illness and medical conditions. The diagnosis of any acute occupational illness depends in part on the history of work-related

symptoms, prior medical conditions, and concurrent associated personal risk factors. For building-associated illness, it is necessary to determine several points in the history of current illness and past medical conditions, including the following:

- Nature, duration, and severity of respiratory, skin, CNS and gastrointestinal symptoms
- Time of onset of symptoms in relation to work, both within the building as a whole and within specific parts of the building
- Variation in symptoms (e.g., do symptoms worsen at work, improve away from work, or get worse over the course of the workday or workweek)
- Use of any medications, such as prescription or over-the-counter medications for allergies, asthma, or skin rashes
- Patient or family history of previous allergies, atopy, or asthma
- History of previous or current associated skin, gastrointestinal, or CNS conditions
- Current medical treatment by health care providers

Questions about respiratory and allergic symptoms and the patient's medical history should cover productive cough, wheeze, exertional dyspnea, chest pain, and history of acute respiratory illnesses; history of cardiovascular or restrictive lung and airway obstructive diseases (emphysema, chronic bronchitis, bronchiectasis, asthma); history of other cardiopulmonary diseases; history of allergy and sinusitis; history of abnormal chest x-ray films; and hospitalizations for chest problems or thoracic surgery.[77] A careful smoking history should be obtained as well. Standardized respiratory questionnaires have been developed and are useful for clinical, as well as epidemiologic, evaluation of chronic respiratory symptoms.[3] Daily symptom diaries are also useful to establish the presence of acute respiratory symptoms.[127]

Occupational and exposure history. With building-associated illness, the temporal relationship between symptoms and work exposures is critical to reaching a diagnosis. For ETS, carbon monoxide, and chemical agents, upper respiratory or CNS symptoms should occur within minutes to

Table 23-3 Classification of sick building syndrome

- Most occupants report symptoms
- Symptoms are especially frequent in one building or part of one building
- Major categories of reported symptoms include eye, nose, throat, and skin irritation; neurologic or general health symptoms (fatigue, reduced memory or concentration, lethargy, headache, dizziness, nausea); odor and taste complaints; and nonspecific hypersensitivity reactions (runny nose, worsening of preexisting asthma)
- Symptoms of upper respiratory irritation most common
- No obvious association with specific exposures

Adapted from Molhave L: Controlled experiments for studies of the sick building syndrome, *Ann NY Acad Sci* 641:46, 1992.

hours and generally abate within a few hours after exposure has ceased. The acute symptoms of fever, chills, myalgia, and shortness of breath associated with hypersensitivity pneumonitis or humidifier fever occur within 4 to 8 hours after exposure at work. Symptoms of work-related asthma (e.g., chest tightness, wheezing, shortness of breath, or coughing) may occur immediately on exposure to the offending agent or over the course of hours during the work shift, or they may be delayed for hours after exposure at work. The nasal congestion, discharge, itching, and sneezing with allergic or vasomotor rhinitis generally is reported during the workday or shortly thereafter. Infectious agents produce clinical illness over days of exposure, with delayed onset of symptoms, depending on the incubation period of the disease. In sick building syndrome, symptoms are reported on entry into the building and worsen over the course of the workday or workweek.

A careful occupational history should be obtained, including major jobs and work responsibilities before present employment. Any history of work-related injury or illness should be noted, particularly those cases in which building-associated complaints or lost work time has resulted. A detailed description of current work responsibilities should be obtained, with an explanation of any use of a chemical product or exposure to chemicals, dusts, or fumes. Any relevant Material Safety Data Sheets (MSDS) or written product information should be obtained and reviewed, along with results of building industrial hygiene investigations or ventilation studies. A history should be noted of recent building or office renovation, installation of new furnishings such as carpets or furniture, pesticide application, visible water damage or leakage, unusual odors, or visible dust on work surfaces or ventilation grates. In some cases, no specific causative agent is suspected, and thermal discomfort or "stuffiness" may be the only complaint.

Physical examination. The physical examination should be performed as soon as possible after the onset of building-associated symptoms and should focus on the respiratory tract (both upper and lower airways), skin, and central nervous system. The physical examination may be helpful in establishing a diagnosis of building-related illness with a specific etiology, but it is rarely helpful in cases of sick building syndrome in which symptoms are nonspecific and are not associated with clinical abnormalities. Nevertheless, a physical examination is critical for detecting other, nonoccupational disorders that may manifest with similar symptoms.

Examination of the respiratory tract may show erythema of the conjunctivae, pharynx, or nasal mucosa consistent with upper airway irritation or allergic rhinitis. The presence of fever, tachypnea, and bibasilar or diffuse crackles and wheezing suggests hypersensitivity pneumonitis or humidifier fever, whereas wheezing may indicate asthma (although asthma may occur without wheezing). Fever and rhonchi with signs of pulmonary consolidation suggest legionnaires' disease.

Examination of the skin may show erythema or urticaria consistent with irritant or contact allergic dermatitis. Examination of the central nervous system usually is normal, but it may show focal abnormalities, suggesting an underlying pathologic process that explains common symptoms of dizziness, headache, trouble concentrating, and fatigue. Neurologic screening to assess cognitive function (mental status screening, Digit Symbol, Trail Making) and long motor track and balance function (tandem walk, Romberg's test, nose-to-finger-to-nose testing) may be helpful in clinical evaluations of employee groups.[85]

Diagnostic procedures. Unfortunately, no readily available diagnostic measures can be used to correlate objective findings with the subjective symptoms of upper respiratory irritation caused by building-associated illness. Complaints of eye irritation from the indoor environment have been associated with an absence of foam in the eye canthus, decreased stability of the precorneal tear film, and epithelial damage documented by slit-lamp technique.[47] Evaluation of symptoms of upper respiratory irritation (nasal congestion, rhinorrhea, sneezing) after ETS exposure has been assessed in experimental studies using measures of nasal resistance, and acoustic rhinometry has also been used to assess changes in the upper airway.[11,12] Experimental exposure to VOCs resulted in a significant increase in nasal passage neutrophils.[68,69] However, none of these techniques is readily available.

Carbon monoxide toxicity should be evaluated immediately after suspected work exposure with quantitative carboxyhemoglobin levels. There is an excellent correlation between symptoms of carbon monoxide exposure and carboxyhemoglobin level.

For the diagnosis of asthma, the patient's report of symptoms should be coupled with objective evidence of disease. Reversible or variable airway obstruction should be documented by serial spirometry, response to inhaled bronchodilator, or nonspecific inhalation challenge testing with methacholine or histamine. When pulmonary function tests are normal, a positive challenge to methacholine or histamine is a sensitive and fairly specific indicator of airway responsiveness. Serial measurements of peak expiratory flow can also be used to objectively document the presence of variable airway obstruction, with excessive diurnal variability (greater than 20%) correlating with both exacerbation of symptoms and increases in nonspecific airway responsiveness. The diagnosis of *occupational asthma* is made by showing variable airway obstruction in relation to workplace exposure, typically by measuring cross-workshift forced expiratory volume in 1 second (FEV_1). Serial measurements of nonspecific airway responsiveness or peak flow can also document increased responsiveness in relation to workplace exposures. Peak-flow meters are cheap, relative easy to use and can produce several measurements over the course of a workday, including time away from work. Specific inhalation challenge with the suspected causative agent is difficult, should be performed in a hospital setting, and fortunately is rarely necessary to establish a diagnosis of occupational asthma (see Chapter 18).

For the diagnosis of *acute HSP,* the chest x-ray film often shows small, poorly defined, reticulonodular opacities that usually are diffuse but occasionally are symmetrically sparing of the apices or bases. In severe cases a pulmonary edema–like pattern can occur. However, the chest x-ray film may be normal, even in symptomatic patients, and patchy or unilateral patterns have been reported. In the chronic fibrotic form of HSP, lung opacities tend to be more linear and the peripheral lung zones more prominently involved. Pulmonary function studies show a restrictive pattern, with decreased compliance and impairment of diffusion during periods of acute pneumonitis. These changes are reversible in acute HSP, whereas they are not in the chronic form. Leukocytosis, an elevated sedimentation rate, and increased rheumatoid factor and immunoglobulins may be present after acute exposure. Precipitin antibodies may be detected against a suspected antigen, although both false-negative and false-positive results occur, and correlation of antibody results with the clinical picture is essential. Inhalation of aerosolized antigen extract in individual patients may support the diagnosis, but these tests are difficult to perform and are not standardized. Although HSP has been associated with T-cell lymphocytosis in bronchoalveolar lavage (BAL) fluid, bronchoscopy with BAL is not recommended as part of the routine work-up for HSP. In patients without sufficient clinical evidence for HSP, an open lung biopsy may be indicated to show bronchocentric mononuclear cell infiltration of both alveolar and interstitial spaces, with some granuloma formation.

Antibody markers have been used with varying success in the diagnosis of building-associated illness. In a study of printing company employees, including two cases of humidifier fever, there was a significant correlation between the presence of allergen-specific IgG antibodies and workplace exposure, although antibody levels did not correlate with the presence of symptoms.[14] In one outbreak of SBS thought to be related to mineral wool fibers, no employees showed positive, reproducible results on scratch tests and none had allergic positive results on patch tests.[122] Antibodies to albumin conjugates of formaldehyde, toluene diisocyanate, trimellitic anhydride, and VOCs were found in employees of a remodeled office building,[123] but the clinical significance of this finding is uncertain. Carefully designed studies to account for confounding factors, along with rigorously standardized laboratory methods, are needed before immune biomarkers are routinely used in the evaluation of building-associated outbreaks.[128] Routine laboratory studies, such as serum chemistries or blood counts, are not recommended as part of a routine diagnostic work-up.

Neuropsychologic test batteries may be helpful in the evaluation of cognitive complaints, although interpretation of individual results may be problematic without baseline data before occupancy of the building, and tests should be interpreted in view of many other factors (concurrent medical conditions, age, gender, depression or anxiety disorders).[19] Further research is needed before it can be concluded that current behavioral performance tests used in neurobehavioral batteries are routinely useful in evaluating the potential adverse health effects of indoor contaminant sources that emit concentrations well below the threshold limit values of constituent VOCs.[97]

Management and follow-up. The key step in treating a patient with building-associated illness is to modify the work environment to substantially reduce or eliminate the exposure or working conditions that led to the symptoms. If necessary, the clinician should take an active role in contacting the appropriate supervisor or building manager to obtain vital information about suspected environmental or ventilation problems. If a diagnosis of building-associated illness is made, with documentation of exposure or deficiencies in the heating, ventilation, or air-conditioning (HVAC) system, the clinician should advise work relocation until the problem can be corrected. If no building-related problem has been identified and the patient continues to complain of work-related symptoms, a brief period of work relocation may be indicated on an empiric basis. Placing the symptomatic employee in an office with greater room air changes or an open window or cross-draft often leads to improvement in symptoms. Alternatively, individuals may not require work relocation or removal, but rather can be given the option of leaving the work environment for brief periods throughout the workday until any environmental problems are corrected. It is important to rapidly identify and correct any environmental sources of the symptoms because prolonged uncertainty may lead to unnecessary anxiety and lengthy absence from work. Timely follow-up visits are essential to evaluate any worsening or improvement of symptoms, particularly if the individual has been relocated or removed from work.

Employers often require medical documentation to substantiate the symptoms of an individual with building-associated illness, or they ask the clinician to provide individual work restrictions or preclusions. Clinicians should state the diagnosis and basis for any work restrictions or preclusions but should not provide detailed clinical information that infringes on the patient's confidentiality. Likewise, confidential medical records may not be released to workplace supervisors or managers without written authorization from the patient.

Visits by the clinician to the patient's building, work station, or office may sometimes be helpful in identifying specific exposures. Most often, however, work site visits are appropriate as part of a team approach in solving building-related problems or conducting a formal epidemiologic investigation (see later). In cases of SBS, it is unusual to identify putative exposures from work site visits, and therefore data from building maintenance or industrial hygienists are more critical in evaluating clinical treatment strategies.

Although efforts are being made to correct any adverse environmental conditions, pharmacologic treatment may be necessary to relieve symptoms of respiratory diseases (e.g., rhinitis, sinusitis, asthma, or hypersensitivity pneumonitis) or skin conditions. Unless a specific disorder is present, drug treatment should be avoided for work-related, nonspecific symptoms such as headache, nausea, fatigue, or difficulty concentrating. Individuals with allergies or asthma probably are more susceptible to the effects of indoor irritant exposures, although data to substantiate this clinical impression are lacking.[78] The odor of cleaning products, paints, and petroleum products has been implicated in the triggering of asthma attacks.[112] Individuals with preexisting allergies or asthma aggravated by indoor building exposures or adverse environmental conditions should be considered to have work-related illness, and more aggressive pharmacologic treatment may be needed for worsening of underlying symptoms.

Generally, acute respiratory or skin conditions resolve over days to weeks after cessation of exposure. In a small minority of individuals, new-onset asthma may persist even after removal from exposure, or preexisting asthma may require prolonged therapy for several months. Likewise, nonspecific symptoms such as headache, nausea, fatigue, difficulty concentrating, and memory impairment usually resolve after exposure has ceased or environmental conditions have improved. However, a few individuals may note persistent symptoms on exposure to low-level environmental irritants or may develop symptoms on reentry to any office building. *Multiple chemical sensitivities* (MCS) is a controversial syndrome characterized by recurrent symptoms, referable to multiple organ systems, that occur in response to demonstrable exposure to many chemically unrelated compounds at doses far below those established in the general population to cause harmful effects.[37] Many of the symptoms of MCS, such as headache, fatigue, upper respiratory irritation, and difficulty concentrating are similar to those reported during outbreaks of SBS. The etiology of MCS is controversial, but this syndrome has been associated with occupants of "tight" buildings, including office workers.[7] MCS has been reported to occur after pesticide exposure among employees in a casino,[35] and among several office workers following a large-scale outbreak of SBS.[132] Individuals with recurrent symptoms such as headache, nausea, and dizziness after odorant concentrations of chemicals are thought to have atypical posttraumatic stress disorder, "acquired solvent intolerance," or "odor-triggered panic attacks."[112] It is not known to what extent these disorders occur in individuals following outbreaks of building-associated illness.

INVESTIGATION AND CONTROL OF BUILDING-ASSOCIATED ILLNESS
Epidemiologic investigation

In some cases individual patient complaints may suggest the need for additional epidemiologic investigation to determine the pattern and extent of building-associated illness among a group of employees. Having identified a single patient or group of patients with building-associated illness, the clinician may play a key role in initiating such an investigation through contact with local, state, or federal agencies. Often several clinicians are involved in the care of employees from a single employer or office building, and common symptoms are not recognized until an epidemiologic evaluation is conducted. Likewise, the individual clinician who is evaluating several employees from a single building may not appreciate common symptoms unless a standardized questionnaire is completed and an examination is performed.

Detailed protocols for conducting a comprehensive evaluation of building-associated illness have been published,[41,101,134] including guidelines for medical investigation of indoor air quality complaints. A medical investigation of indoor air quality complaints should generally be a part of a multidisciplinary team approach that encompasses epidemiology, industrial hygiene, and ventilation and building maintenance personnel. Standardized questionnaires are helpful in identifying patterns of complaints localized to particular building areas or associated with certain environmental conditions and can identify individuals who may need additional follow-up.[53]

Environmental assessment and control

Although it is not necessary for the clinician to have a detailed understanding of HVAC systems, it is important to have a basic grasp of possible deficiencies in these systems that may cause adverse health effects. Detailed reviews of ventilation systems and their design are available.[40,88] Many building-associated problems can be corrected by recognizing common HVAC deficiencies. Unfortunately, published standards for workplace exposure to airborne contaminants, such as the OSHA Permissible Exposure Limits or the guidelines produced by the American Conference of Governmental Industrial Hygienists (ACGIH), probably are not applicable to the indoor air environment, and the clinician must be guided by voluntary guidelines published by other organizations. The American Society of Heating, Refrigerating, and Air-Conditioning Engineers (ASHRAE), the World Health Organization (WHO), and the Canadian government have published guidance documents for indoor air quality standards.[8,102,138] The most recent ASHRAE standard recommends that, regardless of smoking status, a minimum of 15 cubic feet per minute (cfm) per person of fresh air be provided when interior spaces are occupied. Higher ventilation rates are recommended for offices (20 cfm per person) and patient rooms in hospitals and nursing homes (25 cfm per person). Smoking areas should have at least 60 cfm per person of outdoor air.

A comfortable thermal environment is present if the temperature falls between 20° and 23.6° C (68° to 74.5° F) in the winter and 22.8° to 26.1° C (73° to 79° F) in the summer; relative humidity should range between 30% and 60%. ASHRAE recommends that carbon dioxide concentrations in indoor environments not exceed 1000 ppm to satisfy occupant comfort needs (equivalent to a ventilation rate of 15 cfm per person). Thus carbon dioxide often is used as a surrogate measure to determine whether an adequate outdoor ventilation rate is maintained. Acceptable indoor air quality is defined by ASHRAE as "air in which there are no known contaminants at harmful concentrations as determined by cognizant authorities and with which a substantial majority (80% or more) of the people exposed do not express dissatisfaction."[8] However, in most cases of building-associated illness, symptoms occur at concentrations of air contaminants below harmful concentrations as defined by recognized authorities such as OSHA or the ACGIH.

Common HVAC deficiencies include combustion products entering outdoor air inlets or occupied spaces as a result of negative pressure; excessive moisture; poor air circulation caused by blockage of return air; poor preventive maintenance, with dust and debris accumulation; inadequate outdoor air, contaminated insulation, and excessive thermal loading from building occupants.[88] These problems may be corrected by a variety of strategies, such as relocation of air intakes, correct building pressurization, good energy management, preventive maintenance programs, improved air circulation, externalizing HVAC system insulation, improving interior temperatures, or increasing the fresh air supply. Specific solutions depend on the nature of the problem, but all hinge on source control, modification of ventilation, or air cleaning.[41] Increasing air humidification may alleviate symptoms of dry skin, eyes, nose, and throat, and nasal congestion.[103] Odors also may be a source of gastrointestinal or CNS symptoms, and strong or unpleasant odors may be accompanied by somatic symptoms at levels below irritant thresholds.[34] Contributions to odors in the indoor environment include human occupant odors (body odor), ETS, volatile building materials, bioodorants, air fresheners, deodorants, and perfumes. Experimental studies have indicated that symptoms of irritation (eye and throat irritation, headache, and drowsiness) remain constant as perceived odor intensity declines, suggesting that VOCs may stimulate trigeminal nerve receptors independently from the olfactory nerve and that symptoms are not simply a psychosomatic response to odor.[65] Aside from ETS, there are no specific regulations regarding odorants in indoor air. Nonetheless, eliminating odors may reduce symptoms of discomfort.

Bioaerosols can be sampled by a variety of techniques that may identify putative agents responsible for building-associated illness and that are most useful when bioaerosol exposure is strongly suspected on clinical grounds, or when these tests are performed for research purposes. Routine bioaerosol sampling is not recommended.[2] Isolating the source of common indoor pollutants on the basis of indoor measurements is also difficult because of the common emission profiles of VOCs from many office materials. Furthermore, VOC measurements often are well below levels normally associated with adverse health effects.[51] As a result, additional techniques have been developed to characterize emissions from indoor materials and furnishings.[125] For example, office materials can be studied by appropriate sampling (e.g., syringe, canister and sorbent techniques) and analysis (e.g., gas chromatography) to derive information about the content or emissions of organic chemicals. Dynamic chamber studies can be performed to determine the impact of indoor sources on indoor air quality, and indoor air quality test houses can quantify pollutant levels under a variety of conditions (e.g., temperature, humidity, air exchange rates, and operation of the HVAC system).

Most authorities stress the need for effective communication with employees as a cornerstone of any solution to building-associated illness. Essential to effective communication is acknowledgement of the legitimacy of complaints, regardless of cause, along with the understanding that beliefs and perceptions of the problem are the keys to enlisting employees in the solution.[21,75] The clinician can play a key role in communicating information about the health effects of indoor exposures, interpreting the clinical significance of air sampling or ventilation evaluation results and responding to the health concerns of building occupants. Frequent meetings with building occupants, attended by a health professional who can outline possible health effects of building-associated illness and answer individual questions, often are an effective means to respond to concerns about the potential health impact of exposures or ventilation deficiencies.

Evaluation of the effectiveness of intervention for outbreaks of sick building syndrome often is based on empiric evidence of a reduction in employee symptoms, physician visits, or lost work time. More carefully controlled measures, such as a double-blind, cross-over design to study changes in ventilation rates and employee symptoms, are suitable for research studies but are not typically applied to clinical management.[121] A randomized crossover trial of experimental manipulation of outdoor air supply in four office buildings with good air supply failed to demonstrate that further increasing the supply of outdoor air resulted in either improved environmental ratings or a reduction in the number of symptoms reported by participants.[84] This is consistent with epidemiologic studies that have also shown that symptoms correlate poorly with ventilation rates, and it implies the presence of other preventable factors of SBS, such as moisture associated with air conditioning systems.[74] Nonetheless, in the absence of additional evidence as to the cause of SBS, most experts recommend increasing the fresh air supply in buildings with a high prevalence of the syndrome.

REFERENCES

1. Aisner J, Schimpff SC, Bennett JE et al: *Aspergillus* infections in cancer patients: association with fireproofing materials in a new hospital, *JAMA* 235:411, 1976.
2. American Conference of Governmental Industrial Hygienists: *Guidelines for the assessment of bioaerosols in the indoor environment,* Cincinnati, Ohio, 1989.
3. American Thoracic Society: Epidemiology standardization project, *Am Rev Respir Dis* 118:1, 1978.
4. Anderson K, McSharry CP, Boyd G: Radiographic changes in humidifier fever, *Thorax* 40:312, 1985.
5. Arnow PM, Fink JN, Schleuter DP et al: Early detection of hypersensitivity pneumonitis in office workers, *Am J Med* 64:236, 1978.
6. Arnow PM, Anderson RL, Mainous DP et al: Pulmonary aspergillosis during hospital renovation, *Am Rev Respir Dis* 118:49, 1978.
7. Ashford NA, Miller CS: *Chemical exposure: low levels and high stakes,* New York, 1990, Van Nostrand Reinhold.
8. American Society of Heating, Refrigerating, and Air-Conditioning Engineers, Standard 62-1989: Ventilation for acceptable indoor air quality, 1989.
9. Baker DB: Social and organizational factors in office building–related illness, *Occup Med* 4:607, 1989.
10. Bansazak EF, Thiede WH, Fink JN: Hypersensitivity pneumonitis due to contamination of an air conditioner, *N Engl J Med* 283:271, 1970.
11. Bascom R: The upper respiratory tract: mucous membrane irritation, *Environ Health Perspect* 95:39, 1991.
12. Bascom R: Differential responsiveness to irritant mixtures, *Ann NY Acad Sci* 641:225, 1992.
13. Bauer RM, Greve K, Besch EL et al: The role of psychological factors in the report of building-related symptoms in sick building syndrome, *J Consult Clin Psychol* 60:213, 1992.
14. Baur X, Richter G, Pethran A et al: Increased prevalence of Ig-G–induced sensitization and hypersensitivity pneumonitis (humidifier lung) in nonsmokers exposed to aerosols of a contaminated air conditioner, *Respiration* 59:211, 1992.
15. Bayer CW, Black MS: Building-related illness involving formaldehyde and other volatile organic compounds, *Exp Pathol* 37:147, 1989.
16. Berardi BM, Leoni E, Marchesini B et al: Indoor climate and air quality in new offices: effects of a reduced air-exchange rate, *Int Arch Occup Environ Health* 63:233, 1991.
17. Bernstein RS, Sorenson WG, Garabrant D et al: Exposures to airborne *Penicillium* from a contaminated ventilation system: clinical, environmental and epidemiological aspects, *Am Ind Hyg Assoc J* 44:161, 1983.
18. Bloch AB, Orenstein WA, Ewing WM et al: Measles outbreak in a pediatric practice: airborne transmission in an office practice setting, *Pediatrics* 75:676, 1985.
19. Bolla KI: Neuropsychological assessment for detecting adverse effects of volatile organic compounds on the central nervous system, *Environ Health Perspect* 95:93, 1991.
20. Boxer PA: Occupational mass psychogenic illness: history, prevention, and management, *J Occup Med* 27:867, 1985.
21. Boxer PA: Indoor air quality: a psychosocial perspective, *J Occup Med* 32:425, 1990.

22. Brandt-Rauf PW, Andrews LR, Schwarz-Miller J: Sick hospital syndrome, *J Occup Med* 33:737, 1991.

23. Brooks BO, Utter GM, DeBroy JA et al: Indoor air pollution: an edifice complex, *Clin Toxicol* 29:315, 1991.

24. Brundage JF, Scott RM, Lednar WM et al: Building-associated risk of febrile acute respiratory diseases in army trainees, *JAMA* 259:2108, 1988.

25. Burge HA: Indoor air and infectious disease, *Occup Med* 4:713, 1989.

26. Burge PS, Finnegan MJ, Horsfield N et al: Occupational asthma in a factory with a contaminated humidifier, *Thorax* 40:248, 1985.

27. Burge S, Hedge A, Wilson S et al: Sick building syndrome: a study of 4373 office workers, *Ann Occup Hyg* 31:493, 1987.

28. Centers for Disease Control: Employee illness from underground gas and oil contamination, *MMWR* 31:451, 1982.

29. Centers for Disease Control: Respiratory illness associated with carpet cleaning at a hospital clinic—Virginia, *MMWR* 32:378, 1983.

30. Centers for Disease Control: *Mycobacterium tuberculosis* transmission in a health clinic—Florida, *MMWR* 38:256, 1988.

31. Colligan MJ, Murphy LR: Mass psychogenic illness in organizations: an overview, *J Occup Psychol* 52:77, 1979.

32. Colligan MJ: The psychological effects of indoor air pollution, *Bull NY Acad Med* 57:1014, 1981.

33. Committee on Passive Smoking: Environmental tobacco smoke, Washington, DC, 1986.

34. Cone JE, Shusterman D: Health effects of indoor odorants, *Environ Health Perspect* 95:53, 1991.

35. Cone JE, Sult TA: Acquired intolerance to solvents following pesticide/solvent exposure in a building: a new group of workers at risk for multiple chemical sensitivities, *Toxicol Ind Health* 8:47, 1992.

36. Conwill DE, Werner SB, Dritz SK et al: Legionellosis: the 1980 San Francisco outbreak, *Am Rev Respir Dis* 126:666, 1980.

37. Cullen MR: Multiple chemical sensitivities: an overview, *Occup Med* 2:655, 1987.

38. Dondero TJ, Rendtorff RC, Mallison GF et al: An outbreak of legionnaires' disease associated with a contaminated air-conditioning cooling tower, *N Engl J Med* 302:365, 1980.

39. Donnell HD, Bagby JR, Harmon RG et al: Report of an illness outbreak at the Harry S Truman State Office Building, *Am J Epidemiol* 129:550, 1989.

40. Ellenbecker MJ: Engineering controls for clean air in the office environment, *Clin Chest Med* 13:193, 1992.

41. Environmental Protection Agency: Building air quality: a guide for building owners and managers, Washington, DC, 1991, US Government Printing Office.

42. Finnegan MJ, Pickering CAC: Work-related asthma and humidifier fever in air-conditioned buildings. Proceedings of the Third International Conference on Indoor Air Quality and Climate. In Berglund B, Lindvall T, Sundell J, editors: *Recent advances in health sciences and technology,* Stockholm, 1984, Swedish Council for Building Research.

43. Finnegan MJ, Pikering CAC, Burge PS: The sick building syndrome: prevalence studies, *Br Med J* 289:1573, 1984.

44. Finnegan MJ, Pickering CAC: Building related illness, *Clin Allergy* 16:389, 1986.

45. Fink JN, Banaszak EF, Baroriak JJ et al: Interstitial lung diseases due to contamination of forced air systems, *Ann Intern Med* 84:406, 1976.

46. Flachsbart PG, Ott WR: A rapid method for surveying CO concentrations in high-rise buildings, *Environ Int* 12:255, 1986.

47. Franck C: Eye symptoms and signs in buildings with indoor climate problems ("office eye syndrome"), *Acta Opthalmol (Copenh)* 64:306, 1986.

48. Ganier M, Lieberman P, Fink J et al: Humidifier fever: an outbreak in office workers, *Chest* 77:183, 1980.

49. Glick TH, Gregg MB, Berman B et al: Pontiac fever: an epidemic of unknown etiology in a health department. I. Clinical and epidemiological aspects, *Am J Epidemiol* 107:149, 1978.

50. Gold DR: Indoor air pollution, *Clin Chest Med* 13:215, 1992.

51. Goyer N: Chemical contaminants in office buildings, *Am Ind Hyg Assoc J* 51:615, 1990.

52. Guidotti TL, Alexander RW, Fedoruk MJ: Epidemiologic features that may distinguish between building-associated illness outbreaks due to chemical exposure or psychogenic origin, *J Occup Med* 29:148, 1987.

53. Guirguis S, Rajhans G, Leong D et al: A simplified IAQ questionnaire to obtain useful data for investigating sick building complaints, *Am Ind Hyg Assoc J* 52:A434, 1991.

54. Hall EM, Johnson JV: A case study of stress and mass psychogenic illness in industrial workers, *J Occup Med* 31:243, 1989.

55. Harrison J, Pickering CAC, Faragher EB et al: An investigation of the relationship between microbial and particulate indoor air pollution and the sick building syndrome, *Respir Med* 86:225, 1992.

56. Hodges GR, Fink JN, Schleuter DP: Hypersensitivity pneumonitis caused by a contaminated cool-mist vaporizer, *Ann Intern Med* 80:501, 1974.

57. Hodgson MJ, Morey PR, Attfield M et al: Pulmonary disease associated with cafeteria flooding, *Arch Environ Health* 40:96, 1985.

58. Hodgson MJ, Block GD, Parkinson DK: Organophosphate poisoning in office workers, *J Occup Med* 28:434, 1986.

59. Hodgson MJ, Morey PR, Simon JS et al: An outbreak of recurrent acute and chronic hypersensitivity pneumonitis in office workers, *Am J Epidemiol* 125:631, 1987.

60. Hodgson MJ: Clinical diagnosis and management of building-related illness and the sick building syndrome, *Occup Med* 4:593, 1989.

61. Hodgson MJ: Environmental tobacco smoke and the sick building syndrome, *Occup Med* 4:735, 1989.

62. Hodgson MJ, Frohliger J, Permar E et al: Symptoms and microenvironmental measures in nonproblem buildings, *J Occup Med* 33:527, 1991.

63. Hodgson MJ: Field studies on the sick building syndrome, *Ann NY Acad Sci* 641:21, 1992.

64. Hoffman RE, Wood RC, Kreiss K: Building-related asthma in Denver office workers, *Am J Public Health* 83:89, 1993.

65. Hudnell HK, Otto DA, House DE et al: Exposure of humans to a volatile organic mixture. II. Sensory, *Arch Environ Health* 47:31, 1992.

66. Karol MH: Allergic reactions to indoor air pollutants, *Environ Health Perspect* 95:45, 1991.

67. Kohler PF, Gross G, Salvaggio J et al: Humidifier lung: hypersensitivity pneumonitis related to thermotolerant bacterial aerosols, *Chest* (suppl69):294, 1976.

68. Koren HS, Graham DE, Devlin RB: Exposure of humans to a volatile organic mixture. III. Inflammatory response, *Arch Environ Health* 47:39, 1992a.

69. Koren HS, Devlin RB: Human upper respiratory tract responses to inhaled pollutants with emphasis on nasal lavage, *Ann NY Acad Sci* 641:215, 1992b.

70. Kreiss K, Gonzalez MG, Conright KL et al: Respiratory

irritation due to carpet shampoo: two outbreaks, *Environ Int* 8:337, 1982.

71. Kreiss K, Hodgson MJ: Building-associated epidemics. In Walsh PJ, Dudney CS, Copenhaver ED, editors: *Indoor air quality,* Boca Raton, 1984, CRC Press.

72. Kreiss K: The epidemiology of building-related complaints and illness, *Occup Med* 4:575, 1989.

73. Kreiss K: The sick building syndrome: where is the epidemiologic basis? *Am J Public Health* 80:1172, 1990.

74. Kriess K: The sick building syndrome in office buildings: a breath of fresh air, *N Engl J Med* 328:877, 1993.

75. Kroll-Smith JS, Couch SR: As if exposure were not enough: the social and cultural system as a secondary stressor, *Environ Health Perspect* 95:61, 1991.

76. LaForce FM: Airborne infections and modern building technology, *Environ Int* 12:137, 1986.

77. Lebowitz MD: Methods to assess respiratory effects of complex mixtures, *Environ Health Perspect* 95:75, 1991.

78. Lebowitz MD: Populations at risk: addressing health effects due to complex mixtures with a focus on respiratory effects, *Environ Health Perspect* 95:35, 1991.

79. Lessenger JE: Five office workers inadvertently exposed to cypermethrin, *J Toxicol Environ Health* 35:261, 1992.

80. Lyles WB, Greve KW, Bauer RM et al: Sick building syndrome, *South Med J* 84:65, 1991.

81. Main DM, Hogan TJ: Health effects of low-level exposure to formaldehyde, *J Occup Med* 25:896, 1983.

82. Melius J, Wallingford K, Keenlyside R et al: Indoor air quality: the NIOSH experience, *Ann Am Conf Gov Ind Hyg* 10:3, 1984.

83. Mendell MJ, Smith AH: Consistent patterns of elevated symptoms in air-conditioned office buildings: a reanalysis of epidemiologic studies, *Am J Public Health* 80:1193, 1990.

84. Menzies R, Tamblyn R, Farant JP et al: The effects of varying levels of outdoor air supply on the symptoms of sick building syndrome, *N Engl J Med* 328:821, 1993.

85. Middaugh DA, Pinney SM, Linz DH: Sick building syndrome: medical evaluation of two work forces, *J Occup Med* 34:1197, 1992.

86. Molhave L, Bach B, Pedersen OF: Human reactions during controlled exposures to low concentrations of organic gases and vapours known as normal indoor air pollutants. In Berglund B, Lindvall T, Sundell J, editors: *Indoor air.* Vol 3. Sensory and hyperreactivity reactions to sick buildings, Stockholm, 1984, Stockholm Council for Building Research.

87. Molhave L: Controlled experiments for studies of the sick building syndrome, *Ann NY Acad Sci* 641:46, 1992.

88. Morey PR, Shattuck: Role of ventilation in the causation of building-associated illnesses, *Occup Med* 4:625, 1989.

89. Morgan MS, Camp JE: Upper respiratory irritation from controlled exposure to vapor from carbonless copy forms, *J Occup Med* 28:415, 1986.

90. National Research Council: *Environmental tobacco smoke: measuring exposures and assessing health effects,* Washington, DC, 1986, National Academy Press.

91. Norback D, Michel I, Widstrom J: Indoor air quality and personal factors related to the sick building syndrome, *Scand J Work Environ Health* 16:121, 1990.

92. Norback D, Torgen M, Edling C: Volatile organic compounds, respirable dust, and personal factors related to prevalence and incidence of sick building syndrome in primary schools, *Br J Ind Med* 47:733, 1990.

93. Norback D, Edling C: Environmental, occupational, and personal factors related to the prevalence of sick building syndrome in the general population, *Br J Ind Med* 48:451, 1991.

94. O'Mahoney MC, Lakhani A, Stephens A et al: Legion-

naires' disease and the sick building syndrome, *Epidemiol Infect* 103:295, 1989.

95. O'Mahoney MC, Stanwell-Smith RE, Tillett HE et al: The Stafford outbreak of legionnaires' disease, *Epidemiol Infect* 104:361, 1990.

96. Otto DA, Hudnell HK, House DE et al: Exposure of humans to a volatile organic mixture. I. Behavioral assessment, *Arch Environ Health* 47:23, 1992.

97. Otto DA: Assessment of neurobehavioral response in humans to low-level volatile organic compound sources, *Ann NY Acad Sci* 641:248, 1992.

98. Parrott WF, Blyth W: Another causal factor in the production of humidifier fever, *J Soc Occup Med* 30:63, 1980.

99. Pestalozzi C: Febrile Gruppenerkrangungen in einer Modellschreinerei durch Inhalation von mit Schimmerpilzen Kontaminiertem Befeuchterwassee, *Schweiz Med Wochenschr* 89:710, 1959.

100. Pickering CAC, Moore WKS, Lacey J et al: Investigation of a respiratory disease associated with an air-conditioning system, *Clin Allergy* 6:109, 1976.

101. Quinlan P, Macher JM, Alevantis LE et al: Protocol for the comprehensive evaluation of building-associated illness, *Occup Med* 4:771, 1989.

102. Rajhans GS: Report of the Interministerial Committee on Indoor Air Quality, Health and Safety Support Services Branch, Ministry of Labour, Toronto, Canada, 1988.

103. Reinikainen LM, Jaakkola JJK, Seppänen O: The effects of air humidification on symptoms and perception of indoor air quality in office workers: a six period cross-over trial, *Arch Environ Health* 47:8, 1992.

104. Remington PL, Hall WN, Davis IH et al: Airborne transmission of measles in a physician's office, *JAMA* 253:1574, 1985.

105. Riley EC, Murphy G, Riley L: Airborne spread of measles in a suburban elementary school, *Am J Epidemiol* 107:421, 1978.

106. Robertson AS, Burge PS, Hedge A et al: Comparison of health problems related to work and environmental measurements in two office buildings with different ventilation systems, *Br Med J* 291:373, 1985.

107. Robertson AS, Burge PS, Hedge A: Relation between passive cigarette smoke exposure and "building sickness," *Thorax* 43:263P, 1988.

108. Ryan CM, Morrow LA: Dysfunctional buildings or dysfunctional people: an examination of the sick building syndrome and allied disorders, *J Consult Clin Psychol* 60:220, 1992.

109. Samet JM, Marbury MC, Spengler JD: Health effects and sources of indoor air pollution. I, *Am Rev Respir Dis* 136:1486, 1987.

110. Samet JM, Marbury MC, Spengler JD: Health effects and sources of indoor air pollution. II, *Am Rev Respir Dis* 137:221, 1988.

111. Sarubbi FA, Kopf HB, Wilson MB et al: Increased recovery of *Aspergillus flavus* from respiratory secretions during hospital construction, *Am Rev Respir Dis* 125:33, 1982.

112. Shusterman D: Critical review: the health significance of environmental odor pollution, *Arch Environ Health* 47:76, 1992.

113. Sick building syndrome, Lancet 33:1493, 1991 (editorial).

114. Sim MR, Abramson MJ: Indoor air quality and sick buildings, *Med J Aust* 155:651, 1991.

115. Skov P, Valbjorn O, Danish Indoor Climate Study Group: The "sick" building syndrome in the office environment: the Danish town hall study, *Environ Int* 13:339, 1987.

116. Skov P, Valbjorn O, Pedersen BV: Influence of indoor cli-

mate on the sick building syndrome in an office, *Scand J Work Environ Health* 16:363, 1990.

117. Skov P: The sick building syndrome, *Ann NY Acad Sci* 641:17, 1992.

118. Sterling DA: Volatile organic compounds in indoor air: an overview of sources, concentrations, and health effects. In Gammage RB, Kaye SV, editors: *Indoor air and human health,* Chelsea, Mich, 1984, Lewis.

119. Stolwijk JAJ: Sick building syndrome, *Environ Health Perspect* 95:99, 1991.

120. Stolwijk JAJ: Risk assessment of acute health and comfort effects of indoor air pollution, *Ann NY Acad Sci* 641:56, 1992.

121. Tamblyn RM, Menzies RI, Tamblyn RT et al: The feasibility of using a double-blind, experimental cross-over design to study interventions for sick building syndrome, *J Clin Epidemiol* 45:603, 1992.

122. Thestrup-Pedersen K, Bach B, Petersen R: Allergic investigations in patients with the sick building syndrome, *Contact Dermatitis* 23:53, 1990.

123. Thrasher JD, Madison R, Broughton A et al: Building-related illness and antibodies to albumin conjugates of formaldehyde, toluene diisocyanate, and trimellitic anhydride, *Am J Ind Med* 15:187, 1989.

124. Tichenor BA, Mason MA: Organic emissions from consumer products and building materials to the indoor environment, *J Air Poll Cont Assoc* 38:264, 1988.

125. Tichenor BA: Characterizing materials sources and sinks, *Ann NY Acad Sci* 641:63, 1992.

126. US Department of Health and Human Services, Public Health Office, Office on Smoking and Health: The health consequences of involuntary smoking: a report of the surgeon general, Washington, DC, 1986, US Government Printing Office.

127. Utell MJ, Samet JM: Assessment of acute effects in controlled human studies, *Ann NY Acad Sci* 641:37, 1992.

128. Vogt RF: Use of laboratory tests for immune biomarkers in environmental health studies concerned with exposure to indoor air pollutants, *Environ Health Perspect* 95:85, 1991.

129. Wallace LA: Carbon monoxide in air breath of employees in an underground office, *Air Pollut Control Assoc* 33:678, 1983.

130. Wallingford KM: NIOSH indoor air quality investigations: 1971 through 1985, Cincinnati, 1986, National Institute for Occupational Safety and Health.

131. Welch LS: Severity of health effects associated with the building-related illness, *Environ Health Perspect* 95:67, 1991.

132. Welch LS, Sokas R: Development of multiple chemical sensitivity after an outbreak of sick building syndrome, *Toxicol Ind Health* 8:47, 1992.

133. Wechsler CJ, Shields HC, Rainer D: Concentrations of volatile organic compounds at a building with health and comfort complaints, *Am Ind Hyg Assoc J* 51:261, 1990.

134. Whorton MD, Larson SR, Gordon NJ et al: Investigation and work-up of tight building syndrome, *J Occup Med* 29:142, 1987.

135. Winn WC: Legionella and legionnaires' disease: a review with emphasis on environmental studies and laboratory diagnosis, *CRC Crit Rev Clin Lab Sci* 21:323, 1985.

136. Woods JE, Drewry GM, Morey PR: Office worker perceptions of indoor air quality effects on discomfort and performance. In Seifert B, Edsdorn H, Fischer M et al, editors: *Indoor air '87.* Proceedings of the Institute for Water, Soil and Air Hygiene, 1987.

137. Woods JE: Cost avoidance and productivity in owning and operating buildings, *Occup Med* 4:753, 1989.

138. World Health Organization: Air quality guidelines for Europe, European series no 23, 1987, WHO Regional Publications.

24 Infectious Disorders

The acquired immunodeficiency syndrome (AIDS) pandemic has focused greater attention on the issues surrounding all occupational infectious diseases. From this international medical crisis has evolved a series of new policies and procedures, frequently accompanied by legislation, which has influenced medical and dental practices in an unprecedented fashion. Although some of these new guidelines are well founded in proper infection control practices (e.g., hepatitis B vaccination), other proposed regulations are being driven by fear and an incorrect perception of risk.

However, the new challenges in this field are not limited to the problems posed by the human immunodeficiency virus (HIV). The development of an assay for hepatitis C and the emergence of multidrug-resistant tuberculosis reflect some of the many evolving concerns that face clinicians dealing with these issues.

Recent advances in vaccine development also continue to change the practice of medicine in this area. The hepatitis B vaccine, introduced in the 1980s, has had a dramatic impact on disease prevention among health care workers. Other vaccines, such as those developed against the varicella-zoster and hepatitis A viruses, will further add to treatment considerations in many occupational and nonoccupational groups.

Several occupational groups, such as veterinarians, animal handlers, and laboratory researchers, have specific infectious disease concerns. Some of these diseases (e.g., brucellosis and leptospirosis), while important, are not commonly seen in the general occupational health clinic and will not be discussed in this chapter.

HEPATITIS B VIRUS

Hepatitis B virus (HBV) remains the single most important infectious disease organism transmitted through blood or blood products. As such it remains the strongest single justification for universal precautions when handling any human blood–derived material. Although estimates vary on how many health care workers contract hepatitis B, the number may be as high as 12,000 a year. Of these approximately 500 to 600 are hospital-

ized, and 250 die as a result of acute or chronic effects of the disease.[2] These deaths are related to fulminant hepatitis, superinfection with delta-hepatitis, and cirrhosis and hepatocellular carinomas, all secondary to hepatitis B infection.

Several factors account for the high rates of (HBV) transmission. High viral titers, ranging from 10^8 to 10^{13} viral infective units per milliliter are found in individuals with hepatitis B. HBV is also known to remain infective for many weeks on dried surfaces, posing long-term hazards to health care workers.

A nonimmunized person who sustains a needle-stick injury from an individual with hepatitis B faces a 6% to 30% risk of contracting the disease. Serologic studies for hepatitis B in selected health care workers have shown rates exceeding 20% in specific groups, including some emergency and operating room personnel. Many of these seropositive individuals have had no specific exposure to hepatitis B and no history of acute hepatitis. A substantial number of these individuals will also be chronic carriers for hepatitis B.

The introduction of the hepatitis B vaccine has proved a major advance in eradicating this disease from the health care arena. The initial vaccine was prepared from pooled human blood products, which included three separate processes to inactivate biologic contaminants.[14] These techniques also have been shown to inactivate representatives of all classes of pathogenic human viruses, including HIV. The vaccine currently used has been developed through recombinant deoxyribonucleic acid (DNA) technology, using yeast cells to produce hepatitis B surface antigen. Because this does not involve any viral or human blood product, there is no risk of transmitting a biologic agent.

Some institutions may find it cost effective to prescreen certain health care workers (e.g., veteran workers with past exposure to blood or workers coming from endemic areas) to avoid unnecessary vaccinations. Although most institutions currently use hepatitis B surface antibody (HB_sAb) as a screen, testing hepatitis B core Ab is an alternative that identifies all previously infected individuals, including carriers and noncarriers. Testing for HB$_S$Ab identifies only previously infected noncarriers. The Centers for Disease Control (CDC) recommend that individuals who spend a significant amount of time working with human blood products undergo a hepatitis B core Ab test before they are given the vaccine. When the core antibody is positive, indicating previous HBV infection, it is important to check for both the surface antigen and the surface antibody for hepatitis B, to determine if the individual is a chronic carrier or if the infection has resolved.

The federal Occupational Safety and Health Association (OSHA) requires that the hepatitis B vaccine be given to all health care workers with significant exposure to human blood or blood products. This should considerably reduce the incidence of hepatitis B in the United States. However, not all recipients of the vaccine develop antibodies against hepatitis B surface proteins (as measured with titers above 10 sample ratio units [SRU] by radioimmunoassay for hepatitis B surface antibodies, or anti-HB$_S$). Studies have shown that certain human lymphocyte antigen (HLA) subtypes (e.g., HLA-B8, SC01, and DR3) show diminished or no response to the vaccine.[1] Postvaccination testing for antibodies has been advised for those with an occupational risk for HBV; this is done routinely in many medical centers and clinics.

Anti-HB$_S$ antibodies can be measured in 80% to 95% of normal, healthy adults who are tested 1 to 6 months after receiving the third dose of the vaccine, *provided the vaccine is administered in the deltoid muscle of the arm* (administering the vaccine into the gluteal muscle produces a significantly reduced response[2]).

Factors that influence immune response to the HBV vaccine, other than the site of administration and genetically determined antibody response, are an immunocompromised state, age over 50 years, and an improperly stored vaccine.

For those who do not respond to the three-dose series, the current recommendation is one to three additional doses. Approximately 15% to 25% of recipients will show an antibody response after one additional dose, and 30% to 50% should respond after three additional doses.[14] Individuals who have completed only a portion of the initial series should complete only the three doses, picking up where the next dose would be given (e.g., giving dose two and waiting 5 months for dose three).

Individuals who continue to fail to mount an antibody response after six doses of vaccine often are counseled about alternative lines of work that do not involve significant exposure to human blood or body fluids. Obviously, strict adherence to universal precautions should be followed. Those who do not respond to the vaccine should also be treated with two doses of hepatitis B immune globulin (HBIG), given a month apart, after exposure to HB$_S$Ag-positive blood if reassignment to work avoiding blood contact is not possible. HBIG should also be used for individuals exposed to known HB$_S$Ag-positive blood who either have not received or have not completed the hepatitis B vaccine series. If hepatitis B vaccination is initiated concomitantly, a second dose of HBIG is not required. Because HBIG is expensive, its use should await the results of HB$_S$Ag studies on the source, as long as these results can be determined within 72 hours of exposure. If testing cannot be performed within this time, HBIG should be administered when the source has risk factors for hepatitis B.

After demonstrable antibodies to HBV have developed, approximately 24% to 42% of responders lose measurable antibodies by 5 years. However, it appears that protection against hepatitis B continues for up to 7 years based on two studies evaluating long-term immunity.[4,16] A rapid antibody response following booster doses of the vaccine given in experimental studies has indicated the presence of long-term, cell-mediated immunity. Because more studies are needed to assess the need for and timing of booster doses, they are not recommended at this time.

HBV-infected health care workers are an important consideration, because transmission of HBV to patients has been documented in numerous outbreaks in the world.[6,9] Many institutions have established policies preventing HBV-infected workers from performing invasive procedures. The higher infectivity associated with those who are "e"-antigen positive can be used to further define a high-risk individual when restrictions would be appropriate.

HEPATITIS A VIRUS

Hepatitis A virus (HAV) generally is not a problem for most occupational groups. For health care workers treating HAV-infected patients, strict adherence to proper handwashing techniques and infection control procedures should eliminate most potential infectious routes of exposure. Sanitation workers, sewage treatment employees, plumbers, and other individuals who work with untreated sewage have not been found to have an increased risk of HAV infection or typhoid fever and do not need routine administration of immune globulin, or HBV and typhoid vaccinations.

HEPATITIS C VIRUS

Hepatitis C virus (HCV) until recently was considered one of the non-A, non-B (NANB) hepatitis viruses. The advent of an enzyme-linked immunosorbent assay (ELISA) for antibody to a nonstructural peptide of this ribonucleic acid (RNA) virus (anti-HCV) has established HCV as the responsible agent for more than 75% of cases of posttransfusion hepatitis. Patients with HCV often have a history of blood transfusions, parenteral drug abuse, or percutaneous exposure to human blood products.

Although the transmissibility of this virus after occupational exposure to blood products has not yet been established, it appears that HCV has been passed through needle-stick injuries and other percutaneous exposures in approximately 3% of cases where the patient was positive for antibodies to HCV using the first-generation tests.[7]

The antibody to HCV can be detected $3\frac{1}{2}$ to 6 months after infection and 5 to 20 weeks after the onset of symptoms. Thus anti-HCV serves as a marker for chronic infection but is less useful as a marker for acute disease. A polymerase chain reaction (PCR) assay to detect and quantify HCV may be developed in the near future to identify early infections.

A significant number of HCV-infected individuals go on to develop chronic infections (as many as 50%), and as many as 20% of those with chronic infections may develop cirrhosis. It also appears that chronic HCV infections lead to an increased incidence of hepatocellular carcinoma.

The treatment for acute and chronic HCV infections remains controversial. Some evidence supports the use of alpha-interferon for those with chronic infections, although the high rate of recurrence of these infections, along with the high cost of the treatment, do not warrant widespread use of this therapy outside clinical trials. Antiviral agents, such as ribavirin, have also looked promising in recent studies, although more data are needed.

Investigation of immunoprophylaxis for HCV exposure also has failed to identify an effective agent. The use of immunoglobulin (or gamma-globulin) remains controversial, but some centers use it when the source is a known or probable HCV-positive individual (e.g., an intravenous drug user), because it is a relatively benign, inexpensive treatment that may be partially protective. However, with the virtual elimination of any significant HCV titer from donor screening, this practice should be discontinued.

Because sexual activity is not a well-established route for transmitting HCV infection, sexual precautions probably are not warranted in health care workers exposed to or infected with the virus. However, more information is needed about the potential for transmitting HCV through sexual activity before this issue can be clarified.

HUMAN IMMUNODEFICIENCY VIRUS

The issues surrounding exposure to the human immunodeficiency virus (HIV) in the workplace have been the focus of attention ever since bloodborne transmission of this virus was first demonstrated. Fortunately, HIV infection in health care remains a relatively uncommon occurrence. However, as the number of HIV-infected individuals in the community continues to grow, the incidence of accidental exposure to blood products from HIV-positive sources also will increase.

Among the health care workers who have had documented HIV seroconversions, many have been exposed to large quantities of infected blood or blood products through percutaneous incidents. Needle-stick injuries have been found to transmit much smaller quantities of blood, averaging approximately 0.001 ml. When needle-stick injuries occur through protective gloves, the amount of blood and body fluid transferred is reduced by more than 50%.[10]

The most recent data on HIV transmission after a needle-stick injury from a known HIV-positive patient shows that seroconversion occurs in approximately 0.3% (or 1:300) of cases.[5] Interestingly, these numbers have continued to decline over time as more data become available. This risk probably is so much lower than that for hepatitis B following exposure to a known seropositive patient, because the viral counts found in HIV infected individuals is lower. Studies have shown counts ranging from 10^1 to 10^4 viral colony units per milliliter. The lower concentrations are found in asymptomatic HIV-positive patients and the higher counts in individuals with documented AIDS.

A 1991 survey on HIV involving 3,420 orthopedic surgeons attending a national conference failed to demonstrate a single case of occupationally derived infection in this group (the two positive cases were among 109 with risk factors).[13]

Despite the seroconversions that have occurred from an HIV-infected dentist, studies performed on other HIV-infected health care providers have failed to demonstrate similar patterns of transmission. This suggests that significant breaks in standard infection control procedures may have been involved in this case, although further studies clearly are warranted.

MANAGEMENT OF EXPOSURE TO HUMAN BLOOD PRODUCTS

All exposure to blood products initially should address immediate cleansing of the wound or irrigation of the affected skin or mucous membranes. Some advocate using agents such as povidone-iodine or hydrogen peroxide for contaminated areas of skin, but rapid cleansing with soap and water probably should be the first line of response, because they usually are readily available and probably highly effective. Use of caustic agents such as bleach or concentrated disinfectants should be discouraged, because they can cause additional medical problems and may disrupt intact skin, leading to more avenues for entry of biologic material. Wounds should be cleansed thoroughly and managed appropriately.

Splash injuries to intact skin and mucous membranes should be washed, although blood contact with intact skin should not be considered a significant injury, because this does not allow the transfer of biologic agents. Splash injuries to the eyes and intact mucous membranes also have not been found to transfer viruses such as HIV.

An evaluation or estimation of the amount of blood transferred should be made. If any blood could have been transferred, a risk assessment of the patient (if known) should be performed. Risk factors should be determined for HIV, HBV, and HCV, including any history of percutaneous drug abuse; transfusion of blood or blood products (especially between 1978 and 1985); male homosexual or bisexual contacts; previous diagnoses for HIV, HBV, or HCV; or sexual contacts with any high-risk groups. Inquiries should also be made about contacts with multiple sexual partners or with prostitutes.

This evaluation of the patient usually can be expedited by a tactful explanation of the reasons for the interview and by explaining that a health care worker was injured while caring for that individual. It also is important to have an established system for ensuring confidentiality of the interview and an alternative method of payment for any laboratory tests.

Testing of the patient for HIV and HBV usually is attempted after informed consent has been obtained. This is particularly important if the patient has any of the risk factors listed previously. HCV testing usually is performed only if the patient has risk factors for HCV. (See Table 24-1.)

Zidovudine (azidothymidine, AZT) is an antiviral agent that acts as a competitive inhibitor of reverse transcriptase, which is involved in replication of HIV. Zidovudine has been widely used to treat patients with AIDS, but no clinical trials have demonstrated efficacy of this drug for prophylaxis following exposure to HIV. The clinical trial to assess this effect was discontinued for lack of sufficient numbers when participants refused to receive a placebo. Animal studies have shown that early use of zidovudine may reduce the antibody response after inoculation with HIV.[11] Several case reports have shown failure of the drug after accidental inoculation in humans, although larger quantities of blood were involved in these incidents.[8]

Another consideration in the use of zidovudine is the potential for toxic side effects. Most of the serious complications (bone marrow depression with anemia, neutropenia, and thrombocytopenia) occur with high-dose regimens, usually after several months of treatment. More common are the less serious but occasionally disabling symptoms of headache, nausea, vomiting, insomnia, restlessness, and agitation, which occur with early treatment. Some of these symptoms can be controlled with medications such as ibuprofen, antiemetics, and benzodiazepines.

Treatment with zidovudine is begun with 200 mg every 4 hours for 4 weeks. Usually we include the nighttime dose for the first 3 days, dropping to five doses per day (dosed every 4 hours while awake) on day 4. During this time complete blood counts (CBCs) and liver function tests are monitored every week, and therapy is discontinued when white blood cell (WBC) counts fall below 50% of the baseline count, or when anemia, thrombocytopenia, peripheral neuropathy, hepatitis, or other severe reactions occur. Dosage reduction is also considered when incapacitating side effects occur.

The long-term safety of zidovudine has also been questioned, because a carcinogenic effect has been demonstrated in animals. This drug should not be used during pregnancy.

Cost is another factor, because a course of treatment can range from $700 to $1,200. To avoid having bills sent for zidovudine prophylaxis (thereby indicating a possible HIV exposure), we have arranged for direct, confidential funding for these cases through the institutions where the exposure occurred. Although such arrangements are not always possible in advance, they can avoid breaks in confidentiality for the health care worker.[14]

If the patient refuses an interview for risk factors or serologic testing or has any of the risk factors listed previously, serial testing of the health care worker for HIV and any of the other potential viral agents is begun. HIV antibody tests are per-

Table 24-1

CONFIDENTIAL

Protocol for Blood/Body Fluid Exposures

Date and time of injury: _____

Medical record #: _____

Code Name: _____

Job Title/Responsibilities: _____

Phone: work (___)_____ home (___)_____

Description of injury:

    Description of sharp object: _____

    Depth of injury: _____

    Estimate of quantity of fluid exposed: _____

    Location of exposure: _____

    Description of task causing accident: _____

    Duration of time between direct contact with source and the time of accident: _____

Area of exposure:

    Description of baseline skin/mucous membranes: _____

    Type of protective equipment used at time of accident (e.g. mask, gloves, gowns, and etc.): _____

    _____

Vaccination status:

      for hepatitis B (# of doses and date of last dose): _____

      for tetanus: _____

Patient source (where applicable):

    Code name: _____

    Chart #: _____

    Diagnosis: _____

    Attending physician: _____

Risk factors of patient source (Donor if known)

    HIV/AIDS diagnosis: _____

    HIV/AIDS associated illness: _____

    IV drug abuse: _____

    Transfusions/blood products (1978-1985): _____

    Bisexual/homosexual practices: _____

    Sexual contact with above groups: _____

    Multiple sexual partners: _____

    Hepatitis status and type (include LFTs): _____

    Country of origin (if not U.S. born): _____

Patient:

    HIV/AIDS diagnosis: _____

    HIV/AIDS associated illness: _____

    IV drug abuse: _____

    Transfusions/blood products (1978-1985): _____

    Bisexual/homosexual practices: _____

    Sexual contact with above groups: _____

    Multiple sexual partners: _____

    Hepatitis status and type (include LFTs): _____

    Country of origin (if not U.S. born): _____

formed in these circumstances at the initial visit and at 6 weeks, 3 months, and 6 months after exposure. Occasionally testing is extended to 12-month intervals in high-risk situations. Test results should be released to only one provider involved in management of the incident (or to a designated provider in her absence).

Testing of both the patient and the health care worker in our institution is sent out using a coded name and a nonidentifiable medical record number that has been established and accepted by all involved departments. All contact and documentation of information collected must be kept strictly confidential and is stored in a locked cabinet outside the medical record. Alternatively, some institutions have adopted a coded system that is still placed in the health care worker's chart with instructions that this information is not to be copied without the written permission of the patient and the attending physician. These measures can prevent confidentiality from being compromised for health care workers employed within the institution. Documentation in the formal medical record should list only the basic information about the nature of the injury (e.g., "needle-stick") and "possible exposure to infectious diseases."

A written protocol should accompany all bills to workers' compensation insurance carriers. It should detail the procedures followed in all percutaneous exposures to human blood products. Many hospitals and clinics cover the costs for prophylaxis with AZT from a private fund to keep claim experience ratings down.

Counseling is an important and often time-consuming component of all exposure evaluations. It is not uncommon to have an extremely distraught and confused individual or spouse involved in these incidents. Often the perception of risk of acquiring HIV infection with any percutaneous injury is extraordinarily high, even in relatively low-risk exposures.

Health care workers need to have lengthy and detailed information about the data related to these injuries. Time must be allocated to answer all questions and concerns expressed by the health care worker and his family. It is important to recognize the stress associated with the long waiting period for results of serial testing (if recommended), because empathy and compassion are crucial. Occasionally referral for further counseling is needed, and a knowledge of skilled therapists with this expertise is helpful. Sexual precautions, including the use of condoms, should be recommended when the source has identifiable risk factors for HIV. Because this directly affects the health care worker's sexual partner or spouse, counseling of that individual also is often required.

TUBERCULOSIS

Mycobacterium tuberculosis, the causative agent in pulmonary tuberculosis (TB), has seen a resurgence in recent years. Occupational infections have long been a hazard associated with medical care of individuals with active pulmonary infections. These infections are transmitted almost exclusively through airborne respired droplets.

A recent increase in TB has been attributed to infections from HIV-infected individuals. In these immunosuppressed patients, TB can progress to active infection and death in only a few months.

Concomitant with the increase in TB cases has been an increase in organisms resistant to both isoniazid (INH) and rifampin (RIF), to date the two most effective drugs used for TB infections. A more serious problem also has arisen with institutional outbreaks of multidrug-resistant tuberculosis (MDR-TB). These organisms are uniformly resistant to INH and RIF, and some are resistant to as many as seven antituberculin medications. Mortality from these infections frequently has exceeded 70%, with documented transmission to health care workers and prison employees. Active infections in these occupational groups also have been shown to occur, with deaths reported in several workers, most with existing HIV infections.[12]

The cause of these new, resistant organisms is believed to be poor compliance with antituberculin therapy and an increase in the number of patients with active disease in close quarters, a situation frequently found in institutional facilities such as hospitals and prisons. These places also have a greater number of HIV-infected individuals.

The management of MDR-TB–exposed occupational groups is especially difficult, given the limited alternative drugs, which generally are expensive and more toxic than the standard antituberculin drugs. Because of this, greater efforts have been directed toward preventing disease transmission through infection control procedures, early identification of resistant organisms, and active surveillance of medical and prison staff.

Infection control procedures include respiratory protection, especially for high-risk procedures such as aerosolized administration of pentamidine and sputum induction. The proper choice of respirator should be established for all procedures in advance and made part of the protocols for that department (see Chapter 34, Personal Protective Equipment). Improved ventilation in these areas, with rapid air exchange, and use of high-efficiency particulate air (HEPA) filters with external exhaust outlets also have been recommended. Respiratory isolation procedures have been established, with the use of surgical masks for those with suspected or confirmed TB and more stringent methods for confirming compliance with medical regimens to avert the development of MDR-TB.

Surveillance of occupational groups exposed to TB should include ongoing monitoring of tuberculin skin test conversions. Generally, those with prolonged, regular contact with patients with suspected or confirmed cases of active TB should undergo purified protein derivative (PPD) testing every 6 months, and all other health care workers should have yearly tests. The Mantoux technique should be used (intracutaneous injections of 0.1 ml of PPD-tuberculin containing 5 tuberculin units), because it is the preferred screening test. A two-step procedure for new health care workers has been advocated to reduce misinterpretation of a boosted reaction as opposed to a true conversion caused by recent infection. This involves repeating the Mantoux test at least 1 week (and no later than 3 weeks) after an initial test when the result is 0 to 9 mm of induration. A reaction larger than 10 mm of induration is considered positive. It is imperative that trained professional staff interpret these tests for induration (not erythema) 48 to 72 hours after application. Skin tests should not be placed on those with previous positive test results.

Testing should be done on individuals who have received bacille Calmette-Guérin (BCG) vaccination but who have not had tuberculin skin testing, because the protective effect of the vaccine is highly controversial. BCG can induce tuberculin sensitivity, although this is thought to be less reactive than naturally acquired infection. A large skin reaction that occurs many years after BCG vaccination therefore should be interpreted and treated as a positive reaction.

Health care workers exposed to a patient infected with active pulmonary TB should be adequately protected in advance with proper respiratory equipment. If inadvertent exposure occurs, baseline Mantoux testing, followed by repeat testing at 10 weeks, should be done to document recent conversion. All health care workers with recent conversions need chest x-ray films to exclude active pulmonary disease, along with medical evaluation for appropriate treatment. Repeat chest x-ray films have not been found necessary when following these individuals unless they have symptoms that suggest pulmonary TB.

The emergence of MDR-TB has dramatically changed the picture of tuberculosis as a benign infectious disease. New efforts to contain, prevent, and eradicate this organism must be taken, along with a concerted drive to identify new safe and effective drugs.

ANIMAL BITES

Bite injuries from animals are relatively common problems in both occupational and nonoccupational settings. Although dog bites account for 60% to 90% of these injuries, other animal bites require special consideration, especially when secondary infection develops.

Human bites following altercations for law enforcement and for child-care workers require consideration for potential HIV transmission, although no transmission from this route has been documented to date. HIV transmission would not be likely, given the extremely low titer of HIV in nonbloody saliva, but human bites can transmit diseases such as hepatitis B, tuberculosis, syphilis, and actinomycosis.

The initial approach to a bite injury should focus on any associated fracture or internal injury. Wounds near the metacarpophalangeal joint (in closed fist injuries) or involving deep penetration or crushing injury should be evaluated with x-ray films for fractures, foreign bodies, or air in the joint, or as a baseline for possible osteomyelitis. Wounds should also be washed out with soap and water (preferably before medical evaluation), as this can effectively remove debris and bacteria and significantly reduce the risk for diseases such as rabies.

The patient's tetanus status should also be evaluated, although tetanus is not a common complication of animal bites. It is always important to check for primary immunization in individuals born in other countries (who need both primary immunization and tetanus immune globulin) and to provide tetanus booster immunization to individuals who have not received tetanus-diptheria toxoid within the last 5 years.

Animal bite injuries must be carefully assessed and treated to prevent subsequent complications. Puncture wounds can appear superficial but can extend deeply. Copious high-pressure irrigation with sterile saline using a blunt needle and 20 ml syringe can effectively remove debris and bacteria. If a needle is used (18 to 19 gauge), the clinician must take care not to infiltrate the tissue. Most physicians do not close the wounds to prevent infection unless the wound involves the head or neck, where scarring is a factor and infection is less likely because of these areas' high vascularity. In other areas of the body, loose approximation of large wounds can be considered as long as wound drainage is not impeded.

Rabies is a common consideration when animal bites are evaluated. Despite frequent use of postexposure rabies vaccination in this country, an average of only one case of rabies occurs each year, with most of these cases imported from other countries. The animals that most commonly carry rabies in this country are skunks, foxes, raccoons, and bats. Domestic animals that have been vaccinated and can be observed for 10 days can be assumed to be nonrabid unless the animal becomes ill or acts erratically during this time. If this occurs, the animal should be killed and the brain analyzed by fluorescent antibody staining for the rabies virus. Wild or domestic rodents and rabbits are rarely infected with rabies and have not been found to cause rabies in this country.

It often is useful to discuss these incidents with local public health officials to assess the likelihood of rabies transmission. Noting whether the bite was provoked, the animal captured or contained, and the animal's rabies vaccination status are among the issues that must be addressed to make this determination.

Wound infection is another important consideration in the management of these injuries. *Pasteurella multocida* often is present in the oral secretions of cats and is also common in dogs. Infections from this gram-negative, aerobic bacteria develop rapidly, usually in less than 24 hours. Other common pathogens in animal bites include *Capnocytophaga canimorsus,* a microaerophilic gram-negative rod, along with *Staphylococcus aureus,* Enterobacteriaceae, and *Pseudomonas* species. Infections often are mixed and include anaerobic bacteria as well.

The issue of prophylactic antibiotic coverage of these wounds is highly controversial. We generally provide antibiotic coverage for wounds to the hand (particularly to the palmar regions), because these are more serious and potentially disastrous, and to cat bites, because these are more often infected. Plain penicillin is not effective, because significant resistance has been demonstrated in most animal bites. Dicloxicillin, although effective against staphylococci, gram-positive, and some anaerobic bacteria, is only partly effective against *P. multocida.* Amoxicillin-clavulanate (Augmentin) is a reasonable choice, because it covers most of the common oral flora except *Pseudomonas* species. The major drawback is the significant cost of the antibiotic, although this can and must be weighed against the costs of lost work time. A reported side effect with amoxicillin-clavulanic acid is diarrhea, which occurs in approximately 10% of patients. This may be minimized by instructing the patient to take the medication with food, because clavulanate stimulates bowel peristalsis. Alternative antibiotics include cephalosporins, such as cefuroxime, although these are also relatively expensive. Erythromycin can be used in individuals allergic to penicillin, but these cases should be

closely monitored due to some *Pasteurella* resistance.

Hand injuries warrant special consideration, because complications from introduction of bacteria into the tendon sheath can rapidly lead to devastating infections. These wounds should be managed by hand specialists at the early stages of treatment because of their complexity.

It is always important to carefully evaluate those patients with underlying conditions such as prosthetic valves or joints or any type of immunosuppression, including diabetes, alcoholism, asplenia, corticosteroid use, organ transplantation, or use of cytotoxic drugs, because these all increase the chances for significant wound infection. In cases where systemic illness with fever, lymphangitis, and lymphadenopathy are present, parenteral antibiotics and hospitalization should be considered.

Rodent bites seldom become infected, although rat-bite fever, caused by *Streptobacillus moniliformis,* occasionally can develop. Symptoms include fever, chills, headache, vomiting, and severe migratory arthralgia. This is followed by a maculopapular morbilliform rash over the palms, soles, and extremities. The diagnosis is confirmed by culture of the wound or by the presence of specific agglutinins in the serum.

CASE STUDY

A 37-year-old postal worker seeks treatment after he is bitten by a dog in the palmar aspect of the left hand. The dog is well known to the patient, because it has bitten several other postal employees in the past. The postal worker was seen by another physician immediately after the bite incident and was treated with local irrigation of the wound and sent home with a prescription for penicillin VK, which he has been taking. He reports that now, 14 hours later, the wound is tender and swollen, although he currently is afebrile. He had his last tetanus booster 2 years ago. The dog had been vaccinated for rabies and is under surveillance by the local animal control officer.

This injury to the palmar aspect of the hand is particularly worrisome, because infections in this region can lead to severe complications and occasionally permanent dysfunction. Evaluation and treatment by a surgeon trained to manage hand injuries should be contemplated at the initial presentation of the injury. Now that an early wound infection is present, such an evaluation should be expedited. The relatively rapid onset of symptoms in this case suggests that *P. multocida* is a likely etiology. Many clinicians think about this organism in the context of cat bites, but it is important to remember that *Pasteurella* infections are also frequently found in dog bite injuries. This is particularly true because the patient had been given penicillin VK, which is only partly effective against *Pasteurella* infections. Cultures obtained from the wound subsequently grew *P. multocida* resistant to penicillin and sensitive to ampicillin.

INTERNATIONAL TRAVEL

Because of the continued development of global markets for goods and services, international travel and relocation for occupational reasons have increased. This creates a need for medical recommendations for these travelers. Travel to most developed countries does not require special consideration beyond jet lag and motion sickness, but travel to developing countries, where food and water purity and parasitic, bacterial, or viral diseases are factors, requires knowledge of the diseases in those countries.

There usually are very few requirements for entry into developing countries; most regulations involve either cholera or yellow fever immunizations, although cholera currently is rarely required. However, many other preventive measures, including immunizations and medication, should be taken to guard against unnecessary illness or, occasionally, death.

Malaria continues to be a major cause of morbidity and mortality in the world, even though it is virtually absent in the United States. Appropriate antimalarial prophylaxis (see the section on Malaria), along with vaccines to prevent other diseases, should be part of routine medical practice in anticipation of potential exposure. Consideration must also be given to routine immunizations such as measles, polio, and tetanus, because such travel may impose special risks. Hepatitis B is another issue, because several areas of the world, including Asia, Southeast Asia, Africa, and parts of the Caribbean have significantly higher rates of infection among the general population.

Routine immunizations

Measles, mumps, and rubella.   Measles, mumps, and rubella (MMR) are considered as a group, because they are most often administered together during childhood in the United States. Outbreaks of measles have occurred in this country in recent years, in part because of importation of cases from countries where routine immunization is not provided. If primary immunization has been given (and attempts to document this should be made), booster doses of the vaccine should be given to travelers born in or after 1957 who have not received a second dose of the vaccine from age 5 or thereafter or who do not have physician-diagnosed measles or serologic evidence of measles immunity. Those born before 1957 are assumed to have naturally acquired immunity to measles. In addition, those who received MMR immunizations between 1963 and 1967 but cannot identify the type of vaccine administered should also be revaccinated, because some killed strains of vaccine that may not have conferred immunity, were used during that time.

Because MMR is a live attenuated vaccine, it should not be given to a pregnant woman, and women should avoid becoming pregnant for 3 months after receiving the vaccine. Many infectious disease experts recommend use of the trivalent MMR vaccine rather than the monovalent vaccines, because there is no significant additional risk with MMR. Immune globulin should be withheld for at least 2 weeks after MMR administration, because passive antibodies could interfere with the response to the vaccine.

Poliomyelitis.   The polio virus is found more commonly in developing countries with inadequate sanitation and incomplete immunization practices. Primary immunization for all travelers to these areas should be checked and completed before departure. A single booster dose is recommended for all travelers after age 18 who have completed primary immunization. If primary immunization was completed with live oral polio vaccine (OPV) and if the individual is not immunocompromised or is living with an immunocompromised individual, oral polio can be used. If injected polio vaccine was used or if the type of primary immunization is unknown, enhanced-potency, inactivated polio vaccine (eIPV) should be given to prevent the rare case of vaccine-associated paralysis, which is more common in adults.

Tetanus-diphtheria.   Tetanus and diphtheria are present both in the United States and abroad. Most individuals have received primary immunization during childhood. Booster doses are needed every 10 years and should be up-to-date before traveling abroad. In cases involving injuries with dirty or deep wounds that are tetanus-prone, booster doses should be given if more than 5 years have elapsed since the last tetanus immunization. An exception to the 10-year booster schedule can be considered for those traveling for extended periods, particularly to remote locations. To avoid vaccination in developing countries, where sterile conditions and vaccine quality may not be ensured, providing tetanus immunity that will be within 5 years of the last dose can be considered, because this eliminates the need for any additional doses of vaccine while traveling, regardless of the type of injury.

Required immunizations

Yellow fever and cholera are the only vaccinations occasionally required for entry into certain countries. Cholera immunization is rarely required and seldom needed, because this is a highly unusual disease in travelers. Updated requirements for travel are available through the CDC by phone (available 24 hours) by calling (404) 332-4559 or through the annual publication "Health Information for International Travel," available through the U.S. Government Printing Office. The biweekly "Summary of Health Information for International Travel" (or Blue Sheet), available through the CDC, lists countries that currently have areas infected with quarantinable diseases. The Blue Sheet can be obtained by writing to the Centers for Disease Control and Prevention, Center for Prevention Services, Division of Quarantine, Atlanta, Georgia 30333. Both publications should be reviewed to determine which vaccinations will be required.

It is important to reiterate that many useful vaccinations and medications are not required for entry into a foreign country, but they should be recommended to prevent debilitating or fatal diseases (see the section on Optional Vaccinations).

Yellow fever. Yellow fever is a viral disease transmitted by mosquitos that occurs in parts of tropical Africa, South America, and Panama. Immunization can be required for entry into countries in these regions or for entry into other countries (even if only in transit) if the traveler is coming from yellow fever–endemic areas. Yellow fever vaccination should *never* be given to children under 4 months of age, and preferably should be deferred to 9 months of age to avoid adverse reactions. Because this is a live attenuated vaccine, it has a relative contraindication for pregnant women and immunosuppressed individuals. However, if the risk of exposure to yellow fever is high, vaccination should be considered. Booster doses of the vaccine are needed every 10 years.

Cholera. The World Health Organization (WHO) and the CDC do not consider the current cholera vaccine necessary for international travel. Cholera vaccination should be contemplated only when it is required for entry into a country, or when a second country requires it for entry when the traveler is coming from an area where cholera is present. Vaccination probably is needed only for individuals lacking gastric acid (e.g., those taking H_2 antagonists or antacids), because this natural host defense protects against many ingested pathogens.

Cholera is a self-limited disease transmitted through fecally contaminated water or food. Because it is caused by an enterotoxin that stimulates adenylate cyclase in intestinal cells, it is not a true dysentery. Oral rehydration has been effective for established infections, along with oral tetracycline.

The recent outbreak of cholera in South America has been associated with raw seafood caught in contaminated waters.

The current vaccine is only about 50% effective and requires booster doses every 6 months following the two-dose initial series (spaced 1 to 4 weeks apart). Protection from this illness is best accomplished through food and water precautions, which also protect against other forms of travelers' diarrhea. A new live attenuated vaccine has been developed and appears promising as a more effective means of protection. However, the new vaccine probably will not be available for several years.

Optional vaccinations

Typhoid. Typhoid fever is caused by *Salmonella typhi,* which is acquired through contaminated food or water. It is found in many countries of Africa, Asia, and Central and South America. Vaccination with either the older parenteral, inactivated vaccine or the newer live attenuated oral vaccine appears to be effective in about 70% to 90% of cases. The oral vaccine is administered on alternate days for four doses, whereas the parenteral vaccine is given in two doses 4 weeks apart or three doses 1 week apart. The reduced side effects seen with the oral vaccine make it the preferred choice, although there are relative contraindications for pregnant women and immunosuppressed individuals, because it is a live bacterial vaccine. Booster doses are required every 5 years with the oral vaccine and every 3 years with the parenteral vaccine.

Meningococcal diseases. Meningococcal meningitis and bacteremia, which are caused by *Neisseria meningitidis,* occur sporadically or in epidemics in various parts of the world, including the United States. Work-related exposure often involves coworkers who are either diagnosed with undefined viral meningitis or with meningococcal meningitis. In cases where household or intimate exposure does not occur, such as in most office situations, prophylaxis with rifampin is not indicated. Although the risk to most travelers is extremely low, vaccination with the inactivated bacterial vaccine is required for pilgrims to Mecca and Saudi Arabia for the annual Haj. This disease also occurs frequently in subSaharan Africa during the dry season (December to June), and vaccination is recommended for travelers who have extensive contact with the local population during these periods. Booster doses are recommended every 3 years.

Rabies. Rabies is a viral disease transmitted by carnivorous animals and bats. It is uncommon in the United States, with an average of one case per year. The usual vectors in this country are raccoons, skunks, foxes, and bats. Dogs are still the most commonly infected animal in other parts of the world. In countries such as India, as many as 25,000 people die each year of rabies.[15] Because rabies is a uniformly fatal disorder, vaccination is critical to the management of potential exposure. Although this is clearly overtreated in this country, the higher incidence of disease in many developing countries makes it a consideration for certain travelers.

Preexposure vaccination can be considered for young children, field workers, animal handlers, spelunkers (cave explorers), people on treks or extended hikes in endemic countries, and people living in high-risk countries (e.g., parts of Central and South America, the Indian subcontinent, Southeast Asia, and the Philippines) for longer than 30 days. Preexposure vaccination with human diploid cell rabies vaccine (HDCV) is administered in the deltoid region or intradermally (using one-tenth the intramuscular dose) on days 0, 7, 21, or 28. The low-dose intradermal route should not be used if chloroquine (for antimalarial prophylaxis) will be taken within 3 to 4 weeks of the third dose of the vaccine, because the immune response is diminished.

Preexposure vaccination serves several functions. For a traveler in remote areas, it provides some protection (through preformed antibodies) against rabies when medical care is not available quickly. It also eliminates the need for rabies immune globulin (RIG), which is not readily available in many developing countries and which is derived from pooled human blood products (which may not be prepared with appropriate procedures and precautions against contamination). Finally, this simplifies the postexposure vaccination series to two additional doses (rather than the full five-dose series) given on days 0 and 3.

It is important to remember that appropriate wound care can play a significant role in reducing or eliminating the risk of rabies. Use of a local anesthetic (if available), followed by thorough cleansing of the bite area with benzalkonium chloride, soap, or povidone-iodine, may be the most important method of reducing the chance of acquiring rabies after a bite injury from a potentially rabid animal.

Japanese encephalitis. Japanese encephalitis (JE) is a mosquito-borne viral disease found in various regions of Asia and Southeast Asia during the summer and autumn months, and during the rainy season in various tropical regions of Southeast Asia, the Indian subcontinent, and the Philippines. The disease is asymptomatic in most individuals but can cause serious CNS infection and death. Although the overall risk to travelers is low, those living in endemic or epidemic rural areas for prolonged periods (arbitrarily set at longer than 4 weeks) should consider vaccination with the JE vaccine. The vaccine is given in three separate doses given on days 0, 7, and 30. It can be given over a shorter period on days 0, 7, and 14, although this may confer less immunity and is not generally recommended.

Hepatitis B. Hepatitis B (previously discussed in the section on bloodborne pathogens) is a significant disease in specific areas of the world. Parts of Asia, Southeast Asia, Africa, and the Caribbean have significantly higher rates of infection, with the prevalence of HBV carriers at roughly 5% to 20% of the general population. Moderate areas of infection include parts of Southern Asia, Israel, Japan, Eastern and Southern Europe, the Soviet republics, and parts of Central and South America. In contrast, the prevalence of HBV carriers in the general population of the United States is less than 1%. Besides health care workers, travelers who should receive hepatitis B vaccination include those living in endemic areas for longer than 6 months, those anticipating sexual or daily physical contact with the local population, and those likely to receive medical or dental care in endemic countries.

Hepatitis A. Because of its fecal-oral route of transmission, hepatitis A is an extremely common disease in developing nations with poor sanitary practices. Prevention is best accomplished by observing food and water precautions and through the administration of immune globulin. Travel for less than 2 to 3 months requires 2 ml of immune globulin intramuscularly (IM) (or 0.02 ml/kg), whereas longer travel requires a dose of 5 ml IM (or 0.06 ml/kg) repeated every 5 months. Immune globulin should be administered as close to departure as possible. Individuals with documented hepatitis A infections (which can be evaluated by measuring IgG antibodies to hepatitis A) do not need immune globulin.

An effective vaccine against hepatitis A has been introduced in other areas of the world and currently is awaiting approval by the Food and Drug Administration (FDA). Introduction of this vaccine may offer a more effective and longer-acting solution for all travelers.

Malaria. Malaria is a parasitic disease carried by the female *Anopheles* mosquito and caused by one of four species of *Plasmodium; P. vivax, P. ovale, P. malariae,* or *P. falciparum.* In recent years, infections caused by *P. falciparum,* the most serious of the four types of malaria, have become increasingly resistant to chloroquine, previously the recommended prophylactic drug for travelers going to malarious regions. Resistant strains of *P.*

falciparum have been found in most areas of South America, Africa, and Asia. Only certain regions of Central America and the Middle East have chloroquine-sensitive strains. Information on malaria recommendations for specific countries can be obtained by calling the CDC 24-hour malaria hotline at (404) 332-4555.

Mefloquine, which is a quinoline methanol drug, has proved effective against most forms of chloroquine-resistant malaria except in areas of Thailand and Indonesia. Like chloroquine, it can be used for malaria prophylaxis on a weekly dosing schedule beginning 1 to 2 weeks before entering malarious zones, weekly while in these regions, and for 4 weeks after leaving these areas. The usual dose of mefloquine for adults is 250 mg. Relative contraindications to mefloquine include known hypersensitivity to the drug, children under 15 kg (30 pounds), individuals taking beta blockers, those requiring fine motor skills (e.g., pilots), pregnant women, and those with seizure disorders or significant psychiatric disorders.

Alternatives to mefloquine include chloroquine (500 mg salt taken weekly) with three doses of Fansidar (pyrimethamine-sulfadoxine) to be taken for presumed chloroquine-resistant malaria if medical care is not available. Doxycycline can also be used as a single agent taken in daily doses of 100 mg beginning 1 to 2 days before travel, daily while in malarious regions, and for 4 weeks after leaving these regions.

It is important to recognize that the risk of malaria can be effectively reduced by avoiding outdoor activity during the evening hours (when the *Anopheles* mosquito bites), by wearing long-sleeved clothing and applying DEET-containing mosquito repellents during these times, and by using mosquito netting on beds. Permethrin can also be sprayed on clothing, and a pyrethrum-containing insect spray may be applied in living quarters as additional methods to repel mosquitos. Travelers should also be told to seek medical attention immediately for any unexplained febrile illness so that malaria can be ruled out.

Travelers' diarrhea. Travelers' diarrhea is caused by various agents, principally infectious pathogens. These include enterotoxigenic *Escherichia coli* (ETEC), *Shigella* species, *Campylobacter jejuni, Aeromonas* species, *Plesiomonas shigelloides, Salmonella* species, and noncholera *Vibrio* organisms.[3] Viral agents include Norwalk-like virus and rotavirus, whereas parasitic causes include *Giardia lamblia, Entamoeba histolytica,* and *Cryptosporidium* organisms. Prophylactic use of antibiotics is not recommended by most infectious disease specialists because of the increased risk of side effects and the generation of resistant

organisms. Bismuth subsalicylate, found in Pepto-Bismol, is 40% to 60% effective in preventing travelers' diarrhea for shorter trips (less than 3 weeks) when taken in a dosage of two tablets four times a day.

Recent studies have shown that use of an antibiotic with an antimotility agent can dramatically shorten the duration of symptoms. For travel to Mexico and Central America, trimethoprim-sulfa (Septra/Bactrim) with loperamide (Imodium) is an effective combination. In many parts of the developing world, resistance to trimethoprim-sulfa is becoming more common. In these situations, use of ciprofloxacin (Cipro) with loperamide has proved a reasonable alternative. Treatment with trimethoprim-sulfa is dosed at one double-strength tablet as a single dose for mild diarrhea, or the same dosage taken twice daily for 3 days for more severe illness. Ciprofloxacin recently has been found effective when given as a single 500 mg dose for diarrhea without blood or fever (temperature over 38.1° C [100.5° F]), although many treat the condition with a 3-day course of 500 mg twice a day. Treatment is usually recommended after the third loose stool, and loperamide can be used concomitantly. When bloody diarrhea or fever (or both) are present, treatment with 500 mg of ciprofloxacin twice daily for 3 days without loperamide is preferred. Symptoms that do not resolve must be evaluated in a medical clinic to rule out other causes of diarrhea.

Travelers must also be strongly encouraged to observe proper food and water precautions. These include avoiding tapwater and ice (choosing instead bottled water or water that has been properly treated by boiling or chemical disinfection). Improperly handled food should also be avoided, especially food from street vendors, who lack proper cleaning facilities and maintain food at warm, incubating temperatures. Travelers should also avoid poorly cooked meats or fruits or vegetables that have been washed or peeled; travelers should peel their own fruits or vegetables to avoid problems. Above all else, those with diarrheal illnesses should adhere strictly to proper rehydration (including the World Health Organization's oral rehydration formula), because dehydration is the most common severe complication in these situations. Individuals who traveled for a prolonged period should also consider stool samples for ova and parasite studies upon their return, for these often reveal pathogens in the absence of symptoms.

Returned travelers should also be evaluated by those familiar with tropical diseases if they develop medical problems either during or after foreign travel. Many treatable diseases have been missed by physicians who did not consider these infectious agents in their differential diagnoses.

In summary, many diseases can and should be prevented before traveling by a thorough review of the diseases present in the countries that will be entered. Although most host countries require few immunizations for entry, many diseases can be avoided by appropriate use of specific vaccines, proper instructions on disease prevention, and judicious use of medications before travel begins.

REFERENCES

1. Alper CA et al: Genetic prediction of nonresponse to hepatitis B vaccine, *N Engl J Med* 321:708-712, 1989.
2. Centers for Disease Control: Guidelines for prevention of transmission of human immunodeficiency virus and hepatitis B virus to health care and public safety workers, Atlanta, 1989, US Department of Health and Human Services.
3. DuPont HL, Ericsson CD: Prevention and treatment of travelers' diarrhea, *N Engl J Med* 328:1821-1827, 1993.
4. Handler SC et al: Long-term immunogenicity and efficacy of hepatitis B vaccine in homosexual men, *N Engl J Med* 315:209-214, 1986.
5. Henderson DK et al: The risk for occupational transmission of human immunodeficiency virus type 1 (HIV-1) associated with clinical exposures: a prospective evaluation, *Ann Intern Med* 113:740-746, 1990.
6. Kane MA, Lettau LA: Transmission of HBV from dental personnel to patients, *J Am Dent Assoc* 110:634-636, 1985.
7. Kiyosawa K et al: Hepatitis C in hospital employees with needle-stick injuries, *Ann Intern Med* 115:367-369, 1991.
8. Lange JMA et al: Failure of zidovudine prophylaxis after accidental exposure to HIV-1, *N Engl J Med* 322:1375-1377, 1990.
9. Lettau LA et al: Transmission of hepatitis B virus with resultant restriction of surgical practice, *JAMA* 255:934-937, 1986.
10. Mast S, Gerberding JL: Factors predicting infectivity following needle-stick exposure to HIV: an in vitro model, *Clin Res* 58A:39, 1991.
11. McCune JM et al: Suppression of HIV infection in AZT-treated SCID$_{hu}$ mice, *Science* 247:564-566, 1990.
12. Multidrug-resistant tuberculosis, *MMWR* 41:5-71, 1992.
13. Preliminary analysis: HIV serosurvey of orthopedic surgeons, *MMWR* 40:309-312, 1991.
14. Protection against viral hepatitis: recommendations of the Immunization Practices Committee (ACIP), *MMWR* 39:5-23, 1990.
15. Steele J: Rabies in the Americas and remarks on global aspects, *Infect Dis* 10:S535, 1988.
16. Taylor PE, Stevens CE: Persistence of antibody to hepatitis B surface antigen after vaccination with hepatitis B vaccine, *J Med Virol* 21:90A, 1987 (abstract).

25 Chemical Exposures

Evaluation of a chemically exposed patient is one of the most challenging areas of occupational medicine. The types of chemical exposures possible in industry are unlimited. Processes normally safe for workers can go awry in many ways, causing unusual releases or allowing uncontrolled reactions to form novel chemical exposures. Nevertheless, primary care physicians see most of these cases and have to manage them. The goal of this chapter is to outline an approach that enables practitioners to avoid some of the pitfalls of evaluating chemical exposure.

PREPARATION

Most practitioners are unaccustomed to evaluating chemical exposures. The best way to avoid being caught by surprise is to give some advance thought to the types of industries in the community and the support services for that industry. For example, an oil refinery supports hundreds of its own employees, as well as environmental consultants, hazardous waste haulers, machinists, and so forth. Information on local industries can be obtained from the local Chamber of Commerce or simply by looking out the window and identifying the plants within view. Some industries are invisible because of their small unit size (e.g., restaurants in the tourist industry) or because we do not traditionally identify them as an industry (municipal services such as the police, fire, and public works departments).

The clinician should take advantage of everyday patient encounters to educate herself on local occupations. She should ask her patients what type of work they do. If there is time, she should find out whether their jobs involve any hazards and the names of their employers. Workers often deny that they face any daily job hazards, but they are quick to recount the exposures or accidents of other workers. Another clue to the presence of chemical hazards is whether the employer requires periodic physical examinations for the work or respirators for protection; these usually are signs that regulated hazardous chemicals are present in the workplace.

After informing herself about the primary hazards of local occupations, the clinician can start gathering meaningful data about the magnitude and route of hazardous exposures. Common routes of exposure are inhalation, skin absorption, and ingestion. The amount of inhaled chemicals is affected by the respiratory rate during work and the airborne concentration of the chemical. Air concentration levels usually are measured by industrial hygienists (e.g., measuring benzene levels in parts per million). These measurements are compared with government standards (federal or state occupational safety and health agencies) or privately developed standards (e.g., those of the American Conference of Governmental Industrial Hygienists). The chemical form is important in determining how easily a chemical may become airborne. Processes involving phase transformations (such as liquid evaporation) should receive particular attention because they can generate high levels of exposure.

Obtaining an exposure history

The goal of an exposure history is to survey the spectrum of an individual's chemical exposures and obtain qualitative or quantitative information on the identity, form, concentration, and duration of chemical exposure.

The identity and form may be available from a Material Safety Data Sheet (MSDS). The MSDS is usually two to three pages long and contains standardized information about the chemicals contained in a product, along with a brief description of the toxic effects of the chemicals. According to federal law, MSDS sheets must be kept at the workplace, accessible to workers. There is usually a telephone number on the sheet that can be used to gather additional information. Some poison control centers can also help with information about the constituents and toxicities of brand-name chemical products.

Estimating the concentration of airborne chemicals is difficult from a patient history alone. Descriptions of odor concentration are unreliable, because people vary greatly in their ability to detect and identify odors. In addition, some patients with chronic exposure develop olfactory fatigue, which impairs their ability to smell. Sometimes suspended dusts or mists create visible clouds whose density can be described. How the chemical is used gives important clues. Generally, heating, spraying, or coating processes increase the potential for exposure. An estimate of the amount of chemical used often is helpful. The clinician should ask about controls used to reduce exposure, such as local exhaust ventilation, general workplace ventilation, use of barriers (e.g., glove boxes), and personal protective equipment. This equipment includes gloves, respirators, safety glasses, aprons, and so on. The physician should talk to the plant industrial hygienist or safety officer, if there is one (see the chapters on Personal Protective Equipment and on Safety).

Once the clinician has a feel for the chemicals present in the workplace, priority should be given to chemicals present in the greatest quantities, those undergoing phase transformations, those with the highest reactivities (acids, caustics, and some catalysts), and those capable of causing allergic sensitization.

Anatomy of a chemical exposure

To produce toxic effects, chemicals must get onto or into the body. The organs of primary interest are the lungs, the gastrointestinal tract, and the skin.

Respiratory exposure is of obvious concern for airborne chemicals. The amount of chemical inhaled varies with the respiratory rate and depth of breathing. Some chemicals, such as chlorine gas, are so irritating that workers stop breathing before pulmonary absorption occurs. For acute or accidental exposure, measurements of airborne concentrations probably will not be available. Daily exposure in an industrial process may have been measured by an industrial hygienist. For some chemicals, it is possible to predict the clinical effects by knowing the airborne concentration.

Ingestion and gastrointestinal absorption is a surprisingly common route of chemical exposure. Most airborne particles are captured in the respiratory tract mucus and eventually swallowed. In addition, workers often eat, drink, and smoke in their workplaces, providing additional opportunity for ingestion. This type of exposure is virtually impossible to quantify. Lead poisoning is often caused by inadvertent ingestion of lead dust.

Skin contact with chemicals can cause local effects, transdermal absorption with systemic effects, or ingestion from fingers during eating or smoking in the workplace. Most workers have a good idea if skin contact occurs. For most toxic chemicals, immediate skin decontamination by flushing the skin with copious amounts of water is the primary treatment. Hydrofluoric acid is a special case, calling for unique topical treatments and injection of calcium gluconate, or both. Transder-

mal absorption has been of theoretical interest in the past, but the increasing use of glycol ethers and dimethylsulfoxide indicates a trend toward the use of skin-soluble chemicals capable of causing systemic effects.

Clinical examination

Unlike localized physical injuries, chemical exposures often cause systemic reactions. For this reason, it is important to assess the chemically exposed worker on an overall basis. An excellent reference for primary clinicians is *Proctor and Hughes' Chemical Hazards of the Workplace.*[6]

Vital signs should be measured carefully. Even body temperature can be affected by some chemical exposures (e.g., pentachlorophenol, which is used in wood preservation). Many chemical exposures are unusually frightening events and occur under exciting circumstances. Pulse and blood pressure are expected to be slightly elevated the day of the chemical exposure. One pattern that needs to be watched for is a rapid heart rate in a calm worker. This may represent pesticide exposure to a cholinesterase-inhibiting compound. Treatment of vital sign abnormalities is generally supportive, except for organophosphate pesticides, which have specific antidotes.

A critical physical assessment in a chemically exposed worker is assessing signs of eye, nose, and throat irritation. Most chemical exposures are irritating to some degree, and the presence of conjunctivitis, pharyngitis, laryngitis, and cough are significant. First, they can help indicate the severity of exposure during triage. Second, these findings help establish that chemical exposure actually occurred, rather than that the patient simply was in the vicinity of a chemical release. However, one should expect variations in individual response among similarly exposed workers because of the interindividual variation in sensitivity (see Chapter 18 on Respiratory Injuries).

Cardiac examination can reveal tachycardia and even angina from anxiety. Some chemicals, such as fluorocarbons, have been reported to increase cardiac irritability, leading to dysrhythmias.[2,16] Chemical asphyxiants inhibit oxygen utilization in the cardiac muscle and, especially with coronary artery disease, can lead to angina or even myocardial infarction.[13]

Pulmonary examination can be misleading because some chemical exposures cause pulmonary damage in a delayed fashion. Oxides of nitrogen produce pulmonary edema 12 to 24 hours after exposure. If these exposures are suspected, it may be necessary to observe the patient in the hospital overnight.[11] Wheezing and other signs of asthma that begin during working hours may be work related. Clinicians should be aware that chemical allergens found in some workplaces may precipitate severe asthma in a previously asymptomatic person[7] (see Chapter 18, Respiratory Injuries).

Abdominal examination generally is unimportant in a chemically exposed worker, other than to rule out other underlying illness. It is rare these days for lead-exposed workers to develop the abdominal cramping called "lead colic," but it does still occur, particularly in foreign-born employees working in lead battery or radiator operations.[8]

Neurologic examination of acutely exposed workers is difficult. They generally are excited and show signs of anxiety unrelated to the chemical itself. Most often there is no baseline available to assess whether a worker has impaired reflexes, cognition, or peripheral nervous function. General obtundation is obviously a serious finding and should prompt questioning of coworkers about possible exposure to an asphyxiant or central nervous system (CNS) neurotoxin (many solvents have anesthetic effects at high doses). Similarly, hyperexcitability may be related to cholinesterase inhibition from organophosphate pesticides. Chronically exposed workers often show more subtle symptoms, such as a headache that occurs only during the workweek and worsens until the weekend offers some relief. Chronic limb numbness and tingling are characteristic of some neurotoxins, such as arsenic poisoning.[1]

Skin examination shows acute chemical irritant effects easily. However, a chronic dermatitis caused by an allergy to a specific workplace chemical can be very difficult to diagnose, requiring sophisticated selection of chemicals for patch testing. A dermatologist with an interest in occupational dermatitis often is needed to identify the offending agent. The skin can also show manifestations of systemic toxicity, including cyanosis from oxygen deprivation or the "cherry red" hyperoxygenation caused by carbon monoxide poisoning.[10]

HAZARDS OF CHEMICAL EXPOSURE

The following conditions represent a spectrum of chemical hazards in terms of time to onset of symptoms, mechanism of injury, and severity of effect.

Asphyxiation

Conditions allowing for an oxygen-deprived atmosphere are relatively common in industry. Often these injuries are doubly devastating because not only is the initial victim killed, but the would-be rescuer entering the atmosphere often is a second victim. Oxygen-deprived atmospheres can be generated by oxygen consumption in an enclosed space or by displacement of oxygen by another gas. Lack of oxygen has no warning properties, and usually a worker falls unconscious without warning.

Most industries have confined-space entry procedures calling for a standby person outside the confined space with equipment to rescue an overcome worker out of the confined space. Brain damage from anoxia can begin within 5 minutes. Rescues rarely go smoothly, and delays often are encountered.[15]

Chemical asphyxiants interfere with oxygen delivery to tissues, causing toxic effects even with adequate amounts of atmospheric oxygen. Carbon monoxide binds to hemoglobin 200 times more avidly than oxygen, reducing the amount of hemoglobin available for oxygen transport. Carbon monoxide also shifts the oxygen dissociation curve, causing less oxygen to be released from hemoglobin to the tissues. Carbon monoxide poisoning usually results from combustion in an enclosed space. The enclosed space can be as large as a warehouse: sufficient rates of combustion generate toxic levels of carbon monoxide in even large spaces.[5]

Hydrogen sulfide and cyanide gas are both cellular toxins that bind to the oxidative enzymes in cellular mitochondria. This causes cells to lose their ability to oxidize metabolites and forces them into anaerobic metabolism. Carbon monoxide, hydrogen sulfide, hydrogen cyanide, and oxygen-deficient atmospheres can cause tissue damage. The organs that use the most oxygen are most susceptible to injury. Myocardial and CNS damage usually are most evident.[3]

Heavy metal poisoning

Heavy metal poisoning is unique in many respects. First, heavy metals are excreted slowly from the human body and, with daily exposure, gradually rises to higher and higher levels if intake exceeds excretion. Second, some heavy metals are often deposited in skeletal bone, causing extremely long excretion half lives. Third, the symptoms caused by heavy metal poisoning often can be correlated to blood levels and/or urine of heavy metals, allowing an unusually integrated assessment of history, symptoms, and laboratory findings.

The most common heavy metal encountered is lead, which is used in automobile batteries and lead-based paint. Most paints currently in use contain no lead; however, sandblasting of old outdoor painted surfaces often generates significant amounts of lead dust. Lead is also found in connections of automobile radiators, resulting in exposure during radiator repair. Contrary to popular perception, the use of lead-based solder in the electronics industry does not often result in lead poisoning.

Lead accumulates in the body following even low-level exposure. The most common routes of exposure to lead are inhalation of lead dust or fume and ingestion. Ingestion occurs inadvertently when beverages or food are consumed in a lead-contaminated workplace. Preventive measures include shower and changing facilities for lead workers to prevent cross-contamination of eating areas. As little as 1 mg of lead consumed per day can result in a gradually increasing blood level in adults. Children are even more susceptible to the neurotoxic effects of lead.[8]

Lead poisoning has a specific treatment. Chelating agents (such as EDTA) can bind to lead in the peripheral bloodstream and hasten its excretion. However, these agents are not effective in cleaning lead from skeletal bone. The side effects of EDTA treatment reserve it for symptomatic individuals. EDTA should never be used during ongoing lead exposure.[14]

Organophosphate pesticide poisoning

The agricultural industry applies tons of pesticides, usually by spraying. Most pesticides are purchased in concentrated solutions, which are diluted by a trained technician before spraying. Spraying may be done by airplane, and large numbers of workers can be accidentally exposed in a short period. In addition, exposure often occurs when workers are sent into a recently sprayed field. Evaluation of pesticide exposure follows the steps described previously. The exposure history should assess the route of exposure and whether skin contact occurred. Most pesticides and their solvents have chemical odors, which are somewhat helpful in determining the extent and duration of exposure.

Physical examination of organophosphate exposures should look for the tachycardia, agitation, blurred vision, nausea, and muscle twitching of cholinergic stimulation. Laboratory evaluation of plasma and red blood cell cholinesterase activity gives an indication of recent and distant exposure effects. Lack of baseline levels impairs interpretation of an individual's results because of significant population variation in cholinesterase activity.[4]

Hydrocarbon solvent exposure

Hydrocarbon vapor exposure is common because of the widespread use of hydrocarbon solvents as cleaning agents and paint solvents. It is difficult to generalize about the effects of hydrocarbon exposure because of their variety, but common symp-

toms include headache, dizziness, nausea, and an intoxicated feeling with higher levels of exposures.[12]

The exposure history should include some details about the process using the hydrocarbons, such as whether the solvents are spread onto a surface, heated, or sprayed. Ventilation is of paramount importance, with confined spaces representing the most likely situation causing an overexposure.

Physical assessment should include looking for signs of irritation. Neurologic evaluation is important to check for signs of solvent intoxication, such as dizziness, tremors, or ataxia. Other causes of intoxication should also be considered. Laboratory evaluation usually is disappointing because levels of exposure sufficient to cause symptoms do not usually cause abnormal liver function tests. Solvent-specific biologic monitoring is possible for some chemicals, but it is often impractical because of its specialized nature.[9]

CASE STUDIES

Chemical injuries are not common. The most common day-to-day exposures involve the use of solutions for cleaning or coating surfaces. The most direct contact is skin contact. However, as outlined below, industrial processes create some unique situations that result in chemical exposure.

Case 1

An assembler at a surgical device manufacturer complains of episodic dizziness every 1 to 3 months. She works in a large room with 20 other employees assembling small hollow probes. The final step in assembly is flushing the channels with a fluorocarbon solvent. The flushed solvent is sprayed beneath the table onto the floor. No specific ventilation or protective equipment is provided for this purpose. No industrial hygiene data are available. At the time of physical examination, no dysrhythmia is present, orthostatic blood pressure changes are absent, and no other cause of dizziness is identified.

Overexposure to fluorocarbon solvents could be occurring, possibly causing dizziness directly from the CNS effects of the solvent, or possibly from cardiac dysrhythmias generated by fluorocarbon exposure.[2] Other medical causes should be considered. Holter monitoring to detect cardiac dysrhythmias may be helpful. Industrial hygiene evaluation of the exposure (including better chemical identification) must be performed to determine whether the occupational exposure is toxicologically significant. If a link to the workplace is established, treatment would include temporary restriction from the area until appropriate exhaust ventilation is installed.

Case 2

An older wood shop supervisor has complained of progressive dyspnea for the past 6 months. The dyspnea occurred in the late evenings and early mornings. His work involved extensive use of particleboard and thermoplastic glues for veneer lamination. The worker was loaned a Wright peak flow meter to measure his peak expiratory flow rate throughout the workday and evening. His graph showed significant reductions in flow rate in the evenings after work, which correlated with his subjective complaints.

Despite his lifelong history of work with wood, this patient developed new occupational asthma to one of the woods or chemicals used in his shop. He attempted to work wearing a respirator but was unable to do so. An intercurrent illness caused him to leave the workplace, and further studies were not possible.

DIAGNOSTIC PEARLS

- Workers unaccustomed to chemical exposure are more difficult to evaluate and treat than experienced chemical workers. In my experience, some of the worst levels of anxiety are encountered in office workers and schoolteachers who are exposed to chemicals.
- Unfamiliar exposure upsets even sophisticated chemical workers. I have seen refinery workers upset by sewage spills and sewer workers upset by chemical spills, each unconcerned with the exposures they face daily.
- Chemical odor has only limited value as a guide for assessing possible chemical exposure. Interindividual variation in odor detection capability is great in the general population.

REFERENCES

1. Allen N: Chemical neurotoxins in industry and environment. In Tower DB, editor: *The nervous system,* vol 2. The clinical neurosciences, New York, 1975, Raven Press.
2. Antti-Poika M, Heikkila J, Saarinen L: Cardiac arrhythmias during occupational exposure to fluorinated hydrocarbons, *Br J Ind Med* 47:138-140, 1990.
3. Becker CE: Gases. In *Occupational medicine.* LaDou J, editor: East Norwalk, Conn, 1990, Appleton & Lange.
4. California Department of Health Services: Medical supervision of pesticide workers: guidelines for physicians — 1988, Sacramento, Calif, 1988, The Department.
5. Fawcett TA et al: Warehouse workers' headache: carbon monoxide poisoning from propane-fueled forklifts, *J Occup Med* 34:12-15, 1992.
6. Hathaway GJ et al: *Proctor and Hughes' chemical hazards of the workplace,* New York, 1991, Van Nostrand Reinhold.
7. Lam S, Chan-Yeung M: Occupational asthma: natural history, evaluation, and management. In *State of the Art Reviews,* Occupational Medicine, Volume 2, Number 2, Philadelphia, 1987, Hanley & Belfus. 1987.
8. Landrigan PJ: Occupational and community exposures to toxic metals: lead, cadmium, mercury, and arsenic, *West J Med* 137:531-539, 1982.
9. Lauwerys RR, Hoet P: *Industrial chemical exposure: guidelines for biological monitoring,* ed 2, Boca Raton, Fla, 1993, Lewis.
10. Mathias CGT, Maibach HI: Perspectives in occupational dermatology, *West J Med* 137:486-492, 1982.
11. National Institute for Occupational Safety and Health: Criteria for a recommended standard: occupational exposure to oxides of nitrogen (nitrogen dioxide and nitric oxide), US Department of Health, Education, and Welfare, HEW (NIOSH) 76-149, Washington, DC, 1975, The Department.
12. National Institute for Occupational Safety and Health: Criteria for a recommended standard: occupational exposure to alkanes (C5-C8), US Department of Health, Education, and Welfare, (NIOSH) 76-151, Washington, DC, 1977, The Department.
13. Radford EP: Carbon monoxide and human health, *J Occup Med* 18:310, 1976.
14. Rempel D: The lead-exposed worker, *JAMA* 262:532-534, 1989.
15. Sahli BO, Armstrong CW: Confined-space fatalities in Virginia, *J Occup Med* 34:910-917, 1992.
16. Speizer FE, Wegman DH, Ramirez A: Palpitation rates associated with fluorocarbon exposure in a hospital setting, *N Engl J Med* 292:624-626, 1975.

26 Temperature-related Disorders

This chapter discusses disorders associated with exposure to extreme temperatures. The heat-related illnesses covered include skin disorders, heat edema, heat syncope, heat cramps, heat exhaustion, and heat stroke. Cold-related conditions includes chilblains (perniosis), trench foot and immersion foot, frostbite, and hypothermia. The physiology of temperature regulation is reviewed, and the pathophysiology, predisposing factors, clinical presentation, and treatment are discussed for each injury.

PHYSIOLOGY OF TEMPERATURE REGULATION

The human body maintains its temperature by means of a complex, multisystem mechanism. The generally accepted normal temperature of 98.6° F does not always obtain; rather, "normal" can range from below 97° F to above 99.5° F.[30] Rectal temperatures generally are 1° F higher than oral temperatures and can rise as high as 107.6° F during stenuous exercise or fall below 97° F with exposure to cold.[28,30]

The body should be thought of as two compartments, the shell and the core. The shell is the outer layer of skin, which acts as either a radiator or an insulator. Muscular arteriovenous anastomoses in the subcutaneous tissue control the blood flow to the skin, maintaining a stable temperature for the underlying core tissue. The shell temperature rises and falls with the surrounding temperature, but the core temperature, in the absence of disease, remains remarkably stable, varying by no more than 1° F.[27]

Several sites may be used to measure the core temperature. The esophageal temperature provides an indirect measurement of the temperature of the blood leaving the heart and therefore probably most accurately reflects the true core temperature. However, measurements from the mouth, rectum, and auditory canal are most accessible and most commonly used. They have been shown to vary in

an individual, and the difference between each site and the esophageal temperature has been described by a mathematical model.[21] Although each site has its drawbacks in different clinical situations, measurements carefully taken from any of the previously mentioned sites can be used to assess a patient's status. The advantages and disadvantages of each site are shown in Table 26-1.

A balance must constantly be maintained between heat production and heat loss. The physiology of temperature regulation is outlined in Fig. 26-1. Temperature receptors are found primarily in the skin, but also in the spinal cord and abdominal viscera, and in or around the great veins. Although the body has both cold and warmth receptors, cold receptors far outnumber warmth receptors, by up to 10 times as many in parts of the skin.[30] Besides triggering a direct local response by the blood vessels and sweat glands, these temperature receptors transmit impulses to the hypothalamus via the spinothalamic tract. The hypothalamus also has temperature-sensitive neurons that react directly to changes in blood temperature.[6] The hypothalamus functions as a temperature control center, attempting to maintain a constant temperature by means of two mechanisms: immediate control, through the autonomic nervous system, and delayed control, through the endocrine system. Shivering, sweating, vasodilation, vasoconstriction, changes in skeletal muscle tone and thyroxine output are the results of this control.[15]

Heat loss

Heat is lost from the body through radiation, conduction, convection, evaporation, and warming of respired air. Approximately 60% of heat loss occurs in the form of infrared heat rays or radiation.[15] Conduction accounts for only a 2% to 3% loss; however, heat loss may increase fivefold in wet clothing and 25-fold in cold water.[38] Convection, or the movement of air currents, produces an average heat loss of 12%, but this amount can greatly increase with wind speed. We are all aware of the windchill factor (Table 26-2). The cooling effect of the wind at low velocities is approximately proportional to the square root of the wind velocity.[30] For example, a wind of 9 mph is about

" The views expressed in this article are those of the author and do not reflect the official policy or position of the Department of the Navy, Department of Defense, nor the U. S. Government."

Table 26-1 Sites for temperature measurement

Site	Advantage	Disadvantage
Mouth (T_o)	Accessible, not embarrassing to patient; approximates esophageal temperature under neutral and hot conditions during rest; suitable for routine estimates	Affected by ambient temperature and mouth breathing; overestimates rectal temperature during work in heat
Esophagus (T_e)	Closely correlates with core temperature	Uncomfortable; learned skill; unsuitable for routine measurement
Auditory canal (T_{ac})	Approximates hypothalamic temperature; accessible; not embarrassing to patient	May be painful; technical problems; influenced by temperature of head skin
Rectum (T_r)	Approximates core temperature during steady state; accessible	Embarrassing to patient; overestimates core temperature during leg exercise

Modified from Kielblock AJ, Schutte PC: Physical work and heat stress. In Zenz C, editor: *Occupational medicine: principles and practical applications,* ed 2, Chicago, 1988, Mosby.

three times as effective for cooling as a wind of 1 mph. Evaporation accounts for about 20% of heat loss, and the rest is lost heating inspired air.[30] Other factors that affect heat loss are clothing and relative humidity. As relative humidity approaches 100%, the ability to dissipate heat through evaporation approaches zero. This can be an important consideration for workers who must use vapor-proof garments, even at mild or low temperatures. Children cool faster than adults because they have a greater ratio of surface area to mass.[8]

Heat gain

Heat sources can be thought of as internal or external. Internal sources include (1) heat generated as a by-product of basal cellular metabolism or of increased metabolism caused by thyroxin, catecholamines, or sympathetic stimulation, and (2) heat produced by exercise.[30] Hard work can increase internal heat production up to twelve times.[8] Environmental sources can add to this thermal load. When ambient temperature is greater than body temperature, heat accumulates.

Another external heat source is radiant energy.

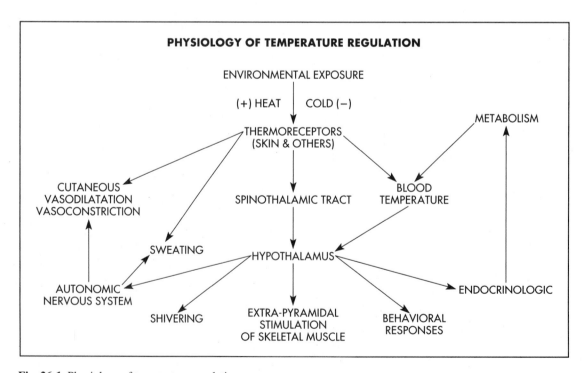

Fig. 26-1 Physiology of temperature regulation.

Table 26-2 Windchill index

Estimated windspeed (mph)	Actual thermometer reading (° F)											
	50	40	30	20	10	0	−10	−20	−30	−40	−50	−60
Calm	50	40	30	20	10	0	−10	−20	−30	−40	−50	−60
5	48	37	27	16	6	−5	−15	−26	−36	−47	−57	−67
10	40	28	16	4	−9	−24	−33	−46	−58	−70	−83	−95
15	36	22	9	−5	−18	−30	−45	−58	−72	−85	−99	−112
20	32	18	4	−10	−25	−39	−53	−67	−82	−96	−110	−124
25	30	16	0	−15	−29	−44	−59	−74	−88	−104	−118	−133
30	28	13	−2	−18	−33	−48	−63	−79	−94	−109	−125	−140
35	27	11	−4	−21	−35	−51	−67	−82	−98	−113	−129	−145
40	26	10	−6	−21	−37	−53	−69	−85	−100	−116	−132	−148
Risk of frostbite		Mild				Moderate				Severe		

Modified from Prevention and treatment of heat and cold stress injuries, NEHC-TM: 92-6, June, 1992, (technical manual).

An unclothed person exposed to bright sun can gain 150 kcal/hour, or about twice the body's basal rate of heat production.[35] Radiant heat loads accumulate regardless of the ambient temperature in such places as boiler rooms, engine rooms, sun-exposed metal vehicles, saunas, and hot tubs. Jobs involving hot metals and masonry materials are other sources of radiant heat.[8]

HEAT-RELATED ILLNESS

Heat-related illnesses consist of an array of maladies that range from relatively minor abnormalities, such as prickly heat, to the life-threatening disorder of heat stroke. The obvious predisposing factors of high ambient temperature, high humidity, and heavy work make these common illnesses in many occupations.

Pathophysiology

The primary determinants of heat stress are ambient temperature, humidity, air movement, and exercise. Environmental heat stress is best measured by the wet bulb globe temperature (WBGT) index.[8] This index, which is somewhat complex, consists of a weighted combination of three determinants: 70% of the index is derived from a wet bulb temperature, measuring the effect of humidity; 20% comes from a black globe temperature, measuring radiant energy; and 10% comes from a shaded, dry bulb temperature.[4] If a WBGT index is not available, a sling psychrometer, or Botsball, measures the wet bulb temperature and gives a simple alternative. This device consists of a wetted thermometer that is rapidly twirled in a sling.[25]

Several agencies use the WBGT index to make recommendations on activity levels. Table 26-3 gives the criteria for light, moderate, and heavy work; Table 26-4 shows activity levels recommended by the American Conference of Governmental Industrial Hygienists (ACGIH). Studies of South African gold miners have shown that work can be maintained without performance decrement up to about 77° F WBGT for an acclimatized worker.[56] Loss of productivity increases progressively, from 1.08% at 79° F to 3.79% at 80.6°; 7.86% at 82.4°; 13.96% at 84.2°; 22.76% at 86°; 33.6% at 87.8°; 50.54% at 89.6°; and 70.19% at 91.4°. Ninety percent of heat stroke cases occur at a WBGT over 86° F (30° C).[34]

Heat loads must be dissipated by radiation, convection, conduction, or evaporation. In extremely hot environments, heat loss through the production and evaporation of sweat becomes crucial to preventing heat illness. Each liter of sweat that vaporizes relieves the body of 580 kcal of heat.[64] The maximum rate of sweating may vary from 1.5

Table 26-3 Work rate categories

Criteria	Light work	Moderate work	Heavy work
Watts	<232	231−340	>340
Heart rate (beats/min)	75−100	101−125	126−150
Oxygen consumption (L/min)	<1.0	1−1.5	>1.5

Modified from Kielblock AJ, Schutte PC: Physical work and heat stress. In Zenz C, editor: *Occupational medicine: principles and practical applications*, ed 2, Chicago, 1988, Mosby.

Table 26-4 Threshold limits for wet bulb globe temperature (WBGT) index*

Work-rest cycle (% of each hour)		Temperature at which productivity declines (° F)		
Work	Rest	Light work	Moderate work	Heavy work
Continuous		86	80	77
75	25	87	82	79
50	50	89	85	82
25	75	90	88	86

* Assumes acclimatization; values provided by the American Conference of Governmental Industrial Hygienists (ACGIH).
Modified from Kielblock AJ, Schutte PC: Physical work and heat stress. In Zenz C, editor: *Occupational medicine: principles and practical applications,* ed 2, Chicago, 1988, Mosby.

L/hour in unacclimatized men to 2.5 L/hour in acclimatized men.[35] Although sweat is always a hypotonic solution of sodium chloride, the concentration of ions may vary greatly as a result of conditioning.[30] As humidity approaches 100%, evaporation is no longer effective in dissipating heat.

The body's ability to tolerate and work under heat stress is a function of the cardiovascular system. Nearly all heat loss takes place at the skin-air interface. Intense cutaneous vasodilation can produce a local blood flow rate of 8 L/minute.[64] During hard work, blood flow to exercising muscles can increase 20 to 40 times.[35] Glycolysis in exercising muscles can consume water at a rate that may result in losses of 10% of inflowing arterial volume.[52] Intense splanchnic vasoconstriction occurs to compensate for the large volume of blood shunted to the skin and muscles.[48] Renal blood flow decreases up to 50%.[8] The ability to increase and maintain the necessary cardiac output becomes crucial.

Repeated exposure improves tolerance to work in hot environments, a process called *acclimatization.* Acclimatization is accomplished by sweating at a lower core temperature, increasing the volume of sweat, and decreasing the salt content of sweat.[18] Cardiac output and stroke volume increase while peak heart rate decreases.[49] These cardiovascular changes are the result of an increase in plasma volume that occurs with exposure to heat and exercise.[64] Exercising in the heat for about 100 minutes a day for 7 to 10 days will result in acclimatization.[8]

Predisposing factors

Anything that adversely affects the ability to sweat or the integrity and responsiveness of the cardiovascular system predisposes a person to heat illness. Cardiovascular disease, obesity, old age, and dehydration can impair cardiac output. Skin disorders such as heat rash, burns, scleroderma, and cystic fibrosis are risk factors because they impair sweating.[8] Anticholinergic drugs (e.g., tricyclic antidepressants, antihistamines, antispasmodics, phenothiazines, monoamine oxidase (MAO) inhibitors, and atropine) inhibit sweating and are dangerous.[64] Vasoconstrictors, beta blockers, and diuretics are risk factors because they may reduce cutaneous blood flow or cause dehydration. Drugs that stimulate muscle activity (cocaine, amphetamines, PCP, and LSD) increase the endogenous heat load.[11] Salicylates uncouple oxidative phosphorylation, and standard doses may produce hyperthermia if taken during exercise.[63] Other risk factors include chronic illnesses such as diabetes mellitus, alcoholism, fatigue, lack of sleep, and previous episodes of heat stroke.[64] Of course, any restrictive or vapor-proof clothing retards heat loss.

Two rare causes of heat illness are neuroleptic malignant syndrome and malignant hyperthermia. An adverse reaction to antipsychotic medication, especially haloperidol, causes neuroleptic malignant syndrome. This syndrome is characterized by fever, diffuse muscular rigidity, altered level of consciousness, and autonomic instability. Physical exhaustion and dehydration may be predisposing factors in some cases.[10] Malignant hyperthermia is related to increased skeletal muscle activity during anesthesia, which may be triggered by potent inhalation agents and by succinylcholine and decamethonium.[45]

Clinical problems

Skin disorders. A variety of cutaneous maladies caused by heat have been described in the literature and are commonly called *miliaria.* They go by many other names as well, such as prickly heat, heat rash, and lichen tropicus. These disorders are caused by sweat retention. *Miliaria crystallina* occurs when the ducts in the stratum corneum close, causing small, clear vesicles to form, usually on the palms and in intertriginous areas. These vesicles most often are asymptomatic. Closure deeper in the epidermis causes *mil-*

iaria rubra, which may develop in a few days but usually is seen after months of exposure to heat. This condition manifests as pruritic, erythematous macules and vesicles, especially on the trunk and in intertriginous areas, with sparing of the palms and soles. These lesions may become pustular and are commonly infected with staphylococci. Even deeper obstruction causes *miliaria profunda,* which is characterized by small, white papules that produce few symptoms. If widespread, these inactive sweat glands may predispose the individual to heat exhaustion. Wearing light, clean, nonocclusive clothing and avoiding prolonged periods of sweating help prevent miliaria. The acute phase can be treated with cool compresses of Burow's solution and antibacterial lotions such as chlorhexidine. Occlusive ointments should be avoided. Systemic and topical steroids are not useful, but parenteral antibiotics such as dicloxacillin may be required for severe, pustular disease. The individual must also avoid hot, humid conditions.[33]

Heat edema. Heat edema is a benign condition characterized by mild swelling of the hands and feet. It is thought to be caused by vasodilation of cutaneous vessels and possibly by increased production of aldosterone in unacclimatized individuals.[64] Serious causes of edema should be ruled out, but an extensive diagnostic evaluation usually is not necessary. Treatment can include elevating the legs, using support hose, or offering reassurance because this self-limiting condition resolves with acclimatization or removal from the hot environment.

Heat syncope. Heat syncope is seen in unacclimatized individuals who must stand for a prolonged period or perform strenuous work in a heat stress environment.[8] Loss of vasomotor tone and venous pooling causes hypotension rather than true dehydration. Individuals quickly regain consciousness when supine, but anyone who falls must be examined for more serious injuries. Treatment consists of rest, removal to a cool environment, and fluids. People at risk for heat syncope should be cautioned to avoid standing for long periods, to flex the leg muscles repeatedly, and to sit down when prodromal signs of syncope occur.

Heat cramps. Heat cramps occur in muscles that are subject to intense exertion, often the calves, thighs, or hamstrings. These cramps are intense and last a few seconds to a few minutes. They often occur near the end of the work shift or later when the person is relaxing. Individuals at high risk for heat cramps typically are highly fit and acclimatized. They can produce a large amount of sweat, and they consume adequate amounts of water, but they do not replace the lost

salt.[35] The diagnosis is made by the history and physical examination, and treatment involves administering an oral 0.1% to 0.2% salt solution (made by mixing ¼ to ½ teaspoon of table salt or two to four 10-grain salt tablets in 1 quart of water), which usually relieves the cramp. Intravenous normal saline is effective for severe cases. Salt tablets are not recommended because they irritate the stomach.[64] Supplemental salt in the diet can prevent these cramps.

Exposure to heat alone does not cause heat cramps, but it may cause heat tetany. Hyperventilation with respiratory alkalosis in response to heat exposure can cause carpopedal spasm.[35] It is seen after short but intense periods of heat stress and is related to the rate of rise in blood pH rather than the absolute pH value. This condition is self-limiting and resolves when the person is removed from the heat stress and hyperventilation declines.[36]

Heat exhaustion. The term "heat exhaustion" has no clear definition and constitutes a spectrum of disorders that range from mild fatigue to frank heat stroke. Symptoms include weakness, fatigue, malaise, nausea, vomiting, headache, muscle cramps, anxiety, and impaired judgment. Body temperature may be normal or moderately elevated, up to 104° F.[64] The patient has hypotension, tachycardia, and moist, clammy skin. Hyperventilation may cause a respiratory alkalosis. The only symptom consistently quoted that differentiates heat exhaustion from heat stroke is the lack of severe cerebral impairment. If sweating ceases and cooling and rehydration measures are not instituted, the person quickly progresses to heat stroke.

Heat exhaustion often is categorized as due predominantly either to water depletion or salt depletion, although it usually is caused by a combination of the two.[35] Individuals working in hot environments usually fail to adequately rehydrate themselves voluntarily.[46] If water replacement is not convenient, palatable, and encouraged, hypertonic dehydration occurs. This condition is seen in athletes, military personnel, and laborers. Exhaustion stemming from salt depletion occurs when large volumes of sweat are replaced with adequate water but not salt.[41] This condition usually develops after several days of heavy work in a hot environment and continued inadequate salt intake. It is rarely seen in industrial settings.[20]

Initial assessment should focus on the history and physical examination, with particular attention to the degree of cardiovascular stress and cerebral impairment. Because quick access to laboratory testing usually is not available, except in a hospital emergency department, it may not be possible to discern the exact loss of salt relative to water. However, this does not mean most cases must be sent to the hospital. A review of heat exhaustion seen in aluminum smelters found that hospitalization was necessary in only 5 of 343 cases (1.5%).[20] Clinical judgment, the treatment facility's capability for monitoring the patient for several hours, and access to more advanced care must be considered when deciding to treat or transport. Certainly any patient with unstable vital signs, complicating factors such as old age or chronic disease, or evidence of organ damage should be transported for definitive care.

Treatment should consist of rest in a cool environment. If the person has an elevated temperature, using fans and keeping the skin moist will aid evaporative cooling. In mild cases that do not involve orthostatic changes in vital signs, oral rehydration with 1 to 3 L of an electrolyte solution (e.g., 0.1% salt solution) may be adequate, but individuals usually voluntarily drink only about 65% of the total loss. Gastric emptying is enhanced by large volumes (500 to 600 ml) and cool temperature (50° to 60° F); it can reach a rate of 25 ml/minute under such conditions.[51] In more severe cases, intravenous rehydration is necessary. A good initial choice is a solution of 5% dextrose in 0.45% saline. Fit young people may require several liters over 6 to 8 hours. Overzealous intravenous hydration can cause congestive heart failure, pulmonary edema, or seizures and must be monitored. A patient who does not feel well or have normal vital signs after 2 to 3 hours of treatment must be hospitalized.[8]

Heat stroke. Heat stroke is a true medical emergency, with a mortality rate as high as 80%.[35] It is caused by thermoregulatory failure, and death is due to tissue damage and organ failure.[8] Cerebral damage and cardiovascular collapse are of primary importance.[35] Although it may be the result of progressive heat exhaustion, heat stroke has a sudden onset in most cases.[54] The classic presentation of heat stroke includes hyperpyrexia (core temperature over 106° F), severe central nervous system (CNS) dysfunction, and hot, dry skin.[64] However, this triad is not always seen, by any means. Heat stroke has been reported in patients with an initial rectal temperature of only 103° F.[54] Sweating is maintained in as many as 50% of victims.[35] Cerebral dysfunction (delirium, coma, or seizures) is seen, but initially only confusion may be present.[8] Because of the dire consequences of this condition, a high degree of suspicion must be maintained when evaluating victims of heat stress.

Two forms of heat stroke have been described. Classic heat stroke is seen during heat waves and commonly develops over days in the elderly, invalids, and alcoholics.[58] Exertional heat stroke is seen in young, healthy individuals such as athletes, military personnel, and miners.[16] The incidence of heat stroke in military recruits and also pilgrims to Mecca during hot weather has been reported to be 0.18%.[13,60]

The prodromal symptoms of heat stroke are the same as those of heat exhaustion. Severe CNS dysfunction is the key difference. Mental impairment ensues at 100.4° F, with complete deterioration of neural function at 107.6° F and above, resulting in coma or seizures.[35] Besides a rise in core temperature, tachycardia, hypotension, and hyperventilation with respiratory alkalosis may occur.[8] Myocardial, hepatic, renal, and bleeding disorders are seen.[24]

Once the diagnosis has been made or if it is even suspected, the patient must be transported to a hospital, but treatment must begin immediately to lower the core temperature and stabilize vital signs. Lowering body temperature typically has involved either ice water baths or evaporative cooling. Although ice water immersion has been used successfully, it has many disadvantages: it is uncomfortable; it causes profound vasoconstriction; it provokes shivering; it makes CPR nearly impossible; and it makes assessment of the patient difficult.[64]

Evaporative cooling is the preferred method of heat reduction. It can be effective in the field,[3] and it has been shown to produce five times the cooling rate of ice water baths.[60] In this method the body is stripped of clothing, suspended in a hammock, and kept moist with warm water to prevent shivering. A fan or any other available means is used to blow air over the body and promote evaporation. Care must be taken to avoid overcooling. Of course, simultaneously the airway should be secured, oxygen administered, an intravenous line established, and the bladder catheterized. Though hypotension often is present, it usually represents high output failure and responds to cooling and cutaneous vasoconstriction.[8] Therefore, fluid replacement should be judicious and closely titrated to vital signs.

Prevention

Preventing heat-related illnesses requires a multidimensioned approach. Individuals in high-risk jobs should be carefully screened for preexisting medical conditions and use of medications. Workers should be trained to recognize early signs of distress, and they should be counseled about the need for adequate fluid intake, nutrition, proper clothing, and rest. The WBGT index and level of acclimatization should be taken into consideration when assigning work schedules. Fluid must be readily available. Cool, flavored water results in greater intake than does warm tap water. Salt tablets should be avoided.[32]

CASE STUDIES
Case 1

A 38-year-old sandblaster was transported to the dispensary complaining of severe fatigue. He had been working in a confined space onboard a ship that was undergoing a scheduled overhaul. He had been wearing complete personal protective equipment, including an air-fed hood, rubber boots and gloves, and an impermeable suit that was cooled by a vortex cooling unit. After working 3 hours of a normal 4-hour shift, he felt poorly and left the space. At the dispensary he complained of extreme weakness, nausea, light-headedness, and headache. His medical history was remarkable for a recent cold, and he had been taking an over-the-counter decongestant for 2 days.

Physical examination showed a young man who answered questions appropriately but was in moderate distress. Vital signs showed a rectal temperature of 103.5° F, pulse of 150, blood pressure of 100/65, and a respiratory rate of 20 per minute. His skin was flushed and covered with sweat. The rest of the examination was normal, and he showed no neurologic deficits. A diagnosis of acute heat exhaustion was made. Laboratory analysis showed a hematocrit value of 53.3, white cell count of 8900, and a platelet count of 220,000. Urinalysis showed a specific gravity of 1.030 with trace protein and ketones, and no myoglobin. A chemistry panel, liver function tests, creatinine phosphokinase (CPK), and clotting studies were ordered.

The patient's clothes were removed, and he was placed on a canvas cot. He was sprayed with warm water, and two large fans were used to cool him. An IV line was placed, and 2 liters of normal saline solution were infused over 1 hour. After 45 minutes his temperature was 101.8° F, and the fans were turned down. After 1 hour the patient felt better but was still weak and nauseated and produced only 100 ml of dark urine. His IV fluid was changed to D5 ½ normal saline and infused at 1 L/hour. After 2 hours his temperature was 100.0° F, and he felt much better. The fans were turned off, he was allowed to drink water ad lib, and the IV infusion was reduced to TKO. After 3 hours, his temperature was 99.2° F, he had consumed 1500 ml of water, and his pulse was 80 with a blood pressure of 130/80. He was sent home and told to rest and drink fluids.

On follow-up the next day, he felt fine and the previous laboratory tests were all normal. Repeat urinalysis and serum glutamic–pyruvate transaminase (SGPT), lactate dehydrogenase (LDH), and CPK values were also normal. Further questioning revealed that he had been on vacation for the previous 2 weeks. He also admitted that he did not hydrate himself before work to avoid having to urinate while suited up. An industrial hygiene investigation showed the WBGT was 72° F on the day of the incident. Examination of the suit showed a leak in the air supply hose, which reduced the air flow rate.

This man had heat exhaustion secondary to poor acclimatization, use of medication, self-induced dehydration, and a faulty air-cooled suit. He was restricted from working in heat stress areas for 1 week and then was gradually reintroduced to that work environment without difficulty.

Case 2

A 44-year-old foundry worker went to the plant's occupational health nurse complaining of a headache, fatigue, and nausea. He requested aspirin. He had been pouring molten metal for 3 hours that morning and finally felt too poorly to continue. He had been seen for a heat rash twice in the past 3 weeks, and he also had a history of hypertension and was taking atenolol.

Physical examination showed a moderately obese man in moderate distress from his headache. He was somewhat confused at times while answering questions. His vital signs showed an oral temperature of 100° F, pulse of 80, blood pressure of 120/75, and a respiratory rate of 20. His skin was flushed and damp with sweat. There was a diffuse, erythematous, macular rash with numerous small, white papules over his trunk. The rest of the examination was normal. He was given aspirin and after resting in the office, he felt better and went to lunch.

The man returned to work and resumed his job. After about 90 minutes he began acting sluggish and then collapsed. His coworkers carried him from the area, an ambulance was summoned, and he was transported to the emergency room. His vital signs there were a rectal temperature of 105.6° F, pulse of 90, blood pressure of 105/50, and a respiratory rate of 30. He was conscious but oriented to person only. His physical examination was remarkable for hot, dry skin and extreme weakness. The patient's clothes were removed, and his temperature was lowered by evaporative cooling with fans and warm water mists. Intravenous normal saline solution was judiciously infused, with frequent monitoring to prevent fluid overload. As his temperature slowly came down, the patient's sensorium cleared. He was admitted to the hospital with a diagnosis of heat stroke.

This man was suffering from heat exhaustion when he first saw the nurse. His obesity and use of beta blockers depressed his cardiovascular system's ability to respond to increased demand. Miliaria profunda also inhibited his ability to sweat. The use of aspirin may have added to the heat load by uncoupling oxidative phosphorylation. On the initial examination his temperature was taken orally, and this probably did not accurately assess the true core temperature. This case shows the importance of recognizing early symptoms and the need to be aware of factors that predispose to heat-related illnesses.

COLD INJURIES

Without proper protection, humans are susceptible to the cold. The two most common and worst injuries are hypothermia and frostbite. Two other nonfreezing injuries, chilblains and trench foot, are also discussed.

Chilblains (perniosis)

Chilblains is a condition that results from intermittent exposure to cool, windy, humid conditions with temperatures ranging from 33° F to 60° F.[17] It is usually seen in young women and children. The patient has reddish blue, warm, swollen patches that itch and burn.[53] The fingers, toes, nose, and anterior surfaces of the legs are commonly affected.[29]

Some people develop a chronic form of chilblains, with the lesions appearing perennially as cold weather approaches and subsiding as warm weather returns.[17] These individuals may have predisposing conditions such as Raynaud's disease, collagen-vascular diseases, macroglobulinemia, dysproteinemias, or a genetic predisposition.[29]

The etiology of chilblains is believed to be related to edema of the papillary dermis and vasculitis of the dermal vessels secondary to intermittent or prolonged cold-induced vasoconstriction.[17] Chilblains is often misdiagnosed, and a subsequently extensive medical investigation may result. The differential diagnosis includes Raynaud's syndrome, lupus erythematosus, erythromelalgia, polycythemia vera, embolism, and purple toe syndrome from anticoagulation therapy. The laboratory work-up should include a complete blood count, antinuclear antibody titer, serum chemical profile, and cryoglobulin/cryofibrinogen analysis.[29]

Treatment of acute chilblains should consist of warm water immersion, not to exceed 108° F.[17] Rewarming increases the pain and itching and may require analgesia. Nifedipine has proved to be an effective treatment.[50] The dosage is 20 mg three times a day, but it may need to be reduced because of side effects. Bland, soothing topical creams or ointments may provide symptomatic relief, but topical steroids should be avoided.[7] Chilblains is self-limiting and resolves spontaneously in 3 to 4 weeks without treatment.[29] Prevention consists of proper protection from the cold.

Trench foot and immersion foot

Trench foot and immersion foot are similar forms of nonfreezing cold injuries that have primarily been seen in military settings. The former can develop with prolonged exposure to cold, wet conditions, such as in trench warfare. Direct immersion in water below 50° F for longer than 10 to 12 hours, especially if associated with dependency and immobility of the lower limb, can result in immersion foot.[61]

These injuries have three phases. Initially there is vasospasm and ischemia, producing tissue anoxia and nerve and blood vessel damage. The extremity is cold, swollen, and white or blue, and pulses are diminished or absent. On rewarming, the extremity is warm, dry, red, swollen, and painful. The pulses are bounding. This phase lasts 4 to 10 days and may result in atrophy, ulceration, or gangrene. In the last phase the extremity returns to normal; however, depigmentation, cold hypersensitivity, hyperhidrosis, and pain with weight bearing may develop, persisting for years. Treatment consists of rewarming, elevation, and supportive care.[17]

Frostbite

Frostbite has been a well-documented problem of past military campaigns. The experience gained in the Korean War and in treating civilian injuries in the Arctic has shaped our current concepts about the treatment of frostbite. Freezing injuries can be a threat to anyone working in the Arctic, northern United States, and many mountainous regions.[43]

Frostbite develops when tissue freezes.[26] Temperature, of course, is an important factor, but frostbite usually develops over several hours. It was found in Korea that 90% of frostbite occurred at temperatures below 20° F and after exposure of 7 to 18 hours.[53] The windchill index is important in predicting the risk of frostbite (see Table 26-2).

Pathophysiology. The pathophysiology of cellular death and damage caused by frostbite occurs as a result of two mechanisms: (1) the direct cellular effects of ice crystal formation, and (2) the effects of vascular stasis.[26] Unless freezing occurs rapidly, crystallization occurs extracellularly. The remaining fluid becomes hypertonic and draws water from the cell. This damage is reversible until more than one third of the intracellular fluid is lost. Cell injury occurs secondary to dehydration and disruption of enzymatic processes.[19]

Tissue freezing causes endothelial cell damage in the microvasculature.[26] Within minutes after thawing, increased capillary permeability causes fluid loss and intravascular aggregation of platelets and erythrocytes. Complete vascular stasis can occur within 2 hours.[53] These clogged vessels and arterioles disappear from the microvasculature, and if these tissues do not subsequently slough, they retain a distorted vascular pattern.[5]

Predisposing factors. Frostbite usually occurs in people who are unexpectedly caught in storms, suffer from injuries or exhaustion, or are mentally impaired. Predisposing factors included use of drugs or alcohol, diabetes mellitus, previous cold injury, and peripheral vascular diseases.[53] Studies of the military have shown that soldiers who are black and were born and raised in a warm climate have a greater risk of frostbite. Interestingly, cigarette smoking has not been consistently shown to be a risk factor.[42,57]

Clinical presentation. Frostbite most often involves the fingers, toes, ears, and nose, and in more severe injuries the hands and feet.[26] It has been classified in the same manner as burns (i.e., first degree, second degree, and third degree), but because early clinical evaluation often is inaccurate and tends to overrate the injury (and has led to unnecessary surgical amputation), a more appropriate method is to classify an injury as superficial or deep.[44] Even this is not important at the time of presentation because the initial treatment is the same.

The early stage of frostbite is often called "frostnip" and does not involve actual freezing of tissue or tissue loss.[53] This is characterized by initial stinging followed by loss of sensation, but the skin blanches. After rewarming, the affected part is red and tingles for a short time, and then the signs and symptoms resolve without sequelae.

Superficial frostbite involves the skin and subcutaneous tissue. Initially there is pain as the tissue freezes, and this progresses to numbness. The area is white, waxy, and does not blanch, but it is resilient when depressed. After thawing the tissue is flushed, edematous, and develops a purple color. Impressive blistering develops within 24 hours and resolves over 4 to 10 days. As these blisters dry, a hard, black eschar develops that may appear to be gangrenous. If the injury is superficial, this eschar sloughs over 3 to 4 weeks and new skin replaces the damage. The affected skin is sensitive to heat and cold and may exhibit hyperhidrosis for months.[26,44]

Deep frostbite manifests as a white, solid block that cannot be depressed. After rewarming, the tissue remains cold, dusky, and mottled, and there is little edema and no blistering. Eventually a line of demarcation forms, and spontaneous amputation occurs.[26,44] Patients may seek treatment after thawing has taken place. At this stage it is difficult to estimate the degree of injury.[43] Favorable signs include warmth of tissue, relatively normal color, intact sensation, edema persisting longer than 24 to 48 hours, and large, clear blebs that extend to the tips of the digits. Signs of severe damage include complete absence of edema, cyanotic tissue, complete loss of sensation, and late appearance of small, dark-colored blebs that do not extend to the tips of the volar pads of the digits.[26,44]

Treatment. Treatment consists of rapid rewarming of the frozen tissue because there is a direct correlation between the length of time tissue is frozen and ultimate tissue damage.[55] However, in the field it may be best to keep the part frozen because slow or partial thawing, or refreezing of previously thawed tissue, may result in even greater damage. Also, in the case of foot or toe injuries, once thawed, the pain may make walking out to a point of safe evacuation impossible.[44]

Patients with frostnip can be treated and released. All cases of deep frostbite must be hospitalized, and all but the most superficial and limited injuries should be referred for surgical consultation. When examining a patient, the physician must rule out other serious injuries such as fractures and especially hypothermia.

The cornerstone of treatment of frostbite is rapid rewarming in a whirlpool bath at a temperature between 100° F and 108° F for 20 to 30 minutes.[44] If the tissue is already thawed, rewarming provides no benefit.[26] Rewarming is painful and may require analgesia or sedation. Theoretically, alcohol may serve as a peripheral vasodilator and as a sedative, as long as hypothermia is not present.[53]

Once rewarmed, the tissue should be elevated and protected from pressure and infection. Treatment should be open and nonocclusive, avoiding ointments and dressings. Whirlpool baths with a mild antiseptic soap twice a day for 20 minutes provide debridement and improve circulation. Antibiotics generally are not needed, but tetanus prophylaxis should be given. Blebs should be left intact. Constant, active motion of the digits is mandatory. If eschars develop and restrict motion, they must be slit along the dorsum or lateral borders. Surgical debridement or amputation must be avoided, and the tissue must be given maximum time to recover.[44]

Hypothermia

Hypothermia is present when the core temperature is 95° F (35° C) or lower.[47] Obviously, the more a person is exposed to cold, wet, windy conditions, the greater the risk of hypothermia. Although the condition is more commonly seen in far northern latitudes, hypothermia occurs even in southern locations, such as Florida.[1] With proper protection and knowledge, hypothermia can be prevented. It is most commonly seen in infants, the elderly, the unconscious, the immobile, in drug-intoxicated persons, or those who become exhausted while working in cold environments.[47] The maritime occupations are at particular risk because of the possibility of immersion in cold water, which produces a conductive heat loss 25 times greater than that of air.[38]

Pathophysiology. As thermosensors in the skin and hypothalamus detect a drop in temperature, the core temperature is maintained by vasoconstriction and behavioral responses.[30] When these heat conservation mechanisms fail, heat production is supplied by an increase in the basal metabolic rate, endocrinologic thermogenesis, and shivering. Shivering is especially important because it can increase heat production two to five times.[37] Shivering reaches a maximum when the core temperature drops to 95° F, but it cannot be sustained for long periods, and it ceases when the core temperature falls below 88° F, leaving individuals incapable of restoring body temperature without external help.[15]

As body temperature drops, nearly all organ systems are affected. Table 26-5 outlines these physiologic changes. The body's need for oxygen drops as the basal metabolic rate falls to 50% of normal at 82° F.[47] The CNS becomes depressed as cerebral blood flow decreases 6% to 7% for each 1.8° F (1° C) at temperatures between 95° F and 77° F. Short-term memory and calculation speed are significantly diminished at temperatures below 95° F.[12] The pupils often are dilated below 86° F, and the EEG is flat below 68° F.[23]

The cardiovascular affects of hypothermia include an initial tachycardia followed by gradual declines in heart rate, blood pressure, and cardiac output.[31] A blood pressure measurement may be difficult or impossible to obtain below 87° F.[47] Atrial fibrillation is common, and myocardial irritability is an extreme problem because ventricular fibrillation is resistant to defibrillation and pharmacotherapy below 86° F.[9] The electrocardiogram

Table 26-5 Three zones of hyperthermia

Stage	Core temperature ° F	° C	Characteristics
Mild	99.6 ± 1	37.6	Normal rectal temperature
	98.6 ± 1	37	Normal oral temperature
	96.8	36	Metabolic rate increases
	95	35	Urine temperature 94.6° F (34.8° C); maximum shivering thermogenesis
	93.2	34	Amnesia, dysarthria, poor judgement; blood pressure normal; maximum respiratory stimulation
	91.4	33	Ataxia, apathy
Moderate	89.6	32	Stupor; 25% decrease in O_2 consumption
	87.8	31	Shivering thermogenesis stops
	86	30	Atrial fibrillation, other dysrhythmias; poikilothermia; pulse, cardiac output 66% of normal; insulin ineffective
	85.2	29	Progressive decline in pulse, respiration, level of consciousness; pupils dilated
	82.4	28	Decreased ventricular fibrillation threshold; 50% decline in pulse, O_2 consumption
	80.6	27	Reflexes, voluntary motion absent
Severe	78.8	26	Major acid-base disturbances; no response to pain
	77	25	Cerebral blood flow 33% of normal; cardiac output 45% of normal; possible pulmonary edema
	75.2	24	Significant hypotension
	73.4	23	Corneal and oculocephalic reflexes absent
	71.6	22	Maximum risk of ventricular fibrillation; 75% decrease in O_2 consumption
	68	20	Lowest temperature for resumption of cardiac electro-mechanical activity; pulse 20% of normal
	66.2	19	Flat EEG
	64.4	18	Asystole
	60.8	16	Lowest temperature for adult survival of accidental hypothermia
	59.2	15.2	Lowest temperature of infant survival of accidental hypothermia
	50	10	92% decrease in O_2 consumption
	48.2	9	Lowest temperature for therapeutic survival of hypothermia

Adapted from Danzl DF, Pozos RS, Hamlet MP: Accidental hypothermia. In Auerbach PS, Geehr EC, editors: *Management of wilderness and environmental emergencies,* ed 2, St Louis, 1989, Mosby.

(ECG) may show the characteristic J wave or "Osborn wave" at the terminal portion of the QRS complex.[40] This reversible feature may occur at any temperature below 90° F and increase in size with decreasing core temperature.[15]

Respiratory depression occurs and acid-base disturbances are complex but usually result in acidosis.[15] Although renal blood flow is greatly reduced, the kidneys excrete large amounts of urine in what is known as cold diuresis. This condition is most likely due to peripheral vasoconstriction, which causes relative central hypervolemia.[9] Hematologic effects include an increase in hematocrit level, a decrease in white blood cells and platelets, and an increase in blood viscosity.[47] Hyperglycemia results from inhibition of insulin production and reduction of glucose use.[14]

Predisposing factors. Conditions that diminish heat production, increase heat loss, or impair thermoregulation can predispose or actually be the cause of hypothermia.[15] These conditions are outlined in Fig. 26-2. A review of euthyroid hypothermic patients noted that the most common associated medical illnesses were cerebrovascular disease, congestive heart failure, and pneumonia.[62]

Evaluation. Although many cases of hypothermia are obvious from the history, this diagnosis must be kept in mind because of the wide variety of potential presenting symptoms. The most important point the physician must remember is to measure the core temperature with a thermometer capable of reading below 94° F, the limit of many standard thermometers.[47] This is especially important in profoundly hypothermic patients because they may have no recordable heart rate, blood pressure, heart sounds, or deep-tendon reflexes and may appear apneic with dilated pupils. Death can be diagnosed only with irreversible cardiac arrest in a warm patient. Because many hypothermic patients have been pronounced dead only to recover subsequently with warming, the clinician should remember the old adage, "No one is dead until they're warm and dead."[22] This is especially important in drowning victims because they may survive after prolonged submersion as a result of the diving reflex.[15]

Early symptoms may often include fatigue, sluggishness, incoordination, apathy, and confusion. Early recognition and treatment in the field may avert severe hypothermia. As the temperature drops, judgment becomes impaired, placing the victim at increased risk of injury and making self-help less likely. Sometimes bizarre behavior results, such as paradoxic undressing.[59]

Treatment. The treatment of hypothermia has been extensively studied, but because it is obviously unethical to conduct controlled experiments

Endocrinologic factors
Hypothyroidism
Hypoadrenalism
Hypopituitarism
Hypoglycemia

Central nervous system dysfunction
Cerebrovascular disease
Tumors
Trauma
Anorexia nervosa

Drug toxicity
Alcohol
Barbiturates
Phenothiazines
Organophosphate poisoning

Skin disorders
Burns
Erythrodermas

Sepsis
Miscellaneous
Previous hypothermia
Pneumonia
Uremia
Malnutrition
Vascular insufficiency
Cardiopulmonary disease

Fig. 26-2 Conditions predisposing to hypothermia.

on subjects with more than mild hypothermia, there is still considerable controversy over the best method to treat severe cases. The methods generally are classified as passive rewarming, active external rewarming, and active internal or core rewarming. These methods are outlined in Fig. 26-3. The choice of treatment must consider the duration and degree of hypothermia, the available resources and the time it takes to mobilize them, and possible complications from each procedure.[47] It also is important to remember that the mortality rate from hypothermia is more closely related to the underlying pathologic condition than to the actual method of rewarming.[9]

Mild hypothermia can be treated in most clinics, if they are properly staffed and equipped. Certainly any moderate to severe case needs to be treated in a hospital. If shivering is present, active rewarming is not necessary, and the focus should be on preventing further heat loss. Cold, wet clothing should be removed, and the patient should be insulated with warm blankets. Because dehydration is common, taking warm fluids by mouth is

Passive rewarming

Removal from environmental exposure
Insulation measures to prevent further loss from conduction, convection, radiation evaporation, and respiration

Active external rewarming

Heated water bath immersion
Electric blankets or pads
Heated objects (e.g., hot water bottle, piped suit)
Radiant warming

Active core rewarming

Heated inhalation
Heated IV fluids
Gastrointestinal irrigation (intragastric balloon, colonic)
Bladder irrigation
Mediastinal irrigation via thoracotomy
Peritoneal lavage/dialysis
Extracorporeal rewarming
Diathermy

Fig. 26-3 Rewarming methods in hypothermia.

fine as long as the patient is neurologically stable
and can tolerate them. Otherwise, an intravenous
solution of 5% dextrose in $\frac{1}{2}$ normal saline should
be used. The IV fluid should be heated to 104° to
108° F. Three 1 L bags can be heated from room
temperature in 3 minutes with a microwave oven.
This does not affect the solutions, but "hot spots"
are possible.[2] Other active external rewarming
methods can be used safely in mild hypothermia.[15]

Anything more than mild hypothermia must be
treated in a hospital emergency department if possible. When a patient must be transported, she
should be handled gently and immobilized. Passive external rewarming is appropriate, but active
external rewarming should be avoided unless definitive treatment can be provided. Moderate to severe hypothermia may have a high mortality rate,
and the early stages of rewarming are especially
dangerous for three reasons: (1) cardiac output is
reduced, and shock may ensue when peripheral
vessels dilate in response to surface heating; (2) an
"after drop" usually is seen in the core temperature
as cool peripheral blood released by vasodilation
flows centrally, further cooling the heart and possibly provoking dysrhythmias; and (3) prolonged
peripheral stagnation causes biochemical abnormalities in the blood, which may affect the heart.
These problems may be minimized by means of
active core rewarming.[39]

When definitive care is available, therapy can
be divided into general supportive care, drug therapy, and rewarming methods. Accurate core temperatures, as well as the ABCs (airway, breathing,

circulation) must be constantly monitored. In light
of the reduced metabolic demands, depressed hemodynamic indices may be misleading, and iatrogenic fibrillation is easily induced. Ventilatory requirements are also reduced. Clinical judgment
must be used when assessing fluid needs, but most
severe cases are those in which the patient is dehy-
drated. A fluid challenge, naloxone, thiamine, and
administration of D50 are appropriate for obtunded patients. Antibiotics should be used as indicated. Laboratory evaluation includes serum glucose, arterial blood gases, complete blood count,
chemistry panel, clotting studies, amylase, and a
toxicology screen. Thyroid function tests, cardiac
isoenzymes, and serum cortisol may be indicated.
X-ray studies should include chest and abdominal
films, as well as cervical spine films if the patient
is not alert.[15]

CASE STUDY

*A 27-year-old painter slipped while working on a
bridge and fell approximately 20 feet into the water.
While falling, she struck a girder, injuring her right
arm. A flotation device was thrown to her, and she was
immersed in 55° F water for about 20 minutes before
being rescued. After a 15-minute transport, she arrived
at the local hospital. She was weakly shivering and
somewhat stuporous but answered questions slowly and
accurately. She complained of arm and neck pain. Her
coveralls were torn at the right upper arm, where a
blood-soaked dressing had been placed. She was placed
in a cervical collar, and after all her wet clothing was
removed, an examination showed a rectal temperature
of 90° F, a pulse rate of 60, a blood pressure of 110/50,
and a respiratory rate of 10. The skin was mottled, and
there was a 6 cm laceration over the right upper arm
with a bony deformity present. The rest of the examination was unremarkable except for dysarthria and impaired short-term memory. Warm blankets were placed
over the patient, an IV line was placed in the left arm,
and the cardiac rhythm was monitored. The right arm
wound was cleaned, dressed, and splinted. The patient
was given warmed oxygen by mask. X-ray films of the
spine, chest, and right arm revealed a fracture of the
midhumerus, but no other fractures. An ECG showed sinus bradycardia with a rate of 56. The patient felt better
but was not shivering vigorously despite a rectal temperature of 90° F. D5 $\frac{1}{2}$ normal saline heated to 104° F
was infused, and the trunk was warmed with heating
pads. After 30 minutes the temperature fell to 89.4° F
but then slowly began to rise. After 60 minutes the temperature was 91° F, and in 3 hours it was 94.1° F. At
this point the patient's sensorium was totally clear, and
she was allowed to drink warm fluids and consume
high-carbohydrate foods. After 6 hours her temperature
was 98.2° F.*

REFERENCES

1. Altus P et al: Hypothermia in the sunny South, *South Med
   J* 73(11):1491, 1980.
2. Anshus JS, Endahl GL, Mottley JL: Microwave heating of
   intravenous fluids, *Am J Emerg Med* 3:316, 1985.

3. Barner HB et al: Field evaluation of a new simplified method for cooling of heat casualties in the desert, *Mil Med* 149:95, 1984.

4. Barthel HJ: Exertion-induced heat stroke in a military setting, *Mil Med* 155:116, 1990.

5. Bellman S, Strombeck JO: Transformation of the vascular system in cold-injured tissue of rabbit's ear, *Angiology* 11:108, 1960.

6. Boulant JA, Dean JB: Temperature receptors in the central nervous system, *Ann Rev Physiol* 48:639, 1986.

7. Burry JN: Adverse effects of topical fluorinated corticosteroid agents on chilblains (letter), *Med J Aust* 146(8):451, 1987.

8. Callahan M: Heat illness. In Rosen et al, editors: *Emergency medicine: concepts and clinical practice,* ed 2, St Louis, 1988, Mosby.

9. Carden D et al: Hypothermia, *Ann Emerg Med* 11:497, 1982.

10. Carson SN: The neuroleptic malignant syndrome, *J Clin Psychiatry* 41:79, 1980.

11. Cohen R: Injuries due to physical hazards. In LaDou, editor: *Occupational medicine,* Norwalk, Conn, 1990, Appleton & Lange.

12. Coleshaw et al: Impaired memory registration and speed of reasoning caused by low body temperature, *J Appl Physiol* 55(1):27, 1983.

13. Costrini AM et al: Cardiovascular and metabolic manifestations of heat stroke and severe heat exhaustion, *Am J Med* 66:296, 1979.

14. Curry DL, Curry KP: Hypothermia and insulin secretion, *Endocrinology* 7:750, 1970.

15. Danzl DF: Accidental hypothermia. In Rosen et al, editors: *Emergency medicine: concepts and clinical practice,* ed 2, St Louis, 1988, Mosby.

16. Delaney KA: Heatstroke (underlying processes and lifesaving management), *Postgrad Med* 91(4):379, 1992.

17. DeLapp TD: Taking the bite out of frostbite and other cold weather injuries, *Am J Nurs* 80:56, 1980.

18. Dill DB, Hall FE, Edwards HT: Changes in composition of sweat during acclimatization to heat, *Am J Physiol* 123:412, 1938.

19. Dinep M: Cold injury: a review of current theories and their application to treatment, *Conn Med* 39(1):8, 1974.

20. Dinman BD, Horvath SM: Heat disorders in industry, *J Occup Med* 26(7):489, 1984.

21. Edwards HA et al: Apparent death with accidental hypothermia, *Br J Anaesth* 42:906, 1970.

22. Edwards RJ, Beyyavin AJ, Harrison MH: Core temperature measurement in man, *Aviat Space Environ Med* 49(11):1289, 1978.

23. Ehrmantraut WR, Ticktin HE, Fazekras JF: Cerebral hemodynamics and metabolism in accidental hypothermia, *Arch Intern Med* 99:57, 1957.

24. Eichler AC, McFee AS, Root HD: Heat stroke, *Am J Surg* 118:855, 1969.

25. Engerbretson D: Too hot to trot, *Backpacking J* 3:22, 1977.

26. Gage AM, Gage AA: Frostbite, *Trauma Emerg Med* 7(9):25, 1981.

27. Gale CC: Neuroendocrine aspects of thermoregulation, *Ann Rev Physiol* 5:391, 1973.

28. Gilat T, Shibolet S, Sohar E: Mechanism of heat stroke, *J Trop Med Hyg* 66:204, 1963.

29. Goette DK: Chilblains (perniosis), *J Am Acad Dermatol* 23:257, 1990.

30. Guyton AC: Body temperature, temperature regulation, and fever. In Guyton AF, editor: *Textbook of medical physiology,* ed 8, Philadelphia, 1991, WB Saunders.

31. Harnett RM, Pruitt JR, Sias FR: A review of the literature concerning resuscitation from hypothermia. II. Selected rewarming protocols, *Aviat Space Environ Med* 54:487, 1983.

32. Hubbard RW et al: Voluntary dehydration and allesthesia for water, *J Appl Physiol Respir Environ Exercise Physiol* 57:868, 1984.

33. Kanerva L: Physical causes of occupational skin disease. In Adams RM, editor: *Occupational skin disease,* ed 2, Philadelphia, 1990, WB Saunders.

34. Kew MC: Temperature regulation in heat stroke in man, *Isr J Med Sci* 12:759, 1976.

35. Knochel JP: Environmental heat illness, *Arch Intern Med* 133:841, 1974.

36. Lampietro PF: Heat-induced tetany, *Fed Proc* 22:884, 1973.

37. Lampietro PF et al: Heat production from shivering, *J Appl Physiol* 15:632, 1960.

38. Levinson R et al: Comparison of the effects of water immersion and saline infusion on central hemodynamics in man, *Clin Sci Molec Med* 52:343, 1977.

39. Marcus P: Laboratory comparison of techniques for rewarming hypothermic casualties, *Aviat Space Environ Med* 49(5):692, 1978.

40. Martinez-Lopez JI: A cool-inary problem, *J La State Med Soc* 144(7):299, 1992.

41. McCance RA: Experimental sodium chloride deficiency in man, *Proc R Soc London Biol* 119:245, 1936.

42. Miller D, Bjornson DR: An investigation of cold-injured soldiers in Alaska, *Mil Med* 127:247, 1962.

43. Mills WJ: Frostbite and hypothermia: current concepts, *Alaska Med* 15(2):56, 1973.

44. Mills WJ: Out in the cold, *Emerg Med* 8:134, 1976.

45. Nelson TE, Flewellen EH: The malignant hyperthermia syndrome, *N Engl J Med* 309(7):416, 1983.

46. Pitts GC, Johnson RE, Consolazio FC: Work in the heat as affected by intake of water, salt, and glucose, *Am J Physiol* 142:253, 1944.

47. Reuler JB: Hypothermia: pathophysiology, clinical settings, and management, *Ann Intern Med* 89:519, 1978.

48. Rowell LB et al: Redistribution of blood flow during sustained high skin temperature in resting man, *J Appl Physiol* 28:415, 1970.

49. Rowell LB et al: Reductions in cardiac output, central blood volume, and stroke volume with thermal stress in normal men during exercise, *J Clin Invest* 45:1801, 1966.

50. Rustin MHA et al: The treatment of chilblains with nifedipine: the results of a pilot study, a double-blind, placebo-controlled, randomized study, and a long-term open trial, *Br J Dermatol* 120:267, 1989.

51. Ryan AF, moderator: Balancing heat stress, fluids, and electrolytes, *Physician Sportsmed* 1:43, 1973.

52. Schlein EM, Jensen D, Knochel JP: The effect of plasma water loss on assessment of muscle metabolism during exercise, *J Appl Physiol* 34:568, 1973.

53. Shaw JF: Frostbite. In Rosen et al, editors: *Emergency medicine: concepts and clinical practice,* ed 2, St Louis, 1988, Mosby.

54. Shibolet S, Lancaster MC, Dannon Y: Heat stroke: a review, *Aviat Space Environ Med* 47(3):280, 1976.

55. Smith DJ, Robson MC, Heggers JP: Frostbite and other cold-induced injuries. In Auerbach PS, Geehr EC, editors: *Management of wilderness and environmental emergencies,* ed 2, St Louis, 1989, Mosby.

56. Smith O: Effects of a cooler underground environment on safety and labour productivity. In Howes MJ, Jones MJ, editors: Proceedings of the third mine ventilation congress (Harrogate), London, 1984, The Institution of Mining and Metallurgy.

57. Sumner DS, Criblez TL, Doolittle WH: Host factors in human frostbite, *Mil Med* 139:454, 1974.

58. Vicario SJ, Okabajue R, Haltom T: Rapid cooling in classic heatstroke: effect on mortality rates, *Am J Emerg Med* 4:394, 1986.

59. Wedin B, Vanggaard L, Hirvonen J: "Paradoxical undressing" in fatal hypothermia, *J Forensic Sci* 24:543, 1979.

60. Weiner JS, Khogali M: A physiological body cooling unit for treatment of heat stroke, *Lancet* 1:507, 1980.

61. White JC, Scoville WB: Trench foot and immersion foot, *N Engl J Med* 232(15):415, 1945.

62. Whittle JL, Bates JH: Thermoregulatory failure secondary to acute illness, *Arch Intern Med* 139:418, 1979.

63. Wyndham CH: The physiology of exercise under heat stress, *Ann Rev Physiol* 35:193, 1973.

64. Yarbrough BE, Hubbard RW: Heat-related illnesses. In Auerbach PS, Geehr EC, editors: *Management of wilderness and environmental emergencies,* ed 2, St Louis, 1989, Mosby.

27 Occupational Hearing Loss

The National Safety Council lists noise-induced hearing loss in the top ten of work-related illness and injuries. Although occupational noise-induced hearing loss has been recognized since before the industrial revolution (with described syndromes such as blacksmith's ear), little was done to prevent noise-induced hearing loss in industry until the passage of Occupational Safety and Health Administration's (OSHA's) Hearing Conservation Act in 1983.

It is difficult to determine the exact number of workers exposed to noise levels that can induce hearing loss. 1987 statistics estimate the following figures:

1. 7,449,000 workers were exposed to an 8-hour, time-weighted average (TWA) of 80 decibels (dB) or greater
2. 4,685,000 workers were exposed to a TWA of 85 dB or greater
3. 2,707,000 workers were exposed to a 8-hour TWA of 90 dB or greater
4. 1,164,990 workers were exposed to a TWA of 90 dB or greater, and
5. 407,000 were exposed to an 8-hour TWA of 100 dB or greater (see Table 27-1).

It is also estimated that if all industries complied with the 1983 OSHA hearing conservation amendment, 34% of the work force would be enrolled in a hearing conservation program.[2]

Noise-exposed workers often injure their hearing mechanisms before any problem is perceived. Workers can comfortably perform tasks in areas as loud as 95 dB. Sound does not become physically uncomfortable until approximately 120 dB. It is therefore incumbent for the physician who works in the primary care occupational setting to obtain a work history that includes noise exposure. Tinnitus, trouble understanding telephone conversations, difficulty understanding *ph, th,* and *p* sounds are all clues for the physician that a worker's ears may be injured from noise.

Noise-induced hearing loss is socially isolating and treatment modalities are inadequate at best; it is, however, for the most part preventable. Occupational medicine physicians should be at the forefront in preventing and diagnosing this disease. It is incumbent for the occupational medicine physician to ask patients about noise-induced hearing loss and to take a noise exposure history when indicated. If the history suggests hearing loss, the physician should obtain a screening audiogram and refer to the appropriate otologist.

This chapter will attempt to relate to the occupational physician a basic understanding of noise induced hearing loss so it will be both looked for and recognized in practice. Only if noise-induced hearing loss is recognized as a problem can the appropriate preventive steps be taken, including education of both the worker and company, promotion of hearing protection use, and, if necessary, aural amplification.

ANATOMY AND PHYSIOLOGY OF HEARING

The ear consists of three major parts—the external, middle, and inner ear. The external ear is made up of the auricle and external auditory meatus. The external auditory canal terminates at the tympanic membrane, which is also the border between the middle and outer ear (Fig. 27-1).

Sound waves enter the external meatus and strike the tympanic membrane. The vibration of the tympanic membrane against the malleolus (attached to the tympanic membrane) causes it to strike the incus that, in turn, strikes the stapes. The stapes then moves against the oval window, the entrance to the inner ear.

The ossicles of the middle ear increase the efficiency of sound transfer from air to liquid. Without the exact impedance matching of the ossicles, 99.9% of the sound energy would be reflected as the sound waves go from air in the middle ear to fluid in the inner ear. When the stapes strikes the oval window, the transfer of the sound energy from air to fluid is completed.

The oval window is the entrance to the inner ear. The inner ear consists of the bony and membranous labyrinth. The bony labyrinth, part of the temporal bone, has three parts—the vestibule, the cochlea, and the bony semicircular canals.

The vestibule is the central portion of the bony labyrinth. It contains the oval and round windows that are the openings to the middle ear. Also in this

Table 27-1 Percentage of noise-exposed workers for each industry within the manufacturing group

Manufacturing group	Estimated percentage of exposed workers				
	≥80 dB	≥85 dB	≥90 dB	≥95 dB	≥100 dB
Manufacturing (Total)	53.1	35.4	19.3	8.3	2.9
Food	47.0	28.0	16.0	6.0	1.0
Tobacco	28.0	10.0	7.0	3.0	1.0
Textiles	87.0	75.0	52.0	33.0	14.0
Apparel	20.0	1.0	0.0	0.0	0.0
Lumber and wood	97.0	94.0	72.0	35.0	8.0
Furniture	53.0	30.0	12.0	2.0	0.0
Paper	59.0	40.0	21.0	6.0	0.4
Printing	66.0	45.0	19.0	4.0	0.0
Chemicals	55.0	37.0	20.0	6.0	0.1
Petroleum	82.0	74.0	52.0	31.0	14.0
Rubber and plastic	40.0	20.0	9.0	2.0	0.3
Leather	20.0	1.0	0.0	0.0	0.0
Stone, clay and glass	42.0	16.0	5.0	2.0	1.0
Primary metals	81.0	63.0	38.0	20.0	0.8
Fabricated metals	56.0	34.0	19.0	11.0	4.0
Machines, nonelectric	48.0	26.0	13.0	6.0	3.0
Electric machines	27.0	7.0	2.5	0.5	0.1
Transportation equipment	42.0	23.0	13.0	7.0	3.0
Utilities	89.0	74.0	30.0	0.0	0.0

Used with permission, Franks JH, Numbers of workers exposed to occupational noise, *Seminars in Hearing* 9 (4): 291.

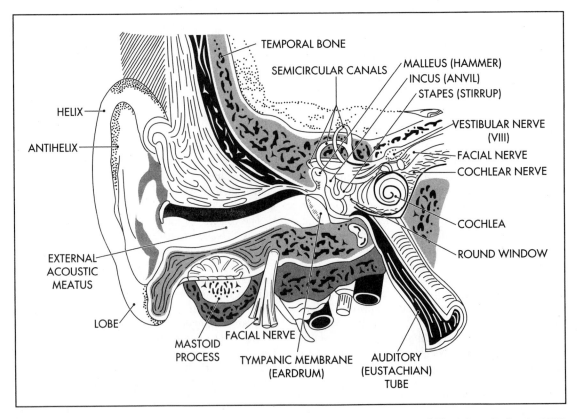

Fig. 27-1 Components of the ear. Used with permission, Thibodeau, GA: *Anatomy and Physiology,* St. Louis, 1987, Mosby-Year Book p 378.

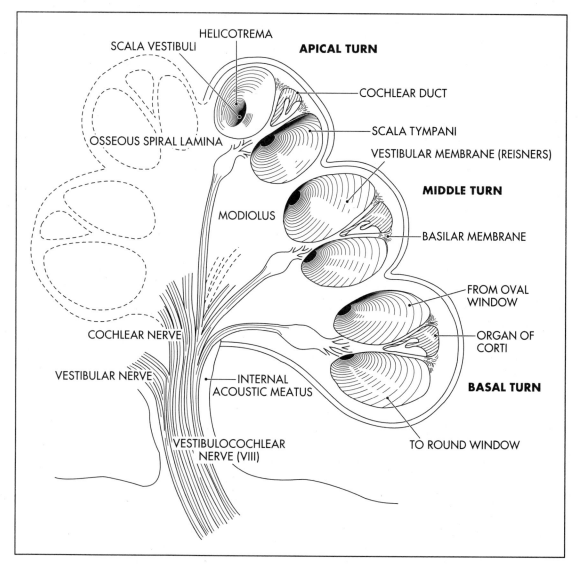

Fig. 27-2 Cross-section of the cochlea. Used with permission, Meyerhoff, W: *Diagnosis and Management of Hearing Loss,* Philadelphia, 1984, W.B. Saunders p 10.

portion of the labyrinth are the utricle, which contains endolymph, and the macula, the equilibrium sense organ.

The cochlea, located in the labyrinth, is the portion of the ear concerned with hearing. The membranous cochlear duct forms a shelf inside the bony cochlea that divides it into upper and lower sections. The upper section or scala vestibula is bounded by Reissner's or the vestibular membrane. The scala tympani is the lower section of the cochlear duct whose floor is the basilar membrane (Fig. 27-2).

The organ of Corti in the cochlea is the organ of hearing and contains approximately 17,000 hair cells. These sensory cells are bathed in endolymph and are bordered apically by the tectorial membrane. Surrounding the hair cells are the afferent sensory neurons of the cochlear nerve. The hair cells are arranged with the higher frequency sensitivities at the top and the lower frequency sensitivities at the bottom.

After the stapes strikes the oval window, waves are transmitted through Reisner's (vestibular) membrane to the endolymph inside the membranous cochlear duct. The fluid wave is transmitted to the organ of Corti and terminates at the round window. The fluid wave stimulates the hair cells, enabling the fluid energy to be transformed into electrical energy by the sensory afferent nerve fibers. How the movement of hair cells against the tectorial membrane stimulates the afferent dendrites of the auditory nerve is unclear, but it results in the nerve sending the auditory impulses to the brainstem and the temporal lobe of the brain.

COMMON TYPES OF HEARING LOSS

Primary care occupational medicine physicians should have a basic understanding of the types of hearing loss based on the anatomy and physiology.

Conductive hearing loss

Conductive hearing loss occurs when the transmission of sound waves from the outer ear to the inner ear is prevented. The defect can be in the external auditory canal from otitis externa, excess cerumen, or cholesteoma, a collection of dead skin cells that accumulate near the tympanic membrane and cause pressure erosions. The defect can be in the middle ear as a result of serous otitis or otosclerosis, an arthritis of the ossicles of the middle ear. Conductive hearing losses, unlike sensorineural hearing losses, are often readily correctable by antibiotics, antihistamines, and/or surgery.

Although cerumen is often implicated as a reason for conductive hearing loss, it is rarely a significant cause. If any part of the tympanic membrane is visualized on otoscopic exam, the hearing loss should not be attributed to cerumen. If the tympanic membrane is totally obscured by cerumen, then the cerumen should be removed. If the hearing loss completely resolves on audiometric testing, only then can one attribute the hearing loss to cerumen.

Industrial causes of conductive hearing loss include impulse noise after an explosion or a rise in baropressure during diving or an airplane descent. These events may cause tympanic membrane rupture along the anterioinferior quadrant or pars flaccida. A blow to the head can also cause a tympanic membrane rupture or hemotympanum (blood behind the tympanic membrane).

Impulse noise can cause a sudden temporary or permanent conductive hearing loss. The tympanic membrane can rupture at a sound pressure level of 180 dB. The ossicles of the middle ear can fracture, resulting in blood in the middle ear and loss of impedance matching of the ossicles. If severe enough, impulse noise can affect not only the conduction system, but the sensorineural system of the inner ear.

Another etiology of industrial-related conductive hearing loss is a tympanic membrane burn. During welding or soldering, a spark can hit the eardrum causing a severe burn. When this occurs, the entire tympanic membrane is usually destroyed and hearing loss can be as high as 60 dB. Oral antibiotics and an urgent referral to an ear, nose, and

throat (ENT) specialist is required. A myringoplasty is electively performed with almost total restoration of hearing. Ear protectors to prevent such burns should be mandatory in industries where such an accident is possible.

Foreign bodies that become lodged in the ear can be a source of conductive hearing loss and may be seen in an occupational setting. The worker will often complain of pain and irritation in the ear where the foreign body is lodged. Tinnitus may also be present. Removal of a foreign body from the ear is best performed by an otolaryngologist because the patient's total cooperation is required and the ear canal is sensitive. Without proper local anesthesia and appropriate tools, including a suction tip, a blunt hook, and a small alligator forceps, an inexperienced physician can rupture the tympanic membrane and dislocate the bones of the middle ear.

Sensorineural hearing loss

Sensorineural hearing loss is a broad term that includes any hearing loss that is due to a failure of the inner ear or auditory nerve. Unlike conductive hearing loss, it is difficult to pinpoint the precise cause of the hearing loss anatomically because the cochlea is extremely small and intricate.

The causes of sensorineural hearing loss are many, but the most common causes include presbycusis (the hearing loss of old age), infections (including meningitis), ototoxic drugs, hereditary factors, and, of course, noise-induced hearing loss either from occupational or nonoccupational causes.

Noise and noise-induced hearing loss (NIHL)

Noise is generally defined as discordant or unwanted sound. Noise is not only a nuisance problem but, depending on its intensity and duration, it is also a health hazard. Among its other effects, noise can irreversibly damage the inner ear. Although the noise a person experiences at work is probably the most common cause of noise-induced hearing loss, there is nothing particularly special about industrial noise. Other nonindustrial noise sources such as rock concerts, portable radios with headsets turned up too loud, hunting, and carpentry can contribute significantly to noise-induced hearing loss.

There is a wide variation in an individual's susceptibility to hearing loss from noise. There is also disagreement among experts on the threshold intensity level for significant speech frequency hearing loss caused by noise (anywhere from 85-92 dB). There is no doubt, however, that the higher the intensity and the longer the duration of exposure to that high intensity noise, the more likely and profound the hearing loss. Frequency is also an element in noise-induced hearing loss. It is believed that lower frequency sounds are less damaging to the inner ear then higher frequency sounds.

When the sound is loud enough and prolonged enough, changes take place in the ear mechanism itself. One of the first is a temporary threshold shift that occurs when the auditory threshold increases after an exposure to noise. If the exposure to noise is not too prolonged or loud, the hearing loss will return to the person's baseline usually within 12 to 24 hours. It is believed that a temporary threshold shift is due to edema or to a metabolic disturbance to the hair cells that eventually recover as the sensory input to the hair cells decreases after a person removes himself from noise. A permanent threshold shift occurs when the person's sensory hair cells do not recover from the acoustic insult, resulting in permanent hearing loss at the frequency affected. A permanent threshold shift signifies loss of sensory hair cells at a particular frequency.

Noise does not affect all frequencies equally. Noise damages the higher frequencies especially at 3000, 4000, and 6000 hertz (Hz). Small but measurable hearing threshold losses can be demonstrated in persons exposed to continuous noise of 80 dB over time. A 10 dB threshold loss at 3000, 4000, and 6000 Hz is typical when a person is exposed to 85 dB of continuous noise for 8 hours over years. With exposure to 90 dB, a 20 dB threshold drop typically occurs at the above frequencies, but even at that sound level the speech frequencies of 500, 1000, and 2000 Hz are not affected.[4]

What are the hallmarks of noise-induced hearing loss?

As stated previously, noise-induced hearing loss presents with a permanent threshold shift in the higher frequency ranges. As a result a person will complain that although speech may be heard, it is often not readily understood. Consonants are mainly high-frequency sounds (Fig. 27-3), and a person with NIHL may have difficulty distinguishing between the sounds, *p, t, th,* and *ph.* A telephone has less fidelity at the higher frequency ranges, so this same person may have difficulty understanding telephone conversations.

Noise-induced hearing loss also causes a phenomenon called recruitment. Recruitment occurs when the loudness of the noise perceived increases more rapidly after exceeding that person's auditory threshold. This perception of loudness in the hearing impaired ear is much greater than the perception of loudness in the normal ear. The phenomenon of recruitment can impede the use of au-

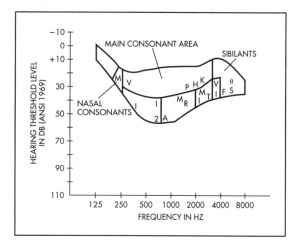

Fig. 27-3 Part of audiogram indicating area of conversational speech and levels at which specific sounds are heard. Used with permission, from Noise and Hearing Loss, *Postgraduate Medicine,* p. 120, permission through Mayo Foundation.

ral amplification for people with noise-induced hearing loss. Amplified sound will often be perceived as unpleasant and flat.

People with NIHL may also experience paracusis. Paracusis is a shift in pitch that occurs when a specific frequency of hair cells on the basilar membrane of the cochlea is totally destroyed. When this specific pitch enters the cochlea, the hair cells that are closest in frequency to that pitch will act as the sensory receiver. When a wide frequency range of hair cells is damaged, many frequencies will be perceived at the same pitch. Aural amplification cannot mitigate paracusis, but selective compression amplification may be of some benefit if some hair cells in a particular frequency survive.

Tinnitus, a buzzing or ringing in the ear, is another consequence of NIHL. The cause of tinnitus is not known, but noise-related tinnitus is always accompanied by a hearing loss in that ear.

Occupational-related noise-induced hearing loss

As one moves from NIHL in general to occupational-related NIHL, certain characteristics must be kept in mind.

The first concept is asymptotic hearing loss. This means that a specific job will induce a maximum degree of hearing loss that is unique and reproducible in different individuals. For example, jack hammer operators develop a severe high frequency loss but rarely develop significant low frequency loss. Workers in the weaving industries usually develop no greater than a 40 dB loss in the speech frequencies. Employees exposed to 92 dB of noise rarely experience greater than a 20 dB loss in the lower frequencies.[4]

Intermittent noise may have different effects on the inner ear than does continuous noise. Those exposed to high intensity intermittent noise experience mainly high frequency loss. The speech frequencies do not become affected even after many years.

Industrial noise-induced hearing loss is bilateral. If the hearing loss is due to noise, there should not be a significant asymmetry in auditory thresholds between the two ears. On audiometric testing, if an employee has a substantial hearing difference in one ear compared with the other, a nonoccupational source needs to be investigated. In rifle-shooting, for example, the ear closest to the barrel sustains more hearing loss than the other, which also sustains hearing loss.

Occupational hearing loss develops gradually over the first few years of exposure and worsens maximally over 8 to 10 years. Occupational NIHL hearing loss usually does not progress significantly after 10 years of exposure. After 4 or 5 years of continuous noise exposure, a worker who does not develop high-frequency hearing loss is unlikely to develop progressive hearing loss from noise.

Employees with occupational hearing loss generally have good speech discrimination scores in quiet environments, often 75% or better. If an employee complaining of NIHL tests low on speech discrimination, other causes of hearing loss must be sought.[4]

Industrial hygiene data is crucial to evaluate NIHL. Without data, it is often impossible to determine whether a worker was exposed to enough noise to account for the hearing loss. A perception of working in a noisy environment is not confirmation that one has worked in an environment that is noisy enough to damage the inner ear. Certain occupations by definition, however, have severe exposure to noise. Jack hammer workers, riveters, and sheet metal workers are only a few occupations that by their very nature a physician can assume noise of sufficient intensity and duration to produce hearing loss.

OSHA mandated an 85 dB 8-hour, time-weighted average for workers as the action level for hearing conservation programs in industry. As previously stated, exposure to that action level will not cause debilitating hearing loss in the speech frequencies. If an employee presents with severe hearing loss in the speech frequencies, other causes for the hearing loss must also be explored.

HISTORY AND PHYSICAL EXAMINATION IN NIHL

It is important to take a good history. Even when noise has been implicated in the hearing loss, other factors may play a role. Presbycusis, hobbies, exposure to ototoxic drugs, and viruses, to name a few, can complicate what at first appears to be a straightforward case of NIHL.

A physician should ask certain standard questions of anyone who presents to the office with hearing loss. The answers to will give the physician diagnostic clues as to the etiology of the hearing loss.

The physician needs to know whether the hearing loss is unilateral or bilateral and whether the hearing loss is stable or fluctuates over time. It is important to know if the onset was sudden and whether the hearing is getting worse. The physician needs to know whether the patient can hear better in a noisy or quiet environment. A history of tinnitus is important to elicit because it may also be a diagnostic clue. A history of taking ototoxic medication must also be sought (Table 27-2).

Previous infections including frequent episodes of otitis media as a child, meningitis, viral infections, and previous ear surgery may give important diagnostic clues. A systemic disease history for entities such as diabetes, hypothyroidism, vascular disease, hypertension, and hyperlipidemia that may affect hearing should be obtained. A history of previous trauma especially to the head must also be sought. Stroke, multiple sclerosis, and

Table 27-2 Medications causing hearing loss

Aminoglycoside antibiotics	
Gentamicin	Kanamycin
Neomycin	Streptomycin
Amikacin	Tobramycin
Other antibiotics	
Erythromycin	Vancomycin
Analgesics/Antiinflammatories	
Aspirin	NSAIs
Loop diuretics	
Furosemide	Ethacrynic acid
Antineoplastics	
Cisplatin	Bleomycin
Mechlorethamine	Methotrexate
Others	
Chloroquine	Quinidine

Used with permission, Brechtelbauer, DA: Adult hearing loss in Volt, BH, editor: *Primary care: disorders of the ears, nose, and throat,* 17:2, p 251, Philadelphia, 1990, WB Saunders.

other central nervous system (CNS) disorders may also affect hearing.

In addition, a careful noise history is crucial. The patient should be questioned about occupational noise, and a thorough recreational noise history should be taken that includes exposure to rock music, wood working, hunting, etc. Portable radios with headsets or those held close to the ear can also contribute significantly to NIHL.

If the patient has a history of significant recreational gun use, one must ask about hearing protection. If appropriate ear protection is worn when shooting, the contribution of guns to the hearing loss is minimal. If a rifle is used, it is important to know which shoulder is used to support the rifle. Knowing this information may help account for some but not all of the asymmetry seen between the left and right ears on audiogram.

Although the contribution of recreational noise exposure is important (for example a rock concert can routinely measure sound levels at 99 dB or greater), it must be emphasized that the length of exposure may not be cumulatively long enough to result in significant hearing loss compared with the daily exposure at work. If one has a second job with significant noise exposure or spends considerable time at noisy hobbies, those experiences should be factored in when determining the cause of the hearing loss.

The employment history is extremely important. By asking about an employee's noisiest job and the duration of that job, a physician can often estimate the degree of noise exposure (Table 27-1). Included in the employment history is whether and what type of ear protection was used. If ear protection was worn, the physician needs to ascertain whether it was worn consistently or sporadically. The type of ear protection worn is also important because different types of ear protection have different attenuation factors. The physician must also question whether the ear protection devices were well maintained and worn properly. Ear muff seals can crack with age and decrease in effectiveness. Earplugs must be inserted properly for maximum attenuation. (See Chapter 34, Personal Protective Equipment.)

Lastly, if the patient has been exposed to impulse noise, it is important to identify any complaint of vertigo. Although dizziness is not a common complaint, true vertigo is.

Why are these questions important? The history helps direct the primary care physician and specialist regarding further testing and often allows the physician to determine whether the hearing loss is work-related. For example, sudden hearing loss can be caused by Ménière's disease, mumps, explosions with rupture of the round window, or even an acoustic neuroma. NIHL, presbycusis, hereditary nerve deafness, and otosclerosis often occur gradually.

Certain disease processes are also known to cause deafness. Cytomegalovirus, measles, herpes, scarlet fever, mononucleosis, and mycoplasma pneumoniae have been associated with both a sudden or a gradually progressive hearing loss. Fungal and bacterial meningitis may cause deafness but viral meningitis rarely causes such problems. Systemic diseases such as sarcoid, tuberculosis (TB), syphillis, and rheumatoid arthritis can also cause hearing loss.

Allergies can be associated with a conductive hearing loss, especially in children (serous otitis media). Hyperlipoproteinemia may be responsible for a fluctuating hearing loss that is sensorineural in pattern but mainly in the lower speech frequencies. An increase in lipids can be associated with several systemic diseases that include diabetes, hypothyroidism, and obesity. High-frequency hearing loss can also be found in renal failure.

Patients with advanced atherosclerosis and a history of myocardial infarction have a higher incidence of high-frequency hearing loss than the rest of the population. It is believed that this hearing loss may be due to problems with the blood supply to the inner ear. Stroke can cause deafness, as can multiple sclerosis, which may first manifest itself as high-frequency bilateral hearing loss.

Ototoxic drugs are common. It is therefore important to get a complete drug history from each patient. An entity called streptomycin-induced hypersensitivity is genetically determined. In sensitized persons, even small doses of streptomycin can cause hearing loss.

Fluctuating hearing loss may point to Ménière's syndrome. A person hearing better in a noisy environment probably has a conductive hearing loss. If the patient hears better in quiet areas, a sensorineural hearing loss is the more likely choice. Tinnitus and vertigo can point to Ménière's disease. Tinnitus alone can point to NIHL.

The history is essential for the differential diagnosis of hearing loss because there are many etiologies of hearing loss and some are correctable. Therefore, an accurate diagnosis is critical.

PHYSICAL EXAMINATION IN NOISE-INDUCED HEARING LOSS

A primary care physician with an otoscope and tuning fork can obtain basic information regarding the possible etiologies of the hearing loss.

Otoscopy should be carefully done in all cases

to see whether any structural abnormality may be contributing to the hearing loss. The tympanic membrane should be examined for perforation, retraction, or signs of tympanosclerosis. In impulse noise, one should look for blood or fluid behind the tympanic membrane. The primary care physician should be familiar with the pneumatic otoscope to test the mobility of the tympanic membrane.

A nasal exam should also be performed. One should note the state of the mucous membranes and whether there is any purulent discharge. The mouth should be examined; however, information obtained from the examination of the mouth is usually more helpful if the patient has ear pain. The thyroid should be palpated. If tinnitus is a complaint, one should auscultate the carotid arteries.

A tuning fork can give the primary care occupational physician an idea of the extent of hearing loss and whether the hearing loss is conductive or sensorineural. At best, however, a tuning fork can only diagnose a hearing loss that is at least 25 dB. Otherwise, the test is not sensitive.

To test for hearing, the physician strikes the tuning fork until it can barely be heard and puts it next to the patient's bad ear. If the patient cannot hear it, the physician puts the tuning fork next to the good ear. Afterwards, the physician listens to the tuning fork to make sure that it is still vibrating and audible.

Air conduction is tested by placing the vibrating tuning fork near but not touching the pinna of the ear. Bone conduction is tested by placing the tuning fork on the mastoid, forehead, or incisor, thereby bypassing the middle ear.

The physician will want to determine whether a patient's hearing loss is conductive or sensorineural. Screening audiometry will not differentiate between the two because it relies on air conduction only. The Rinne test however can help the physician differentiate between the two.

A tuning fork (either a 1024 Hz or perhaps a 2048 Hz) should be struck in such a way that the patient hears it well. The physician then moves the tuning fork back and forth between the pinna and mastoid bone until the patient is able to discriminate in which position the tone is louder. If the tone is louder on the mastoid, the patient has a conductive defect. If, on physical examination, the external auditory canal and tympanic membrane appear normal, the problem is probably with the ossicles. One should repeat the process with the opposite ear.

The Weber test is used to confirm the findings of the Rinne test. The tuning fork is struck and placed on the center of the patient's head. The sound will lateralize to the ear with the conductive hearing loss.

The Schwabach test is less commonly known. One strikes a tuning fork and places it on the mastoid bone by the ear with the hearing loss. Then the tester puts the tuning fork on his own mastoid bone. A person with a conductive hearing loss will hear the tone longer on the mastoid bone than will a person without such a loss.

These simple tests with a tuning fork can also help differentiate between sensorineural hearing loss and a conductive defect. A patient with a sensorineural hearing loss will hear better with air conduction rather than bone conduction. During the Weber test, the sound will lateralize to the patient's good ear rather than the one with the loss. The physician will hear the tone on the mastoid bone longer than will the patient with a sensorineural loss during the Schwabach test.

Despite the usefulness of the tuning fork tests, it is sometimes difficult to determine the patient's exact type of hearing loss. That is why more advanced testing is always required either to determine or confirm the patient's type of hearing loss.

ADDITIONAL TESTING
Audiometry

Screening audiometry is the backbone test for the clinical occupational specialist. A basic understanding of the audiometer and interpretation of its results is essential to help diagnose occupational NIHL.

The audiometer gives quantifiable information of a patient's response to different pure tone sounds at varying intensities. Hearing levels are usually tested from 250 to 8000 Hz. At a given frequency is a hearing threshold that is the number of decibels the patient hears above the 0 threshold reference for that particular frequency. Audiometers are calibrated so that 0 dB corresponds to the reference threshold. (This threshold is calculated by averaging the hearing thresholds at each frequency of young adults with normal hearing). A normal auditory threshold result at any given frequency on audiometeric testing is anywhere from 0 to 25 dB.

Audiometry screening is an air conduction test only. Bone conduction audiometry is beyond the scope of the primary care occupational medicine physician and should be performed by trained audiologists only. Screening audiometry can only determine that a hearing impairment exists. It cannot determine the type of hearing impairment.

When performing screening audiometry, it is essential that the audiometer is in good working order and meets American National Standards Institute (ANSI) standards. The audiometer must produce pure tones and sound pressure levels within certain specified standard deviations. The type of earphones used during testing should meet the specifications of the brand of audiometer used. Substitute earphones may result in an inaccurate audiogram.

Two basic types of audiograms are available today. One is manual, the other is automatic. The automatic audiometer is programmed to take the patient through the different testing frequencies and auditory thresholds. With today's computer chips, the automatic audiometer is a highly valid way of testing and is recommended for screening tests in most occupational medicine facilities.

An audiometer is just a machine and screening audiometry is just a test. Its validity depends on the accuracy of the audiometer, the testing site, and the tester. The machine must be biologically calibrated for validity either by a device created for such a purpose or by a person who is known to have normal stable hearing preferably before testing is performed each day. The audiometer must be calibrated yearly to check the accuracy of the frequency and the validity of sound pressure levels. An exhaustive calibration should be performed every 5 years.

Where the screening test takes place is crucial. A hearing booth is essential and it should be placed in a quiet area, away from any loud or distracting noises that will affect the outcome of the test. If the area is not quiet, the conditions will not allow a test that accurately reflect the patient's hearing status or threshold shifts.

It is also important that the person who performs audiometeric testing be familiar with the machine and be certified. Certification is provided through courses approved by the Council for Accreditation in Occupational Hearing Conservation. These courses are approximately 20 hours long and focus on pure tone audiometric testing and basic hearing principles. Certification is recognized by OSHA and tests performed by certified technicians stand up legally before the Workers' Compensation Appeals Board. More important, however, is the fact that without appropriate training on potential problems with the audiometer or the test itself, factors that may help the interpreter understand the validity of test results will never come to light. An untrained or poorly trained technician can therefore greatly affect the accuracy of these tests.

Bone conduction audiometry

Bone conduction audiometry is similar to air conduction audiometry, but the test bypasses the middle ear by placing a vibrator behind the ear.

A complex noise is placed next to the nontest

ear to prevent it from aiding the test ear (masking). One needs to mask the good ear especially when hearing between the two ears differs significantly. Bone conduction audiometry then proceeds in the same way as the air conduction test, with the vibrator rather than pure tones. Different auditory threshold values in the air and bone audiometric tests (such as a better hearing test with bone conduction than with air conduction) signifies an air-bone gap, which represents a conductive hearing loss.

If the audiogram is abnormal on air conduction audiometry and corrects to normal on bone conduction, the hearing loss is a pure conductive defect. If the audiogram shows no difference between air and bone conduction, the hearing loss is sensorineural. In the mixed type of hearing loss, there is an improvement in hearing during bone conduction but the hearing does not return to normal. This is called mixed hearing impairment and indicates both conductive and sensorineural problems.

Speech reception threshold test

A speech reception threshold test uses a speech audiometer and quantifies the decibel level at which speech is understood. A live or recorded voice recites each spondee (two-syllable words spoken with equally accented syllables such as "birthday," "eardrum," and "sunset"). The patient is asked to repeat the words after each one is presented. A normal hearing person has a speech reception threshold at anywhere from 0 to 10 dB. It is at this decibel level that a normal hearing person will get at least 50% of the spondees correct. A speech reception threshold score of 25 dB or less usually means there is no benefit in wearing aural amplification. Above the 25 dB auditory threshold for speech reception, hearing aids may be beneficial.

The speech reception threshold test results should mirror the pure tone audiogram. Discrepancies between the two tests can be caused by a patient's problem with discrimination or emotional state.

Word recognition or discrimination testing

Word recognition or discrimination testing determines if a given patient can discriminate complex sounds. A patient is asked to repeat a word that is presented at a 30 to 40 dB range. These words, spoken through a microphone, are 5 monosyllabic and phonetically balanced words. Examples include "twins," "day," "toe," and "low." Two points are given for each correct answer. A person with normal hearing should be able to repeat 90% to 100% of these words correctly.

Discrimination testing does not give a clinical

indication of a person's speech discrimination in a noisy atmosphere. Speech discrimination always deteriorates in that environment because noise masks consonants. If a person demonstrates a profound speech discrimination loss under ideal testing conditions, other causes for the hearing loss should be sought. Mίeniìere's disease and acoustic neuroma are two conditions that will produce a profound loss in word recognition.

Brainstem and cortical-evoked response tests

Both brainstem and cortical-evoked response tests are rarely used in occupational NIHL except when malingering is suspected. Neither test requires the patient's cooperation. The first test measures electrical activity at the brainstem level while cerebrocortical auditory response measures electrical activity at the cerebral cortex along the auditory pathway. These tests are helpful in locating a lesion in the auditory pathway. These tests can aid in diagnosing an acoustic neuroma or a demyelinating illness such as multiple sclerosis.

Other tests

Other audiometric tests that are useful but beyond the scope of this chapter are impedance audiometry including tympanometry (which is similar to pneumatic otoscopy); static compliance (which measures the acoustic reflex compliance of the middle ear); and the stapedius reflex. The acoustic reflex decay test helps to determine whether there is a retrocochlear tumor such as an acoustic neuroma.

DIAGNOSIS OF OCCUPATIONAL-RELATED NIHL

The patient needs to give a history consistent with continuous exposure to noise at a significant intensity. The patient will often complain of tinnitus, will state that the hearing loss came on gradually, and often will complain of difficulty understanding people on the telephone and in noisy environments. The patient also may complain of difficulty understanding young children. The patient may have problems with comprehending the sibilant consonants such as "f" and "s" (Fig. 27-3). With impulse noise, a patient may complain of a unilateral hearing loss when the intensity of the noise is relatively mild. If the noise is intense enough, the patient will complain of hearing loss in both ears. Vertigo is also a relatively common complaint.

In continuous NIHL, the physical examination of the ears, nose, and throat is typically normal unless other nonnoise-related factors contribute to the hearing loss. In impulse noise, the physical findings can range from a mild injection of the tympanic membrane to hemotympanum. The tym-

panic membrane can be intact; can have a small rupture at the pars flaccida; or can have a complete rupture with fracture of the middle ear ossicles.

On pure tone audiogram, the hearing loss at the speech frequencies is usually minimal with a drop in auditory threshold levels at 3000 and 4000 Hz. In a classic NIHL audiogram, some recovery at the higher frequencies of 6000 and 8000 Hz will be noted (Fig. 27-3).

Although all occupational NIHL literature discusses the 4000 Hz dip, this dip is not unique for NIHL. The 4000 Hz frequency is vulnerable in many disease entities that can cause hearing loss. Examples include viral infections such as respiratory viruses, herpes, mumps, measles, and CMV. Skull trauma, hereditary hearing loss, ototoxicity, and even acoustic neuroma may also initially manifest as a 4000 Hz dip.[3] The audiogram is not the gold standard; there is no substitute for a good history. Only with a history of noise exposure of sufficient duration and intensity can a 4000 Hz dip on audiogram be attributed to industrial noise.

Presbycusis or hearing loss as a result of aging may also complicate the picture. Many patients that present with the possibility of noise-induced hearing loss are over 50 years of age. Presbycusis is the most common form of hearing loss and is prevalent in the possible NIHL age group. Presbycusis can often be distinguished from NIHL because the higher frequencies of 6000 and 8000 Hz are affected first, rather than the 3000 and 4000 Hz typical of NIHL.

With presbycusis, the greatest auditory threshold losses on audiogram should be at 6000 and 8000 Hz. There is typically no 4000 Hz dip with recovery at 6000 and 8000 Hz. When interpreting audiograms on patients with a good noise exposure history and an auditory threshold loss at 3000 Hz with no recovery at 6000 Hz or upwards, one must consider the possibility of presbycusis as the contributing factor. Further complicating the picture is the fact that some people with prebycusis initially lose their hearing at 4000 to 6000 Hz. These patients have an audiogram consistent with NIHL. As always, the history is paramount to help distinguish the two entities.

What other problems confront the evaluating physician when diagnosing occupational-related NIHL?

One particularly vexing problem is that many employees will not have had a baseline audiogram. The hearing conservation amendment was not enacted until 1983, so many companies with significant industrial noise problems did not initiate a hearing conservation program until then. Some employees may have worked for a company for 20 years or more without audiometric testing or adequate hearing protection. It is up to the evaluating physician to make the best guess regarding that employee's baseline audiogram, based on the history. The physician also needs to determine whether the audiograms truly reflect noise induced hearing loss or hearing loss from some other etiology.

Audiometry performed in the industrial setting may not have been taken under ideal testing conditions. Often employees were exposed to significant noise within 12 hours before the audiograms were taken, undermining the test's validity. Noise standards for both the booth and the room are often exceeded and may falsify true test results.

NIHL is not progressive. The physician must determine which audiograms are valid and reliable and which are not. To properly interpret audiograms, the physician needs to know when an employee retired or was moved to a quiet environment. Any increase in hearing loss after retirement or transfer is unrelated to occupational exposure.

In cases of asymmetric hearing loss, the physician must make a reasoned estimate if the asymmetry is due to work conditions or other causes. For example, a fire engineer who drives the fire engine has one ear closer to the engine exhaust, air horns, and sirens. Asymmetry in noise levels between the two ears may help explain different auditory thresholds in the fire engineer's left and right ears. However, asymmetry in hearing loss can be due to nonindustrial causes such as an acoustic neuroma.

Diagnostic clues that may aid the physician include asymmetric hearing loss caused by noise, a condition in which the auditory threshold loss of the poorer ear should mirror the audiometric auditory threshold pattern of the better one. Also, differences in auditory thresholds should not be extreme. For example, one ear should not have moderate hearing loss while the other ear exhibits severe hearing loss. The exception to this rule may occur when the asymmetry in hearing loss is due to an explosion. It is essential to take a complete history and make a complete diagnostic evaluation in asymmetric hearing loss.

When baseline preplacement and retirement or termination audiograms are available and the audiograms and noise exposure history are consistent with NIHL, the diagnosis of NIHL is easy. When the testing is consistent with a mixed conductive sensorineural-picture, however, there can be many different reasons for the hearing loss. It is up to the physician to make the best judgment on the basis of known facts and established norms for hearing loss based on age, occupation, and other factors. Of course in any complicated hearing loss case a referral to an ENT specialist with experience in occupational hearing loss is indicated.

Once it is determined that occupational-related hearing loss has occurred, the American Academy of Otolaryngology has devised a formula to determine the percentage of disability that has occurred from the hearing loss. The formula uses the frequencies of 500, 1000, 2000, and 3000 Hz to determine disability. In the workers' compensation system, states use different formulas to determine the percentage disability. Unless the primary care occupational physician has a special interest in occupational NIHL, disability determination should be made by an ENT specialist after appropriate audiologic testing. Disability status is allowed only if there is substantial impairment in the speech frequencies. In California, for example, there is no reward for disability in the frequencies 4000 Hz and above.

Sataloff and Sataloff, in *Occupational Hearing Loss,* state that NIHL is not occupational unless seven criteria are met.[4]

1. The hearing loss must be sensorineural with damage chiefly to the cochlear cells.
2. The patient must have a history of long-term exposure to intense noise levels sufficient to cause the degree and pattern of hearing loss evident in audiologic findings.
3. The hearing loss must develop gradually over a period of years.
4. The hearing loss must have developed over the first 8 to 10 years of exposure.
5. The hearing loss must initially have started in the higher frequencies (generally 3000 to 6000 Hz) and be almost equal in both ears. (This rule may not be true if the noise source is consistently directed to one ear over another, but both ears should show some hearing loss).
6. Speech discrimination scores, even with substantial high frequency losses, are generally good (over 75%).
7. The hearing loss should stabilize if the patient is removed from the noise exposure.

TREATMENT OF OCCUPATIONAL HEARING LOSS
Impulse noise

Hearing loss as a result of impulse noise will gradually improve over days. Any hearing loss that persists over several weeks should be considered a permanent hearing loss. In most cases of acoustic trauma or impulse noise, however, the hearing returns to normal over several hours or days. If the intensity of the noise is great enough, the actual auditory nerve fibers will be permanently affected.

Patients with significant acoustic trauma should be removed from noise so that hearing will recover. The physician must prevent patient exposure to noise after an explosion. The ear is already fatigued and further noise could permanently damage the hearing apparatus.

Most perforations caused by impulse noise heal spontaneously. Nose blowing should be avoided as much as possible to prevent further rupture from an increase in pressure. Some perforations heal without scarring; others leave thick white scars. These scars do not produce measurable hearing loss, and any hearing loss in such an individual should not be attributed to the scarring.

Perforations should not be closed until the middle ear is free of infection and dry for at least several months. The perforation can be closed by the ENT specialist either by cauterization or myringoplasty.

In patients who sustain a hemotympanum after impulse noise, myringotomy and suction are usually unnecessary. The ear has remarkable ability to clear itself. A myringotomy may introduce infection. One should refer all cases of hemotympanium to the otolaryngologist because there can be disruption of the ossicles of the middle ear that may not be immediately obvious.

In general, if there are any structural abnormalities in the ear or if a worker sustains a significant hearing loss, an urgent referral to an otolaryngologist is appropriate.

Continuous noise

Once a permanent threshold shift has occurred, hearing will not recover. Prevention is the key because treatment is inadequate.

Engineering controls are essential to protect an employee's ear from hearing loss. Muffling engines, placing covers over noisy machines, maintaining equipment, substituting quieter machines, and reducing the vibration of a machine are only a few ways that a noisy environment can be made less so, even below the damaging frequencies of 85 to 90 dB.

The occupational physician, however, can only work with a company and an industrial hygiene team to suggest these types of controls. Realistically, the physician often has little influence on engineering controls in a company. It is therefore important to educate noise-exposed employees about hearing loss before it happens and, once hearing loss has manifested itself, prevent further progression. Because a substantial amount of hearing loss occurs before the employee is even aware that the loss has occurred, it is incumbent on the physician,

as part of a hearing conservation program, to talk to each employee after reviewing audiograms that demonstrate early NIHL.

The conference should include more than handing out pamphlets on NIHL. The physician should sit down with the employee, explain the repercussions of not protecting the ear from noise both in and out of the workplace and stress the importance of wearing ear protection. The physician should have a basic familiarity with the different types of hearing protection so recommendations can be made. If an employee is not wearing hearing protection, the physician should find out why. Complaints about hearing protection usually include the employee's stated inability to hear with protection, problems with discomfort, or the development of otitis externa with the use of earplugs. Alternatives are available.

The physician or occupational health nurse should educate the employee on the signs of early hearing loss, including episodes of tinnitus with hearing loss (a temporary threshold shift), difficulty in hearing high pitched sounds, understanding telephone conversations, or hearing in noisy environments.

Having hearing-impaired employees from the same industry talk to an employee group is extremely effective. Those employees will speak of the problems of being hearing-impaired and the social isolation that is often the result of such a loss in a way that is more effective than a health professional's admonitions.

The physician also should talk to family members about the patient's hearing loss. Family members can aid a hearing-impaired person's comprehension by using appropriate visual cues and other methods. For example, a person talking to a hearing-impaired person should keep the hands away from the face so the hearing-impaired person can take advantage of lip reading. The pace should be moderate, and the speaker should pause at the end of sentences. Pointing to an object or the person of discussion is also helpful. When the hearing-impaired person cannot comprehend the meaning of the sentence, one should change the words to convey the same meaning rather than shouting or repeating the same words. To get the attention of the hearing-impaired person, one should start a sentence with her name rather than placing the name at the end of the sentence, such as "Paul, how are you?"[1]

The hearing-impaired person should tell people that she has a problem and stand in front of the person to watch for visual clues. If she goes to a restaurant a quiet table should be requested. The hearing-impaired person should sit both at a restaurant or at meetings so she faces as many

Table 27-3 Hints for communicating with the hearing impaired

For the speaker
  Provide good visual contact: stand still, face the patient, keep hands away from face
  Reduce background noise
  Use pointing and gestures
  Speak at a moderate rate and volume
  Pause at end of sentences
  Inform the person of changes in the topic
  If you are not understood, change your wording rather than repeating
  Avoid appearing frustrated
  Use portable amplification
For the hearing-impaired person
  Watch the speaker's face for clues
  Be assertive, let people know what makes conversation better and worse for you

Used with permission, Brechtelbauer, DA: Adult hearing loss in Vogt, BH, editor: *Primary care: disorders of the ears, nose, and throat* 17:2, p 259, Philadelphia, 1990, WB Saunders.

speakers as possible. The hearing-impaired person should always have as few auditory distractions as possible. For example, conversations should not be attempted with the television or radio on (Table 27-3).[1]

When the hearing loss is significant in the speech frequencies, aural amplification can be recommended. Hearing aids do not restore hearing, so realistic expectations about them are important. The hearing-impaired employee must understand the limitations of such aids.

Different types of hearing aids are beyond the scope of this book; however, a primary care occupational medicine physician should have the names of reputable hearing aid specialists. Hearing aids can be adjusted for frequency response, output limitations, and gain settings. For maximum effectiveness, a hearing aid's frequency response needs to be set by a formula that is based on the patient's audiogram.

Also available are assisted listening devices including telephone aids that increase the acoustic intensity of the telephone signal, devices that allow the person to know when the doorbell or telephone rings, selective amplification of the audio portion of the television signal, and receivers for hearing impaired people at meetings, theater, and other events.

HEARING PROTECTION

The physician needs to educate all employees who are at risk for NIHL about hearing protectors. There are basically two types, each with its own advantages and disadvantages.

Hearing protection reduces noise levels so the intensity reaching the ear will be at safe levels. First and foremost, hearing protection must provide adequate attenuation. If adequate attenuation can not be achieved by one type of device, two different types of devices (such as earplugs and muffs), may be necessary to protect the ear from hearing loss.

Insert-type hearing protectors (earplugs) are easily portable and do not interfere with eyeglasses, safety helmets, and other equipment. Most people find them comfortable and they are ideal for work in confined spaces. The disadvantages include that they need to be inserted properly for maximum attenuation, and they can only be inserted into a healthy ear canal. Canals must be free of eczema and infection. Because earplugs are not readily visible when worn, it is difficult for the supervisor to monitor compliance.

Ear muffs can be worn even if the employee has otitis media. Muffs are easier than earplugs to put on correctly, and they can be seen at a distance so the supervisor can monitor compliance. Ear muffs are bulky and hot, however, and they cost more than most earplugs. The attenuation factor is reduced by wear and tear and deliberate bending of the frame. They can also become loose when someone is talking or chewing.

Many non–hearing-impaired workers also do not accept the concept that, with hearing protection, speech discrimination actually improves in a noisy environment. This is because speech-to-noise ratios are kept constant and the protected inner ear hair cells do not fatigue. With lower overall noise levels, the ear will not distort the speech perceived.

Hearing protectors reduce both the noise and voice levels so the ear can operate more efficiently. With hearing protection, speech is dulled in a quiet environment but not in noisy environments. The physician needs to convince the employee that one's speech discrimination will be more acute with hearing protection than without it.

Hearing protective devices and potential medical problems

Every worker's ear should be visually inspected before hearing-protective devices are issued. Medical problems that may preclude a worker from wearing hearing protection include ear tenderness or inflammation, sores externally or in the ear canal, eczema of the pinna or of the canal, and any congenital or surgical malformations of the external ear. The physician or other health professional should note cerumen impaction and/or excessive cerumen. Although it is widely believed that earplugs increase cerumen production and the possibility of impaction, there are few studies on the effects of earplugs on cerumen formation.

Although good hygiene and routine cleaning of ear protection to prevent ear infection is a good general policy, there is no good epidemiologic data linking the use of hearing-protective devices and otitis externa or infections of the pinna.

The physician or other health professional should never assume that ear irritation or infection is caused by the patient wearing hearing protective devices. A good history is essential. Other causes of ear infections include swimming, hot tub use, water skiing, excessive scratching or picking at the ear with cotton applicators or bobby pins, and various causes of dermatitis unrelated to hearing protection use.

When hearing protection is implicated, caustic or irritative materials contaminating the muffs or earplugs are often the problem. Foreign material from the workplace can get caught in the protective device. Irritation from the concrete, fiberglass, acid, coolants, and other material is the primary problem, not the actual hearing protective device itself. When examining a patient whose chief complaint is ear irritation from wearing hearing protective devices, the physician should ask the employee to bring in the device for visual inspection.

There is little likelihood of an inserted earplug doing damage to the tympanic membrane. The ear canal becomes increasingly sensitive the closer it is to the tympanic membrane. At the first sensation of pain the worker will be alerted to stop pushing the plug in, long before any damage can occur.

Earplugs that form an airtight seal can be a problem. These earplugs are usually premoulded and manufactured out of vinyl or cured silicones. Foam and fibrous earplugs do not form a pneumatic seal. In those that do, however, the worker must be instructed to withdraw the plugs slowly with a twisting motion to break the seal. Rapid removal of the earplug may build up pressures so high that the tympanic membrane can rupture.

CASE STUDIES
Case 1

A 39-year-old male has worked in heavy industry for 15 years, mainly as a machinist, and has infrequently worn his hearing protection. Before working as a machinist, he was in the military but denies being in combat or working around large aircraft or machinery. He states that he participated in shooting practice on the rifle range but ear muffs were provided. His hobbies include going to rock concerts and doing carpentry. He denies tinnitus. He states that in a noisy environment he occasionally has difficulty understanding his young daughter.

He denies frequent ear infections as a child and denies hospitalizations, receiving intravenous antibiotics,

or taking any ototoxic medications. The company wants to know if the hearing loss is related to his work or to his recreational activities.

An otoscopic examination was normal with no evidence of tympanic membrane scarring. There was no fluid behind the ear drum. An audiogram was normal in the speech frequencies. His right ear had a 40 dB auditory threshold at 4000 Hz and a 50 dB auditory threshold at 6000 Hz. His right ear was normal until 4000 Hz with a 40 dB threshold. The auditory threshold at 6000 Hz was 45 dB.

Fortunately a date-of-hire baseline audiogram was available and was normal. A review of the industrial hygiene data from the plant showed that the patient had been exposed to an 8-hour TWA of 90 decibels since working for this company.

On further questioning, the patient denied ever having ringing in his ears, either after rock concerts or during his carpentry work. He stated he rarely used power saws but sawed manually and mainly did hammering and nailing.

This case typifies NIHL. His hearing loss is bilateral with the characteristic auditory threshold loss at 4000 Hz. In early NIHL, the auditory threshold recovers at 6000 Hz but as time progresses the characteristic notch at 4000 Hz is lost. Although uncertainty remains whether his attendance at rock concerts and carpentry work contributed to his hearing loss, the unequivocal industrial hygiene data and his lack of earplugs at work make work-relatedness more likely. By history there were no other likely causes for his hearing loss. No treatment is needed at this time but he must be required to wear earplugs in noisy areas. If he does not, his hearing may continue to deteriorate.

Case 2

A 30-year-old male was near the explosion of an air-filled gasket at work. After the blast he experienced vertigo and tinnitus in the left ear which resolved over 24 hours. He now complains of hearing loss in the ear (left) that was closest to the gasket and blames his hearing loss on the explosion. He also plays bass guitar in a band and worked as a sheet metal operator and in a noisy paper recycling plant for many years before being hired 2 years ago at this present company. He never wore ear protection until he came to work at his present company.

Physical examination was positive for a Weber test that lateralized to the left. The ENT examination was otherwise normal.

Results of audiogram in the office were as follows:

	500	1000	2000	3000	4000	6000
Left ear	0	10	0	0	30	40
Right ear	0	0	0	0	15	15

A baseline audiogram obtained from the company's file was unchanged from 1989, two years before the explosion. The unchanged audiogram rules out the possibility that the left ear hearing loss is due to the explosion. Etiologies that could explain the asymmetry of his hearing loss include damage from the placement of the bass amplifier next to his left ear while he played, an acoustic neuroma, or a past viral infection.

The primary care occupational medicine physician should refer this patient on a private (not occupational-related basis) for an ENT evaluation. The ENT evaluation may include such studies as an auditory-evoked response study or, at the very least, comprehensive audiometric testing. Based on history, he probably did sustain a temporary threshold shift after the explosion that manifested itself by tinnitus and acute hearing loss. His hearing, however, recovered to baseline after the incident.

Case 3

A 51-year-old male is complaining of hearing loss. He has significant difficulty understanding people in noise and must look at people directly to comprehend them. Besides working as a sheet metal operator at his present company for 20 years, he also has a history of multiple ear infections with drainage. He underwent a right tympanoplasty for closure of a right tympanic membrane perforation and a tympanomastoidectomy for a cholesteoma. On physical examination, he had a small perforation of the left tympanic membrane with a large mastoid bowl on the right ear. The Weber tuning fork test lateralized the sound to the right ear. The Rinne test was normal in the left ear but reversed in the right ear.

Results of the audiogram in the office compared with the baseline audiogram are as follows:

	500	1000	2000	3000	4000	6000
Left ear, office	20	35	40	45	40	50
Left ear, baseline	25	20	10	15	20	30
Right ear, office	50	50	45	45	50	55
Right ear, baseline	25	30	40	30	30	25

Because of the complexity of the case and the fact that he has both a conductive as well as a sensorineural loss, a complete ENT and audiologic evaluation will be needed to determine any industrial component to his hearing loss. Both bone and pure tone air conduction studies are needed. The evaluator will also need to correct for presbycusis.

After a complete evaluation it was found that he had a moderate-to-severe mixed hearing loss in his right ear, but it appeared to be due to his surgeries. The left ear, however, tested for a mild sensorineural hearing loss without significant conductive impairment. The left-sided hearing loss is therefore an occupational compensable injury. The small left-sided tympanic membrane perforation did not appear to contribute to his hearing loss on bone conduction audiogram.

This man needs annual audiograms and would benefit from hearing aids. He needs to wear hearing protection in noise and keep his left ear free of water. He also needs follow-up with his private doctor for the tympanic membrane perforation.

This case demonstrates the fact that although it appeared as if the patient had other reasons for his hearing loss due to his multiple surgeries, infections, and a tympanic membrane perforation, he still had a compensable workers' compensation injury.

CONCLUSION

The occupational physician has a responsibility to prevent NIHL. Many workers are unaware of the problems associated with noise and are unaware of the preventative measures that should be taken if one is exposed to noise. By taking a good occupational history, the physician can identify the employees at risk for noise-induced hearing loss and initiate a prevention program with the patient and the company.

The physician must work with employers and, when appropriate, recommend that noise levels be measured in a given department. If an employee tells the physician that he has to raise his voice for a person to hear him 3 feet away, noise levels should be measured in that area. If the noise levels are consistent with the 85 dB 8-hour TWA action level for OSHA's hearing conservation program, then education and hearing protection will be provided and audiograms will be taken yearly.

It is the responsibility of the physician to reinforce the importance of hearing protection and to work with the employee on any problems with hearing protection devices until a satisfactory solution is found.

When a physician is asked to consult on whether an employee sustained an occupational-related NIHL, the history is the key. The patient's history, appropriate noise exposure records, and audiograms are necessary. One must always keep in mind other causes of noise-induced hearing loss and other explanations for why an audiogram that may look consistent with noise-induced hearing loss really is not.

An appropriate referral means referring to an otolaryngologist who is familiar with noise-induced hearing loss. The otolaryngologist must also work with an audiologist who also has an interest in occupational otology. With occupational physicians, otolaryngologists, and audiologists working together, perhaps noise-induced hearing loss from occupational injury will become a thing of the past.

REFERENCES

1. Brechtelbauer DA: Adult hearing loss. In Vogt BH, editor: *Primary care: Disorders of the Ears, Nose, and Throat* 17:2, 1990, 249-265, Philadelphia, 1990, WB Saunders.
2. Franks JH: Number of workers exposed to occupational noise, *Seminars in hearing* 9 (4): 287-296.

3. Satoloff RT: The 4,000 Hz audiometric dip, *Ears, Nose, and Throat Journal,* 59:June 1980, 24-32.
4. Sataloff RT, Sataloff J: *Occupational hearing loss,* New York, 1987, Marcel Dekker, Inc.

SUGGESTED READINGS

Basmajian V, Slonecker C: *Grant's method of anatomy,* ed 11, Baltimore, 1989, Williams and Wilkins.
Browning GG: *Clinical otology and audiology,* London, 1986, Butterworths & Co.
Busis S: Noise-induced hearing loss: the sixth question, *The American Journal of Otolaryngology,* 12(2):81-82, March 1991.
Cantrell RW: Noise–Its effects and control, *The Otolaryngologic Clinics of North America* 13:3, 1979.
Consensus Conference: Noise and hearing loss, *JAMA* 1990 263:3185-3190.
Doyle TJ editor: *Council for accreditation in occupational hearing conservation manual,* Associated Management Corporation, Cherry Hills, NJ, 1988, Fischler's.
Guidotti T, Novak R: Hearing Conservation and Noise, *AFP* 28(4):180-186.
Hamernik RP, Davis RI: Noise and hearing impairment. Levy BS, Wegman DH, editors: *Occupational health, recognizing and preventing work related disease,* Boston, 1990, Little, Brown and Company.

Lipscomp DM: The prevention of noise induced hearing impairment, *Ears, Nose and Throat Journal* 12(2):131-138.
Lipscomp DM, editor: *Hearing conservation in industry, schools, and the military,* Boston, 1989, College-Hill Press.
Martin H, Gibson ES, Lockington JN: Occupational hearing loss between 85 and 90 dBA, *Journal of Occupational Medicine* 17(1):13-18, Jan 1975.
Meyerhoff W: *Diagnosis and management of hearing loss,* Philadelphia, 1984, WB Saunders Company.
Mills H: Relationship of noise to hearing loss, *Seminars in Hearing* 9(4):255-266.
Moller AR: Noise as a health hazard. In Last JM, Wallace R, editors: *Preventative medicine,* E. Norwalk, CT, 1992, Appleton and Lange, 523-531.
Osguthorpe JD, Melnick W, editors: *Clinical Audiology* 24(2) 1991.
Phaneuf B, Hetu R: An epidemiological perspective on the causes of hearing loss among industrial workers, *Journal of Otolaryngology* 19(1):31-38, 1990.
Rose DE: Noise and hearing loss, *Postgraduate Medicine* 70(2):117-128, 1982.
Sataloff RT et al: Intermittent exposure to noise: effects on hearing, *Annals of Otorhinolaryngology,* 92:623-628, 1983.
Sataloff RT, Sataloff J: *Occupational hearing loss,* New York, 1987, Marcel Dekker, Inc.
Thibodeau GA: *Anatomy and physiology,* St. Louis, 1987, Mosby-Year Book.

28 Vibration-related Occupational Injuries

Vibration is a physical stressor to which many people are exposed at work, in the home, or in social activities. For an understanding of the physics of vibration and the pathophysiologic changes that result in humans, the reader must refer to other textbooks, because this chapter is restricted to a review and an evaluation of the injuries resulting from vibration exposure.[1-3]

The health effects of whole-body vibration (WBV), infrasound that is vibration-related, and hand-arm vibration (HAV) that causes the hand-arm vibration syndrome (HAVS) are reviewed. The latter has three components: vascular, sensorineural, and musculoskeletal. The diagnosis, treatment, and management of HAVS is reviewed, and the respective safety standards for WBV and HAV are referenced and briefly described.

Humans and physical structures respond characteristically to certain critical vibration frequencies at which maximum energy transfers from source to receiver. The vibration may even be enhanced. At specific resonant frequencies, depending on the different organs in the body, the adverse effects from exposure are exacerbated. In general the larger the system mass the lower the resonant frequency. For humans, the principal whole-body resonance when sitting occurs at 5 Hz. For the chest, it is in the 4 to 6 range; with the eyes, in the 20 to 25 Hz range. The existence of resonance always means particularly high strain for the tissue involved.[4]

It is common to distinguish two different types of vibration exposure in humans: whole-body vibration when the body is supported on a vibrating surface (usually a seat or floor), and hand-arm vibration (segmental) when contact with the source is through the fingers and hands. Both are discussed separately.

WHOLE-BODY VIBRATION (WBV)

To suffer health effects from whole-body vibration exposure, the frequency range 1 to 100 Hz is critical. In the occupational situation several vibration frequencies are usually present simultaneously in the spectrum, and one or more are predominant. Depending on the magnitude, direction (axis), frequency, and duration of exposure to vibration, the health effects will range from sensations of pleasure, discomfort or pain; to interference with performance (reading and hand control); to acute or chronic illness with physiologic and pathologic changes.

Health effects

The occupational groups most exposed to WBV are:[5-11]

1. Drivers of tractors, heavy trucks, earth-moving equipment, construction vehicles, and other similar equipment. (Drivers of buses, light vehicles, forklift trucks, cars, and motorcycles are only at increased risk if the road surface is rough.)
2. Workers on vibrating stationary or quasi-stationary equipment, such as cranes, excavators, and drilling platforms.
3. Pilots of helicopters. Helicopters vibrate in all major axes at frequencies related to both rotor speeds and flight conditions, while further vibrations are produced by the engines, gearboxes, and rotors.

Studies on the subjective assessment of vibration levels have permitted reliable comparison of the discomfort produced by most common vibration exposures; this information is used by vehicle designers. The lowest subjective discomfort level occurs around the 5 Hz resonant point. The effects of vibration on performance are known to be highly dependent on the activity, so any adverse effect can usually be reduced by redesigning the task so as to make the worker less susceptible.[12]

Knowledge of the health effects of whole-body vibration is less certain and incomplete.[13] Ship motion studies have shown that WBV exposure in the region of 0.1 to 0.5 Hz is generally associated with motion sickness (Kinetosis) in susceptible people. The incidence is at a maximum after 2 to 3 hours at sea, and the incidence increases as the frequency decreases at a constant acceleration.[14] Acclimatization occurs as days at sea increase.[15] Heavy-equipment operators do not suffer motion sickness at these levels because of the short-term nature of the motion. Transient disequilibrium, postural sway, and tremor may occur after exposure to excessive levels of vibration, for example, after long drives over bumpy roads, turbulent flights, or sea journeys.

The most frequently associated long-term effects of WBV exposure are low back pain and degenerative changes in the spine. The symptoms and signs may be aggravated or caused by adverse ergonomic factors with respect to machine design and seating, or bad driving posture, so these factors must be considered and explored. Sitting flattens the normal lumbar curve (lordosis) and shifts the spine's line of force to a point posterior to the effective pivot point of the ischial tuberosities.[16] Sitting also increases the posterior disc height which may mechanically strain the posterior and postero-lateral collagen fibres of the annulus fibrosus.[17] Additional stress factors that may induce or contribute to low back pain are as follows:

1. Work activity requiring forward flexed motion of the spine, because the facets disengage and allow more anterior-posterior motion.[18-20]
2. A seated posture, because this will significantly increase lumbar intradiscal pressures.[21-23]
3. Repetitive loading and vibration, which tends to soften polymers in disc collagen fibres.[24-26]
4. Lifting activity after vibration exposure, because back muscle fatigue occurs with vibration exposure and mechanical damage to the disc is more likely.[27]

All these factors and the worker's operating movements in some situations enhance the likelihood of the spine to buckle and degenerate.[28] Experimental data have shown that the human spinal system has a characteristic response to compressive vibrational input in a seated posture and that the response is most apparent at 4.5 to 6 Hz, with the peak vibratory input occurring at 5 Hz. At this resonant frequency, marked enhancement of vibrational input occurs as vibrations pass through the spinal system.[29] The degenerative changes occur most frequently in the middle and lower thoracic spine, the upper lumbar, and to a lesser extent in the lower lumbar spine. Changes are usually localized in one part of the spine, a feature that is generally in favor of an external cause. Reported symptoms in the cervical spine are more likely to be caused by a forced posture rather than vibration. Although many years of exposure are usually considered as a prerequisite for WBV-related pathology in the spine, some reports indicate that a few years of exposure suffice to cause a higher health risk. In such situations the magnitude of WBV (intensity measured as acceleration in metres per second squared [m/sec^2]) at the critical frequencies is an important factor. Standing workers exposed to intense WBV at 40 to 50 Hz have experienced osteoporosis and arthrosis of the feet.[30]

A patient's exposure to WBV from sport or recreational activity (such as power boats, water skiing, snowmobiles, dirt track bikes) can be a problem in the differential evaluation of any injury ascribed to vibration exposure at work. Objective tests including radiographs, magnetic resonance imaging (MRI), and computerized tomography (CT) will not distinguish vibration from noninduced vibration injury. A comprehensive work and leisure history of source (Table 28-1) and length of exposure is, therefore, important in the evaluation.

In vibration-induced back injuries it is necessary to correct the environment as well as to treat the patient. Steps must be taken to reduce exposure to vibration of high magnitude or long duration at work by vibration isolation or attenuation, and/or reduction in exposure time. The worker must also be advised to reduce weight as necessary; use a hard seat and support the back as much as possible; take frequent breaks from driving and

Table 28-1 Examples of potentially harmful sources of vibration

Whole-body	Hand-arm
Vehicles	*Tools*
Agricultural—tractor, tree fellers, back-hoe	*Air-compressed drills*—jack hammer, jack leg, stoper, concrete
Construction—bulldozer, grader	*Air compressed grinders*—disc, rotatory, jitter-bug
Transport—bus, train, helicopter, jeep, truck, motorcycle, motorboat, snowmobile	*Air-compressed impact*—impact wrench, hilte gun, riveting gun
Mining—jumbo drill, trucks, trains	*Air-compressed hose*
Work platforms—drilling, crane	*Electrical*—drills, saws
	Combustion engine—chain saw, brush saw
	Vehicles—snowmobile, motorcycle

get out of the vehicle to walk around; avoid lifting and bending after driving for an hour; participate in a back exercise and work hardening program; and wear shoes with shock-absorbing soles.

A higher incidence of inguinal hernia, muscular insufficiency, scoliosis (mainly lumbar), and disorders of the digestive system including lower bowel and anal complaints have been reported. Apparently, exposures with frequencies mainly above 20 Hz do not cause many disorders of the digestive system.[30]

Women exposed to WBV show a distinct increase in blood volume during the phases of ovulation and menstruation, and there seems to be a higher risk of menstrual disorders, proneness to abortion, and other complications of pregnancy including hyperemesis gravidarum and varicose veins.[30] These conclusions have been derived from weak epidemiologic studies with dubious data and statistical analysis, so they may not be relevant. Realistic safe exposure limits for WBV cannot be derived from the literature, hence there is no reason to restrict women from risk occupations at this time, even during pregnancy, unless there is some clinical indication or personal history of associated problems.

After long-term exposure in both sexes there is decreased vestibular excitability and a higher incidence of other vestibular disturbances, including subjective complaints of dizziness. The interaction with noise could be an important factor. The question of long-term exposure to WBV below 20 Hz on the central nervous system (CNS) remains open.[30]

With respect to the circulatory system a variety of symptoms and diseases have been reported including varicose veins, hemorrhoids, varicoceles, ischemic heart disease, and hypertension.[30] Although there is an association between WBV and these conditions, the evidence at present does not permit the conclusion that WBV is a direct cause. Little data available indicates higher morbidity with higher intensity, longer duration of exposure, or longer daily exposure time.[31]

Finally it is well recognized that after an intense period of WBV exposure, a general morbidity with malaise, lassitude, and temporary disablement occurs. Full recovery usually occurs within a period of days or weeks after exposure has ceased.

ISO Standard 2631

The International Organisation for Standardisation (ISO) in Geneva, Switzerland has established a number of Technical committees with scientific representatives from member states to develop guides or codes for the health protection of workers.[32,33] For WBV, the International Standard 2631 (originally published in 1974 and republished with minor changes in 1978 and 1985) specified recommended exposure levels for vibrations transmitted to the human body in the frequency range 0.5 to 80 Hz for periods from 1 minute to 24 hours. The exposure time had to be reduced as the intensity of vibration increased (time dependency). Levels were specified for (1) the preservation of health and safety (exposure limit); (2) the preservation of working efficiency (fatigue-decreased deficiency boundary); and (3) the preservation of comfort (reduced comfort boundary).

Because of the difficulty recognizing and quantifying WBV-induced health effects in the work environment, the majority of the data used to derive the standard were performance data from laboratory and field studies. This was clearly unsatisfactory, so in the revision of ISO 2631, now awaiting approval by the technical committee, vibration limits based on such data are not included. In the revision, methods are defined to encourage precise measurement, and guidance is provided on the levels of WBV likely to affect comfort. Because 50% of alert, fit persons can just detect weighted vibration with a peak magnitude of 0.015 m/s^2, the likely values of vibration magnitude for comfort are specified (Table 28-2), but no limits are defined. Two alternative methods of calculating a motion sickness dose value are described.

CASE STUDIES
Case 1

A trucker and his codriver journeyed for days on end across the continent. As the weeks progressed in his work schedule, the truckdriver would notice that he could sleep less well, his appetite would deteriorate, and he would become less tolerant and more aggressive with his contacts. He would feel fatigued and, on occasion, nauseous. When he sought advice from his attending physician he was told that he was not suffering from any disease and that he was fit for full duties. He had no respite from trucking work or these symptoms until an opportunity arose to work as a temporary cab driver in his home town. Over the succeeding weeks, while driving the cab, he realized that his sense of well-being, vigor, and vitality had returned. When he recommenced

Table 28-2 Guidance for acceptable values of whole-body vibration for comfort

Vibration magnitude comfort	
Less than 0.315 m/s^2	Not uncomfortable
0.315 − 0.63 m/s^2	A little uncomfortable
0.5 − 1.0 m/s^2	Fairly uncomfortable
0.8 − 1.6 m/s^2	Uncomfortable
1.25 − 2.5 m/s^2	Very uncomfortable
Greater than 2.0 m/s^2	Extremely uncomfortable

trucking he had a recurrence of the earlier symptoms, although he preferred this activity. Self-preservation persuaded him to alternate trucking with 3 months cab driving. He is now able to remain symptom free.

Case 2

A school bus driver working in an agricultural area began to experience increasing back discomfort after her work shift. Her physician could detect no obvious cause and x-ray films of her spine were normal. When her concerns were raised as a health and safety issue the work station was examined and WBV measurements were taken on the driver's seat. These were found to be above the ISO fatigue-decreased deficiency boundary level. By modifying the driver's seat with the use of damping materials and isolation to reduce WBV transmission, the levels were satisfactorily reduced. She was then able to continue working without stress.

Infrasound

Closely related to WBV is infrasound, defined as airborne sound in the frequency range below 20 Hz. Infrasound is generated at low levels by several natural phenomena such as thunder, air turbulence, volcanic activity, winds, large waterfalls, or ocean waves. Manmade sources, which are increasing in terms of intensity and incidence of exposure, include airplanes, helicopters, cars, buses, lorries, trains, ships engine rooms, compressors, and ventilation systems.[34] This type of noise can cause annoyance, interfere with task performance, and cause biological damage.[35] Perception to infrasound is contingent on hearing and vibration. The vibrations sufficient to induce perception will occur only at relatively high pressure levels, 20 to 40 dB above the thresholds of auditory perception. The threshold of hearing rises rapidly as the frequency drops; for example, from approximately 65 dB at 32 Hz, to 95 dB at 16 Hz, 100 dB at 3 Hz, and 140 dB at 1 Hz.

The adverse effects of aural pain (related to displacements in the middle ear system), speech interference, and temporary threshold shift (TTS), normally appear at levels 30 to 40 dB above the hearing threshold.[36] In addition sound at 10 to 75 Hz may cause resonant vibration of the abdomen, chest, and throat. The chest wall vibrations may interfere with respiratory activity. Intense levels of infrasound at 130 to 150 dB may give rise to tickling and choking sensations in the throat. The subjective sensations are unpleasant and are often described as a pressure build-up. From investigations of noise annoyance complaints in environments where the noise energy was at 32 Hz or lower, a type of adverse reaction such as disturbance or unease was noted.[37] This description was also used by subjects in a work situation where a level of 99 dB at 34 Hz was recorded. Additional symptoms

were occipital headaches and giddiness.[38] Exposure to infrasound thus appears to become an environmental problem when the pressure exceeds the threshold of hearing perception.

Reduction in wakefulness during periods of infrasonic exposure above the hearing threshold has been identified through changes in electroencephalogram (EEG), blood pressure, respiration, hormonal production, performance, and heart rate. The reduction in wakefulness is based on hearing perception because deaf subjects have an absence of weariness.[39-42] In a work situation such as train driving, the environment is usually a combination of many factors such as seat comfort, visibility, instrumentation, vibration, and noise. Any one or a combination could be the critical stress factor, so caution is necessary before ascribing workplace symptoms and signs to infrasound exposure just because the levels are found to be significantly raised.

Thus, although exposure to infrasound at the levels normally experienced by humans does not tend to produce any dramatic health effects, exposure above the hearing perception level will produce headaches and vestibular symptoms together with weariness, annoyance, and unease. This may precipitate safety concerns in some environmental and many work situations.

CASE STUDY

Several staff in a small laboratory within a foundry began to experience occipital headaches, general unease, and some giddiness during and at the end of a day's work. Specialist examinations did not reveal any abnormality of their ears or sinuses. When their complaints were raised as a health and safety issue, the work situation was investigated. It was found that the vibration from a descaler in the foundry was being transmitted through the concrete flooring to the laboratory, and the infrasound levels in the laboratory were significantly raised. When the concrete linkage was broken, the laboratory staff became symptom free.

HAND-ARM VIBRATION
Health Effects

Adverse health effects from exposure to hand-arm vibration (HAV) have been recognized since 1911 when Loriga reported dead fingers among the Italian miners who used pneumatic tools.[43] Such tools had been introduced into the French mines in 1839 and were being extensively used by 1890. In the United States pneumatic tools were first introduced into the limestone quarries of Bedford, Indiana, about 1886. The health hazard from their use was subsequently investigated by Dr. Alice Hamilton and her colleagues in 1918.[44]

Since then there have many reports in the literature from all over the world.[45] It is now evident that adverse health effects can result from almost any vibrating source in contact with the hands (and the feet in some situations) if the vibration is sufficiently intense over the frequency range 4 to 5000 Hz for a critical period. The time exposure necessary may range from 1 month to 30 years. The most important sources of HAV are air-compressed and electrical pneumatic tools (Table 28-1). High risk examples are drills, fettling tools, im-pact wrenches, riveting guns, jack hammers, grinders, and chain saws. Moderate risk tools include brush saws, cement vibrators, and levelers; and low risk examples include floor buffers and dental drills.

The predominant health effect is known as the hand-arm vibration syndrome (HAVS), a disease entity with the following separate peripheral components:[46]

- Circulatory disturbances (vasospasm with local finger blanching white finger);
- Sensory and motor disturbances (numbness, loss of finger coordination and dexterity, clumsiness and inability to perform intricate tasks); and
- Musculoskeletal disturbances (muscle, bone and joint disorders).

The vasospasm, also known as Raynaud's phenomenon, is precipitated by exposure to cold and/or damp conditions and sometimes HAV exposure itself. The period between first exposure to HAV and its onset is termed the latent interval. The shorter this period the greater the risk to workers, but there is considerable variation because of individual susceptibility. The blanching is accompanied by numbness, and as the circulation to the digits recovers there is usually tingling and pain. In many subjects, tingling and paraesthesia may precede the onset of blanching.[47]

The blanching is initially restricted to the tips of one or more fingers but progresses as the vibration exposure time increases. The thumbs are usually the last to be affected. The existence of both

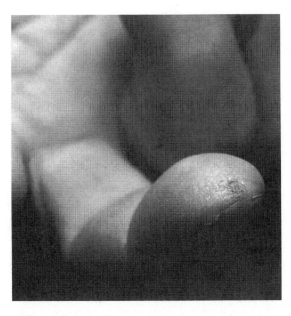

Fig. 28-1 With advanced HAVS, circulation becomes very sluggish, giving a cyanotic tinge to the skin of the digits. In very severe cases, trophic skin changes (gangrene) will appear at the finger tips.

sensory and vascular components in HAVS lead to the adoption of the Stockholm grading,[48,49] which is based on the subjective history supported by clinical test results to stage the severity (Table 28-3). The vascular and sensorineural symptoms and signs are evaluated separately and for both hands.

In addition to tactile, vibrotactile, and thermal threshold impairment, which may be less evident in some subjects but marked in others, impairment of grip strength is a common symptom in the longer exposed worker. Discomfort and pain in the upper limbs is also a frequent complaint. These latter symptoms, although similar to those experienced by patients with reflex sympathetic dystrophy, will lessen and resolve when the vibration exposure ceases.

Table 28-3 The Stockholm Workshop Scale for the classification of cold-induced Raynaud's phenomenon in the hand-arm vibration syndrome*

Stage	Grade	Description
0		No attacks
1	Mild	Occasional attacks affecting only the tips of one or more fingers
2	Moderate	Occasional attacks affecting distal and middle (rarely also proximal) phalanges of one or more fingers
3	Severe	Frequent attacks affecting all phalanges of most fingers
4	Very severe	As in stage 3, with trophic skin changes in the finger tips

* The staging is made separately for each hand. In evaluating the subject, the disorder's grade is indicated by the stages of both hands and the number of affected fingers on each hand; for example, 2L(2)/1R(1), –/3R(4).

The toes may be affected if directly subjected to vibration from a local source (such as vibrating platforms), or they may suffer with reflex spasm in subjects with severe hand symptoms.[50-55] Reflex sympathetic vasoconstriction may also account for the increased severity of noise-induced hearing loss in HAVS subjects.[56-62] Bone cysts and vacuoles, although often reported, are more likely to be caused by biodynamic and ergonomic factors. Working while leaning on vibratory tools, for example a jack hammer, may result in abdominal injuries.[63-65]

Carpal tunnel syndrome (CTS), an entrapment neuropathy affecting the median nerve at the wrist, is often associated with HAVS.[66,67] In most instances the critical factors are the weight, torque, and operating requirements of the tool plus the repetitive nature of the work. Vibration as the primary cause is due to the vibration-induced oedematous reaction in the nerve itself and in the tissues around the nerve. In most instances both the ergonomic factors and HAV contribute. In CTS patients without HAV exposure, it is unusual for the ulnar nerve to be involved, whereas with HAV exposure a neuropathy of the ulnar nerve is usually present as well. It is important to distinguish a median nerve neuropathy caused by CTS from that caused by HAV exposure because the response to treatment will differ.[68] Surgical decompression is usually advantageous in the former when conservative therapy has failed, but this is invariably not so in the latter because symptoms are rarely completely relieved and the reduction in grip strength is an additional burden to the worker. (See chapter on hand and elbow occupational disorders for further discussion of CTS.)

Whether smoking accelerates the onset of HAVS has not yet been proved conclusively, but this aggravating factor has been shown to increase the risk in several studies.[69]

The association of Dupuytren's contracture with HAV exposure is not conclusive,[70] but cases are being reported.[71]

Diagnosis

The diagnosis of HAVS is initially based on a history of HAV exposure and the exclusion of other causes of Raynaud's phenomenon, such as primary Raynaud's phenomenon (Raynaud's disease or constitutional white finger), local trauma to the digital vessels, thoracic outlet syndrome, drugs, peripheral vascular and collagen diseases, including scleroderma. The diagnosis and the severity staging (Tables 28-3 and 28-4) of HAVS need to be confirmed with the results of laboratory tests,[72,73] because, with compensation available for work-induced illness, the patient's assessment of his severity is not reliable. Statistical analysis has

shown that agreement between the history and diagnostic Stockholm grading is low, less than 40% for both vascular and sensorineural effects.[74]

The required laboratory tests have been described elsewhere.[73] The vascular tests may include Doppler and Duplex studies (to check the patency and the blood pressure ratios in the peripheral vessels); plethysmography (to evaluate the pulse waves before and after cold stress); finger systolic pressure measurement (to compare the blood pressure of an affected digit pre- and post-cold stress with the thumb, which is not usually affected); and cold water provocation tests (immersion of the digits in water at 10° C for 2 to 10 minutes with recording of skin temperature) to note any reactive hyperemia while immersed, and delay in recovery afterward to verify that vasospasm does occur on cold exposure. When the plethysmography wave forms are abnormal, the patient has to be at least stage 1; the severity of the findings in the remaining vascular tests will determine the patient's more advanced grading, stages 2 to 4 vascular.

The sensorineural tests may include depth sense and two-point discrimination (using von Frey hair, Semmes-Weinstein monofilaments, callipers or plastic blocks with split levels and widening groves);[75] finger tip vibration thresholds (8 to 500 Hz with vibrometer instrumentation);[76] thermal hot/cold perception (using Minnesota thermal discs[77] or instrumentation);[78] current perception threshold (CPT) test (detection of a 0 to 10 milliamperes current at 5, 250, and 2000 Hz);[79] and objective nerve conduction tests[80] to confirm the presence and severity of the neuropathy. When the depth sense and/or two-point results are abnormal the patient is at least stage 1; if the vibration, thermal, or CPT test results are abnormal she should be stage 2; and if the nerve conduction test result is abnormal she must be considered to be in stage 3 sensorineural.

In a family or occupational physician's office the only feasible vascular tests are Allen's, to check the effectiveness of the circulation in the superficial and deep palmer arches, and immersion of the hands in cold water to stimulate blanching. Often the latter will be unsuccessful because central body cooling is usually required as well. The sensory tests that are feasible are depth sense and two-point discrimination, together with vibrometry or current perception threshold measurement in the better equipped offices. When HAVS is suspected, the patient should be referred for a complete clinical and laboratory evaluation.

Pathophysiology

The pathophysiology of HAVS is still under investigation because the basic mechanism is not fully understood. Because of the mechanical stimulus, specific anatomic changes occur in the digital vessels — vessel wall hypertrophy and endothelial cell damage. In the initial stages there is extrusion of fluid into the tissues. This edema, together with the subsequent spasmodic ischemia from the cold-induced vasospasm, damages the mechanoreceptor nerve endings and nonmedullated fibers. Subsequently a demyelinating neuropathy of the peripheral nerve trunks, median and/or ulnar, develops.

The vascular response to cold is complex because in addition to the diversity of receptor systems (adrenergic, cholinergic, and serotonergic), there are several subtypes of specific receptors. The differential distribution and functional significance of the various receptor types are largely unknown. It is probable that the cold-induced pathologic closure of the digital arteries and end vessels is mainly mediated by alpha-2 adrenoceptors in the wall of the arterioles and veins. Although arterial spasm is necessary to stop the blood flow, vasospasm in the skin arterioles is essential to produce the blanching. For a more complete understanding the reader should read a recent review by Gemne.[69]

Treatment

To reduce the frequency of blanching attacks, the central body temperature must be kept high, and cold exposure must be avoided. Mitts rather than gloves should be worn, if it is feasible to do so, to permit the digits to warm each other. Discontinuation of smoking is a further essential requirement, because of the adverse action of nicotine and carbon monoxide on the digital arterial system. To reverse the pathology and achieve recovery in the worker aged less than 40 years, further HAV exposure must be avoided. If this is not possible a modified work routine should be practiced to reduce HAV exposure to slow progression.

Recent advances in drug therapy have focused on three aspects: (1) use of calcium channel blockers to produce peripheral vasodilation; (2) use of drugs such as pentoxiphylline, to improve the flexibility of red blood cells and promote platelet deaggregation in combination with the previously mentioned factors; and (3) drugs such as isosorbide dinitrate with prostaglandin E_1, to reduce platelet deposition and increase platelet survival.

The necessity for and extent of drug therapy increases with the severity of the Raynaud's phenomenon and the age of the subject. The ability of drugs to dilate blood vessels selectively is still being researched, and although the use of these therapeutic agents was not encouraging initially because of drug intolerance, the more recent long-acting calcium channel blockers felodipine and nifedipine show promise. Their use should be en-

couraged and the patients advised that treatment will be lifelong, unless their condition is mild and will reverse.[81] Surgical cervical sympathectomy has proven not to be beneficial in these cases and can no longer be justified.

There is no specific treatment for the median and ulnar neuropathy other than wrist splints at night, if sleep is disturbed, together with analgesics and a nonsteroidal agent such as naproxen. Physiotherapy with wax baths and ultrasonography is merely palliative and can rarely be justified; likewise the use of vitamin B6 or cortisone cannot be justified. Recovery, if at all, is slow; however, if the peripheral circulation is improved by drug therapy the neuropathy may benefit. Surgical intervention to relieve CTS symptoms should not be attempted if there has been HAV exposure. The results are invariably disappointing, and the further loss of grip strength will increase the worker's handicap. Surgery should be restricted to retired workers who have not responded to prolonged conservative treatment.

Prevention

Because the development of HAVS is dose-related, effective control measures should first be directed at reducing the intensity of vibration at the source, followed by the use of isolation and damping techniques to reduce transmission. Only antivibration tools conforming to recommended safety limits should be used.[82]

Tools should also be ergonomically designed to place minimum strain on the user. They should also have a high power-to-weight ratio; have low torque with a cut-off rather than slip-clutch mechanism; and the handles should have a nonslip surface to reduce the need to grip tightly. These ergonomic needs have been fully reviewed and illustrated by Radwin et al.[83]

The wearing of leather gloves or mitts at all times when using vibratory tools at work is recommended. They will maintain hand temperature, reduce the risk from cuts and abrasions, and attenuate some of the high frequency vibration. Until recently the antivibration gloves available for use in the workplace have been unsatisfactory because they were either too bulky to use or left the fingers exposed. The more recent products have been designed to avoid these faults and may be used with advantage.

Administrative controls should be introduced in high-risk situations to reduce exposure time by means of job rotation or rest periods. Alternative vibration-free work should be made available to workers who have HAVS at stage 2.

All workers should be advised of the potential hazard and receive training on the need to service their tools regularly; to grip the tools as lightly as possible within the bounds of safety; to use the protective clothing equipment provided; to undergo periodic medical surveillance; and to report all signs and symptoms of HAVS as soon as they develop.

CASE STUDY

A 55-year-old mechanic has been exposed to HAV from 3/8'' to 2'' impact wrenches (60%), disc grinders (30%), and air drills (10%) for about 2 hours a day, 5 days a week, 48 weeks a year, for 27 years. Before this he did not have any HAV at work and has not had any significant exposure at home. He does not wear gloves at work. He has not had any significant injuries to his upper limbs. Apart from mild diabetes, controlled by oral chlorpropamide for the past 10 years, he has enjoyed good health. There is no history of Raynaud's phenomenon in the family. He has never smoked and no longer consumes alcohol. He first noticed blanching of his fingers on exposure to cold about 12 years ago and it now extends to the MP joints of all fingers. The fingers are numb when blanched or cold, and they tingle on recovery. His hands ache at times but he has not had any sleep disturbance. Stockholm grading (history): Vascular 3R(4); 3L(4). Sensorineural 1 SN both hands.

At examination the patient's hands were warm and the skin was moist. (a) Vascular—blood pressure 130/70 both arms. Adson's and Allen's tests normal. Duplex scan and Doppler study of upper and lower extremities normal. Digital plethysmography of fingers revealed mild abnormal wave forms after cold stress. Following cold water immersion at 10° C for 7 minutes, recovery of skin temperature was moderately prolonged in all digits of both hands except for the right thumb and index finger, which were slightly delayed. (b) Sensorineural—arm reflexes present and equal. Tinel's test negative both wrists. Phalen's test positive both hands, with all fingers. Depth sense appreciation slightly impaired. Two-point discrimination normal. Grip strength right, 43.0 kg; left, 42.5 kg. Vibration perception: decreased sensitivity bilaterally with index and little fingers. Neurometer current perception: the distal digital branches of the right median and ulnar nerves have a very severe, and the left median and ulnar nerves, a severe hypoesthetic condition. Nerve conduction: latencies of the sensory components of both the median and the right ulnar nerves were moderately prolonged; some action potentials reduced; calculated velocity of the motor component of the left median nerve was significantly reduced. All hematology and biochemistry results normal, except for glycosuria 280 umol/L.

Diagnosis and conclusion: This patient is suffering from the hand-arm vibration syndrome. The diabetes is mild and is not believed to be a significant factor contributing to the severity of the peripheral circulation impairment or neuropathy. The vascular impairment is moderate/severe stage 2 both hands, and the sensorineural impairment is severe stage 3 SN both hands. The grip strength is below normal for his age. Treatment with felodipine 5°mg daily was prescribed to improve the peripheral circulation. He was advised to use A/V gloves and to grip the tools as lightly as possible.

Standards

Currently two human exposure to HAV standards or guides are used in the United States: American Conference of Governmental Industrial Hygienists (ACGIH-) Threshold Limit Value and American National Standards Institute (ANSI) S3.34. There is one United Kingdom standard (BS 6842) and one International standard, International Standards Organization (ISO) 5349.[84]

ISO/DIS 5349: 1986. The frequency range of measurement shall be at least 5 to 1500 Hz. The measurements, taken on the handle of the tool or with a knuckle grip, in the three perpendicular directions (X,Y,Z) shall be presented in terms of a weighted vibration level. The dominant axis is used to determine the daily weighted vibration exposure. This can then be compared with the dose-effect relationship graph in the standard to determine the likely onset of HAVS vascular symptoms as a percentage of the exposed population. ISO chose not to recommend acceptable human vibration intensity (acceleration) levels for exposure times in a work day. The critical issue is whether the basic ISO dose-response curves are totally valid for all work tools because they were mainly derived from chain saw data. Furthermore some doubt now exists on the application of these curves because of the high-frequency spectra of many tools and the removal of this high-frequency component through the use of weighted measurements.

ANSI S3.34: 1986. This is similar to ISO, in that ANSI requires weighted vibration measurements and a spectrum analysis in three perpendicular axes. For each axis a determination is then made to see if the standard has been exceeded for various exposure times. The overall weighted measurement is compared with a 4 hour-per-day exposure in each axis to predict the latent interval.

ACGIH-TLV. Triaxial weighted vibration measurements are required to be compared with the threshold limit value (TLV) table using the appropriate daily exposure times. The intent of the guideline is to prevent HAVS from progressing beyond stage 1. None of the measured acceleration levels should exceed the given levels. This standard covers frequencies from 5.6 to 1400 Hz.

BS 6842: 1987. The standard has ISO-type curves for daily exposures of 150 and 400 minutes, the former established at 1 ms[2] and the latter at 10 ms[2]. The standard includes a table showing the frequency weighted acceleration level values likely to produce stage 1 finger blanching in 10% of persons exposed.

NIOSH Criteria Document 1989. The National Institute for Occupational Safety and Health (NIOSH) document is not a standard in that it does not recommend a safe level for HAV exposure.[85] It voices concern, however, over the shape of the weighted curves and their adequacy to protect workers principally exposed to high-speed tools. It chose not to issue a recommended exposure level until further epidemiological study results become available. Recommendations are given for engineering controls, work practices, worker training, and so forth, and NIOSH urges the collection of both weighted and unweighted data over frequencies from 5.6 to 5000 Hz.

REFERENCES

1. Wassermann DE: *Human aspects of occupational vibration.* Amsterdam: Elsevier, 188, 1987.
2. Griffin MJ. *Handbook of human vibration.* London: Academic Press, 988, 1990.
3. Pelmear PL, Taylor W, Wasserman DE, editors: Hand-arm vibration: a comprehensive guide. New York: Van Nostrand Reinhold, 226, 1992.
4. Dupuis H, Zerlett G. *The effects of whole-body vibration.* Berlin: Springer-Verlag, 162, 1986.
5. Boshuizen HC, Bongers PM, Hulshof CTJ: Self-reported back pain in tractor drivers exposed to whole-body vibration. *Int Arch Occup Environ Health* 62:109-115, 1990.
6. Wassermann DE, Doyle TE, Asburry WC: *Whole-body vibration exposure of workers during heavy equipment operation.* DHEW (NIOSH) Publication No. 78-153, 1978.
7. Gruber GJ, Ziperman HH: *Relationship between whole-body vibration and morbidity patterns among motor coach operators.* HEW Publication No. (NIOSH) 75-104, 1974.
8. Helmkamp JC, Talbott EO, Marsh GM: Whole-body vibration - a critical review. *Am Ind Hyg Assoc J* 45(3):162-167, 1984.
9. Bongers PM, Boshuizen HC, Hulshof CTJ, Koemeester AP: Long-term sickness absence due to back disorders in crane operators exposed to whole-body vibration. *Int Arch Occup Environ Health* 61:59-64, 1988.
10. Harding RM, Mills FJ: Special forms of flight. II: Helicopters. *BMJ* 287:346-349, 1983.
11. Dupuis H, Zerlett G: Epidemiological research on professional groups exposed to vibration. In Dupuis H, Zerlett G, editors: *The effects of whole-body vibration.* 91, 1986.
12. Griffin MJ: Activity interference caused by vibration. In Griffin MJ, editor: *Handbook of human vibration.* London: Academic Press, 125-169, 1990.
13. Griffin MJ: Whole-body vibration and health. In Griffin MJ, editor: *Handbook of human vibration.* London: Academic Press, 171-220, 1990.
14. Dupuis H, Zerlett G: Acute effects of mechanical vibration: kinetosis. In Dupuis H, Zerlett G, editors: *The effects of whole-body vibration.* Berlin: Springer-Verlag, 66-69, 1986.
15. Kanda H, Goto D, Tanabe Y: Ultra-low frequency vibrations and motion sickness. *Ind Health* 15(1-2):1-12, 1977.
16. Chaffin DB, Andersson GBJ: *Occupational biomechanics,* ed 2, New York: Wiley & Sons, 518, 1991.
17. Krag MH, Seroussi RE, Wilder DG, Pope MH: Internal displacement distribution from in vitro loading of human lumbar motion segments: experimental results and theoretical predictions. *Spine* 12:1001-1007, 1987.
18. Panjabi MM, Krag MH, White AA, Southwick WO: Effects of preload on load displacement curves of the lumbar spine. *Orthop Clin North America* 8:181-192, 1977.
19. Schultz AB, Warwick DN, Berkson MH, Nachemson AL: Mechanical properties of human lumbar spine motion seg-

ments–Part I: responses in flexion, extension, lateral bending and torsion. *ASME J Biomech Eng* 101:46-52, 1979.
20. Tencer AF, Ahmed AM, Burke DL: Some static mechanical properties of the lumbar intervertebral joint, intact and injured. *ASME J Biomech Eng* 104:193-201, 1982.
21. Nachemson AL, Morris JM: In vivo measurements of intradiscal pressure. *J Bone Joint Surg* 46-A; 1077-1092, 1964.
22. Okushima H: Study on hydrodynamic pressure of lumbar intervertebral disc. *Arch Jap Chir* 39:45-57, 1970.
23. Betschko T, Kulak RF, Schultz AB, Galante JO: Finite element stress analysis of an intervertebral disc. *J Biomech Eng* 7:177-285, 1974.
24. Fung YC. *Biomechanics: mechanical properties of living tissues.* New York: Springer-Verlag, 433, 1981.
25. Weisman G, Pope MH, Johnson RJ: Cyclic loading in knee ligament injuries. *Am J Sports Med* 8:24-30, 1980.
26. Hertzberg RW, Manson JA: *Fatigue of engineering plastics.* New York; Academic Press, 64, 1980.
27. Hansson T, Magnusson M, Broman H: Back muscle fatigue and seated whole body vibrations - an experimental study in man. *Clin Biomechan* 6(3):173-178, 1991.
28. Wilder DG, Pope MH, Frymoyer JW: The biomechanics of lumbar disc herniation and the effect of overload and instability. *J Spinal Disorders* 1:16-32, 1988.
29. Wilder DG, Woodworth BS, Frymoyer MD, Pope MH: Vibration and the human spine. *Spine* 7(3):243-254, 1982.
30. Seidel H, Heide R: Long-term effects of whole-body vibration: a critical survey of the literature. *Int Arch Occup Environ Health* 58:1-26, 1986.
31. Gruber GJ, Ziperman HH: *Relationship between whole-body vibration and morbidity patterns among interstate coach drivers.* Report, contract no. HSM-99-72-o47. NIOSH Cincinnati, 56, 1976.
32. Griffin MJ: Whole-body vibration standards. In Griffin MJ, editor: *Handbook of human vibration.* London: Academic Press, 415-451, 1990.
33. Griffin MJ: Measurement and evaluation of whole-body vibration at work. *Int J Ind Ergonomics* 6:45-54, 1990.
34. Landström U: Occupational aspects of infrasound and whole body vibrations. *Arh Hig Rada Toksikol* 34:287-293, 1983.
35. Johnson DL: The effects of high level infrasound. In Conference on low frequency noise and hearing. Aalborg 1980.
36. Gierke von HE, Nixon CW: Effects of intense infrasound on man. In Tempest W, editor: *Infrasound and low frequency vibration.* London: Academic Press, 114-150, 1976.
37. Tempest W: Loudness and annoyance due to low frequency sound. *Acoustica* 29:205-209, 1973.
38. Pelmear PL. Noise and health. In Tempest W, editor: *The noise handbook.* London: Academic Press, 31-46, 1985.
39. Landström U, Liszka L, Danielsson A, Lindmark A, Lindquist M, Söderberg L: Changes in wakefulness during exposure to infrasound. *J Low Freq Noise Vib* 1(2):79-87, 1982.
40. Landström U, Lundström R, Byström M: Exposure to infrasound–perception and changes in wakefulness. *J Low Freq Noise* 2(1):1-11, 1983.
41. Landström U: Laboratory and field studies on infrasound and its effects on humans. *J Low Freq Noise Vib* 6(1):29-33, 1987.
42. Danielsson A, Landström U: Blood pressure changes in man during infrasonic exposure: an experimental study. *Acta Med Scand* 2317:531-535, 1985.
43. Loriga G: Il lavoro con i martelli pneumatici. *Boll Inspett Lavoro* 2:35-60, 1911.
44. Hamilton A: A study of spastic anaemia in the hands of stonecutters. *Ind Accident Hyg Services Bulletin 236,* No.

19. U.S. Dept. of Labor, Bureau of Labor Statistics 53-66, 1918.

45. Behrens VJ, Pelmear PL: Epidemiology of hand-arm vibration syndrome. In Pelmear PL, Taylor W, Wasserman DE, editors: *Hand-arm vibration: a comprehensive guide for occupational health professionals.* New York: Van Nostrand Reinhold, 105-121, 1992.

46. Gemne G, Taylor W: Hand-arm Vibration and the central autonomic nervous system. In Gemne G. Taylor W, editors: *J Low Freq Noise Vib Special Volume* XI, 1983.

47. Pelmear PL, Taylor W: Clinical picture (vascular, neurological, and musculoskeletal). In Pelmear PL, Taylor W, Wasserman DE, editors: *Hand-arm vibration: a comprehensive guide for occupational health professionals.* New York: Van Nostrand Reinhold, 26-40, 1992.

48. Gemne G, Pyykkö I, Taylor W, Pelmear PL: The Stockholm workshop scale for the classification of cold-induced Raynaud's phenomenon in the hand-arm vibration syndrome. *Scand J Work Environ Health* 13:275-278, 1987.

49. Brammer AJ, Taylor W, Lundborg G: Sensorineural stages of the hand-arm vibration syndrome. *Scand J Work Environ Health* 13:279-283, 1987.

50. Hedlund U. Raynaud's phenomenon of fingers and toes of miners exposed to local and whole-body vibration and cold. *Int Arch Occup Environ Health* 61:457-461, 1989.

51. Sakakibara H, Akamatsu Y, Miyao M, Kondo T, Furuta M, Yamada S, Harada N, Miyake SM, Hosokawa M: Correlation between vibration induced white finger and symptoms of upper and lower extremities in vibration syndrome. *Int Arch Occup Health* 60:285-289, 1988.

52. Sakakibara H, Hashiguchi T, Furuta M, Kondo T, Miyao M, Yamada S: Circulatory disturbances of the foot in vibration syndrome. *Int Arch Occup Environ Health* 63:145-148, 1991.

53. Hashiguchi T, Sakakibara H, Yamada S: Changes of skin blood flow in the finger and dorsum of the foot during chain saw operating. In Okada A, Taylor W, Dupuis H, editors: *Hand-arm vibration.* Kanazawa, Japan: Kyoei Press, 133-135, 1990.

54. Toibana N, Ishikawa N: Ten patients with Raynaud's phenomenon in fingers and toes caused by vibration. In Okada A, Taylor W, Dupuis H, editors: *Hand-arm vibration.* Kanazawa, Japan: Kyoei Press, 245-248, 1990.

55. Sakakibara H, Hashiguchi T, Furuta M, Kondo T, Miyao M, Yamada S: Skin temperature of the limbs in patients with vibration syndrome. In Okada A, Taylor W, Dupuis H, editors: *Hand-arm vibration.* Kanazawa, Japan: Kyoei Press, 249-251, 1990.

56. Pyykkö I, Starck J, Färkkilä M, Hoikkala M, Korhonen O, Nurminen M: Hand-arm vibration in the aetiology of hearing loss in lumberjacks. *Brit J Ind Med* 38:281-289, 1981.

57. Iki M, Kurumatani N, Moriyama T: Vibration induced white fingers and hearing loss. *Lancet* 282-283, 1983.

58. Iki M, Kurumatani N, Hirata K, Moriyama T: An association between Raynaud's phenomenon and hearing loss in forestry workers. *Am Ind Hyg Assoc J* 46(9):509-513, 1985.

59. Iki M, Kurumatani N, Hirata K, Moriyama T, Satoh M, Arai T: Association between vibration-induced white finger and hearing loss in forestry workers. *Scand J Work Environ Health* 12:365-370, 1986.

60. Miyakita T, Miura H, Futatsuka M: Noise-induced hearing loss in relation to vibration-induced white finger in chain saw workers. *Scand J Work Environ Health* 13:32-36, 1987.

61. Pelmear PL, Leong D, Wong L, Roos J, Pike M: Hand-arm vibration syndrome and hearing loss in hard rock miners. *J Low Freq Noise Vib* 6(2):49-66, 1987.

62. Iki M, Kurumatani N, Satoh M, Matsuura F, Arai T, Ogata A, Moriyama T: Hearing of forest workers with vibration induced white finger: a five year follow up. *Int Arch Occup Environ Health* 61:437-442, 1989.

63. Kron MA, Ellner JJ: Buffer's Belly. *N Eng J Med* 318(9):584, 1988.

64. Shields PG, Chase KH: Primary torsion of the omentum in a jackhammer operator: another vibration injury. *J Occup Med* 30(II):892-894, 1988.

65. Wasserman DE: Jack hammer usage and the omentum. *J Occup Med* 31(6):563, 1989.

66. Weislander G, Norback D, Gothe CJ, Juhlin L: Carpal tunnel syndrome (CTS) and exposure to vibration, repetitive wrist movements, and heavy manual work: a case referent study. *Brit J Ind Med* 46:43-47, 1989.

67. Koskimies K, Färkkilä M, Pyykkö I, Jäntti V, Aatola S, Starck J, Inaba R: Carpal tunnel syndrome in vibration disease. *Brit J Ind Med* 47:411-416, 1990.

68. Pelmear PL, Taylor W: Carpal tunnel syndrome v hand-arm vibration syndrome: a diagnostic enigma. *Arch Neurology* (in press).

69. Gemne G: Pathophysiology and pathogenesis of disorders in workers using hand-held vibratory tools. In Pelmear PL, Taylor W, Wasserman DE, editors: *Hand-arm vibration: a comprehensive guide for occupational health professionals.* New York: Van Nostrand Reinhold, 41-76, 1992.

70. McFarlane RM: Dupuytren's disease: relation to work and injury. *J Hand Surg* 16A(5):775-778, 1991.

71. Roberts FP: A vibration injury: Dupuytren's contracture. *J Soc Occup Med* 31:148-150, 1981.

72. Pelmear PL, Taylor W: Hand-arm vibration syndrome - clinical evaluation and prevention. *J Occup Med* 33(11):1144-1149, 1991.

73. Pelmear PL, Taylor W: Clinical evaluation. In Pelmear PL, Taylor W, Wasserman DE, editors: *Hand-arm vibration: a comprehensive guide for occupational health professionals.* New York: Van Nostrand Reinhold, 77-97, 1992.

74. Pelmear PL, Kusiak R, Dembek B: Cluster analysis of laboratory tests used for the evaluation of hand-arm vibration syndrome. *Proc 7th Int Meeting Noise and Vib 1993* (in press).

75. Carlson WS, Samueloff S, Taylor W, Wasserman DE: Instrumentation for measurement of sensory loss in the fingertips. *J Occup Med* 21(4):260-264, 1979.

76. Lundborg G, Lie-Stenström A, Sollerman C, Strömberg T, Pyykkö I: Digital vibrogram: a new diagnostic tool for sensory testing in compression neuropathy. *J Hand Surgery* 11A(5):693-699, 1986.

77. Dyck PJ, Curtis DJ, Bushek W, Offord K: Description of Minnesota thermal indices and normal values of thermal discrimination in man. *Neurology* 24(4):325-330, 1974.

78. Ekenvall L, Nilsson BY, Gustavsson P: Temperature and vibration thresholds in vibration syndrome. *Brit J Ind Med* 43:825-829, 1986.

79. Katims JJ, Naviasky EH, Rendell MS, Ng LKY, Bleecker ML: New screening device for assessment of peripheral neuropathy. *J Occup Med* 28(12):1219-1221, 1986.

80. Araki S, Yokoyama K, Aono H, Murata K: Determination of the distribution of nerve conduction velocities in chain saw operators. *Brit J Ind Med* 45:341-344, 1988.

81. Pelmear PL, Taylor W: Treatment and management. In Pelmear PL, Taylor W, Wasserman DE, editors: *Hand-arm vibration: a comprehensive guide for occupational health professionals.* New York: Van Nostrand Reinhold, 98-104, 1992.

82. Wasserman DE: The control of hand-arm vibration exposure. In Pelmear PL, Taylor W, Wasserman DE, editors: *Hand-arm vibration: a comprehensive guide for occupational health professionals.* New York: Van Nostrand Reinhold, 175-185, 1992.

83. Radwin RG, Armstrong TJ, VanBergeijk: Hand-arm vibration and work-related disorders of the upper limb. In Pelmear PL, Taylor W, Wasserman DE, editors: *Hand-arm vibration: a comprehensive guide for occupational health professionals.* New York: Van Nostrand Reinhold, 122-152, 1992.

84. Wasserman DE: Hand-arm vibration standards/guides. In Pelmear PL, Taylor W, Wasserman DE, editors: Hand-arm vibration: a comprehensive guide for occupational health professionals. New York: Van Nostrand Reinhold, 164-174, 1992.

85. *Criteria for a recommended standard. Occupational exposure to hand-arm vibration.* 1989 Sept; DHHS (NIOSH) Publication No. 89-106.

Commercial divers and others who work in pressurized environments are at risk for a variety of work-related injuries and illnesses. The first section of this chapter describes acute and chronic illnesses and the diagnosis and treatment of each. Appendix D provides details regarding the physical examination of potential divers. The second half of this chapter describes the diagnosis and treatment of injuries to the ear and sinus.

COMPRESSED GAS ACTIVITIES
Diving

Divers are exposed to several environmental stresses that include cold, lack of visibility, currents, the risk of entanglement, pollution, dangerous marine animals, and isolation. The unique aspects of the underwater environment include the increased ambient pressure and the need to deliver breathing gas at the increased environmental pressure. The breathing gas components (oxygen, nitrogen) may have pharmacologic effects at increased partial pressures. Because the toxicity of a gas is proportional to its partial pressure, subtoxic concentrations of trace contaminants (such as carbon monoxide) can also become dangerous at increased pressure. Additionally, the uptake of inert gas during a dive can result in supersaturation and bubble formation during decompression. Defined ascent rates must be maintained and often interrupted by decompression stops. The depths and durations of these stops are prescribed by decompression schedules or tables and depend on the depth of the dive and the bottom time. Decompression schedules can also be calculated by small, portable decompression computers carried by the diver. These devices continuously record ambient pressure and calculate inert gas partial pressure in theoretical tissue compartments and have been widely accepted in recreational diving.

While recreational divers use a self-contained breathing apparatus with the gas supply carried on the diver's back, commercial divers almost invariably use gas supplied from the surface. Their diving apparatus usually incorporates a helmet or full-face mask, which enables voice communica-

tion with the surface. Thermal protection is provided passively, using an insulated suit, or actively with hot water pumped from the surface along an umbilical conduit (see Fig. 29-1A-D). The diver can be lowered or raised in the water column with the aid of a cable attached to his rig. Alternatively it may be more convenient or safer to use a bell, an enclosed compartment in which one or more divers can sit during ascent and descent. Wet bells open at the bottom, allowing easy access, and a gas space inside automatically maintains pressure equal to that of the water. The diver can remove his helmet for easy communication with the surface or another diver. Using a wet bell requires that the diver make all his decompression stops in the water. Closed bells, on the other hand, can be completely sealed and their pressure adjusted independently of the actual bell depth. At the end of a job the closed bell can be hoisted onto the deck of the dive support vessel where decompression of the divers can occur in a relatively dry, warm environment. Closed bells can also be mated to larger, more comfortable surface chambers for this purpose. (See Fig. 29-2A-B.)

An alternative decompression procedure is for the diver to ascend directly from a predetermined decompression depth and then enter a deck chamber, which is then immediately decompressed to an equivalent depth somewhat greater than the depth of the last stop. A staged decompression can then be performed, often with the diver breathing 100% oxygen to hasten nitrogen elimination. This technique is known as surface decompression ("sur-D" or "sur-D O_2" if O_2 is breathed).

For long jobs that would otherwise require many compressions and decompressions, an alternative technique called saturation diving can be performed, in which divers are compressed in a surface chamber to a storage depth close to that of the working depth. Divers then enter a closed bell, which is lowered into the water. When a hydrostatic pressure equal to the internal bell pressure is reached, the hatch is opened and the diver proceeds to the worksite. He is connected to the bell by an umbilical incorporating breathing gas sup-

Fig. 29-1 One-atmosphere suit (Newt Suit, Can-Dive, Vancouver, BC) which protects the diver from pressure. Because the ambient pressure inside the suit is always 1 ATA, decompression is unnecessary. Suit can be used to a maximum depth of 300 m. Suits are also available that can be used to a depth of 350 m. These suits have a life-support sufficiency of 48-54 hours. **A,** Diver entering suit. **B,** Diver being lowered into the water.

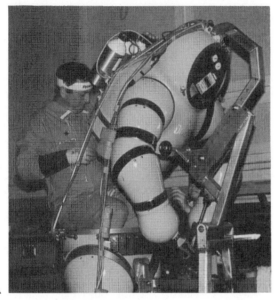

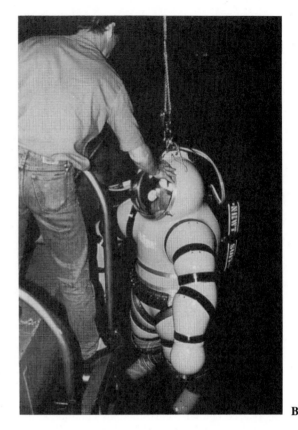

A

B

C, Commercial diver being prepared for a dive. Light and video camera are attached to the helmet. **D,** Diver entering water from the deck of dive-support vessel. Umbilical cables with air supply and communications cables are attached to the diver's belt.

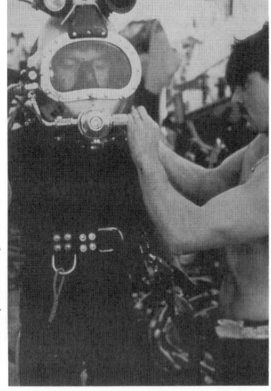

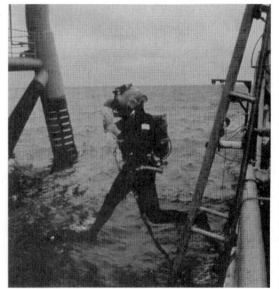

C

D

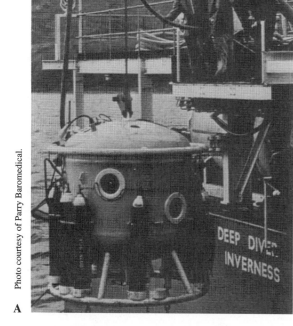
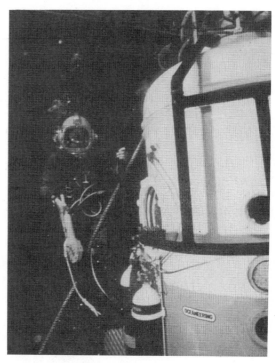

Photo courtesy of Parry Baromedical.

Photo courtesy of Oceaneering International.

A

B

Fig. 29-2 A, Diving bell being lowered into the water. **B,** Diver in water alongside bell.

ply, communication cables, electric power for illumination, and often a video cable connected to a camera on the diver's helmet, which permits the dive supervisor to observe his progress. At least one diver remains inside the bell. At the end of a shift the bell is closed, returned to the surface, and mated with the deck chamber where the divers eat and sleep. At the end of several days or weeks at pressure, the deck chamber can be slowly decompressed. Further details of commercial diving operations can be found in Bevan[8] (see Table 29-1).

Compressed air work

The earliest systematic exposure of humans to increased ambient pressure was in mining and tunneling operations and in building bridge abutments. Elevating the worksite pressure in wet or muddy soil conditions prevents the ingress of water. Caissons are large, hollow, boxlike structures with an open under-surface, used to build bridge peers. The caisson is placed on the bottom, and the bridge peer is built on top. The weight forces the edges into the soft sediment. The water is pumped out and replaced by compressed air, allowing personnel to enter the caisson, scoop out the muck, and enable it to be pumped to the surface. As the caisson slowly sinks, the pressure must be maintained equal to the mud's hydrostatic pressure. The process is continued until bedrock is reached, after

which the interior of the caisson can be filled with concrete. The length of time that men can work in the pressurized environment depends on the ambient pressure. The maximum safe ambient pressure for manned compressed air work is around 4.4 atmospheres absolute (ATA). Automated caisson evacuation systems allow unmanned excavation at greater ambient pressures. Workers only enter the pressurized environment of these high-pressure caissons to conduct maintenance. To minimize nitrogen narcosis at the elevated pressures the workers breathe a mixture called trimix: oxygen, helium, and nitrogen.[55] To minimize the risk of decompression illness, the worker must be decompressed at the end of each shift in accordance with appropriate procedures.

Acute illness

Decompression illness/arterial gas embolism
Gas bubble disease in divers and compressed air workers occurs by way of two main mechanisms. The first is due to pulmonary hyperexpansion during a breath hold or rapid ascent, in which the rate at which lung volume expands in accordance with Boyle's law exceeds the rate at which alveoli are emptied by exhalation. If the pulmonary elastic limit is exceeded, rupture occurs. This allows gas to enter the pulmonary interstitium, pleural space, or pulmonary capillary blood, causing arterial gas embolism (AGE). Pulmonary barotrauma can oc-

Table 29-1 Equivalent pressures

Depth (meters)	Gauge pressure (psi)	Gauge pressure (kPa)	Absolute pressure (atmospheres absolute— ATA)	Absolute pressure (mm Hg)	PO$_2$ (air) (mm Hg)	PO$_2$ (air) (ATA)	O$_2$ content for PO$_2$ = 0.5 ATA* (percent)	Comments
0	0.0	0	1.00	760	158	0.21	50.0	Sea level
10	14.5	100	1.99	1,510	315	0.41	25.2	Decompression illness extremely rare unless pulmonary barotrauma occurs
14	20.3	140	2.38	1,810	377	0.50	21.0	Deepest depth for air saturation diving
44.5	64.5	445	5.39	4,098	854	1.12	9.3	Highest pressure for compressed air work
50	72.5	500	5.93	4,511	940	1.24	8.4	Deepest depth for commercial air diving
150	217.5	1,500	15.80	12,012	2,502	3.29	3.2	Effects of HPNS become evident
305	442.2	3,050	31.10	23,638	4,924	6.48	1.6	Deepest operational dive
534	774.3	5,340	53.70	40,815	8,502	11.19	0.9	Deepest ocean experimental dive
701	1,016.4	7,010	70.19	53,342	11,111	14.62	0.7	Deepest chamber dive (H$_2$-H$_2$-O$_2$ trimix)

*The percentage of O$_2$ necessary to result in an oxygen partial pressure of 0.5 ATA is equivalent to 50% O$_2$ at sea level.

cur after a breathhold ascent to the surface from a depth as shallow as 2 or 3 meters.

After pulmonary barotrauma interstitial gas can track into the mediastinum and dissect upward into the soft tissues of the neck and around the larynx, and be detectable as subcutaneous emphysema or a change in the voice. Pleural gas, and hence pneumothorax, is less common. Intravascular gas usually results in focal neurologic deficits. Neurologic abnormalities in uncomplicated AGE usually follow a cortical distribution with hemianesthesia or hemiparesis. In a diver with significant depth-time exposure, however, arterial gas embolism may produce neurologic abnormalities with spinal cord distribution.[73]

Pulmonary disease may predispose to pulmonary barotrauma during ascent, even in the absence of a breathhold. Bullous lung disease,[66] interstitial, fibrosis, asthma, and unilateral absence of the pulmonary artery[18] have been associated with pulmonary barotrauma in divers.

The second mechanism of gas bubble disease occurs when gas bubbles form in situ within tissues by virtue of supersaturation of inert gas during decompression (decompression sickness [DCS]), in a fashion analogous to CO$_2$ bubble formation when a carbonated drink bottle is opened. Gas formation via this mechanism appears to occur commonly around articular structures, pro-

ducing joint pain, and within the spinal cord producing hypesthesia, paresthesia, dysfunction of urinary and anal sphincters, or frank paraplegia and quadriplegia. In situ bubble formation can occur in the skin, lymphatics, inner ear, cornea, and also peripheral nerve.[29,40]

Gas can also form asymptomatically and be transported into the venous blood (venous gas embolism or VGE), where bubbles can be detected in the right side of the heart or pulmonary artery using ultrasonography.[74] VGE are usually cleared from the blood when they enter the pulmonary capillary network. When they occur in large numbers, however, they can produce cough, dyspnea, or pulmonary edema (chokes).[109] If the rate at which they impinge on the pulmonary vascular bed is sufficiently high to exceed the ability of pulmonary capillaries to clear them from the circulation, or, if there is an intracardiac right-to-left shunt, VGE can enter the arterial circulation, causing AGE.[107]

Decompression syndromes have conventionally been classified as DCS type I (skin, lymphatic, or pain-only bends), type II (neurologic, vestibular/auditory, cardiorespiratory [chokes] or with accompanying shock), AGE, and other barotrauma (see Table 29-2).

Table 29-3 enumerates the most commonly observed symptoms.[29] Although pain is the most

Table 29-2 Traditional classification of decompression illness

---

Decompression sickness

Type I*
    Musculoskeletal
    Skin
    Lymphatic
    Fatigue
Type II
    Neurological
    Cardiorespiratory ("chokes")
    Vestibular/auditory
    Shock

Arterial gas embolism

Barotrauma

    Lung
    Sinus
    Inner ear
    Middle ear
    Dental
    Gastrointestinal

---

*Sensory symptoms (numbness, paresthesias) are classified as type I by the United States Air Force.[106]

common initial symptom, neurologic symptoms are more common overall.

If an accurate history of the dive is available it is often possible to infer the mechanism of gas bubble formation (pulmonary barotrauma versus in situ tissue gas). For example, divers with loss of consciousness immediately after a short, shallow dive with breathhold or rapid ascent are most likely suffering from AGE secondary to pulmonary barotrauma. On the other hand, a history of a deep, prolonged dive, with paresthesias and limb weakness 1 hour after surfacing is more likely due to in situ tissue gas formation (DCS). In evaluating divers with possible DCS, standard decompression tables (such as the U.S. Navy Air Decompression Tables[102]) may serve as a guide to the degree of the depth-time exposure; however, DCS cannot be reliably excluded on this basis. In many cases, it is impossible to distinguish DCS from AGE, and both mechanisms can exist in the same patient. Moreover, the treatment algorithms are usually the same. Therefore many diving physicians consider more appropriate the term "decompression illness" (DCI), which encompasses both mechanisms.

Neurologic symptoms usually have a short latency after surfacing. More than 50% of patients have symptoms within 10 minutes; 90% have symptoms within 3 hours.[39,40] When pain is the only symptom the onset may be delayed for several minutes or hours after the dive. Ninety percent of individuals have symptoms within 6 hours after surfacing; however, aircraft flight or other altitude exposure can precipitate symptoms of DCI

Table 29-3 Distribution of symptoms in 1,249 cases of decompression illness in recreational divers

Initial symptom	%	Symptom at any time	%
Pain	40.7	Pain	56.7
Altered skin sensation	19.2	Altered skin sensation	52.1
Dizziness	7.8	Weakness	22.4
Extreme headache	5.7	Dizziness	18.6
Headache	5.7	Extreme fatigue	17.1
Weakness	4.8	Headache	16.1
Nausea	2.9	Nausea	13.9
Difficulty breathing	2.5	Difficulty walking	10.2
Altered level of consciousness	2.1	Difficulty breathing	8.7
Itching	1.6	Altered level of consciousness	6.9
Visual disturbance	1.5	Visual disturbance	6.4
Rash	1.1	Paralysis	6.3
Paralysis	1.0	Itching	5.0
Personality change	0.8	Restlessness	4.6
Difficulty walking	0.7	Muscle twitching	4.0
Restlessness	0.4	Rash	3.5
Muscle twitching	0.4	Urethral/anal sphincter dysfunction	3.5
Urethral/anal sphincter dysfunction	0.4	Personality change	3.0
Tinnitus	0.2	Speech disturbance	2.8
Speech disturbance	0.2	Tinnitus	1.7
Convulsions	0.2	Hearing loss	1.1
Hearing loss	0.1	Convulsions	1.0
		Hemoptysis	0.7
Total	*100.0*		

Data reported to the Divers Alert Network. Reproduced with permission from Elliott & Moon.[29]

many hours later. In this setting DCI has been reported as long as 3 to 4 days after a saturation dive.[5,45]

Decompression illness can also occur after decompression to high altitude, for example in aviators.[108] The usual threshold for altitude-induced decompression illness is around 5500 m (18,000 ft, 0.74 ATA). Less severe altitude exposure, however, can occasionally result in bubble formation. Most commonly, flying in a commercial aircraft within 24 to 36 hours after a dive can induce decompression symptoms.[105]

Serious cases of decompression illness can be associated with capillary endothelial damage and resulting third space fluid loss. Brunner et al have described two cases in which significant loss of intravascular volume with hemoconcentration was documented with radioactive tagging.[10]

Diagnostic methods. Almost any symptom after a dive should raise the suspicion of decompression illness. The diagnosis is usually made by history, physical examination, and the response to recompression. Laboratory, radiographic, and neurophysiologic evaluation are usually of limited value.

Divers complaining of limb pain should be questioned about musculoskeletal trauma. Unless there are obvious signs of trauma implicating some cause other than DCI, the physical examination is often not helpful. In DCI palpation usually results in no increased pain, although inflation of a sphygmomanometer around the affected area will sometimes result in pain reduction. This sign, however, is neither sensitive nor specific. Because neurologic abnormalities are so common, all patients should have a complete neurologic examination. Characteristically, the patterns of abnormality observed in neurologic DCI are different from those typically seen in other neurologic emergencies such as stroke. Patchy areas of hypesthesia may not be detected with only a cursory neurologic evaluation. One of the most sensitive signs is abnormality of tandem gait, with eyes open or closed, which will often detect ataxia due to spinal cord, cerebellar, or vestibular damage.

Electronystagmography (ENG) and audiometery can be used to detect inner ear damage, which may not be apparent to clinical examination. Psychometric testing has also been reported to be capable of detecting abnormalities caused by decompression illness with greater sensitivity than clinical examination.[16,44] Computerized topography (CT), magnetic resonance imaging (MRI), emission scanning, somatosensory, and brain stem evoked potential studies, and electroencephalography (EEG) have not been shown to be as sensitive or specific as clinical evaluation. A detailed discussion of testing of individuals with decompres-

sion illness can be found in the work of Elliott and Moon.[29]

Treatment of decompression illness should begin with principles of basic life support. While transporting the patient to a definitive treatment facility, oxygen should be administered in as high a concentration as possible. This results in washout of inert gas, and hence an increased rate of diffusion of gas from bubbles into the surrounding tissue. Additionally, higher arterial blood O_2 content may improve oxygenation of ischemic tissue from vascular obstruction. Intravascular volume resuscitation should be initiated using isotonic fluids, preferably not containing glucose. Because hyperglycemia can worsen outcome after neurologic insult, it may be preferable to avoid glucose-containing solutions.[21]

In the past, the head-down position was recommended for the initial management of AGE to avoid further embolization because of buoyancy effects by causing cerebral vasodilatation, and by facilitating the clearance of obstructing bubbles.[4] However, buoyancy effects probably have little or no influence on the distribution of arterial bubbles, and the head-down position can promote the development of cerebral edema.[4,24] The head-down position is therefore no longer recommended unless it is required to maintain arterial pressure.

Recompression therapy is the definitive treatment for DCI. Most cases can be managed successfully by recompression to 18 m equivalent depth (2.8 ATA) and administration of 100% O_2. Typical decompression schedules (tables) last 4 to 6 hours. Serious cases that respond incompletely can be saturated at a stable treatment pressure for several hours or days while breathing oxygen intermittently. Once clinical stability has occurred, slow decompression can be initiated. Further details of treatment of decompression illness can be found in Moon and Gorman[69] and the US Navy Diving Manual.[102]

The risk of decompression illness in commercial diving operations has been reported to average 0.1 to 0.2%, of which 25 to 50% are type II.[67,75] The risk varies with the type of diving. Overland reported only one episode of decompression illness in 15,094 no-stop air dives. In the same period, 10 bends out of 4,548 dives required in-water decompression stops, and 19 bends out of 6,640 dives used surface oxygen decompression (sur-D O_2). Bends are usually observed more frequently in saturation diving. Leitch reported 6 episodes of decompression illness in 458 saturation man-dives at depths of up to 300 m.[59] Because on-site recompression facilities are always available at commercial dive sites, serious sequelae of decompression accidents are rare.

Thermal problems

Divers are susceptible to thermal stress, usually cold, by virtue of conductive and convective heat losses from the skin and respiratory systems. Considerable heat can be lost through the skin because the water in some locations can approach 0° C. At high ambient pressure, even in a dry habitat or bell, considerable heat can be lost through the skin because of the high heat capacity and conductivity of gas at high ambient pressure. In addition, there may be significant convective heat loss through the respiratory tract. To maintain diver comfort it may be necessary to keep the ambient temperature of a saturation diving environment between 30° and 34° C.

Mild hypothermia is defined as a core temperature between 32° and 35° C; moderate hypothermia, 28 to 32° C; severe hypothermia, <28° C. Mild hypothermia induces impaired judgment and shortened attention span. As core temperature drops the individual becomes progressively obtunded. With mild hypothermia shivering initially becomes intense, gradually declines, and is often accompanied by a sensation of warmth. There is usually bradycardia between bouts of shivering. In moderate and severe hypothermia, hypotension develops. An increase in bronchial secretions can occur, particularly if cold gas is breathed, resulting in airway obstruction and audible rhonchi.

Reduction of extremity temperature to 10 to 20° C results in pain. Some individuals then experience an inappropriate sensation of warmth. If fingertip temperature reaches 8 to 10° C or below there is a risk of nonfreezing cold injury (NFCI). Rewarming after NFCI may produce edema, erythema, pruritus, and pain. A permanent alteration in the vascular response to temperature changes often results, and subsequent exposure to low temperatures causes immediate pain as a result of an exaggerated vasoconstrictive response. Exposure to cold sufficient to cause numb digits for 60 minutes will cause NFCI in the majority of divers. No more than 30 minutes of numbness should be allowed.[88]

Prevention of hypothermia includes appropriate thermal protection of the skin using either passively or actively warmed suits. The latter is usually provided by hot water pumped from the surface. During deep diving it is also usually necessary to heat the inspired gas.

Divers being treated for hypothermia should maintain a supine position to prevent hypotension. Warm intravenous fluids should be administered along with peripheral rewarming. Patients with moderate or severe hypothermia may require peritoneal lavage or cardiopulmonary bypass.

Hyperthermia can occur if water temperature exceeds 35° C at rest or 32° C during light exercise. Symptoms of thirst, fatigue, ataxia, impaired judgment, nausea, vomiting, and diarrhea can indicate mild hyperthermia. Heat-induced vasodilatation, often accompanied by dehydration, can result in syncope. Hyperpnea, resulting in respiratory alkalosis, can also be associated with hyperthermia. Treatment includes application of icepacks to the neck, axilla, and groin. Cooled intravenous fluid administration can help to reduce core temperature.

Prevention of hyperthermia includes adequate hydration; gradual, deliberate heat acclimatization; and the use of ice vests or water-cooled diving suits. A comprehensive review of thermal problems in diving has been covered by Sterba[88] (see Chapter 26 on Temperature-related Injuries).

Scuba disease

A syndrome consisting of chills, fever, anorexia, nausea, vomiting, cough, malaise, body aches and headache, followed by fever, signs of pulmonary consolidation, and leukocytosis has occasionally occurred in divers exposed to equipment contaminated by pseudomonas species. Scrupulous cleaning and decontamination of scuba gear prevents this problem. The syndrome has informally been called "scuba disease."[9]

Other barotrauma

Changes in ambient pressure can also affect gas-containing spaces in the gastrointestinal tract, tooth pulp (usually under fillings), and within the diver's mask. Gas pockets in teeth can become painful on descent or ascent. Rupture of abdominal viscera as a result of expansion of intraluminal gas during ascent can occur.[46,63,101] "Mask squeeze" occurs on descent when the diver fails to equalize the pressure of the gas behind the mask with the ambient pressure. This can result in periorbital edema, ecchymosis, and subconjunctival hemorrhage.

Problems caused by breathing mixtures

Inert gas narcosis. During air diving there is a progressive deterioration in mental function, first noticeable in depths of around 20 to 30 m. At depths of 70 to 100 m, intermittent inattention to instructions and amnesia occur[47] and, at depths greater than 90 to 100 m, divers can lose consciousness. These effects are due to the narcotic effects of nitrogen and are almost instantaneously reversible when the pressure is decreased. The narcotic potency of inert gases (see Table 29-4) varies in accordance with their lipid solubility.

Deeper diving requires mixtures of oxygen and helium, which are not narcotic. At shallow depths the nitrogen partial pressure can be reduced somewhat by using an enriched oxygen breathing mix. Using inspired O_2 concentrations higher than 21% O_2 reduces nitrogen narcosis and extends the safe bottom time (or reduces the necessary decompression time) by decreasing the amount of tissue nitrogen uptake. This concept has been implemented

Table 29-4 Relative narcotic potencies of physiologically inert gases

Gas	Relative partial pressure required to produce equivalent narcosis
Helium	4.26
Neon	3.58
Hydrogen	1.83
Nitrogen	1
Argon	0.43
Xenon	0.04

Inert gases are listed in order of potency from helium (least narcotic) to xenon (most narcotic).[6]

in practice by using a fixed O_2 percentage in the supply gas (typically up to 32%). The limiting factor is central nervous system oxygen toxicity, which can occur when the inspired PO_2 exceeds 1.3 to 1.5 ATA (see below). Another approach has been to use a feedback control system to vary the inspired O_2 concentration such that inspired PO_2 is constant (typically 0.7 to 1.4 ATA).[104]

Oxygen toxicity. Toxicity caused by increased partial oxygen pressures is believed to cause toxic tissue effects by generating reactive oxygen species such as hydrogen peroxide, superoxide, singlet oxygen, and hydroxyl radical. Biochemical effects include protein degradation, lipid peroxidation, and nucleic acid damage. The most common clinical effects of these changes are observed in the lung and central nervous system. Pulmonary effects include tracheobronchitis, manifested as a dry cough and inspiratory central chest pain, reduction in vital capacity and lung compliance, increased resistance of small airways, reduced carbon monoxide transfer factor, pulmonary edema, and fibrosis. These changes develop at rates varying considerably with each individual, depending on the inspired PO_2. For instance, changes are rarely detectable at inspired PO_2 of 0.5 to 0.6 ATA or less, whereas breathing oxygen at 2 ATA for an average of 10 hours results in an average 10% decrease in vital capacity.[14]

Pulmonary oxygen toxicity is a limiting factor to prolonged exposure to air at depths deeper than around 20 m. For saturation dives exceeding this depth, oxygen concentration must be reduced to maintain a partial pressure lower than 0.5 to 0.6 ATA (see Table 29-1). If an appropriate atmosphere is breathed, pulmonary oxygen toxicity does not occur under usual diving operations unless supplemental oxygen is used as an aid to inert gas washout during decompression or to treat decompression illness.

Central nervous system oxygen toxicity manifests as nausea, vomiting, muscle twitching and, most severely, convulsions. Less common symp-

toms include euphoria, visual symptoms, acoustic symptoms, olfactory sensations, and changes in respiratory pattern. If oxygen partial pressure is reduced, these symptoms are self limited. No evidence exists that an oxygen convulsion per se has any permanent effect. In-water convulsions, however, can cause drowning unless a full-face mask or helmet is in use. Furthermore, rescue of an unconscious postictal diver who has experienced an in-water convulsion can also result in pulmonary barotrauma if his glottis remains closed during ascent.

The threshold PO_2 for oxygen convulsions in a dry chamber under resting conditions is usually between 2 and 2.5 ATA. Hyperoxic convulsions, rarely occur, for example, at an inspired PO_2 of 2.0 ATA in patients undergoing 2-hour periods of hyperbaric oxygen therapy. Exercise and immersion in water both reduce the threshold for convulsions, and it is inadvisable to allow the inspired PO_2 to exceed 1.5 ATA during operational diving conditions (other than during decompression or for DCI treatment). There has been one observed instance of a convulsion in a commercial diver breathing oxygen at 1.3 ATA.

Both central nervous system and pulmonary O_2 toxicity are reversible. Convulsions and other symptoms and signs of CNS toxicity resolve within a few seconds or minutes after reducing the inspired O_2 partial pressure. Manifestations of pulmonary O_2 toxicity simultaneously resolve, although hours or days of relative normoxia are required. We have observed complete clinical resolution of even pulmonary edema caused by pulmonary O_2 toxicity.

Gas contamination. Toxic gases exert their effects in direct proportion to their partial pressures; therefore, air purity standards for divers must be more stringent than in other industrial settings. Although a carbon monoxide concentration of 50 ppm is considered safe for a multihour exposure at 1 ATA, carbon monoxide poisoning would rapidly result if breathed at a depth of 90 m. It would result in CO exposure equipotent to a 500 ppm exposure at 1 ATA. Breathing gas can become contaminated because of faulty compressors or unsafe procedures, such as allowing the air intake of a compressor to become contaminated by engine exhaust. Welding gases (including CO and particulates) can also pollute the atmosphere in welding habitats (Fig. 29-3) and divers can avoid inhaling the chamber atmosphere by using a separate breathing gas supply (BIBS, or built-in breathing system).

High pressure nervous syndrome (HPNS)
Rapid compression of divers to depths of around 150 to 200 m results in acute diminution of psychometric performance along with nausea, vomit-

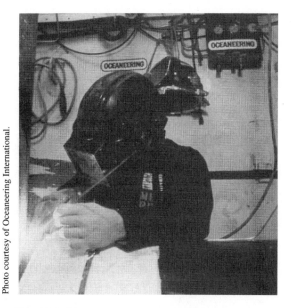

Fig. 29-3 Welding in a dry habitat. Welding is a potential source of toxic gases and burns.

ing, tremor, and ataxia, known as high pressure nervous syndrome (HPNS). If divers are then maintained at a stable depth, there is some adaptation. This syndrome can also be minimized by slow compression and the addition of a narcotic gas to the usual mix of helium and oxygen (for example nitrogen[7] or hydrogen).[83] Despite early indications that HPNS would preclude diving deeper than around 300 m, experimental dives have been conducted to equivalent depths of 686 m breathing He-N_2-O_2 trimix and to 701 m breathing He-H_2-O_2 trimix. HPNS is probably due to a transient change in brain neurotransmitters, and is completely reversible upon decompression.

Chronic illness
Bone necrosis
Exposure to compressed gas during diving or compressed air work can result in necrosis of the long bones.[64] This is believed to be due to disruption of blood supply by virtue of bubble formation in the intramedullary fat, resulting in bone infarction. It most commonly affects femoral and humeral heads, the shaft of the femur, humerus, and the proximal section of the tibia and fibula. Kawashima demonstrated platelet aggregation and thrombosis in proximity to air bubbles in the femoral heads of 4 divers dying from acute decompression illness.[53] Lanphier demonstrated raised intramedullary pressure during decompression of sheep from a dive. He argued that this increased pressure causes both decompression illness and bone necrosis.[57]

Bone necrosis is most prevalent in individuals who have spent long periods under pressure. Table 29-5 shows the relationship between dive depth and a history of decompression illness. In a substantial number of cases of bone necrosis, however, no such history exists. Groups at greatest risk include compressed air workers and saturation divers. Bone necrosis is rare in individuals whose maximum exposure pressure does not exceed 26 pounds per-square-inch gauge (2.8 ATA). In divers it is extremely uncommon unless the diver has spent time at more than 3.4 ATA. Bone necrosis is extremely uncommon in recreational divers, although it has been reported after a single dive.[52]

Bone necrosis is usually asymptomatic initially, although it has been suggested that nonspecific pain may occasionally occur.[64] Despite the absence of early symptoms, lesions that occur adjacent to intraarticular cortical surfaces can result in subchondral collapse and osteoarthritis.

Detection of osteonecrosis has traditionally been accomplished by plain radiography. Findings include radiodense areas, irregular calcification, areas of translucency, cysts, articular collapse, and sequestration of cortex (see Fig. 29-4).[64] Additional diagnostic techniques include computerized tomography, scintigraphy, and magnetic resonance imaging (MRI), which is probably the most sensitive indicator.

Shaft lesions are believed to be of no clinical consequence and require no treatment. Divers and compressed air workers with shaft lesions only are usually allowed to continue diving. Juxtaarticular lesions, on the other hand, are at risk of resulting in collapse of the cortex and secondary osteoarthritis. Most dive physicians will advise such an individual to discontinue diving or compressed air work. The prognosis of osteonecrosis in most cases is good (Table 29-6). Surgery (joint reconstruction) is necessary in only a tiny fraction of cases. Introduction of a free fibular vascularized graft has been used in cases of osteonecrosis from other causes prior to articular collapse, in an attempt to reestablish blood supply and prevent

Table 29-5 Bone lesions in relation to divers' claimed maximum depth and history of decompression illness*

Number of men	Maximum depth dived	Decompression sickness	Number (%) of bone lesions
1,078	<50 m	−	6 (0.6)
71		+	2 (2.8)
74	>200 m	−	7 (9.5)
117		+	25 (21.4)

*MRC Decompression Sickness Registry, November 1980.[65]

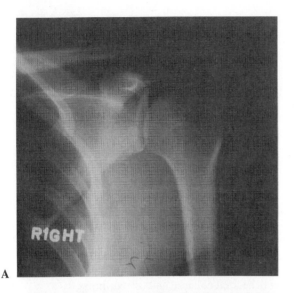

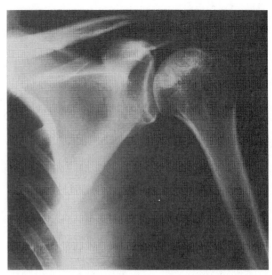

A

B

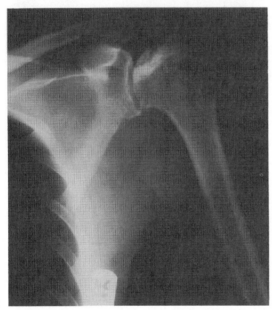

C

Fig. 29-4 Progression of osteonecrosis in a saturation diver. **A,** Baseline, normal shoulder. **B,** Eleven years later, 8 years after his last saturation dive. Lytic areas seen in the head of the humerus and a subchondral area of sclerosis. **C,** Four years after B, there is subchondral collapse of the cortical bone and evidence of osteoarthritis.

degenerative changes.[11] This may also provide a satisfactory means of therapy for divers or compressed air workers with this condition.

Other long-term health effects of diving

A recent review of possible long-term health effects of diving is presented by Elliott and Moon.[29]

Neurologic decompression illness does not necessary resolve completely, even with appropriate treatment. Long-term neurologic effects can exist in individuals with such a history. It is also recognized that the neuropathologic abnormalities may be disproportionate to the clinical manifestations of such residual effects.[77] The possibility that asymptomatic progressive neurologic damage can

occur has also been suggested by Rózsahegyi, who reported observations consistent with a progressive encephalopathy in compressed air workers.[84,85] All of his clinical cases, however, were in individuals who had suffered decompression illness. Evidence for asymptomatic cerebral damage was provided by 3 abnormal EEG studies among 12 compressed air workers who had not suffered decompression illness; however, there were no case controls.

Minor neurologic abnormalities in the absence of reported DCI after saturation dives have been described by a number of authors.[1,96-98] The clinical significance of these findings has not yet been established. Psychometric investigations

Table 29-6 Prognosis of dysbaric osteonecrosis

Category	Total N	Percent
Commercial divers in MRC registry	6961	100.00
Radiographic evidence of osteonecrosis	293	4.21
Head, neck, shaft	216	3.10
Juxtaarticular	77	1.11
Subchondral collapse	12	0.17
Orthopaedic surgery	1*	0.01

From United Kingdom Research Council Registry.[100]
*Of 12 divers with pathological fracture, follow-up information was obtained in 9.

have been performed by a number of authors. Vaernes[103] and Aarli[1] reported behavioral disturbances, including sleepiness and depression in divers after completing saturation dives. Vaernes et al studied 82 commercial saturation divers and found that greater than 10% impairment on some scales could be shown in about one-fifth of divers. The authors admitted that these changes could have been random statistical variations, but could not exclude organic cerebral damage. On the other hand, Thalmann,[91] Torok,[99] and Canvenel[12] failed to find any such abnormalities. Similarly Edmonds and Hayward[26] and Andrews et al[3] failed to demonstrate any statistical evidence of neuropsychologic damage in groups of air-diving fishermen, despite extraordinary depth-time exposures and a high prevalence of decompression illness. Curley demonstrated transient post-dive alterations in neuropsychologic testings of US Navy saturation divers without any evidence of long-term effects.[16]

Electrophysiologic studies include EEG, a technique in which abnormalities may be nonspecific and subject to interobserver variability. Other techniques have included MRI. Fueredi et al observed a higher number of foci of increased T_2 signal in the white matter in 19 compressed air tunnel workers compared with 11 controls.[42] Rinck et al, however, found no differences in MRI studies of the brains between a group of 70 professional divers and 47 nondivers.[82]

Some neuropathologic studies have been reported. Palmer et al reported some evidence of acute tract degeneration in three of eight professional divers in whom the spinal cord was examined using Marchi staining.[75] It is believed that such staining does not become positive until 7 to 10 days after an injury, and remains positive for around 10 weeks. Mork[70] and Palmer et al[76] found some evidence of premature aging changes in the brains of divers, although the clinical significance

of these changes is unknown. Retinal fluorescein angiography was used in a study of divers and nondivers.[81] Pigment epithelial changes were reported in one of 22 nondivers and in approximately half the divers. These changes were more likely in individuals who had experienced decompression illness. There was no evidence of visual loss of any of these individuals, and the clinical significance of the observed retinal changes remains unknown.

Pulmonary effects

Evidence of mild airways obstruction has been reported by Davey et al,[17] Cotes,[15] Elliott et al,[27] and Thorsen.[91,93,95] It is unknown to what extent these effects may have been caused by cigarette smoking, oxygen exposure, or breathing gas contaminants. Thorsen et al demonstrated decrements in spirometry related to cumulative diving exposure, which may be age-related.[93] Reduced pulmonary carbon monoxide transfer (D_LCO) has been observed after saturation dives.[50,89,92-94] Similar findings have been observed after short air dives.[22,23] It is believed that these changes may be due to the cumulative effect of low (subclinical) levels of VGE, although oxygen exposure and welding gas or other contaminants may also play a role. On the other hand, Lehnigk et al[58] reported no significant change after a 450 m saturation dive.[30]

The observed changes tend to resolve within a few weeks and are of such minor degree that no clinical effect has been shown.

Other effects

The various causes of deafness are described in detail in section 2 of this chapter. Other effects include transient liver enzyme abnormalities of uncertain significance;[20] chromosome abnormalities in cultured T lymphocytes;[38] and ventricular hypertrophy (Maehle et al[62]), although this may be a function of physical fitness ("athlete's heart") rather than a specific abnormality related to diving. Instances of azoospermia have been reported, although no cross-sectional studies are presently available.

Dembert et al[19] performed a cross-sectional study of 197 U.S. Navy divers and reported no significant abnormalities. Hoiberg and Blood[48,49] compared a group of divers and nondivers and found no difference on morbidity or mortality. There was a slightly greater number of hospitalizations for joint disorders in the third decade of life in divers, but morbidity was otherwise less in the divers. Among less-experienced diving officers, there was a greater number of hospital admissions for stress-disorders and cardiovascular disease, but no health risks were attributable to diving.[49]

Except for osteonecrosis and hearing loss, the

weight of evidence fails to support the existence of any clinical or subclinical syndrome in divers other than as a result of symptomatic decompression illness.

Returning to diving

Most diving physicians recommend that individuals who have suffered pulmonary barotrauma should never return to diving. There is evidence that recurrent episodes tend to be more likely to involve AGE and are often worse than the initial episode.[60] Some individuals have been allowed to return to diving if an appropriate, preventable explanation for pulmonary barotrauma can be found. Instances of barotrauma associated with uncontrolled ascent, particularly if beyond the divers control, may be classified as excusable. Divers with a previously unidentified anatomic predisposition, such as pulmonary bullae or reactive airways disease, should not be allowed to return to diving. Some physicians who suspect reactive airways disease have advocated using provocative testing (such as exercise, methacholine challenge) to provide greater sensitivity for detection.

The prevailing opinion among dive physicians is that individuals who have suffered skin bends or pain-only bends may be allowed to dive at any time after complete resolution of symptoms, provided that no neurologic abnormalities are detected. Individuals with neurologic decompression illness, on the other hand, should be discouraged from diving for some time.

Several pieces of evidence support this view. Intravascular bubbles have been observed even after successful recompression treatment.[25] Evidence for persistence of bubbles for several weeks after spontaneous resolution of decompression illness has been reported by Acott and Gorman.[2] Coagulation does not return to normal until several days after decompression illness.[79,80] Evidence exists that brain function may remain abnormal for about a month after treatment of decompression illness.[44] Return to diving should also require absence of overt sensitivity to decompression illness, absence of sequelae, and the absence of obvious risk factors for decompression illness.

Although possibly the most common predisposing factor is reactive airways disease, other identifiable risk factors have included patent foramen ovale (PFO), which can provide a mechanism by which VGE can become arterialized and has been identified as a risk factor for serious neurologic decompression illness.[67,103] Divers with a PFO (which can be detected using bubble contrast echocardiography) might be counselled to avoid diving patterns in which VGEs are likely to occur (saturation dives, dives requiring decompression stops).

EAR AND SINUS INJURIES

Multiple descriptions of ear and sinus problems in divers have appeared in the literature since the latter part of the nineteenth century. These and current concepts have been reviewed in several publications.[32-36]

The mechanism of inner ear injuries and their proper treatment differ depending on the phase and type of diving in which the injury occurred. These injuries are classified as:

1. Injuries occurring during descent or compression and largely related to middle ear barotrauma, discussed later in this section
2. Injuries occurring at stable deep depths related to changes in inert gas composition, not reported in recreational divers
3. Noise trauma during diving occurring mostly in military and commercial divers using gas-supplied chambers and helmets

Inner ear decompression sickness
Diagnosis and treatment

The following principles of the diagnosis and treatment of inner ear decompression sickness were proposed by Farmer et al.[37] Thus far these principles seem to be effective; however, adequate reports of such cases are infrequent, and future experience may indicate the need for modifications.

1. Vertigo, nausea, vomiting, and tinnitus (with or without hearing loss) beginning, during, or shortly after the decompression phase should be considered as representing inner ear decompression sickness. Prompt recompression is needed. Commercial or military divers experiencing such symptoms during and after a switch to an air environment during the decompression phase of a deep helium oxygen exposure should be switched back to the presymptom helium oxygen atmosphere and recompressed promptly.
2. The optimum depth of recompression is theoretically the lesser of the depth of relief or the bottom depth. Intralabyrinthine hemorrhages and/or structural deformities from inner ear decompression sickness, particularly those described by Landolt et al,[56] may not be immediately reversed with recompression. Prompt relief may not be seen, even though an adequate depth of recompression to drive the bubbles back into solution is achieved. Also, a return to the bottom depth may result in additional hazards or be impractical. It has been arbitrarily suggested that the optimum treatment depth in such situations should be at least 3 atmospheres deeper than the depth of symptom onset. This seems to be adequate; however, more

precise definitions of optimum recompression profiles for inner ear decompression sickness are needed. In most cases, inner ear decompression sickness, particularly in recreational divers, seems to be recognized immediately or shortly after reaching the surface. Prompt recompression using recompression tables for treating central nervous system decompression sickness should be used.

3. Drugs designed to increase intracranial or inner ear blood flow are not recommended. They are generally ineffective and may result in shunting blood to the periphery. If labyrinthine hemorrhage has occurred as indicated by animal studies, anticoagulants may result in additional intracochlear bleeding. These agents are also not recommended.

4. Diazepam, 5 to 15 mg intramuscularly, has been noted to result in significant relief of vertigo, nausea, and vomiting during diving-related inner ear injuries. Respiratory rate and blood pressure must be monitored after parenteral administration of this drug.

5. Other treatment measures advocated for the management of decompression sickness are needed. These include fluid replacement and the administration of oxygen-enriched treatment gases and other measures such as appropriate recompression schedules and gases described in section 1 of this chapter.

6. A complete otologic examination and follow-up by a specialist is needed as soon as possible after adequate recompression therapy. A history should be taken and a physical examination should include a neurologic examination, audiometry, and electronystagmography. The disappearance of vestibular symptoms several weeks after the injury does not usually mean that inner ear function has recovered. Adequate follow-up over 1 to 3 years is usually needed. Divers who suffer permanent inner ear dysfunction should not return to diving. Further injury to the same ear may be more likely and could result in extreme danger at depth from the associated vertigo and possible nausea and vomiting. Injury to the opposite ear during further diving could result in significant disability for nondiving activities.

Otologic barotrauma

The air-containing middle ear spaces and paranasal sinus cavities are liabilities for humans during diving. Proper pressure equilibration between these cavities in the ambient atmosphere must occur. The absence of sufficient pressure equilibration results in significant injury to the tissues adjacent to these air-containing cavities.

Middle ear barotrauma pathophysiology

Middle ear barotrauma, the most common medical problem encountered in diving, occurs most often during compression or descent when middle ear pressure becomes negative relative to the increase in ambient pressure. The eustachian tube is the only route for adequate pressure equilibration in the middle ear in the presence of an intact eardrum. The nasopharyngeal ostium of the eustachian tube, normally closed, opens with swallowing, primarily through the actions of the levator and tensor muscles of the palate. During the rapid, increasing pressures encountered during descent, insufficient opening frequently occurs, especially if the diver makes no active attempt to open the tube or if local inflammation or swelling, resulting from nasal inflammatory disease, prevents sufficient opening. With increasingly negative middle ear pressure, injury consisting of swelling, congestion, and bleeding of the mucosa lining the middle ear and eustachian tube occurs with subsequent narrowing of the lumen. A nasopharyngeal valve effect is also present (Fig. 29-5B and C).

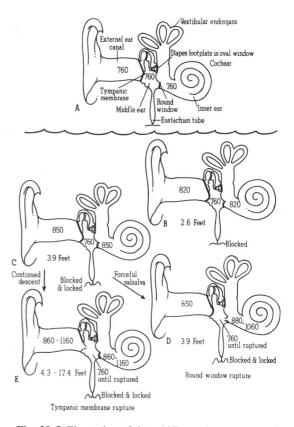

Fig. 29-5 Illustration of the middle ear barotrauma and the pathologic changes that occur during diving. The ear anatomy before diving is shown in A. The effects of continued descent and of increased pressure on the middle ear are shown in B, C, D, and E.

Further pressure equilibration through the eustachian tube and adequate ear clearing is therefore more difficult. This explains why many divers have no difficulty with middle ear pressure equilibration during the first one or two dives only to develop problems with ear clearing during subsequent dives.

The pathologic changes during middle ear barotrauma occur in the entire middle ear and the eardrum. Changes include edema and hemorrhages in the middle ear mucosa plus inflammation and collection of serous fluid or blood or both in the middle ear. Eardrum perforations, if present, may be obvious or small and obscure. Blood in the external ear canal suggests an eardrum perforation. Occasionally, little or no signs of middle ear barotrauma are seen with initial otoscopic examination; more obvious signs of negative middle ear pressure with eardrum retraction and inflammation and/or middle ear effusion develop in the subsequent 24 hours. Tympanic membrane ruptures have been noted at varying pressure differentials ranging from 100 to 500 mm/Hg equivalent to depths of 4.3 to 17.4 feet, 1.3 to 5.3 meters (see Fig. 29-5E).[54]

A forceful Valsalva maneuver during these conditions results in an increase in cerebrospinal fluid pressure and in inner ear fluid pressure. The resulting increase in the pressure differentials between the inner and the middle ear can lead to rupture of the round or oval windows and the intralabyrinthine membranes with inner ear injury (see Fig. 29-5D).

Diagnosis, treatment, and prevention of middle ear barotrauma

The best treatment of middle ear barotrauma is caution and prevention. An adequate prediving otolaryngologic examination that emphasizes nasal and eustachian tube function is needed. Particular attention must be paid to diving candidates with a history or signs and symptoms of middle ear and/or nasal disease. A history of ear infection, drainage, or middle ear surgery, the presence of a healed or unhealed eardrum perforation, and the existence of a cholesteatoma suggest poor eustachian tube function during nondiving conditions. Individuals with these conditions are more likely to have difficulties equilibrating the pressure changes encountered in diving. Other important factors in preventing middle and possible inner ear barotrauma include the avoidance of diving in the presence of significant nasal inflammatory disease, aborting descent without sufficient middle ear pressure equilibration every 2 feet, slow descent rates, descent in a feet-first, head-up posture, and avoiding the performance of a modified Valsalva maneuver at depth. Once middle ear barotrauma has occurred, the first task of the examining physi-

cian is to rule out inner ear dysfunction related to inner ear barotrauma. Nerve deafness, loud tinnitus, or vertigo with nystagmus suggest inner ear injury.

Divers should also be made aware of the various safe maneuvers to aid middle ear pressure equilibration. The simplest and perhaps most effective maneuver for most individuals is a modified yawn and swallowing. This involves thrusting the lower jaw anteriorly and partially opening the jaw while maintaining the lips closed around the regulator. This also may be followed by a swallow if clearing has not occurred. Another nontraumatic method of ventilating the middle ear is called the Frenzel maneuver. This involves closing the glottis, mouth, and nose while contracting the floor of the mouth and the superior pharyngeal constrictor muscles. The mass of the tongue is then strongly driven backward and upward to compress the nasopharyngeal space directly and indirectly through the soft palate. This forces air into the eustachian tube. Another method of middle ear pressure equilibration includes activating the palatal muscles by raising the soft palate. With experience, this technique may be mastered without the need to swallow or move the jaw. The Toyne maneuver consists of swallowing with the mouth and nose closed. It is the inverse of the modified Valsalva maneuver and has more use in relieving middle ear overpressure than underpressure.

These techniques are not likely to induce significant changes in arterial, central venous, or cerebrospinal fluid pressures or in the inner ear. Thus dangerous overpressures with subsequent pulmonary or inner ear barotrauma are less likely than with the modified Valsalva maneuvers. Also, these techniques involve contraction of the tensor muscle of the palate, the major muscle involved in opening the eustachian tube. Thus, less pressure may be required for tubal opening than with the modified Valsalva maneuver.

Diagnosis. After ruling out inner ear injury, the treatment principles depend on the degree of middle ear injury. Teed[90] presented a grading of middle ear barotrauma and included the following categories: grade 0: normal appearance; grade 1: retraction of the eardrum with redness over the pars flaccida and the long process of the malleus; grade 2: retraction and redness of the entire eardrum; grade 3: grade 2 plus evidence of fluid in the middle ear; grade 4: blood in the middle ear, or perforation of the eardrum, or both. This classification is useful in describing the pathology but has limited value for the treating physician. The otoscopic findings in middle ear barotrauma frequently include combinations of changes in different grades, and previous eardrum scarring may obscure the findings. More important, treatment would not closely depend on which grades are present. Therefore, patients with middle ear barotrauma and no signs of inner ear injury (loud tinnitus, nerve deafness, vertigo, and nystagmus) are classified as follows:[33-36]

1. Patients with symptoms but without otoscopic signs
2. Individuals with symptoms and otoscopic signs but without eardrum perforations (most frequently encountered)
3. Those with symptoms and otoscopic signs including eardrum perforations.

Treatment. Three treatment principles of middle ear barotrauma are recommended.

1. **Patients with symptoms but without otoscopic signs.** Avoid further diving until any preexisting nasal symptoms have improved, all ear symptoms have cleared, and the individual can easily autoinflate both ears at the surface. Long-acting topical nose-drops (0.5% oxymetazoline) may be used for 3 to 4 days, twice daily. Systemic decongestant or antihistamine preparations or both are frequently used. Caution should be observed regarding the sedative effects of antihistamines and the possible undesired adrenergic side effects of the decongestant agents.
2. **Divers with symptoms of middle ear barotrauma and otoscopic findings.** Usual findings are a retracted and injected eardrum with possible middle ear effusion, either serous or hemorrhagic, or both, but without eardrum perforation. These individuals should avoid further diving until the otoscopic findings are completely resolved and both ears can be easily autoinflated at the surface. This commonly requires 5 to 10 days and depends on the severity and the presence of nasal disease. Topical nasal decongestants, systemic decongestants, and antihistamines are usually beneficial, provided that the precautions described under number 1 are observed.

   Systemic antibiotics should be considered if signs of bacterial infection such as purulent nasal discharge or cough with purulent sputum production are present. Topical eardrop preparations containing antibiotics, steroids, and/or anesthetic agents are of little or no benefit with an intact eardrum. These substances do not readily cross the outer squamous epithelial layer of the tympanic membrane and commonly contain ototoxic antibiotics which should not be used with a possible eardrum perforation.

3. **Divers with symptoms and otoscopic findings including eardrum perforations.** These individuals should be treated in a manner similar to that described previously for cases of otoscopic findings without eardrum perforations. Diving must be avoided until the eardrum has healed. Antibiotics are usually indicated to prevent secondary infection. Ear irrigation is generally not wise as this may flush debris lying in the external ear canal into the middle ear. As noted previously, commercial antibiotic ear-drop preparations contain ototoxic drugs and should not be used. Most eardrum perforations resulting from middle ear barotrauma will heal spontaneously in 5 to 7 days and surgical repair will not be required. Poor eustachian tube function resulting from nasal disease can delay healing. If otoscopic examination reveals the possibility of a flap of torn eardrum displaced into the middle ear, referral to an otolaryngologist as soon as possible should be done. Also, if the eardrum does not heal after 2 to 3 weeks, referral to an otolaryngologist is indicated.

Middle ear barotrauma during ascent (alternobaric vertigo)

Inadequate middle ear pressure equilibration during ascent with a relative positive pressure in the middle ear does not occur. The eustachian tube usually opens without difficulty in response to a positive middle ear pressure. However, inadequate middle ear pressure equilibration during descent results in swelling and congestion of the eustachian tube with narrowing of the lumen. Frequently this swelling can be sufficient to completely obscure the eustachian tube. This can result in an overpressure in the middle ear during ascent. Indeed, transient vertigo secondary to asymmetrical middle ear pressure equilibration during ascent (alternobaric vertigo) has been described by several investigators and is reviewed by Lundgren et al.[61] During ascent, overpressure has been found to develop in divers in one ear with unequal vestibular endorgan stimulation. Many individuals have described unilateral middle ear pressure equilibration problems during descent. Vertigo occurred during ascent and disappeared by stopping the ascent, descending again, or in association with the sudden hissing of air in one ear.

Prevention of alternobaric vertigo. Middle ear overpressure and vertigo during underwater exposures can be hazardous. Spatial disorientation and accompanying nausea and vomiting can be fatal. The best treatment of this problem is prevention.

1. Divers having difficulty with ear clearing or who experience vertigo when performing a

Valsalva maneuver at the surface should not dive.

2. Ear fullness, blockage, or vertigo during descent should signal divers to halt further compression and ascend until the symptoms disappear.
3. If symptoms are noted during ascent, the ascent should be stopped and the diver should descend until his symptoms disappear if gas supplies and other conditions permit.
4. Divers should dive with a companion.

External ear canal barotrauma

Obstruction of the external ear canal while diving can result in barotrauma to the canal and eardrum during ascent or descent. Congestion, hemorrhage, and displacement of the eardrum or possible rupture with marked pressure changes occur. The best treatment of external ear canal barotrauma is prevention. The use of tight-fitting diving hoods, solid earplugs, or foams that completely seal the external ear canal must be avoided. Accumulated masses of cerumen that can potentially obstruct the ear during diving should be removed by irrigating the ear with water warmed to body temperature. Once external ear canal barotrauma has occurred, it should be treated similarly to the treatment described previously for middle ear barotrauma. If significant ear canal swelling has occurred, the treatment described in a subsequent section for the management of otitis externa is useful.

Inner ear barotrauma

Inner ear injuries occurring in association with relatively shallow diving or inner ear symptoms occurring during the compression phase of deeper diving have been termed inner ear barotrauma. These injuries were first documented by Freeman and Edmonds in 1972[41] and were related to labyrinthine window ruptures by Edmonds et al in 1974. Explosive and implosive mechanisms for such injuries were postulated by Goodhill et al.[43] In addition, Simmons postulated labyrinthine membrane breaks as a cause of barotrauma-related inner ear injury.[86] The human and animal studies of inner ear barotrauma have been reviewed in other literature.[33-35]

Pathophysiology of inner ear barotrauma. The explosive mechanism depicted in Fig. 29-5D occurs when middle ear pressure becomes negative to inner ear fluid pressure with inadequate middle ear pressure equilibration during descent. Any maneuver that results in an increase in spinal fluid pressure, such as a modified Valsalva maneuver, will cause increases in inner ear fluid pressure and a further increase in the pressure differential between the labyrinth and the middle ear.

Rupture of the round or oval window membrane into the middle ear with a subsequent perilymph fistula and/or tearing of intralabyrinthine membranes occur.

The implosive mechanism proposed by Goodhill et al[43] postulates that a sudden forceful Valsalva maneuver can result in a rapid increase in middle ear pressure with rupture of the oval or round windows into the labyrinthine space. Because most diving labyrinthine window ruptures are associated with middle ear barotrauma and relative eustachian tube obstruction, this mechanism is believed to occur infrequently during diving. As noted previously, however, elevated middle ear pressure during ascent can occur, usually after middle ear barotrauma during descent. This can result in an implosive type injury, described by Caruso et al.[13] Another possible implosive mechanism for inner ear barotrauma suggests that in the presence of negative middle ear pressure, the resulting inward displacement of the eardrum, ossicular chain, and stapes footplate can cause the footplate to sublux into the intralabyrinthine space and an oval window fistula occurs. As noted previously in the discussion of inner ear injuries in diving, Money et al described the temporal bones of a diver who died after pulmonary barotrauma caused by ascent while breathholding.[68] Blood in the middle and inner ear with rupture of the round window membrane were noted. The opposite temporal bone was normal.

Diagnosis and treatment of inner ear barotrauma. Optimum treatment of inner ear barotrauma involves preventing middle ear barotrauma as described previously. A diver who experiences persistent vertigo with or without sensorineural hearing loss or loud tinnitus after dives with unlikely decompression sickness may have inner ear barotrauma and a possible labyrinthine window fistula. These divers should not be recompressed because such therapy results in exposure to the same pressure changes that contributed to the injury. Bedrest with head elevation and the avoidance of maneuvers that result in increases in cerebrospinal fluid and perilymphatic fluid pressures are indicated. Anticoagulants, medications that increase intracranial and inner ear blood flow, and eardrops containing ototoxic antibiotics should be avoided for the same reasons discussed in the treatment of inner ear decompression sickness and middle ear barotrauma. A complete evaluation by an otologist, including an otoscopic examination, proper audiometric testing, a complete neurologic examination, and electronystagmographic test of vestibular function, should be accomplished as soon as possible.

The need for exploratory tympanotomy surgery

is controversial. Some authors advocate immediate surgery in all suspected cases of labyrinthine window rupture, and others suggest that surgery should be reserved for those who do not improve after 48 to 72 hours of bedrest with head elevation. This author currently follows the management principles suggested by Singleton et al that include conservative therapy with exploratory surgery reserved for those who show no improvement after 4 to 5 days or worsen in the interim.[87] Parell and Becker suggest that inner ear barotrauma may indeed be unrelated to an active fistula.[78]

Divers who exhibit permanent inner ear deficits upon otologic testing should not be returned to diving for the reasons described above under inner ear decompression sickness. Future injury—especially to the involved ear—can result in significant permanent disability, and it has been suggested that the injured inner ear may be more subject to further damage during future diving.

Differential diagnosis of inner ear barotrauma and inner ear decompression sickness. Most individuals with inner ear injuries related to diving will have inner ear barotrauma with possible labyrinthine window rupture or inner ear decompression sickness. The differential diagnosis of these entities is usually straightforward; however, in some cases the differentiation of inner ear barotrauma and inner ear decompression sickness can be difficult. Methods of diagnosis of these two entities have been previously described.[33-35] These include the following:

1. **Time of symptom onset.** Divers with symptoms starting during or shortly after decompression are more likely to suffer from inner ear decompression sickness. Those having difficulties with middle ear pressure equilibration during descent may have inner ear barotrauma.
2. **Dive characteristics.** Inner ear dysfunction associated with shallow dives in which decompression sickness is unlikely should not be suspected of being related to inner ear decompression sickness. It is likely due to inner ear barotrauma. Also, dives with rapid descents are more likely to result in inadequate middle ear pressure equilibration during compression and inner ear barotrauma, particularly with inexperienced divers. Isolated inner ear decompression sickness can occur with helium and air diving. It appears to be more common after helium dives, but this has not been established.
3. **Associated symptoms.** Divers with ear pain, blockage, or fullness during compression are more likely to have inner ear barotrauma.

Divers with symptoms suggestive of decompression sickness involving other organs or tissues are more likely to have inner ear symptoms related to bubble formation in the inner ear structures and/or microvasculature.

4. **Associated findings.** Divers with signs of middle ear barotrauma including middle ear effusion and/or a retracted hemorrhagic or ruptured eardrum are more likely to have inner ear barotrauma. Divers who have other neurologic deficits should be suspected of having inner ear symptoms on the basis of inner ear decompression sickness or pulmonary overpressure accidents with arterial gas emboli.

An accurate diagnosis can be difficult when the inner ear symptoms are first noted after no-decompression dives close to the no-decompression limits. Diagnosis can also be difficult in deeper dives where apparently adequate decompression schedules were followed. This is particularly the case when divers cannot recall the time of symptom onset. In these instances, major consideration should be given to other factors such as the breathing mixture used and the presence or absence of other associated signs or symptoms. If other signs of decompression sickness and/or acute neurologic deficits are present, recompression therapy should be initiated.

Paranasal sinus barotrauma
Paranasal sinus barotrauma has been well described in divers by Idicula,[51] Neuman et al,[72] and Fagan et al.[31] Inadequate pressure equilibration between the air-containing paranasal sinus cavities can occur during ascent or descent and seems to be more common during descent. It is usually related to secondary inflammation and congestion of the nasal mucosa which blocks the paranasal sinus ostia. Cysts or polyps may be present within the nose or within the sinus cavity, resulting in blockage of the sinus ostia. Negative intrasinus pressure can result during descent in the case of lesions in the nose. Blockage and increased sinus pressure can occur during ascent—the one-way valve effect. When this obstruction occurs during diving, pressure changes within the sinus cavity result in significant mucosal swelling, engorgement, and inflammation with actual hemorrhage into the submucosal layers and sinus cavities.

Treatment of paranasal sinus barotrauma. Steps to prevent paranasal sinus barotrauma, include the recognition that chronic nasal and sinus disease can predispose a diver to sinus and middle ear barotrauma. Common underlying chronic diseases in the nose and sinuses can be classified as being from: allergy—intrinsic or extrinsic;

chronic irritation from smoking; prolonged or excessive use of topical nosedrops, sprays, or possible exposures to irritating chemical fumes; mechanical obstruction from external or internal nasal deformities, polyps, or neoplasia; and vasomotor causes from chronic stress, tension, or anxiety. In patients with chronic nasal and sinus disease, more than one of these underlying etiologies is frequently involved.

Cold dry air exposures can result in increased nasal blood flow and congestion with secretion of increased volume of a more viscous mucous. Therefore, more frequent secondary infections by viruses and bacteria with worsening of the underlying conditions occurs. Thus, nasal and sinus problems are more frequent with cold temperature exposures. The lower respiratory tract is also commonly involved, particularly in patients with allergies or chronic irritation from smoking. Attempts can be made during prediving physicals and during the examination of injured divers to identify and manage the chronic nasal problems found. Individuals who suffer from chronic nasal and sinus disease or middle ear disease do not adequately maintain proper middle ear or sinus cavity ventilation in the absence of diving. These individuals should not be expected to adequately equilibrate pressure in these spaces during diving and should not be cleared to dive.

Systemic and topical adrenergic agents can improve nasal patency and paranasal sinus and middle ear pressure equilibration. Cautious use of such agents may allow a person to successfully equilibrate these pressures during diving. A rebound phenomenon from topical nosedrops, however, can result in greater nasal congestion and increased difficulties with pressure equilibration. Topical nasal decongestants also cause varying degrees of paralysis of the mucosal microscopic cilia and dissolution of the protective mucosal mucous blanket. Thus, prolonged use of these substances results in chronic nasal irritation and mucosal inflammation and even greater pressure equilibration problems during diving. Systemic decongestant and/or antihistamine medications are also used. The adrenergic components can cause side effects such as tachycardia and excessive drying of the respiratory tract mucosa. Antihistamine components can unpredictably cause drowsiness.

The acute treatment of paranasal sinus barotrauma includes the use of topical and systemic decongestants and adrenergic agents with the previously mentioned precautions. If purulent nasal discharge is present, cultures and appropriate antibiotics should be used. Future diving should be avoided until recovery, which usually requires at least 1 to 2 weeks. Most cases do recover with conservative therapy. None of the cases reported by Fagan et al required surgery.[31] Individuals who have a past history of frequent paranasal sinus barotrauma or chronic nasal or sinus disease in the absence of diving or who have other signs of systemic illness should be referred to an otolaryngologist for further evaluation.

Otitis externa

Otitis externa is the second most common diving injury after middle ear barotrauma. It is a painful, sometimes debilitating malady encountered in all types of diving. Cerumen is produced in the outer cartilaginous ear canal and contains water-soluble, bacteriostatic fatty acids in addition to oil-soluble fatty acids. This results in a slightly acid pH of the squamous epithelium that lines the canal. These factors, along with the constant outward migration of the squamous epithelium, provide a natural cleansing mechanism and protection from infection in this skin-lined cul-de-sac. Exposure to water or humid atmospheres produces maceration of the squamous epithelium and leeches out the water soluble fatty acids with a resulting alkaline pH. This provides a good medium for bacterial growth, particularly in the presence of local trauma or seborrheic dermatitis. Bacterial cultures from the ear canals of divers with otitis externa frequently show mixed flora, with pseudomonas and proteus organisms predominating. *Staphylococcus aureus* and other gram-positive organisms are also found. This is similar to the otitis externa encountered in the nondiving population.

Diagnosis of otitis externa. The symptoms include pain that can be severe, with initial itching and burning. Examination shows an inflamed, swollen, and tender external ear canal. A thin or serous discharge may be present. With progression, erythema of the pinna and surrounding skin and cervical lymphadenitis occur. Further progression may result in complete obstruction of the ear canal with abscess formation. Involvement of bone and cartilage can occur, particularly in immunocompromised individuals such as those with poorly controlled diabetes mellitus. Fortunately, these complications are rare in the diving population.

Treatment of otitis externa. The best treatment of otitis externa, a common problem in diving, is prevention with cleansing of ceruminous debris, avoidance of local trauma, and acidification of the ear canals. Control of any seborrheic conditions should be achieved before diving. If ventilated earplugs are to be used, they should be properly fitted and cleansed. A useful, prophylactic topical ear solution to acidify the ear canal during exposures to humid and aqueous environments contains 2% acetic acid and aluminum acetate. These include domeboro otic or vo-sol solutions and should be used daily and after showers and diving. Another possible solution is the mixture of 2 parts of white distilled vinegar with 3 parts of water. Alcohol has been recommended and is used as a prophylactic measure. The author prefers to avoid alcohol because this will dissolve the ceruminous fat soluble fatty acids that are considered to be protective and can irritate the ear canal skin which may be already inflamed.

Treatment principles of otitis externa include relief of pain and may require narcotics. Cleansing of the ear canal is best accomplished with irrigation using 3% hydrogen peroxide mixed with equal amounts of warm tap water so that the temperature of the resulting solution is body temperature. Care should be taken to dry the ear canal afterwards. A stream of warm air from a hair dryer is useful for this purpose. If eardrum perforation exists, irrigation should be avoided and suction or gentle cottonwipes should be used instead.

Commercial eardrops that are neutral or on the acid pH side with topical antibiotics and steroids are useful. These drops should be avoided with eardrum perforation because they usually contain ototoxic antibiotics such as neomycin. Adequate amounts of these agents can be used 3 to 4 times daily. If debris or other material accumulates in the ear canal, cleansing should be repeated before applying the eardrops. If ear canal swelling is such that the medications cannot be easily instilled into the entire canal, a cotton wick or a commercially available methylcellulose sponge wick should be inserted and the medication instilled several times daily. These wicks can usually be removed in 3 to 4 days once the swelling has subsided. All swimming and diving should cease until the otitis externa has cleared.

Otitis externa occurring in immunocompromised individuals is a potentially serious problem with possible osteomyelitis of the temporal bone. These patients should be referred to a specialist. Parenteral antibiotics effective against pseudomonas and proteus are frequently needed long-term.

Otolaryngologic guidelines for diving for sports scuba divers

These guidelines have been previously reviewed by Neblett[71] and Farmer.[33]

Ear guidelines for diving

History. A history of middle ear disease as noted previously indicates poor eustachian tube function and an increased likelihood of middle ear barotrauma. Also, a history of previous ear surgery should alert the physician to possible continuing poor eustachian tube function. Such ear surgery

may include a previous simple repair of an eardrum perforation. These patients may be considered for diving if the eardrum has healed and the ear can be easily autoinflated or cleared at the surface. This may also be the case with those who have undergone a previous simple mastoidectomy. Those who have undergone a more radical mastoidectomy involving removal of the posterior-external auditory canal wall, however, should not undertake diving since a caloric response with vertigo, nausea, and vomiting is more likely if water enters the cavity. Also, these patients are more likely to have inadequate eustachian tube function. A history of stapes surgery should preclude a patient from diving. The possibility of an oval window fistula with inner ear injury increases because of the middle ear pressure changes encountered in diving. A history indicating possible Ménière's disease and recurrent bouts of vertigo, nausea, vomiting, and/or hearing loss with tinnitus or other inner ear disease should preclude such individuals from diving. The occurrence of vertigo with possible nausea and vomiting can result in drowning.

Physical examination. Suitable candidates for diving should exhibit an intact eardrum with the ability to easily autoinflate each ear by a gentle, modified Valsalva or toyne maneuver while the examiner observes the eardrum with the otoscope. Tympanic membrane perforation is a contraindication for diving. Also, the presence or need for ventilation tubes would contraindicate diving. Eardrums that exhibit whitish plaques or tympanosclerotic plaques that are intact and move well with pneumatic otoscopy and autoinflation may not contraindicate diving. A thin, flaccid, or retracted tympanic membrane indicates poor eustachian tube function and the increased likelihood of eardrum perforation or caloric effects with diving. The presence of a cholesteatoma (a skin-lined sac within the middle ear) indicates chronic middle ear disease and is a contraindication for diving. Other physical examination findings such as stenosis and/or atresia of the ear canal should contraindicate diving. Acute or chronic otitis externa should be contraindications until healed. Patients with cerumen impactions should not dive until the cerumen is removed. Patients with narrowing of the ear canal from osteomas should be cautioned about diving.

Laboratory investigations. Suitable candidates for diving should exhibit in both ears a pure tone audiometric air conduction threshold 25 dB or less in the frequency range of 500 to 2,000 Hz plus a speech discrimination score of less than 90%. No abnormalities suggesting possible inner ear vestibular dysfunction should be seen on electronystagmographic testing. Patients who have hearing thresholds higher than those previously mentioned and/or electronystagmographic abnormalities may be more susceptible to future inner ear barotrauma, inner ear decompression sickness, or both. Also, injury to the opposite inner ear during future diving could result in significant disabilities.

Nasal and paranasal sinus qualifications for diving

Patients who have a history suggestive of chronic nasal or sinus disease are more likely to have paranasal sinus and/or middle ear barotrauma and are unlikely to be able to successfully equilibrate middle ear and paranasal sinus pressure during diving. The basic underlying conditions behind such chronic disease may be allergy, chronic irritation from smoking or excessive use of topical nasal decongestants, mechanical obstruction from a deformed septum or polyps, and/or significant vasomotor rhinitis. Frequently the lower respiratory tract is involved. Bronchial asthma is a contraindication for diving. Patients who require the use of decongestants to dive should be cautioned against rebound phenomena and adrenergic side effects. They should be advised to abort dives if adequate middle ear pressure equilibration does not occur every 2 feet of descent. The use of these drugs does not usually allow adequate pressure equilibration in the presence of acute upper respiratory tract infection. Diving should be deferred until the acute episode has subsided.

REFERENCES

1. Aarli JA: Neurological consequences of deep diving: some case studies. In Shields TG et al, editors: *Long-term neurological consequences of deep diving,* Stavanger, 1983, pp 53-59, AS Verbum.
2. Acott CJ, Gorman DF: Decompression illness in a diver following N_2O anesthesia, *Anaes Intensive Care* 20:249-250, 1992.
3. Andrews G et al: Does non-clinical decompression stress lead to brain damage in abalone divers?, *Med J Austr* 144:399-401, 1986.
4. Atkinson JR: Experimental air embolism, *Northwest Med* 62:699-703, 1963.
5. Barry PD et al: Decompression from a deep nitrogen/oxygen saturation dive—a case report, *Undersea Biomed Res* 11:387-393, 1984.
6. Bennett P: Inert gas narcosis. In Bennett PB, Elliott D, editors: *The physiology and medicine of diving,* London, 1993, pp 170-193, WB Saunders Company Ltd.
7. Bennett PB, Coggin R, Roby J: Control of HPNS in humans during rapid compression with trimix to 650 m (2132 ft), *Undersea Biomed Res* 8:85-100, 1981.
8. Bevan J: Commercial diving equipment and procedures. In Bennett PB, Elliott D, editors: *The physiology and medicine of diving,* London, 1993, pp 33-52, WB Saunders Company Ltd.
9. Bradley ME, Bornmann RC: Scuba disease revisited(?). In Bachrach J, Matzen MM, editors: *Underwater physiology VIII. Proc. eighth symposium on underwater physiol-*

ogy (A). Bethesda, 1984, pp 173-180, Undersea Medical Society, Inc.
10. Brunner FP, Frick PG, Bühlmann AA: Post-decompression shock due to extravasation of plasma, *Lancet,* 1:1071-1073, 1964.
11. Buckley PD, Gearen PF, Petty RW: Structural bone-grafting for early atraumatic avascular necrosis of the femoral head, *J Bone Joint Surg* 73:1357-64, 1991.
12. Canvenel P et al: French experience in deep diving. In Shields TG et al, editors: *Long-term neurological consequences of deep diving,* Stavanger, 1983, pp 111-120, AS Verbum.
13. Caruso BG et al: Otologic and otoneurologic injuries in divers: clinical studies on nine commercial and two sport divers, *Laryngoscope* 87:508-521, 1977.
14. Clark JM: Oxygen toxicity. In Bennett PB, Elliott D, editors: *The physiology and medicine of diving,* London, 1993, pp 121-169, WB Saunders Company Ltd.
15. Cotes JE et al: Respiratory effects of single saturation dive to 300 m, *Brit J Med* 44:76-82, 1987.
16. Curley MD, Schwartz MJC, Zwingelberg KM: Neuropsychologic assessment of cerebral decompression sickness and gas embolism, *Undersea Biomed Res* 15:223-236, 1988.
17. Davey IS et al: Does diving exposure induce airflow obstruction, *Clin Sci* 65:480, 1989.
18. Debatin JF et al: MRI of absent left pulmonary artery, *J Computer Assisted Tomogr* 10:641-645, 1992.
19. Dembert ML et al: Multiphasic health profiles of Navy divers, *Undersea Biomed Res* 10:45-61, 1983.
20. Doran GR: Disturbed liver function in divers: further enzymological evidence, *Undersea Biomed Res* 17:(suppl), 70-71, 1990.
21. Drummond JC, Moore SS: The influence of dextrose administration and neurologic outcome after temporary spinal cord ischemia in the rabbit, *Anesthesiology* 70:64-70, 1989.
22. Dujic Z et al: Lung diffusing capacity in a hyperbaric environment: assessment by a rebreathing technique, *Br J Ind Med* 49:254-259, 1992.
23. Dujic Z et al: Effect of a single air dive on pulmonary diffusing capacity in professional divers, *J Appl Physiol* 74:55-61, 1993.
24. Dutka AJ: Therapy for dysbaric central nervous system ischemia: adjuncts to recompression. In Bennett PB, Moon RE, editors: *Diving accident management,* Bethesda, 1990, pp 222-234, Undersea and Hyperbaric Medical Society.
25. Eckenhoff RG et al: Direct ascent from shallow air saturation exposures, *Undersea Biomed Res* 13:305-316, 1986.
26. Edmonds C, Hayward L: Intellectual impairment with diving: a review. In Bove AA, Bachrach AJ, Greenbaum LJ, Jr., editors: *Proc 9th international symposium on underwater and hyperbraic physiology,* Bethesda, 1987, pp 877-886, Undersea and Hyperbaric Medical Society.
27. Elliott C et al: Narrowing of small lung airways in commercial dives. In Sterk W, Geeraedts L, editors: *Proc EUBS annual scientific meeting,* Amsterdam, 1990, pp 197-202, European Undersea Biomedical Society.
28. Elliott DH: Residual effects and return to diving. In Bennett PB, Moon RE, editors: *Diving accident management,* Bethesda, 1990, pp 235-243, Undersea and Hyperbaric Medical Society.
29. Elliott DH, Moon RE: Manifestations of the decompression disorders. In Bennett PB, Elliott D, editors: *The physiology and medicine of diving,* London, 1993, pp 481-505, WB Saunders Company Ltd.
30. Elliott DH, Moon RE: Long-term health effects of diving. In Bennett PB, Elliott D, editors: *The physiology and*

medicine of diving, London, 1993, pp 585-604, WB Saunders Company Ltd.

31. Fagan P, McKensie B, Edmonds C: Sinus barotrauma in divers, *Ann Otol Rhinol Laryngol* 85:61-64, 1976.

32. Farmer JC: Diving injuries to the inner ear, *Ann Otol Rhinol Laryngol* 86:(suppl 36), 1-20, Jan/Feb, 1977.

33. Farmer JC: Ear and sinus problems in diving, In AA Bove, JC Davis, editors: *Diving Medicine,* ed 2, Philadelphia, 1990, pp 200-222, WB Saunders.

34. Farmer JC Jr: Otologic and paranasal sinus problems in diving, In Bennett PB, Elliott DH, editors: *The physiology and medicine of diving,* ed 4, London, 1993, pp 267-300, WB Saunders Company Ltd.

35. Farmer JC Jr, Gillespie CA: Otologic medicine and surgery of exposures to aerospace, diving, and compressed gases, In Alberti PW, Ruben RJ, editors: *Otologic medicine and surgery,* New York, 1988, pp 1753-1802, Churchill Livingstone Inc.

36. Farmer JC, Thomas WG: Ear and sinus problems in diving, In Strauss EM, editor: *Diving Medicine,* New York, 1976, pp 109-133, Grune and Stratton.

37. Farmer JC et al: Inner ear decompression sickness, *Laryngoscope* 86:1315-1327, 1976.

38. Fox DP et al: Chromosome aberrations in divers, *Undersea Biomed Res* 11:193-204, 1984.

39. Francis TJ et al: Central nervous system decompression sickness: latency of 1070 human cases, *Undersea Biomed Res* 15:403-417, 1988.

40. Francis TJR, Gorman DF: Pathogenesis of the decompression disorders. In Bennett PB, Elliott D, editors: *The physiology and medicine of diving,* London, 1993, pp 454-480, WB Saunders Company Ltd.

41. Freeman P, Edmonds C: Inner ear barotrauma, *Archs Otolar* 95:556-563, 1972.

42. Fueredi GA, Czarnecki DJ, Kindwell EP: MR findings in the brains of compressed-air tunnel workers: relationship to psychometric results, *Am J Neuroradiol* 12:67-70, 1991.

43. Goodhill V, Harris I, Brockman S: Sudden deafness and labyrinthine window ruptures, *Ann Otol Rhinol Laryngol* 82:2-12, 1973.

44. Gorman DF et al: Neurologic sequelae of decompression sickness: a clinical report. In Bove AA, Bachrach AJ, Greenbaum LJ, Jr, editors: *Proc 9th international symposium on underwater and hyperbraic physiology,* Bethesda, 1987, pp 993-998, Undersea and Hyperbaric Medical Society.

45. Hamilton RW et al: Saturation diving at 650 feet, *Ocean Systems Technological Memorandum* B-411, Tonawanda, 1966.

46. Hassen-Khodja R et al: Les ruptures gastriques par accident de plongée. A propos de 2 cas, revue de la literature, *J Chir (Paris)* 125:170-173, 1988.

47. Hill L, Phillips AE: Deep sea diving, *J R Nav Med Serv* 18:157-173, 1932.

48. Hoiberg A, Blood C: Age-specific morbidity rates among US Navy enlisted divers and controls, *Undersea Biomed Res* 12:191-203, 1985.

49. Hoiberg A, Blood C: Health risks of diving among U.S. Navy officers, *Undersea Biomed Res* 13:237-245, 1986.

50. Hyacinthe R, Giry P, Brousolle B: Development of alterations in pulmonary diffusing capacity after deep saturation dive with high oxygen level during decompression. In Bachrach AJ, Matzen MM, editors: *Proc VIIth symposium on underwater physiology,* Bethesda, 1987, pp 75-83, Undersea Medical Society.

51. Idicula J: Perplexing case of maxillary sinus barotrauma, *Aerospace Med* 43:891-892, 1972.

52. James CCM: Late bone lesions in caisson disease: three cases in submarine personnel, *Lancet* 2:6-8, 1945.

53. Kawashima M: Aseptic bone necrosis in Japanese divers, *Bull Tokyo Med Dental Univ,* 23:71-92, 1976.

54. Keller AP: A study of the relationship of air pressures to myringorupture, *Laryngoscope* 68:2015-2029, 1958.

55. Kindwall EP: Compressed air work. In Bennett PB, Elliott D, editors: *The physiology and medicine of diving,* London, 1993, pp 1-18, WB Saunders Company Ltd.

56. Landolt JP et al: Inner ear decompression sickness in the squirrel monkey: Observations, interpretations, and mechanisms, In Bachrach AJ, Matzen MM, editors: *Underwater physiology VII, proceedings of the 8th symposium on underwater physiology,* Bethesda, 1984, pp 211-224, Undersea Medical Society.

57. Lanphier EH: What is bends? In Nashimoto I, Lanphier EH, editors: *Proc 43rd UHMS workshop,* Bethesda, 1991, pp 49-53, Undersea and Hyperbaric Medical Society.

58. Lehnigk B et al: *The effects of a single saturation dive on lung function, diffusing capacity and pulmonary gas exchange during exercise* (in press).

59. Leitch DR: Complications of saturation diving, *J R Soc Med* 78:634-637, 1985.

60. Leitch DR, Green RD: Recurrent pulmonary barotrauma, *Aviat Space Environ Med* 57:1039-1043, 1986.

61. Lundgren C, Tjernstrom O, Ornhagen H: Alternobaric vertigo and hearing disturbances in connection with diving: an epidemiologic study, *Undersea Biomed Res* 1:251-258, 1974.

62. Maehle BO, Giertsen JC, Tyssebotn I: Hypertrophy of the left cardiac ventricle in professional divers, *J Hyperbar Med* 4:189-195, 1989.

63. Margreiter R, Unterdorfer H, Margreiter D: Das Postive Barotrauma Des Magens, *Zentralbl Chir* 102:226-230, 1977.

64. McCallum RI, Harrison JAB: Dysbaric osteonecrosis: aseptic necrosis of bone. In Bennett PB, Elliott D, editors: *The physiology and medicine of diving,* London, 1993, pp 563-584, WB Saunders Company Ltd.

65. Medical Research Council Decompression Sickness Panel Report. Bone lesions in compressed air workers with special reference to men who worked on the Clyde Tunnels 1958 to 1963, *J Bone Joint Surg* 48B:207-235, 1966.

66. Mellem H, Emhjellen S, Horgen O: Pulmonary barotrauma and arterial gas embolism caused by an emphysematous bulla in a SCUBA diver, *Avait Space Environ Med* 61:559-562, 1990.

67. Mills HG: American Oilfield Divers, Inc. In Lang MA, Vann RD, editors: *Proc. American academy of underwater sciences repetitive diving workshop,* Costa Mesa, 1992, pp 81-83, American Academy of Underwater Sciences (publ. #AAUSDSP-RDW-02-92).

68. Money KB: Damage to the middle ear and the inner ear in underwater divers, *Undersea Biomed Res* 12:77-84, 1985.

69. Moon RE, Gorman DF: Treatment of the decompression disorders. In Bennett PB, Elliott D, editors: *The physiology and medicine of diving,* London, 1993, pp 506-541, WB Saunders Company Ltd.

70. Mork S: CNS findings from 40 diver autopsies. In *Report of an open meeting of the MRC decompression sickness panel's long-term health effects working group at the University of Hawaii, Second International Symposium on Man in the Sea,* London, 1988, Medical Research Group.

71. Neblett LM: Otolaryngology and sport scuba diving: update and guidelines, *Ann Otol Rhinol Laryngol* 94 (suppl 115):2-12, 1985.

72. Neuman T et al: Maxillary sinus barotrauma with cranial nerve involvement: a case report, *Aviat Space Environ Med* 46:314-315, 1975.

73. Neuman TS, Bove AA: Combined arterial gas embolism and decompression sickness following no-stop dives, *Undersea Biomed Res* 17:429-436, 1990.
74. Nishi RY: Doppler and ultrasonic bubble detection. In Bennett PB, Elliott D, editors: *The physiology and medicine of diving,* London, 1993, pp 433-453, WB Saunders Company Ltd.
75. Overland T: Oceaneering International. In Lang MA, Vann RD, editors: *Proc. American academy of underwater sciences repetitive diving workshop,* Costa Mesa, 1992, pp 89-101, American Academy of Underwater Sciences (Publ. #AAUSDSP-RDW-02-92).
76. Palmer AC, Calder IM, Yates PO: Cerebral vasculopathy in divers, *Neuropathol Appl Neurobiol* 18:113-124, 1992.
77. Palmer AC et al: Spinal cord degeneration in a case of "recovered" spinal decompresion sickness, *Br Med J* 283:888, 1981.
78. Parell GJ, Becker GD: Conservative management of inner ear barotrauma resulting from scuba diving, *Otolaryngol Head Neck Surg* 93:393-397, 1985.
79. Philp PB et al: Changes in the hemostatic system and in blood and urine chemistry of human subjects following decompression from a hyperbaric environment, *Aerospace Med* 43:498-505, 1972.
80. Philp RB et al: Effects of decompression on platelet and hemostasis in men and the influence of antiplatelet drugs (RA233 and VK744), *Aerospace Med* 45:231-240, 1974.
81. Polkinghorne PJ et al: Ocular fundus lesions in divers, *Lancet* 2:1381-1383, 1988.
82. Rinck PA, Svihus R, de Francisco P: MR imaging of the central nervous system in divers, *JMRI* 1:293-299, 1991.
83. Rostain JC et al: Effects of a H$_2$/He/O$_2$ mixture on HPNS up to 450 m, *Undersea Biomed Res* 15:257-270, 1988.
84. Rózsahegyi I: The late consequences of the neurological forms of decompression sickness, *Br J Ind Med* 16:311-317, 1959.
85. Rózsahegyi I: Participation of the central nervous system in decompression, *Ind Med Surg* 35:101-110, 1966.
86. Simmons FB: Fluid dynamics in sudden sensorineural hearing loss, *Otolaryngol Clin N Amer* 11:55-61, 1978.
87. Singleton GT et al: Perilymph fistulas. Diagnostic criteria and therapy, *Ann Otol Rhinol Laryngol* 87:797-803, 1978.
88. Sterba JA: Thermal problems: prevention and treatment. In Bennett PB, Elliott D, editors: *The physiology and medicine of diving,* London, 1993, pp 301-341, WB Saunders Company Ltd.
89. Suzuki S, Ikeda T, Hashimoto A: Decrease in the single-breath diffusing capacity after saturation dives, *Undersea Biomed Res* 18:103-109, 1991.
90. Teed RW: Factors producing obstruction of the auditory tube in submarine personnel, *US Nav Med Bull* 44:293-306, 1944.
91. Thalmann E: US Navy experience from deep diving. In Shields TG et al, editors: *Long-term neurological consequences of deep diving,* Stavanger, 1983, pp 89-95, AS Verbum.
92. Thorsen E et al: Pulmonary mechanical function and diffusion capacity after deep saturation dives, *Br J Ind Med* 47:242-247, 1990.
93. Thorsen E et al: Pulmonary function one and four years after a deep saturation dive, *Scand J Work Environ Health* 19:115-120, 1993.
94. Thorsen E et al: Effects of raised partial pressure of oxygen on pulmonary function in saturation diving, *Report* 45-91b, Bergen, 1992, NUTEC.
95. Thorsen E et al: Divers' lung function: small airways disease?, *Brit J Ind Med* 47:19-523, 1990b.
96. Todnem K et al: Immediate neurological effects of diving to a depth of 360 metre, *Acta Neurol Scand* 80:333-340, 1989.
97. Todnem K et al: Influence of occupational diving upon the nervous system: an epidemiological study, *Brit J Ind Med* 47:708-714, 1990.
98. Todnem K et al: Neurological long term consequences of deep diving, *Brit J Ind Med* 48:258-266, 1991.
99. Torok Z: Recent British simulated deep diving experience. In Shields TG et al, editors: *Long-term neurological consequences of deep diving,* Stavanger, 1983, pp 103-108, AS Verbum.
100. United Kingdom Research Council Registry. Data quoted in Elliott DH: Residual effects and return to diving. In Bennett PB, Moon RE, editors: *Diving accident management,* Bethesda, 1990, pp 235-243, Undersea and Hyperbaric Medical Society.
101. Unterdorfer H: Das positive Barotrauma des Megens beim Sportauchen, *Beitr Gerichtl Med* 34:215-218, 1976.
102. US Navy Diving Manual. Diving Medicine; NAV SEA 0994-LP-001-9010, Rev 1, Dec 15, 1988.
103. Vaernes R: Reversible and possible irreversible CNS changes of diving. A discussion of some empirical studies. In Shields TG et al, editors: *Long-term neurological consequences of deep diving,* Stavanger, 1983, pp 31-47, AS Verbum.
104. Vann RD, Thalmann ED: Decompression physiology and practice. In Bennett PB, Elliott D, editors: *The physiology and medicine of diving,* London, 1993, pp 376-432, WB Saunders Company Ltd.
105. Vann RD et al: Flying after diving and decompression sickness, *Aviat Space Environ Med* 64:801-807, 1993.
106. Weien RW, Baumgartner N: Altitude decompression sickness: hyperbaric therapy results in 528 cases, *Aviat Space Environ Med* 61:833-836, 1990.
107. Wilmshurst PT, Ellis BG, Jenkins BS: Paradoxical gas embolism in a scuba diver with an atrial septal defect, *Br Med J* 293:1277, 1986.
108. Wirjosemito SA, Touhey JE, Workman WT: Type II altitude decompression sickness (DCS): U.S. Air Force experience with 133 cases, *Aviat Space Environ Med* 60:256-262, 1989.
109. Zwirewich CV et al: Noncardiogenic pulmonary edema caused by decompression sickness: rapid resolution following hyperbaric therapy, *Radiology* 163:81-82, 1987.

SUGGESTED READINGS

Aarli JA et al: Central nervous dysfunction associated with deep-sea diving, *Acta Neurol Scand* 71:2-10, 1985.
Alt F: Pathologie der Luftdruckerkrankungen des Gehororgans, *Verh Dtsch Otol Ges* 6:49-64, 1897 (English translation by Mrs A. Woke, NMRI, 1972).
Becker GD: Recurrent alternobaric facial paralysis resulting from scuba diving, *Laryngoscope* 93:596-598, 1983.
Bennett D, Liske E: Transient facial paralysis during ascent to altitude, *Neurology* 17, 194-198, 1967.
Buhlmann AA, Waldvogel W: The treatment of decompression sickness, *Helv Med Acta* 33:487-491, 1967.
Edmonds C, Freeman P, Tonkin J: Fistula of the round window in diving, *Trans Am Acad Ophthal Oto-lar* 78:444-447, 1974.
Ferguson BJ et al: Spontaneous CSF otorrhea from tegmen and posterior fossa defects, *Laryngoscope* 96:635-644, 1986.
Goldman RW: Pneumocephalus as a consequence of barotrauma, *JAMA* 255:3154-3156, 1986.
McCormick JG et al: Sudden hearing loss due to diving and its prevention with heparin, *Otolaryngol Clin North Am* 8(2):417-430, 1975.
Report by the Long-term Health Effects Working Group to the Medical Research Council Decompression Sickness Panel: *Long-term health effects of diving,* London, 1990, Medical Research Council.

Molvaer OL: Alternobaric facial palsy, *Med Aeronaut Spat Med Subaquat Hyperbar* 18:249-250, 1979.

Moon RE: Treatment of gas bubble disease, *Prob Res Care* 4:232-252, 1991.

Moon RE, Camporesi EM, Kisslo JA: Patent foramen ovale and decompression sickness in divers, *Lancet* 1:513-514, 1989.

Palmer AC, Calder IM, Hughes JT: Spinal cord degeneration in divers, *Lancet* 2:1365-1366, 1987.

Smith AH: *The effects of high atmospheric pressure, including the caisson disease,* Brooklyn, 1873, pp 1-53, Eagle Print.

Thorsen E et al: Exercise tolerance and pulmonary gas exchange after deep saturation dives, *J Appl Physiol* 68:1809-1814, 1990.

Vaernes R, Klove H, Ellertsen B: Neuropyschologic effects of saturation diving, *Undersea Biomed Res* 16:233-251, 1989.

Vail HH: Traumatic conditions of the ear in workers in an atmosphere of compressed air, *Arch Otolaryngol* 10:113-126, 1929.

30 Occupational Injuries Caused by Radiation Exposure

Radiation is the processes involved in emission, transmission, and absorption of energy in the form of waves or particles. The sun radiates heat and light, which are forms of radiant energy. Radiant energy is energy traveling as a wave motion; more specifically, it is the energy of electromagnetic waves. Sunlight contains ultraviolet and infrared rays as well as visible light. Radio and television waves, microwaves, radar, gamma rays, and x-rays are other examples of electromagnetic waves. The differences in the characteristics of these various waves are due to their wavelengths. As the wave frequency increases, wavelength is shorter.

Electromagnetic (EM) waves can pass into or through the body and deposit some or all of their energy in the tissues as they pass. The shortest waves are x-rays and gamma rays, which carry enough energy to form ions by displacing or ejecting an orbiting electron from atoms (and molecules) in absorbing material, such as tissue. This process is called ionization. X-rays or gamma rays, and also swiftly moving atomic particles such as cosmic rays and electrons (beta particles), which deliver enough energy to produce ions, are called ionizing radiation. The other electromagnetic waves mentioned do not have enough energy to produce ions; they are nonionizing radiation.

Radiation, both nonionizing and ionizing, is a normal and essential part of our environment. Exposures from these sources are called natural background radiation. Except for sunlight, most nonionizing radiation comes from numerous manmade sources, such as electric power generation and transmission, electric motors, microwave devices, and transmitters for radio, television, and radar. For ionizing radiation it is the reverse. Natural sources such as soil, rocks, and cosmic rays, produce the majority of exposures to man; however, manmade sources, such as x-ray machines, radioactive sources, and nuclear reactors, produce the occasional accidental exposures that need medical attention.

Nonionizing and ionizing radiation are discussed separately because the characteristics, terminology, biological mechanisms, and risk of potential health effects differ.

NONIONIZING RADIATION
Fundamentals

The radio-frequency electromagnetic (RFEM) spectrum includes EM waves at frequencies that range from near zero up to 3 trillion hertz (Hz). Fig. 30-1 depicts the regions of the electromagnetic spectrum. At the bottom end of the range is common household alternating electricity with a frequency of 60 Hz (commonly 50 Hz in Europe) and a wavelength that is many miles long. Frequencies from 30 to 300 Hz are called extremely low frequency (ELF). The ELF region has come into special interest over the past decade because of intense debates as to whether it induces cancer and/or birth defects. The voice frequency (VF), very low frequency (VLF), and low frequency (LF) regions extend up to 3×10 Hz with wavelengths over 1000 m long.[4] Such long length waves have scattering and absorption properties in the body that differ greatly from EM waves that are shorter than a few meters, such as wavelengths that approximate, or are shorter, than the body's physical dimensions (Box 30-1).

Medium frequency (MF) through extra high frequency (EHF) RFEM bands extend from 3×10^5 to 3×10^{11} Hz and include AM/FM radio, shortwave radio, television (VHF and UHF), radar, and microwaves. The wavelengths (in vacuum) range from 1000 to 0.001 meters. Microwave is a descriptive term for RFEM that includes only the highest frequencies (3×10^8 to 3×10 Hz[11]), regions known as ultra-high frequency (UHF), super-high frequency (SHF), and extremely high frequency (EHF). Description of biological effects from RFEM radiation above the medium frequency (MF) region is the subject of the National Council on Radiation Protection and Measurements' (NCRP) Report 86.[22] The mechanisms of interaction with biological materials are complex.

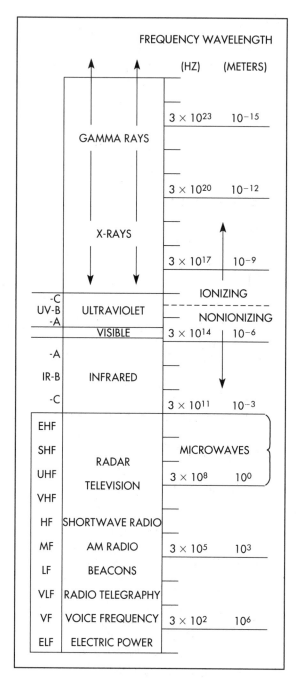

Fig. 30-1 The electromagnetic spectrum.

At high power densities (above 100 mW/cm²), there is no question about the potency of thermal effects from RFEM irradiation. At low power densities (under 10 mW/cm²), various athermal biological effects have been shown, but the interpretation of mechanisms producing these effects remains unclear.

Above the RFEM spectrum are three areas of EM waves that everyone recognizes: infrared radi-ation, visible light, and ultraviolet rays. Fig. 30-2 illustrates various features of this section of the electromagnetic spectrum. Infrared wavelengths are from 1000 to 0.78 mm, or 780 nanometers (nm). Table 30-1 lists the various prefixes, such as micro and nano, commonly used in radiation terminology. Infrared radiation is produced in a wide variety of industrial and domestic sources in-

---

BOX 30-1 GLOSSARY OF TERMS ASSOCIATED WITH NON-IONIZING RADIATION

Angstrom (A): the unit of length equal to one ten-billionth of a meter—used especially for wavelengths of light.

Coulomb (C): a unit of electrical charge; the amount of electrical charge that crosses a surface in one second if a steady current of one absolute ampere is flowing across the surface.

Electric field: a condition of space in the vicinity of an electric charge, manifesting itself as a force of an electric charge within that space. Electric field strength is expressed in units of volt per meter (V/m).

Electromagnetic wave: one of the waves that are propagated by simultaneous periodic variations of electric and magnetic field intensity.

Erg: the centimeter-gram-second unit for work (see joule).

Hertz (Hz): the unit of frequency—the number of complete cycles of the quantity per second (cycles/second).

Joule (J): the meter-kilogram-second unit of work or energy equal to 10^7 ergs or approximately 0.7375 foot-pounds.

Laser: an acronym for "light amplification by stimulated emission of radiation"; a device that generates coherent electromagnetic radiation in the ultraviolet, visible, or infrared regions of the spectrum.

Magnetic field: a condition of space in the vicinity of a magnetic or current-carrying substance, manifesting itself as a force on a moving charge or magnetic pole within that space. Magnetic field strength is expressed in units of ampere per meter (A/m).

Newton: the meter-kilogram-second unit of force, equal to the force that produces an acceleration of one meter per second per second on a mass of one kilogram.

Power density: the amount of energy delivered to unit surface area (mW/cm²).

Watt (W): the meter-kilogram-second unit of power, one joule per second.

Weber (Wb): the meter-kilogram-second unit of magnetic flux.

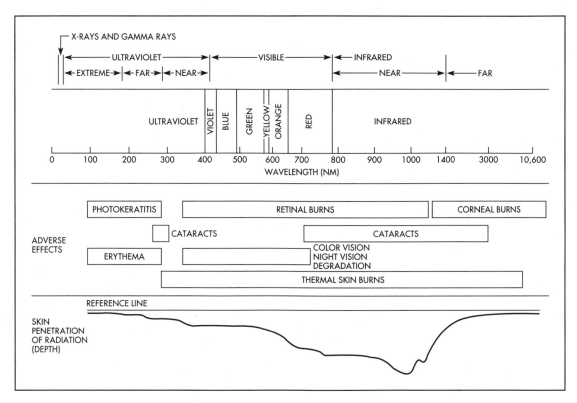

Fig. 30-2 Relationship of possible eye and skin damage to regions of ultraviolet, visible, and infrared electromagnetic waves. Courtesy of Lawrence Livermore National Laboratory, "A guide to eyewear for protection from laser light," report LLL-TB-87, Livermore, Ca, 1987.

volved in heating, baking, and drying processes. The energy of infrared waves is absorbed primarily as heat.

Visible radiation is in a narrow EM band from 780 to 400 nm. Visible light is usually accompanied by some of its neighboring wavelengths: infrared and ultraviolet. Lasers are devices that produce an amplified beam of coherent or synchronized EM radiation in the ultraviolet, visible, or infrared regions of the spectrum.

Table 30-1 Prefixes commonly used with radiation units

Name	Abbreviation	Value
giga	G	10^9
mega	M	10^6
kilo	k	10^3
centi	c	10^{-2}
milli	m	10^{-3}
micro	μ	10^{-6}
nano	n	10^{-9}
pico	p	10^{-12}

Ultraviolet radiation (UVR) is present beyond the visible spectrum at its violet end. By definition, near UV light, also called UV-A or black light, includes wavelengths from 400 to 315 nm; middle or UV-B from 315 to 280 nm; and far or UV-C below 280 nm. UV rays have the shortest wavelengths of the nonionizing spectrum and include the transition zone into the low end of ionizing radiation. The UV-C radiation from the sun is absorbed by the ozone layer in the atmosphere and does not play a role in producing biological effects from that source. Manmade sources of UV radiation include mercury vapor lamps, high intensity lights, special plant growth, and suntanning lamps. Special UV lamps (mostly UV-C) are designed for medical and industrial uses to sterilize instruments and catalyze chemical reactions. UVR is emitted as a byproduct of welding, plasma-torch operations, glass blowing, and glowing hot metal work.

Acute effects from nonionizing radiation

The acute effects from EM fields are well established and provide the bases for restrictions of exposure. The strength of an EM field is measured in power density (mW/cm^2 or W/m^2), electric

Table 30-2 Electromagnetic measurement terms

Term	Unit	Description
Energy	joule (J)	$J = 10^7$ erg
Energy dose	joule/kg	Time integral of dose rate
Specific absorption (SA)		Time integral of SAR*
Power	watt (W)	$W = 1$ J/s
Specific absorption rate (SAR)		Unit of RFEM dose rate*
Power per unit area	watt/m^2	$W/m^2 = 0.1$ mW/cm^2
Electric current	ampere (A)	Flow of 1 coulomb of electric charge/second
Electric potential difference	volt (V)	
Electric current density	ampere /m^2 (A/m^2)	
Electric field strength	volt/m (V/m)	
Magnetic field strength (H)	ampere/m (A/m)	$H = 1$ A/m
Magnetic flux	weber (Wb)	$Wb = 1$ V/s
Magnetic flux density (B)	tesla (t)	$t = 1$ Wb/m$^2 = 10^4$ gauss

* See reference 24.

field (V/m), or magnetic field (A/m). Units and descriptions of measurement terms are given in Table 30-2.

The absorption and distribution of energy deposition of nonionizing radiation in the body varies greatly with frequency. Detailed interpretation of interactions of EM fields and biological systems, including radiation penetration, cellular and molecular reactions, and pathophysiologic considerations, is important to better understanding of the pathophysiology of health effects, particularly potential subtle late effects. Acute EM effects are more easily classified because the skin, eyes, and testes are the primary organs of concern. These effects can be managed clinically by observation and empirical treatment methods.

A special problem is presented by implanted medical devices, which may be adversely affected by EM radiation fields.[11] The implants include orthopedic devices, cardiac pacemakers, and cochlear implants, but exclude dental work. The effect of EM radiation on the devices may increase heat load and produce signal interference; therefore, these special situations require evaluation, special precautions, and management. For example, common practice has been to prohibit pacemaker patients from using electric welding machines. This recommendation is safe but may be overly conservative in some situations. Special testing of work environments for EM interference allows the physician to make a knowledgeable decision regarding return to work for the pacemaker patient in a high EM interference environment.[19] The special testing requires detailed EM measurements of the work environment by a physicist or industrial hygienist experienced in such surveys.

Skin burns and heat

Ultraviolet rays are the cause of acute sunburn, which is the most common and easily recognized burn from EM radiation. UV-B radiation present in sunlight and manmade UV sources (e.g., arc welding, UV lamps) causes an initial skin erythema that largely fades within about 30 minutes. Recurrence of the erythema, accompanied with skin edema and pain, begins within 3 to 12 hours of exposure. These reactions are premonitory to possible vesiculation, bullae formation, desquamation, and itching over a period of 4 to 10 days. The individual responses to absorbed UV radiation vary greatly depending on the skin type, thickness, and melanin content. In severe cases, pain or systemic symptoms of chills, fever, nausea, or delirium will cause the patient to seek medical attention.

Symptomatic treatment with cool topical soaks with water or Burrow's solution may be helpful. Nonsteroidal antiinflammatory drugs are useful early in the course of treatment. Topical steroids are not particularly helpful, but systemic steroids can be used for severe cases with systemic symptoms. A typical treatment regimen would be 40 to 60 mg of oral prednisone with rapid tapering. Steroids are contraindicated in second-degree burn cases because of the risk of infection. Most important, the patient should be advised about the proper future use of sunscreen preparations and physical barriers, such as clothing and wide-brimmed hats. For persons who burn easily, sunscreens with a sun protection factor of 15 or higher and light-screening lipsticks are usually adequate to prevent burning.

The physician should be aware of distinctions between ordinary sunburn and photosensitivity reactions, which occur in the presence of photosensitizing drugs and chemicals.[5,31] The two types of photosensitivity reactions, phototoxic and photoallergic, are almost always due to UV-A exposure. The phototoxic reaction appears like an exaggerated and accelerated sunburn to UV exposure. Oral antimicrobial drugs, such as sulfonamides, declomycin, and nalidixic acid, are inducers of phototoxicity; infrequently, tetracycline and griseofulvin may be involved. Coal tar derivatives, dyes, and furocoumarins (psoralens) are topical photosensitizers. Photosensitivity can be severe in persons with porphyria, especially infants. The second reaction, photoallergy, is much less common and results in an urticarial, papular, or eczematous-type rash. These reactions occur with less UV exposure than do sunburn or phototoxic reactions. Oral photoallergic agents include some diuretics (chlorothiazides, quinethazine), hypoglycemics (chlorpropamide, tolbutamide), phenothiazines, and sulfonamines. Examples of topical photoallergic agents are sunscreens (PABA esters, digalloyltrioleate), topical antimicrobials (sulfathiazole, bithionol, halogenated salicyl-anilides and carbanilides), and some fragrances. A careful history of drug intake and chemical exposure is essential in treating these cases.

Photoallergic dermatitis may be indistinguishable from simple contact dermatitis. Dense perivascular round-cell infiltrate in the dermis is a characteristic finding in photoallergic dermatitis and is helpful in differential diagnosis. Specialized photopatch testing of different agents may be required. Primary treatment is based on identification and elimination of the causative agent. Persons taking medications or using topical agents known to be sensitizing should avoid sun exposure altogether, if possible, and absolutely avoid any form of UV-A from manmade sources.[1]

A less common sunlight-induced skin disease is polymorphous light eruption (PMLE), an idiopathic disease induced by UV-B, or less frequently by UV-A. The onset is often in the first or second decade of life. The lesions begin to appear from a few hours to several days after sun exposure. On exposed skin, these recurring pruritic eruptions range from eczema to small papules or, less commonly, plaques to large nodules. Treatment is photoprotection with sunscreens and avoidance of sunlight. Some relief may be provided by antihistamines and topical corticosteroids.

Laser burns of the skin, other than prescribed medical applications, are rare. They result from rapid large absorption of EV (thermal) energy from a strong laser beam. The resultant burn is a local tissue necrosis similar to that seen after an electrical burn. Topical corticosteroids or antibi-

otics should be used as needed. Experience with laser applications in dermatologic use indicate that hypertrophic scarring and pigmentary changes are occasionally observed.

Infrared radiation results in thermal heating of surface tissues. Skin sensitivity to heat should ordinarily provide adequate warning of high exposures. If a burn occurs, it should be treated the same as thermal burns. Persistent pigmentation may be observed on skin exposed to excessive and repetitive infrared radiation. Prolonged exposure to infrared radiation, along with elevated ambient temperatures, may lead to heat stress.

Microwave and radiofrequency radiation can produce local or general hyperthermia. Metal contacts on skin can absorb microwave radiation and produce a local hot spot. Sensation of skin warmth should provide an early warning mechanism of exposure in advance of a burn. The skin is not usually the major concern here, but rather the heat absorption in internal tissues. In animal experiments, the most sensitive measure of effects from elevated body core temperatures has been teratologic effects. A summary of such studies suggests a maximum body temperature of 39° C or less is most unlikely to produce any measurable biologic effect to occur solely because of heating.[25]

The testes are more heat sensitive than the body as a whole. Temporary sterility is possible, but recovery will occur. Large exposure to testes results in reduction of spermatocytes and damage to the cells lining the seminiferous tubules. Sperm counts may be used for several weeks to detect possible injury. Bonde[5] studied arc welders who had moderate exposure to radiant heat, which raised the skin temperature in the groin an average of 1.4° C. The proportion of sperm with normal shape declined significantly after 6 weeks of exposure. Sperm count and motile sperm count were nonsignificantly reduced among welders in comparison with two different reference groups. The effects were reversible.

Conjunctival and corneal reactions
The thin conjunctival epithelium, unprotected by stratum corneum or melanin, is particularly sensitive to UVR. UV-induced conjunctivitis, such as that seen with sunburn or welder's flash ("flashburn"), is a painful inflammation lasting about 3 days. Treatment generally consists of using cycloplegic drops and keeping on a tight eyepatch until the pain and inflammation subside. Use of ophthalmic anesthetic solutions can be used for pain relief for better diagnostic examination, if necessary. An eyepatch should be used to prevent possible corneal trauma from rubbing. If both eyes are involved, the worst eye may be patched until the patient gets home, at which time the second patch

should be applied. Anesthetic drops should not be dispensed to patients for home use. Oral medication can be used for pain relief if needed. The eyes should be rechecked the next day.

Chronic or repeated exposures will cause thickening and hypervascularity similar to solar dermal hyperkeratosis. Patients should be advised to wear protective eye glasses and side shields when in UVR exposure situations.

The cornea absorbs UV wavelengths below 295 nm and is thus sensitive to UV-B and UV-C. These middle and far UV waves are almost totally absorbed by the cornea and aqueous humor and do not reach the lens of the eye. Excessive exposure will result in a photokeratitis. The reaction is usually temporary, resolving in about 2 days. Near UV waves (UV-A) can penetrate to the lens and retina; thus, the potential ocular pathologic conditions from different UV wavelengths are significantly different.

Intense far IR above 2 mm wavelength (IR-B and IR-C) can cause corneal burns, but these are rarely seen because the heat and pain results in an aversion response that is protective. Near IR (IR-A) penetrates the iris, which is sensitive to thermal effects. Use of protective lenses or goggles by workers working around IR sources will prevent such injuries.

Cataracts

Cataracts have been associated with excessive exposures of UVR, IR, and RFEM at microwave frequencies. Cataract induction is the most prominently reported irreversible effect of RFEM exposure of human beings. Over 50 cases of cataract induction have been attributed to occupational microwave exposures.[22] Although subject to interpretation, the term "cataract" generally refers to lens opacification that results in loss of vision and may proceed to blindness.

Lens fibers are without blood supply, which predispose them to radiation damage by both thermal and athermal mechanisms. Animal experiments indicate that the mechanism of RFEM cataractogenesis is not totally due to thermal effects. Localized elevated temperature alone in the eye does not cause cataracts as does RFEM-induced temperatures of a comparable magnitude.[6] The damage tends to be more permanent in the lens of the eye than other tissues, apparently because of limited capacity for repair or replacement of these fibers.

The initial damage results in early lens opacities located primarily in the posterior subcapsular cortex. The opacities may progress and ultimately involve the anterior cortex and nucleus. In one human case, uveitis and chorioretinitis was observed

in addition to cataracts. At high power RFEM levels (420 mW/cm^2), rabbits have developed lens opacities in as short a time as 5 minutes. If either the power density or the duration of the irradiation are below a certain threshold value, the damage done to the lens is reparable, providing sufficient time elapses before subsequent similar exposures.[6] A National Council on Radiation Protection (NCRP) review indicates that deleterious effects have not been found in epidemiologic studies of ocular changes and occupational RFEM exposure.[22] If the assumption is made that human exposures in occupational environments are generally limited to power densities below 10 mW/cm^2, it may be assumed that this is a practical limit for ocular damage from intermittent exposure in microwave fields.[22]

Intense UV radiation (UV-A and UV-B from 295 to 325 nm) can induce cataracts. Laser light within these frequencies is the most likely exposure source. There is also evidence that repeated exposures to UV-A can result in posterior subcapsular cataracts. A positive correlation is reported between increased cataract formation and decreased latitude, increased UV-B, and total sunlight exposure.[11] Protection of the eyes is important for persons using tanning machines. Protection goggles containing yellow glass lenses that absorb all UV-A, UV-B, and visible light up to 500 nm should be worn; simply closing the eyes, using regular sunglasses, or putting cotton balls over the eyes may not protect against eye damage.[1]

Infrared radiation, especially IR-A wavelengths, has historically been the cause of cataracts among many workers exposed to glowing hot metals or molten glass. Cataracts in such workers have frequently been given names that identify the offending trade: furnaceman's cataract, glassblower's cataract, or bottleworker's cataract. In the United States, use of protective goggles by workers exposed to high infrared radiation has virtually eliminated the problem.

Surgical extraction of cataracts is the only treatment available. Prevention of excessive EM exposure is the objective of occupational medical and safety programs. Proper safety counseling of persons known to be subject to potential EM hazards, especially in their workplaces, is a simple but most valuable practice.

Retinal burns

The amplified energy of laser beams has the ability to induce instantaneous burns of the retina. These burns may occur from direct or reflected beams into the eye. The offending beam may be at a visible or an invisible wavelength. Lasers are classified as to their hazard in accordance to their type (continuous or pulsed), beam power, and wavelength or wavelength range. Some lasers (class 1) emit such low energy beams that no beam hazard exists.

The tissue damage from lasers may be thermal, photochemical, or acoustic (shock wave). Thermal damage, in which absorbed laser energy denatures the tissue proteins, is generally associated with visible and infrared wavelengths. Photochemical damage, in which absorbed laser energy causes chemical reactions and changes within tissue, occurs after exposure to UV and visible wavelengths of less than 500 nm at exposures greater than 10 seconds. Acoustic damage, in which absorbed energy from very short high-power pulses causes an explosive effect that destroys tissue. Such pulses generally occur at pulse durations less than 10^{-7} seconds or < 100 nanoseconds.

Retinal damage is potentially more serious than cataracts because no remedial treatment is available. Safety in workplaces involving lasers (depending on the hazard classification) may require appropriate warning signs, warning lights and interlocks, limited access, trained personnel, standard operating procedures, and appropriate protective glasses and equipment.

Late effects from nonionizing radiation

For years, controversy has swirled around whether late health effects are caused by exposure to nonionizing radiation. There are a number of reasons for this. Some studies have suggested possible effects caused by common services, such as electric power transmission, hair dryers, and electric blankets. The large numbers of persons working long periods of time near video display terminals raise an increasing number of questions and concerns about potential long-term health risks. A lawsuit claiming brain cancer induced by the use of cellular phones is the latest development from these worries. Visibility and importance of the subject is increasing as legal cases and regulatory decisions demand resolution, but research has not yet provided convincing and consistent answers. Newsmedia feed the controversy by presenting results of one or several studies or opinions that represent a limited view of the evidence and serve to stir up emotional reactions.

The controversy centers principally on whether nonionizing radiation induces excess cancers in humans. The entire EM spectrum from ELF (such as, 60-cycle AC electricity) to UV is involved in the question. There are also other important unresolved issues on late effects, such as reproduction and behavior changes. The following four sections provide a few paragraphs on these difficult subjects and may be helpful in counseling patients.

Skin aging and cancer
The subject of the effect of UVR radiation on skin is one area of agreement about the late effects of EMR. Frequent and prolonged exposures to UVR, especially the more penetrating UV-A, contributes to skin aging and an increased risk of skin cancer. Photodamage results in dermal connective-tissue destruction, which produces the coarse, dry, leathery skin with wrinkles seen on exposed parts. Although it has long been held that these changes are irreversible, animal studies indicate that further avoidance of UVR and sunscreen application allows some repair of the damage.[17] There is also preliminary evidence that skin appearance in middle-aged or elderly white people may be improved by long-term application of 0.1% tretinoin cream.[35]

Actinic keratoses (solar keratoses) are also related to photodamage. Squamous cell carcinomas arise in a small percentage of these premalignant lesions.

All three types of skin cancer—basal cell carcinoma, squamous cell carcinoma, and melanoma—relate to UVR exposure, but in somewhat different ways. Basal cell carcinoma, the most common skin cancer, occurs most frequently on men who are outdoors much of the time, sunburn easily, and tan poorly, if at all. Basal cell carcinomas are extremely uncommon in blacks. Squamous cell carcinoma also occurs primarily on skin commonly exposed to sun and has a relatively higher incidence in those persons living near the equator. In general, the risk of squamous cell carcinoma relates more strongly to sun exposure than does basal cell carcinoma.

The risk factors for cutaneous malignant melanoma are much less clear, and the role of UVR as a risk factor is unclear. There is a markedly lower incidence of skin melanoma in races with deeply pigmented skin than in whites. A history of sunburn is more common in persons with skin melanoma than in controls, but melanoma occurs proportionately more often in persons who work indoors rather than in those who work outdoors. Also the distribution of melanoma on the body does not correlate closely with skin areas of greatest UVR exposure.

The increased risk of skin cancer induced by UVR exposures through natural suntanning or use of suntanning lamps is now unquestioned. No form of sunbathing or artificial suntanning can be recommended. Those persons who decide the cosmetic benefits of tanning outweigh the potential risks should be advised that the activity provides no known medical benefits. The key to reducing the risk of skin cancer is to minimize exposure to UVR, avoid mid-day outdoor exposures, beware of reflective surfaces (sand, water, snow, ice), use a sunscreen, protect infants and children, and avoid tanning machines.[1]

Carcinogenesis

The risk of inducing cancer in internal organs is the center of the current controversies. Leukemia, brain cancer, and breast cancer are three diseases where excess risk has been reported among workers engaged in "electrical occupations," but there is no consistency among studies. Two recent publications exemplify the problem. Tornqvist et al conducted a 19-year follow-up study of Swedish workers expected to be exposed to EMR, namely electrical/electronic engineers and technicians.[33] The risk for all leukemias in these workers was increased about 30% (SMR 1.3; 95% CI 1.0 to 1.7). In radio/TV assemblers and repairmen, the risk for all brain tumors was increased 190% (SMR 2.9; 95% CI 1.2 to 5.9). Homogeneous patterns of increased risk of leukemia and brain tumor were not noted in this study, but the hypothesis that electromagnetic fields might play a part in the origin of cancer cannot be rejected. Sahl et al evaluated cancer mortality for leukemia, brain cancer, and lymphoma from 1960 to 1988 in over 36,000 electric utility workers.[30] No statistically significant excess of mortality or support for exposure-response trends was found.

The risk of exposure to ELF (60/50 Hz) fields has been a special concern because everyone has potential exposure. Theriault reviewed the literature on risks resulting from occupational exposure to 60/50 Hz EMF.[32] He found almost all electrical occupations have shown excesses of one cancer or another but no consistent observation has allowed firm conclusions. The size of the excess risk noted so far may seem small, but it is to be regarded seriously in view of the poor estimates used for exposure. The real agent responsible for the excesses of cancer observed in electrical occupations may be something other than EMF, such as chemical exposures. Such associations have not been shown.

Jauchem and Merritt found "no definitive evidence of an association between exposure to EMF and the alleged risks."[15] This review concluded that because of problems and limitations inherent in future studies (misconceptions about exposure levels, uncertainty about field variability, criticisms of surrogate measures), the question of cancer (and abnormal fetal development) risk is unlikely ever to be answered with certainty.

The results of research on cellular and molecular responses to assess carcinogenic potential of electromagnetic fields do not lead to firm conclusions either. Data on early cell signalling events that may lead to changes in gene expression remain far from convincing. A report on the First World Congress for Electricity and Magnetism in Biology and Medicine (1992) concludes that "the growing number of laboratories which have failed to identify a consistent effect on cell proliferation must cast considerable doubt on the significance of any of the reported effects."[7]

Reproduction

Teratogenesis is a well demonstrated effect noted in animals exposed to EMR. In human beings there is no evidence of anomalies after exposure in utero other than a few case reports of a possible or suspected relationship.[22]

With increased use of video display terminals (VDT), questions are raised as to whether working at a VDT affects the risk of adverse pregnancy outcome. A review by Kavet and Tell concludes that epidemiologic studies thus far do not provide a basis for concluding that VDT work and adverse pregnancy outcome are associated.[16]

Behavioral changes

The literature contains much evidence that absorption of microwave energy will lead to behavioral changes in human and laboratory animals. Epidemiologic studies of the problem are few in number and are generally limited in scope. Studies to detect possible effects from occupational exposures have been made of U.S. naval personnel occupationally exposed to radar[29] and of American embassy personnel in Moscow.[18] Both studies failed to detect adverse effects that could be attributed to RFEM radiation.

A NCRP report states several conclusions can be drawn on the behavioral response to RFEM irradiation.[25] These conclusions enjoy a substantial consensus among scientists of many disciplines:

1. Behavior is a highly sensitive index of field-body interactions with a broad spectrum of end points — responses range from changes in perception of warmth and sound to grand mal seizures when the energy absorption is varied over six orders of magnitude.
2. Intermediate endpoints (such as detection of cutaneous warming, radiation field-drug interactions, endurance, impaired performance, and work stoppage) is the area where consensus is lost and controversy begins.
3. The greatest void of scientific knowledge, where experiments are yet to be performed, is the systemic and functional responses of the organism that are observed over the long term after intense (acute) or low-level (chronic) exposures to fields that range the

spectrum and that are evaluated for modulation-specific influences.

D'Andrea concludes that thermal changes in human and animals during microwave exposure appear to account for all reported behavioral effects.[8] The specific absorption rates that produce behavioral effects seem to depend on microwave frequency, but controversy exists over thresholds and mechanism of action. In all cases, however, the behavioral disruptions cease when chronic microwave exposure is terminated.

CASE STUDIES

Complaints about video display terminals

A 28-year-old female complains of headaches and sore eyes. She believes these symptoms are due to her job, which requires constant work with video display terminals (VDT). She admits she, as well as others in her office, is concerned about exposure to radiation from VDTs, particularly with regard to possible effects during pregnancy.

The medical history and physical examination should probe for possible causes of headaches. Her medical examination should include testing of near and far vision, including possible need for correction of astigmatism. If physical factors are not apparent, she should be counseled that studies indicate that levels of physical discomfort experienced by VDT operators are in most offices similar to those experienced by workers who work with old-fashioned paper records. The main physical factors to consider when working with a VDT are the quality of the display (adjustable brightness, sharp focus, and stable); the room lighting (should not be overly bright, place VDTs away from uncurtained windows, shield exposed artificial light sources, and control screen reflections); and the furniture (adjustable seat height, screen height, and keyboard height). If there is a problem with any of these, she should discuss it with her supervisor and see if it can be corrected.

She should be advised that all VDTs are manufactured to specifications that limit the radiation exposure to operators and other office workers. Office workers using VDTs are exposed on average to a magnetic field (about 3.1 mG) only slightly higher than office workers who do not work with VDT (1.1 mG). These exposure levels are within the same range of levels measured in homes. Magnetic levels are frequently somewhat higher at the back of the VDT. In offices with many VDTs, it is usually advisable to have about a 3-foot distance between the back of the VDT and the next permanent full-time operating position. The strength of the magnetic field falls off rapidly as the distance from the source increases. Finally, she needs to know that radiation (both nonionizing and ionizing types) around many different types of VDTs and VDT workplaces have been measured and found to be at safe levels. Furthermore, even at higher levels there is no conclusive evidence that electromagnetic radiation presents a hazard to pregnant women.

Radiation from power lines

During a clinic visit, the young man mentioned to the doctor that he is trying to decide about the purchase of a new house that was attractive to him and his wife. There was one drawback: the house was located close to some overhead powerlines. He was worried about the risk of cancer to the family and possible future children from living close to a power line. Should he just drop the idea of buying a house in such a location?

The physician should point out that if there is extra risk of cancer that results from living near power lines, the studies so far have failed to show it consistently or conclusively. There are many sources of electromagnetic radiation in our lives; power lines are only one of these. Given the inconsistent cancer study results, it is unnecessary to let the power line location be a major factor in his final decision unless it be for esthetics, economics, or some reason other than cancer risk.

IONIZING RADIATION
Fundamentals

Exposures to ionizing radiation can be classified by the position of the radiation source relative to the body: external or internal. External or direct radiation comes from sources outside the body and is usually separated into two general classes. Penetrating radiation includes x-rays, gamma rays, and neutrons; nonpenetrating radiation includes soft (very low energy) gamma rays and beta particles. Penetrating radiation deposits energy or dose throughout the depth of exposed tissue, either whole body or localized exposures. Nonpenetrating radiation is deposited principally in the skin but does not penetrate to deeper tissues, such as skin burns produced by beta radiation.

Internal radiation is delivered by radionuclides taken into the body. Long-lived radionuclides that emit alpha or beta particles present the greatest hazard. Accidental internal exposures require rapid evaluation because medical treatment is much more effective if given in the first few hours.

Definition of types of radiation and some other common terms used in association with ionizing radiation are listed in Box 30-2.

The average person in the United States gets about 15% of her or his total dose of ionizing radiation as a result of medical applications. All other manmade sources, such as consumer products, nuclear industry, nuclear power, and fallout, contribute less than 4%. Nature is the source for over 80% of the ionizing radiation dose to people. Radiation comes from soils, rocks, the sun and natural internal radionuclides, such as potassium-40, and radon/radon progeny.[21] Inhalation of radon and radon progeny account for about two-thirds of the natural radiation dose.

Transportation of radioactive materials is overrated as a potential source of radiation and/or ra-

---

BOX 30-2 GLOSSARY OF TERMS ASSOCIATED WITH IONIZING RADIATION

Absorbed dose: The amount of energy absorbed per unit mass of irradiated material when ionizing radiation passes through the matter. The unit of absorbed dose is the gray (or rad).

Activity: The numbert of nuclear transformations occurring in a given quantity of material per unit time. The unit of activity (radioactivity) is the becquerel (or curie).

Alpha particle: A particle containing two neutrons and two protons and carrying a positive (+2) charge. It is emitted by some radionuclides.

Becquerel (bq): the SI unit of radioactivity defined as one nuclear transformation (disintegration) per second.

Beta particle: An electron with a single negative or positive charge (called a positron) and a mass of 1/1837 of a proton. It is emitted by some radionuclides.

Curie (Ci): the conventional unit of radioactivity. $1 \text{ Ci} = 3.7 \times 10^{10}$ becquerels.

Effective half-life: time required for a specific radionuclide to reduce its activity in a body by half as a result of both radioactive decay and biologic elimination.

Gamma rays: a photon or radiation quantum emitted spontaneously by a radioactive substance.

Gray (Gy): the SI measurement unit of absorbed dose equal to 1 J/kg; 100 rad = 1 Gy.

Ionizing radiation: radiation that produces ion pairs along its path through a substance.

Isotopes: any of two or more species of atoms of a chemical element with the same atomic number and position in the periodic table and nearly identical chemical behavior but with different atomic mass and physical properties.

Neutron: An uncharged elementary particle that has a mass nearly equal to that of the proton and is present in all known atomic nuclei except the hydrogen nucleus.

Photon: a quantum of radiant energy.

Progeny: the decay product produced by the radioactive disintegration of a radionuclide; progeny is often called a daughter or daughter product. The element from which the progeny was produced is called the "parent."

Proton: an elementary particle that carries a positive charge numerically equal to the charge of an electron and has a mass 1,837 times that of an electron.

Rad: refer to Gray.

Rem: refer to Sievert.

Sievert (Sv): the SI unit of dose equivalent; the absorbed dose in gray adjusted by weighting factors to make the long term biological risk per dose equivalent unit approximately equal for different types of ionizing radiation. 100 rem = 1 Sv.

Radionuclide: a radioactive form of an element.

X-rays: penetrating electromagnetic radiation of extremely short wavelength that is nonnuclear in origin.

---

dioactive contamination. Although accidents of transport vehicles carrying radioactive materials occur, they have not been responsible for significant radiation exposures. Of more concern are sealed radioactive sources, such as those used for industrial radiography or oil well logging, which may be lost through careless handling or improper use. Unknown and unannounced radiation exposing patients entering the clinic or emergency room are more likely to arise from such mishandled sealed sources than from transportation accidents.

A total of 357 major radiation accidents have occurred throughout the world from 1944 to 1992.[10] In the United States, 26 radiation-related deaths have been associated with major radiation accidents. Thus, the likelihood of attending a major acute radiation injury is extremely small. By contrast, almost all physicians are queried by pa-tients or friends about potential late radiation effects or about the possibility that some illness may have been caused by past experience around radiation of some unknown magnitude. There are no answers to these questions until a knowledgeable radiation dose estimate can be established.

Dosimetry units for ionizing radiation

The units used to express doses of ionizing radiation are complicated because two systems are currently used interchangeably. Conventional units are still commonly used in U.S. practice, but the SI (Systeme International) metric system is preferred internationally. The principal SI units are used in this section followed by the conventional unit in parenthesis.

The fundamental dosimetric quantity is the absorbed dose. It is the energy absorbed per unit mass of tissue. The gray (Gy) is that quantity of radiation that deposits a joule per kilogram of absorbing material, such as tissues. An absorbed dose cannot be measured directly in tissue without specialized equipment. (The conventional unit of absorbed dose is the rad, which equals 100 ergs per gram of absorbing material. One rad is equal to 0.01 Gy.)

To express a dose for all types of ionizing radiation, (alpha, beta, gamma, or neutrons) on a common scale based on their biological effect, it is necessary to adjust the absorbed dose by a radiation weighting factor, W_R. (This function is performed by the quality factor [QF] in conventional units.) The adjusted dose is called an equivalent dose. The W_R factor is 1 for x-rays, gamma rays, and most beta radiation; 5 for protons; 20 for alpha particles; and from 5 to 20 for neutrons, depending on their energy. These factors are arbitrary values that are judged to make an equivalent dose unit have about the same likelihood of inducing late effects, such as cancer, for the various types of radiation. The sievert (Sv) is the unit of equivalent dose, which is the dose of one joule per kilogram (Gy) weighted by the appropriate W_R. The conventional unit of equivalent dose is the rem. One rem equals 0.01 Sv. Another useful dose conversion is one rem equals 10 millisievert (mSv).

Radiation doses are never uniform throughout the body. The dose may be shielded or collimated so it affects only a part of the body. In addition, the radiosensitivity for acute effects as well as cancer induction is different between organs. To try to account for these variations, a hypothetical whole body dose can be calculated which gives approximately the same health detriment as an actual uniform whole body dose. For this purpose, the ICRP has recommended the use of tissue weighting factors (W_T).[13] These factors (Table 30-3) represent simplistically the relative contribution that various organs or tissues make toward the total health detriment resulting from uniform irradiation of the whole body. The sum of the tissue-weighted equivalent doses in all the tissues and organs of the body is called the effective dose. The unit for effective dose is the sievert (Sv), same as for an equivalent dose.

The strength of a radioactive source or contamination is measured by the number of disintegrating atomic nuclei per second (dps). The becquerel (Bq) is defined as one dps. The unit is frequently modified with a prefix, for example, kilobecquerel. (See Table 30-1 for prefix definitions. The conventional unit for radioactivity is the curie: 3.7×10^{10} dps.)

Table 30-3 Tissue weighting factors*

Tissue or organ	Tissue weighting factors
Gonads	0.20
Bone marrow (red)	0.12
Colon	0.12
Lung	0.12
Stomach	0.12
Bladder	0.05
Breast	0.05
Liver	0.05
Esophagus	0.05
Thyroid	0.05
Skin	0.01
Bone surface	0.01
Remainder	0.05†

* The values have been developed from a reference population of equal numbers of both sexes and a wide range of ages. The definition of effective dose applies to workers, to the whole population, and to either sex.
† For purposes of calculation, the remainder is composed of the following additional tissues and organs: adrenals, brain, upper large intestine, small intestine, kidney, muscle, pancreas, spleen, thymus and uterus. The list includes organs that are likely to be selectively irradiated. Some organs in the list are known to be susceptible to cancer induction.
Reference: ICRP 1990 Recommendations.[13]

Effects of external ionizing radiation

This section discusses exposures from radiation sources located outside the body. In real life, external exposures may also involve contamination of the skin with radioactive material and internal deposition of radionuclides. Mixed exposures occur when the integrity of a sealed radioactive source or equipment containing radioactive material is broken. It is easier to discuss management of external and internal exposure separately, but the radiation doses from the two types of exposure are additive.

Acute radiation syndrome

The person accidentally and highly exposed to ionizing radiation is often aware, or suspects, such an exposure and presents with this history. If there is no history or suspicion of radiation exposure, the presenting symptoms may be diverse. Different accident cases have been initially diagnosed as flu (nausea, vomiting), gastroenteritis, mumps (parotitis), skin ulcerations, burns, or bone marrow depression.

On recognizing an ionizing radiation case, an important action is to get help in estimating the radiation dose. If the owner or operator of the machine (such as accelerator, x-ray equipment, nuclear reactor) or radioactive source is known, it is most helpful to contact them to provide additional information about the accident and equipment. If the individual wore a personal radiation dosimeter, good dose information should be obtained in a few hours to a day. The dose data are useful for prognosis and planning, but it is not critical information for treatment. Careful clinical observation and laboratory tests are adequate to provide good medical management.

Exposure of the entire body to about 1.5 Gy (150 rad) or more in a single exposure results in a progressive series of signs and symptoms known as the acute radiation syndrome. (Doses cited in this section are skin surface doses and are comparable with doses measured on personal radiation dosimetry badges. A body mid-line dose, which roughly represents the average dose to the bone marrow, can be approximated by taking two thirds of the skin surface dose.) The clinical response and prognosis generally depends on the damage sustained by the hematopoietic system. As doses exceed about 3 Gy (300 rad), serious effects on the hematopoietic system become readily apparent. A dose that results in death of about 50% of exposed healthy persons, without treatment, is about 4 to 4.5 Gy (400 to 450 rad). It is important to recognize that these doses are based on a uniform exposure to the whole body delivered over a short period of time. If only one-half of the body is exposed, the doses to produce similar consequences would need to be about 4 times greater. Protraction of the dose over a period of a week or more allows some recovery to occur so that a given dose is tolerated better. A summary of the principal clinical effects in relationship to acute whole-body doses of various magnitudes is shown in Table 30-4.

Initial or prodromal symptoms occur from about 1 to 6 hours after a significant acute exposure. These symptoms are observed in the most radiation sensitive people as the following acute whole body surface doses are exceeded: anorexia, 0.3 Gy (30 rad); nausea, 1.1 Gy (110 rad); vomiting, 1.5 Gy (150 rad); and diarrhea, 2.25 Gy (225 rad).[19] The percentage of exposed people exhibiting these symptoms increases as the magnitude of dose increases. The severity of symptoms is variable and, therefore, their intensity is not very meaningful. The presence of diarrhea is an ominous sign. These initial symptoms subside within a few hours to several days if supralethal doses are not involved. There follows a relatively symptom-free latent period for up to 2 weeks or more; shorter latent periods are present after higherdoses. After the latent period, the characteristic effects of acute radiation damage become evident—anorexia, fatigue, malaise, epilation, fever, infections, stomatitis, and hemorrhagic phenomena.

Table 30-4 Clinical and laboratory findings after acute whole-body irradiation with x-rays or gamma rays

Skin surface dose (gray)*	Clinical and laboratory findings
0.07–0.75	Asymptomatic. Whole blood counts normal. Chromosome aberrations detectable at >0.2 Gy; possible temporary oligospermia at >0.15 Gy after 1 to 2 months.
0.75–1.10	Asymptomatic. Minor depression of leucocytes and platelets may be detectable in some people, if baseline values known.
1.10–1.90	Prodromal symptoms (anorexia, nausea, vomiting) in about 10 to 20% of persons within 2 days. Mild depression of leucocytes and platelets in some people.
1.90–3.0	Symptomatic course (fatigue, weakness, fever, possible infections) with transient disability. About 50% depression of absolute lymphocyte count within 48 hours.
3.75–5.25	Serious, disabling illness in most persons with about 50% mortality, if untreated. About 75+% depression of absolute lymphocyte count within 48 hours.
7.5+	Accelerated version of acute radiation syndrome (fever, infection, hypotension, hemorrhages) and gastrointestinal complications (fluid loss) within 2 weeks. Prognosis is poor.

* Multiply skin surface dose by 0.67 to convert it to an approximate midline (bone marrow) dose.

Another sign of interest after large doses is the presence or absence of skin erythema, which can appear within minutes to hours after a single large exposure. The presence of skin erythema in a person with a known radiation exposure suggests an exposure in excess of several gray. Be aware that skin erythema from sunburn and other causes is indistinguishable from that produced by ionizing radiation. Erythema is not a reliable sign for evaluating the severity of exposure because of variations caused by dose fractionation, dose rate, radiation energy, depth-dose distribution, area size, anatomical region, and the presence of other irritants or trauma. If erythema is present from known exposure to penetrating whole-body radiation, serious system injury is certain.

The most useful early laboratory tests are the total and differential white blood counts, which contribute important information even if normal. Blood counts should be considered even after certain low exposure events: (1) a single acute whole-body exposure is estimated to be in excess of 20 mGy (2 rad), the annual occupational dose limit; (2) a significant radiation dose is possible and when dosimetry or personal monitoring results are not available or possibly inaccurate; and (3) a request for tests is made by a person after a documented exposure event, even if minor. In an acute exposure, a blood sample is usually taken immediately and repeated daily or several times a day over the first 3 days.

An early and important clinical indicator of damage is the response of the peripheral lymphocyte count. If there are 1,200 or more lymphocytes per cubic millimeter at 48 hours after exposure the likelihood of survival is excellent. Lesser counts at this time suggest higher doses and less than 500 lymphocytes/mm^3 at 48 hours suggests a poor prognosis. During the first several days after a high radiation exposure, a fluctuating leukocytosis will usually occur despite the lymphopenia. In the interpretation of lymphocyte counts, especially if the suspected radiation exposure is low, one must also consider possible transient decreases in lymphocyte count that are common with stresses, such as bacterial infections and traumatic injuries.

A mild to moderate reduction in sperm counts has been observed after gonad doses of as low as 80 mGy (8 rad), but any sperm count reduction will not be evident until 1 or 2 months after exposure. In one case involving a dose of about 1.75 Gy (175 rad) to the testes, the individual had a near normal sperm count (over 50 million sperm/mm^3) after 2 months, but developed a temporary aspermia by 6 months. Sperm counts may help assess the relative magnitude of the gonadal dose, but are of little or no value in the early assessment of a radiation exposure.

Cytogenetic analysis of peripheral lymphocytes is the most sensitive laboratory test for detecting a clinical biological response to ionizing radiation. (A 10 ml blood sample, drawn in a sterile vacutainer containing sodium heparin, should be taken as soon after exposure as possible. Reliable dose estimates can be made for up to about 5 weeks after an acute exposure. Immediate consultation with a laboratory familiar with cytogenetic analyses is necessary for proper handling and transportation of the sample. The test requires about 6 days for cell culture and analyses.) The lower limits of sensitivity are about 0.1 to 0.2 Gy (10 to 20

rad) for x-rays or gamma rays and about 0.05 Gy (5 rad) for fission neutrons. Ionizing radiation typically produces dicentric chromosomes. Although many other agents can cause chromosome aberrations, few induce dicentrics. Other aberrations that are scored include acentric and centric rings, reciprocal translocations, and inversions. The rate of aberrations observed can be related to whole body dose by laboratories that have made appropriate calibration studies.

Chromosome analysis reflects an integrated dose to lymphocytes throughout the body and the result will differ from the dose recorded on a personal dosimeter located at one place on the body surface. Thus, this method may be especially valuable in cases in which there is nonuniform distribution of dose in different parts of the body. The presence of increased chromosome aberrations in an irradiated person does not provide a means for estimating the risk of malignancy or other clinical conditions.

Epilation occurs when doses in excess of about 3 Gy (300 rads) are absorbed by hair follicles. This sign occurs rather abruptly beginning on about day 17 to 20 after exposure and is of no value as an early clinical indicator.

Persons exposed to less than 1 Gy (100 rad) do not need to be hospitalized. They can be followed as outpatients and will normally require only counseling and minimal supportive therapy. In most cases, outpatient management is satisfactory up to about 2 Gy (200 rad) whole body dose. The patient should be followed at least weekly for diagnostic hematologic changes during the first month after exposure. The individual can be advised that statistical increases in risk of late effects, such as cancer, that have been identified in large population studies result in relatively small incremental risks in any given individual. It is prudent to advise men with acute gonadal exposures of 0.1 Gy (10 rad) or more that initiation of birth control methods for 6 months is advisable to avoid potential congenital defects in conceptions during this period. After that, further precautions are not needed.

Persons with estimated doses of 2 Gy (200 rad) or more should be hospitalized. Persons with life-threatening doses, such as 3 to 10 Gy (300 to 1000 rad), require close medical observation and probable active treatment during the period of peak bone marrow depression at about 20 to 30 days after exposure. The only initial treatment required may be to provide symptomatic relief of nausea and vomiting, but there is need for prompt planning for future therapeutic measures that may be required. The patient can be transferred to a larger medical center during the first few days, if necessary, after the initial prodromal symptoms have subsided and initial medical evaluation is available.

Treatment techniques of special importance in the management of radiation cases with significant damage to the hematopoietic system are: (1) prevention of infections by reverse isolation and clean room techniques, sterilization of foods and personal items, and bacterial monitoring using culture samples for potential endogenous sources of infection; (2) antibacterial drug therapy especially for prophylaxis against gastrointestinal tract bacilli and other identified infections, leukocyte transfusions as needed, and possible use of immune globulin; and (3) prevention of bleeding by use of platelet or fresh whole blood and protection from trauma. Bone marrow transplantation, performed as soon as possible but no later than about 10 days after exposure, might be considered for a person exposed to over 7.5 Gy (750 rad). Its value in radiation cases is still considered to be uncertain. Bone marrow transplants in 13 patients after the Chernobyl accident proved not to be useful. New therapeutic agents of value are the colony stimulating factors (CSF), which appear to enhance myelopoiesis and the viability of irradiated and/or transplanted marrow. These factors include granulocyte-monocyte CSF (GM-CSF), granulocyte CSF, and macrophage CSF. Additional details on patient management and therapy are available in other publications.[3,9]

If a supralethal exposure of 50 Gy (5,000 rad) or more has occurred, the patient will survive only a few days and medical support for these acute emergencies can be handled at most hospitals. Treatment will consist of pain relief, antiemesis medications, sedation, control of shock, and fluid balance management.

Skin burns
Radiation skin burns may occur from direct contact with a high-level radioactive source or exposure to an intense field or beam of x-rays, gamma rays, neutrons, or electrons. Exposure to such high radiation sources is not always recognized; suspicion of radiation must be high if burn-like pain or a skin burn is present without a known accident or event. Development of burn symptoms and signs occur much more slowly (days) with radiation than with thermal burns.

Clinical classification of acute radiation burns is erythema (first degree), transepidermal injury (second degree), and full-thickness burns (third degree). Erythema, often difficult to identify in the first week, becomes more prominent in the second week. Skin response is variable to the type and energy of the radiation, as well as to the amount of surface area irradiated.

Threshold erythema and epilation begins at about 3 Gy (300 rad) and above for single doses of 100 kVp x-ray. For higher energy x-rays (1000 kVp) or gamma rays, doses of 6 Gy (600 rads) or more may be absorbed with minimal erythema. Erythema that appears within a few hours of exposure indicates an absorbed dose over 20 Gy (2000 rad). Single acute doses of about 10 Gy (1000 rads) or multiple doses over several weeks totaling 30 Gy (3000 rads) will result in dry desquamation. Moist desquamation and ulceration will begin after acute doses in excess of 20 Gy (2000 rads). Fractionation or protraction of the dose results in less skin damage for a given total dose.

Sterile, protective dressings should be used on skin burns. No particular type of local ointment appears to be advantageous in treatment. The extent of whole-body radiation dose should be evaluated by means of history, dosimetry, possibly mock-up dosimetry measurements, and clinical evaluations including blood counts.

Beta rays are less penetrating than higher energy x-rays or gamma rays; thus, beta rays generally produce less underlying vascular damage. Early excision and skin grafting in these cases will spare the patient much discomfort and may permit earlier restoration of function. Early surgical treatment is not advisable for skin burns produced by x-rays or gamma rays. The deeper penetration by these types of radiation does not permit one to make an early accurate evaluation of the extent of the burn and the future adequacy of the underlying circulation. In these cases, surgical repair and grafting of the area should be deferred until the lesion is well demarcated.

Areas of chronic radiodermatitis should be observed periodically for possible neoplasms. Keratoses and ulcerations should be excised and covered with split-thickness skin grafts as necessary.

Cataracts
External ionizing radiation to the lens of the eye at levels above certain threshold values can produce cataracts. The incidence and density of radiation cataracts are dose dependent. A single dose above 5 Gy (500 rad) is needed to produce progressive cataracts.[34] Fractionation or protraction of the dose reduces the damage. The latent period varies from less than one year to 35 years, with an average of 2 to 3 years. Larger doses result in shorter latent periods. Under conditions other than gross accidental overexposure to radiation, it should not be anticipated or speculated that ionizing radiation is the cause of lens changes.

Radiation cataracts form at the posterior pole of the lens as an initial subcapsular plaque and progress to opacification involving the cortex and nucleus of the lens. Many radiation cataracts do not progress beyond partial obstruction of vision. Although in the early stage, a radiation cataract can be readily differentiated from typical senile cataracts, the clinical appearance of a radiation cataract is indistinguishable from cataracts produced by other etiologic agents. Similar posterior subcapsular cataracts have been caused by intense, chronic infrared exposures, high-voltage electrical shocks or lightning shocks, radar and ultrasonic radiation, and certain drugs or toxic agents (such as nitrophenol, naphthalone, steroids, and MER-29). A particularly difficult differential diagnosis exists with complicated cataracts, which form in the posterior subcapsular area of the lens and are indistinguishable from radiation cataracts. These often occur without apparent cause but may be associated with endogenous ocular and systemic diseases.

There is no therapy that will reduce the risk of cataract formation after high-radiation exposure. Surgical extraction of the lens can be performed when and if impairment of vision warrants the procedure.

Prenatal irradiation effects

A fetus is particularly susceptible to ionizing radiation injury. For this reason, additional precautions are taken to reduce exposures to pregnant women in medical practice and at work. Induction of malformations could occur during the period of major organogenesis (weeks 2 to 6 of gestation), but these have not been a problem. From weeks 8 to 25 after conception, a dose-dependent increase in the incidence of mental retardation has been observed in Japanese children exposed in utero by the atom bomb blasts. An increased incidence of small head size is also observed in these children. The data are consistent with a threshold dose of 0.1 to 0.2 Sv even in the most sensitive stage of gestation, which is 8 to 15 weeks postconception. No increase of mental retardation is noted for exposures after 26 weeks postconception. For occupational situations, the National Council on Radiation Protection and Measurement[26] recommends a monthly dose equivalent limit (exclusive of medical exposure and natural background radiation) of 0.5 mSv (50 mrem) to the embryo-fetus once the pregnancy is known. The Council "no longer believes that specific controls are required for occupationally exposed women who are not known to be pregnant."

Carcinogenesis

The major late health effect after ionizing radiation is the increased risk of cancer. It is this risk on which the radiation protection guidelines for workers and the public are based. Estimation of the increased cancer risk depends primarily on human epidemiologic studies of exposed population

tions, for example, atom bomb survivors, radiotherapy patients, and radiation workers. These studies demonstrate a dose/effect relationship between radiation and cancer incidence or mortality, but at high dose rates and high doses, mostly above 0.2 Sv (20 rem). At low doses, the cancer incidence or mortality is not statistically different from that experienced by people without unusual radiation exposure history. Several publications written by prestigious scientific committees have been published recently on these complex issues.[14,27,28]

Radiation-induced cancers are indistinguishable from cancers in persons not exposed to radiation. The latent period between radiation dose and clinical manifestation can be as short as 2 years for leukemia and bone cancers but, for most other cancers, is typically 10 years out to 40 or more. The risk of cancer induction after exposures in infancy or childhood is higher for some types of cancer than it is in adults. This is the case, for example, with leukemia, thyroid cancer, and breast cancer in women exposed under age 20.

Based on human epidemiologic studies, animal experimental data, and use of mathematical models, risk coefficients have been calculated for the excess cancer incidence and mortality that is believed to be attributable to ionizing radiation. The ICRP estimates that a dose of 1 Sv (100 rem) to a population of all ages would produce a nominal 5% lifetime excess of fatal cancer.[13] For a working population of adults aged 20 to 64 years, the same dose would produce a nominal 4% lifetime excess of fatal cancer. A dose of 1 Sv is large—actually much larger than the vast majority of radiation workers would receive cumulatively over a working lifetime. Estimation of overall cancer risk should include consideration of dose, dose rate, and age of the patient. The prospective probabilistic risk on an individual basis turns out to be relatively small for all but the exceptional high accidental exposure. In light of the publicity and media attention given to this subject, the individual patient may find it difficult to accept this news.

Genetic effects

Several decades ago it was thought that the genetic risk from radiation exposure was the limiting factor to consider in determining radiation protection guidelines. Additional research has shown that the genetic risk to a population is less of a problem than the excess cancer risk. Most current estimates of genetic risk come from experimental studies on animals, especially mice. Few data are available on humans. The largest study of genetic effects of exposed humans involves 38,000 Japanese children who had at least one parent exposed to radiation at the Hiroshima or Nagasaki bombings. No statistically significant effect of radiation has been shown.

The BEIR V Committee (Fifth Committee on Biological Effects of Ionizing Radiation, National Academy of Science), after review of human and animal genetic data, concludes that the doubling dose in human is not likely to be smaller than the approximate 1 Sv (100 rem) obtained from studies in mice.[27] A doubling dose is the radiation dose that would double the incidence of spontaneous genetic defects in an exposed population. The committee calculated the estimated genetic effects of an average population exposure of 1 rem/30-year generation. In the first generation, about 15 to 40 additional cases of genetic disorders per million liveborn offspring are estimated, compared with the current spontaneous incidence of about 17,300 cases per million. In addition, about 10 cases of congenital abnormalities are added to a current incidence of 20,000 to 30,000 per million liveborn offspring. These estimates indicate that the likelihood of a genetic disorder stemming from spontaneous processes is much greater than from radiation exposure to an individual.

Sterility

Although sterility is a well-publicized late effect of radiation exposures, it has not been observed after accidental exposures in humans. Permanent sterility has not occurred after accidental whole-body doses up to 3 Sv (300 rem) in the Marshall islanders (fallout), exposed Japanese fishermen (fallout), or industrial accident cases. Temporary periods of sterility do occur after such high doses for up to about 3 years after exposure. The estimated threshold equivalent dose for induction of temporary sterility in the adult human testis is 0.15 Sv; for permanent sterility, it is 3.5 to 6 Sv (350 to 600 rem) when received as a single exposure.[27] In females, permanent sterility results from single doses of 3.2 to 6 Gy (320 to over 600 rads).[34] Conceptions after recovery from temporary sterility have usually resulted in normal healthy children. Whole-body radiation from accidents does not have a long-term effect on potency or libido.

Life-shortening

A nonspecific life-shortening and aging effect has been claimed to be caused by radiation on the basis of gross experimental observations of irradiated animals. This concept is no longer considered to be valid. The United Nations 1982 Committee report concluded that "while the presence of such an effect cannot be excluded for higher doses, there is no firm evidence that diffuse nonspecific mechanisms causing premature death in the irradi-

ated animals may be operating at the low doses and dose rates of significance to the radiation protection of man."[34] The report points out that the long-term radiation effects are essentially carcinogenic under these conditions, and this explains the life-shortening seen in experimental animals. The same conclusion is noted for epidemiologic data in man, such as in the Japanese atom bomb survivors study.

Effects of internal radiation

Radioactive materials can be taken into the body by inhalation, ingestion, and skin or wound contamination. An internal emitter will irradiate surrounding tissues until it is either excreted by some physiologic process (biological half-time), primarily through urine and feces, or it becomes stable through radioactive decay (radiological half-life). Radionuclides taken internally will be metabolized and distributed according to their chemical properties, just the same as their stable isotopes.

The dose from an internal emitter depends on many factors: quantity of radioactivity involved, physical properties of the type of radiation, internal distribution among organs, radiologic half-life, and biological half-time. Obtaining an estimate of radiation dose from internal emitters is complex and should be done by a professional health physicist. The data needed for a dose estimate are obtained by whole-body counting or through multiple measurements of urine and fecal samples.

The psychologic impact from an accidental internal deposition of radioactivity, especially long-lived radionuclides, can be highly significant. The patient knows that the radiation exposure continues as long as radionuclides remain in the body. The situation is different from external radiation accidents where the exposure ends when the accident is over. Thus, it is important in treating persons involved with internal radiation exposure that they are informed by the attending physician about the estimated uptake and its significance.

An accident involving the potential for uptake of radionuclides will by its nature involve transportable or loose radioactive materials in the air or on surfaces. Patients suspected of internal exposure and transported to the hospital from a radioactively contaminated accident may have loose contamination on their clothing and skin. For effective management of such radioactive contamination associated with the patient(s), the hospital staff should prepare an emergency plan (see Box 30-3) to detect, contain, and clean up the contamination.[2,20,23] Experience to date indicates that special respiratory protection (dust or vapor respira-

---

**BOX 30-3 PLANNING CONSIDERATIONS
FOR HOSPITAL MANAGEMENT
OF THE RADIOACTIVELY
CONTAMINATED PATIENT**

---

1. Assemble hospital team of staff persons trained to manage contaminated radiation cases, including physicians, medical physicists, technicians, and nurses. Designate a team leader. Develop a list of consultants for advice—include physicians and health physicists experienced in handling such problems.
2. Use preselected area in hospital that is suitable for decontamination of patients—consider location of room in an area of the hospital having a nearby outside entry, showers, hot and cold water, floor drains, and table suitable for washing patient. Consider also the ease of room cleanup and potential means to stop air flow through air conditioning or heating systems. If special decontamination room is not available, some alternate locations may be a regular emergency room, physiotherapy room, cast room, or autopsy room.
3. Plan to evaluate the patient's medical condition immediately so as to determine priority of need for medical or surgical treatment, important diagnostic procedures, and decontamination procedures.
4. Plan to move patient within the hospital as little as possible so as to minimize hospital contamination. Keep patient in selected work area for medical and minor surgical treatment until loose contamination has been removed.
5. Arrange to have the area entrances and hallways monitored periodically by a health physics technician after the patient is located in the room to prevent tracking to other areas.
6. Be prepared to set up monitoring station(s) at exits from the work area. Personnel should not leave the room (area) unless monitored for radioactivity. Equipment or property should not be removed from the room unless monitored. Designate persons to perform these monitoring tasks at specific locations.
7. Prepare a list of decontamination room supplies and either store them in the room or identify where they are available for quick assembly.

Modified from NCRP Report No. 65.[32]

---

tors) is not needed for the medical staff to deal with contaminated patients. It is necessary to rehearse the plan periodically.

Skin and wound contamination

Skin contamination by radioactive material is a potential problem wherever such materials are being handled. The principal concern is usually not

radiation dose to the skin or body but rather to prevent uptake in the body by absorption, inhalation, or ingestion. Most radionuclides are not absorbed readily through intact skin, but radioactive iodine, tritium (radioactive hydrogen), and some strontium compounds are taken into the body significantly and rapidly via the skin.

The objective of skin decontamination is to remove the radioactive material without injury to the skin. It is usually highly effective to simply wash the skin with a mild detergent and water. Scrubbing with a soft cloth or pad may be necessary. After each washing, the skin is monitored with radiation survey instruments to evaluate the progress. (For alpha surveys, the skin must be dry before monitoring is done.) It is important not to damage the skin by use of scrub brushes, harsh scrubbing agents, or chemicals. The use of complexing (chelating) agents in decontamination solutions is not particularly helpful. If results after washing with detergent and gentle scrubbing are not satisfactory, use of 5% sodium hypochlorite (household bleach) may be effective. It can be used full strength on the hands or forearms of most people. It should be diluted with about five parts of water for use on the face, neck, wounds, or more sensitive skin. Bleach is a skin irritant and some alertness to impending skin damage must attend its use. It is preferable to leave low levels of contamination on the skin rather than to abrade or chemically injure the skin. Certain contaminants attach strongly to hair and refuse to be washed off. Clipping hair is seldom necessary but may be considered if the residual contamination is judged to be unacceptable.

If the contamination proves difficult to remove adequately, limited decontamination efforts performed two or three times during the day or over several days is often more effective than a single overzealous effort. The use of an occlusive dressing (or rubber gloves in the case of contaminated hands) between decontamination efforts may be surprisingly successful because induced sweating helps to bring material to the surface.

Although a special wastewater holding tank is desirable, such a specialized item may not be feasible for hospitals in view of the limited use. The wastewater from skin decontamination activities should be retained in containers to permit monitoring before disposal. In actuality, contaminated water has not presented significant problems because highly contaminated cases have not been handled at hospitals, large dilution factors are present in domestic sewerage systems, and the occurrence of such events is infrequent. Contaminated materials like rags and papers should be collected in plastic bags for subsequent disposal as radioactive waste.

In the event of severe injuries associated with radioactive contamination, the first consideration of the attending physician should be for the patient's physical condition. Emergency procedures to control hemorrhage, restore respiratory and circulatory function, and alleviate pain are a first order of business, even if the contamination levels are high. Most of the contaminated wounds seen in the nuclear industry are trivial injuries and involve low radiation levels.

The first procedure in cleaning a contaminated wound is to rinse the wound with running tap water or use a sterile saline solution irrigation. Use of a pulsating water jet stream may be helpful in larger wounds. Application of a tourniquet frequently is mentioned as a useful procedure to reduce the uptake of radioactive materials but in practice it is seldom used or needed. To the extent possible, the wound area should be treated with conventional aseptic techniques.

The progress of wound decontamination must be measured by means of some type of radiation instrumentation. For beta-gamma radiation, a portable survey meter is usually adequate. Alpha emitters present more difficult monitoring problems and special wound counters are generally necessary. If at all possible, a person with experience in radiation monitoring should assist the medical team in making radiation measurements.

Wound excision has been used primarily to remove long-lived alpha contaminants, such as ^{239}Pu (plutonium-239). Small quantities of alpha contamination in a wound, such as 74 Bq (2 nCi) or less of ^{239}Pu, do not need to be excised. Long-term problems have not been observed in these cases. If more activity is present, it is desirable to obtain complete removal of the contaminant from the wound, if possible. Excision of the area has been the only practical solution. The surgeon should complete the wound excision without creating functional disability if possible. Any significant sacrifice of function is usually not justified.

Beta-gamma emitters in wounds usually do not present as much hazard as alpha emitters. Wound excision has not ordinarily been necessary for beta-gamma type contamination.

Internal deposition of radionuclides

Treatment of internal deposition of radionuclides is much more effective if done within the first 3 hours after exposure. A decision to treat internal contamination at such an early time means that only limited information is available. There are no signs or symptoms relating to the exposure other than those from associated physical injuries. If the exposure occurred at a nuclear facility, the on-site health physicist may have information on the general level of contamination and air concentrations at the accident site.

Measurements of activity on nasal swabs are often used at nuclear facilities to give immediate information as to whether inhalation of radionuclides may have occurred. It has been used most commonly for potential alpha contamination. The swabs should be taken within a few minutes of the accident and before washing the face or showering. They cannot be expected to yield valid information by the time the patient is transported to the hospital. The procedure consists of wiping the nasal membranes of each nostril separately with a moist cotton applicator or a moistened filter paper strip wrapped around a swab stick. Radionuclides on the swab samples are measured with laboratory type counters. If the radioactivity is different in the two nostrils, it may have transferred from contaminated hands or face rather than by an inhalation exposure. A rule-of-thumb used by some health physicists and physicians in the evaluation of cases involving potential inhalation of plutonium, an alpha emitter, is that swab samples greater than 500 disintegrations per minute (dpm) in both nostrils indicate a possible significant inhalation, whereas lower values would suggest no more than a low exposure potential.

Uptake of some radionuclides, such as iodine, tritium, or cesium, may be estimated almost immediately after exposure by measuring the radioactivity in urine samples. By knowing the rate of excretion at different times after exposure, the quantity of the radionuclide within the body can be calculated.

Direct radioactivity measurements of the whole body or organs, such as over the thyroid, can be made if the radionuclide emits gamma rays. Counts in the first day or two may be difficult to interpret because of the likely presence of residual skin contamination.

The decision to treat or not is most likely to be based on a qualitative judgment as to whether an exposure is high or low. At the time, available information may consist only of some scanty information on the details of the accident, possible identification of the major radionuclides by history of the operation, a general idea of the level of contamination involved, and perhaps air concentration levels at the accident site during the exposure. Radioactivity measurements of urine samples or whole body counts, if available promptly, may give more quantitative data on the exposure. For accidents at a nuclear facility, initial decontamination, evaluation, and treatment should be started ideally at the plant's medical facility.

Most of the recommended treatments for internal radionuclide exposure result in little or no risk to the patient. If the potential for a meaningful reduction in radiation dose is thought to be possible, it is probably best to proceed with treatment immediately. The various recommended treatments can reduce the dose by factors of 2 to 10, certainly worthwhile reductions. After the start of treatment, internal dose evaluation should be continued to determine whether continuation of treatment is warranted.

If the mode of exposure is by ingestion, immediate removal of gastric contents will reduce uptake. Fast-acting purgatives may be used to reduce the residence time of radioactive materials in the colon. Gastrointestinal absorption may be reduced for certain radionuclides by use of appropriate agents: 100 ml of an aluminum-containing antacid (aluminum phosphate gel is preferred) reduces uptake of strontium; magnesium sulfate or barium sulfate can be used for radium and strontium; 1 to 3 grams 3 times daily of prussian blue (potassium ferric ferrocyanide) is effective in reducing the gastrointestinal uptake of cesium, thallium, and rubidium. Prussian blue has been used safely for humans at the previously recommended doses, but it is not Food and Drug Administration (FDA)-approved at this time nor is it available commercially in a pharmaceutical grade.

Blocking agents reduce the quantity of radionuclide incorporated in specific organs. Stable iodide is the drug of choice to block the deposition of radioactive iodine in the thyroid. It should be given as soon as possible after exposure because blocking becomes relatively ineffective 6 or more hours after uptake. For individual adult patients, the dose is 300 mg of potassium iodide (crush tablet if enteric-coated) or six drops of saturated solution of potassium iodide in a glass of water. For administration to the general public potentially exposed to radioactive iodine, a dose of 100 mg KI for adults or 50 mg KI for young children is recommended. To continue treatment, these doses should be administered once each day for 7 to 14 days to prevent recycling of the radioiodine into the thyroid.

Diluting agents increase the elimination rates of certain radionuclides by enhancing the turnover rate of the radionuclide. For example, forcing fluids to tolerance (at least 3000 to 4000 ml per day) increases excretion of tritium (radioactive hydrogen) and should reduce the biological half-time from 10 to 12 days to less than 6 days.

The excretion of some radionuclides can be enhanced by use of a chelating agent that binds the nuclide in a soluble complex. Excretion occurs through urine and feces. The most useful chelation drug for treating radionuclides is diethylenetri-aminepenta-acetic acid as either the zinc salt (ZnDTPA) or the calcium salt (CaDTPA). (Physicians needing this investigational new drug should request the drug protocol and permission to use the drug from Radiation Emergency Assistance Center/Training Site [REAC/TS], Oak Ridge Associated Universities, Oak Ridge, TN. [615] 576-3131, office; [615] 481-1000 beeper 241, 24-hour.) A typical daily treatment regimen is to give 1 gram of DTPA (4 ml ampule) intravenously by slow injection over about 5 minutes or to dilute the DTPA in 250 ml of isotonic saline or 5% glucose. Inhalation of 1 gram of DTPA nebulized over 15 to 30 minutes is another convenient method of administration. Do not give more than one treatment per day. DTPA effectively chelates the transuranium metals (plutonium, americium, curium, and californium), the rare earths (such as cesium, yttrium, lanthanum, promethium, and scandium), and some transition metals (zirconium and niobium). If DTPA is not immediately available, the calcium salt of ethylenediaminetetraacetic acid (CaEDTA, calcium disodium edetate, versenate) may be used, but it is much less effective for this application.

There have been no serious side effects from either CaDTPA or ZnDTPA using the recommended doses. CaDTPA is probably more effective than ZnDTPA for the first several days of administration. ZnDTPA is preferred for use over longer periods of administration or for women who are pregnant. In animal experiments, high doses of CaDTPA (about 100 times the clinical dose range) produce severe lesions of the kidneys, intestinal mucosa, and liver. Experiments in dogs have also shown that divided doses of CaDTPA (5 times per day) can produce serious gastrointestinal effects. This side effect is not seen if the same amount of CaDTPA is administered only once each day. The toxic effects are related to reduction of certain essential trace metals in the body.

Chelation therapy with CaDTPA or ZnDTPA is not effective after inhalation of insoluble particulates, such as high fired plutonium oxide. Because solubility characteristics of an aerosol after an accident are almost never known, a clinical trial of chelation is usually warranted to test its effectiveness on the aerosol. In the case of inhaled plutonium, if the urinary excretion is not enhanced by a factor of 30 to 100 times pretreatment levels, the treatment can be discontinued.

Multiple lavages of the bronchopulmonary tree in dogs (usually 10 total procedures were used) have been successful in removing 25% to 50% of inhaled insoluble radioactive particulates if treatment is initiated within 10 days. This technique should be used only after careful consideration of the long-term risk of the radionuclide involved compared with the immediate risk of procedures requiring general anesthesia. It must be performed by a team of specialists experienced in bronchopulmonary lavage.

For additional details on the medical management of internal deposition of radionuclides, the reader is referred to a report prepared by the National Council on Radiation Protection and Measurements.[23]

Late effects from internal emitters

The principal health effect associated with internal radiation is cancer. Excess cancer after internal deposition of radionuclides has been amply demonstrated—lung cancer in uranium miners (radon); bone cancer and sinus/mastoid cancer in radium dial painters; cancers of liver, spleen, and bone, as well as acute myeloid leukemia, in patients injected with thorotrast (thorium); and thyroid cancer in Marshall islanders exposed to radioactive fallout. It should be highlighted that the radiation doses to all these groups are high. Epidemiologic studies of these exposed groups of people have helped to define dose/effect relationships and to assess the radiation risk. In addition, extensive experiments have been conducted on animals exposed to internal emitters. These studies contribute much information on the biological mechanisms, health effects, and potential risks. These data, especially the human radiation risk data, are used to establish appropriate radiation protection guidelines for internal emitters in the same manner as for external radiation doses. A report by the National Research Council of the National Academy of Sciences summarizes the health effects and risks associated with exposure to internally deposited alpha emitters.[28]

The attending physician, by following the principles of treatment for decontamination and treatment of internal emitters, will have reduced future risks from radiation as much as is possible. The general perception of the risks after internal radiation exposures is much higher than has been observed in practice. Radiation exposures in the nuclear industry, in terms of dose as well as the number of persons exposed, have been principally from external radiation.

CASE STUDIES

Case 1: Unknown exposure to a sealed radioactive source

A state policeman reports to a hospital emergency room as a result of possible exposure to radiation. He had responded to an accident involving an overturned van that had burned up. The driver indicated that there was a radioactive source in a lead shielded container in the van. In the course of roping off the area to prevent possible exposure to bystanders, the policeman spotted

a small shiny object on the ground. He picked up the object to examine it more closely. It occurred to him immediately that this might be the source itself, so he promptly dropped it to the ground and left the area. He has noticed no ill effects during the intervening 6 hours, but is worried about his situation. He had no radiation monitoring badge on him.

The medical objective is to observe the patient for possible radiation effects and to try to assess the radiation dose. The history should collect details on how long had he held the object in his hand, the kind of radionuclide, and how much radioactivity was in the source. Where is it now? Was "the object" the source? Note that the policeman will not know the answers to some of these questions. History taking will involve talking to the driver and radiation monitors who were called to the scene.

White blood cell counts (absolute lymphocyte counts) are used to determine whether a high whole body radiation dose is involved. A heparinized blood sample is taken for chromosome analyses and sent to an appropriate laboratory in an insulated box (including a cold pack). White counts are repeated daily for at least 3 days and then weekly for 2 weeks. His hands are examined on each visit to detect any possible local burn. All of this can be done on an outpatient basis, and he may continue his regular work if there is no evidence of unusual symptoms or signs developing. The likely major risk here is a local radiation burn of his fingers, which should be apparent within 2 weeks. The likelihood of a high whole-body radiation dose is small given this accident scenario. If a burn appears, a protective sterile dressing is applied. The patient should be informed on the findings as they develop, and he should be encouraged to ask questions about his situation. Reassurance should be given if normal test results are obtained.

Case 2: High-external radiation exposure

A 30-year-old male operator of a gamma irradiation research facility entered the irradiation vault to fix some malfunctioning equipment. Within less than a minute, he recognized that the large ^{60}Co sources were out of their shielded positions and he fled the room. He reported the event immediately to his supervisor who arranged to have the operator's personal radiation badge sent immediately to the processing vendor for a reading. They went over the details of his accidental exposure and began to investigate why the safety systems and procedures had failed to alert the operator that radiation was present. At about 4 hours the operator felt nauseated and vomited once. At this time, the supervisor sent the operator to the hospital for medical evaluation.

The supervisor told the physician that the operator may have been exposed to 200 rads, up to 750 rads or more. His estimate was based on the time the operator thought he might have been in the radiation field. The patient was having some continued waves of nausea. Physical examination was normal. No skin erythema was evident. Five hours after the accident, a complete blood count was normal, although the absolute lymphocyte count of 1700 cells/mm³ was marginally low. It was decided to hospitalize the patient for further studies. He *was put into a private room, but without reverse isolation or clean room facilities at this time. A blood chemistry profile was ordered for baseline values. A blood sample for chromosome analyses was obtained and arrangements were made to send it to a laboratory equipped to make radiation dosimetry estimates.*

The next morning the patient was feeling reasonably well, but somewhat tired and anxious. The absence of diarrhea was favorable. No significant change in the blood count had occurred. A dosimetry report on his personal dosimetry badge from the vendor indicated a gamma dose of 260 rads. An approximate bone marrow dose is estimated by multiplying the 260 rads times .67, or about 175 rads. It was decided to keep him in the hospital at least 1 more day for complete blood counts twice a day. After 2 days, his lymphocyte count was 1400 cells/mm³ and he was feeling better. He was discharged home at this point with daily blood counts to be done on an outpatient basis for the first week and then reduced in frequency if no significant changes occurred. He was instructed to be sedentary for the next week and not to return to work. He was counseled on the wisdom of employing birth control measures for the next 6 months and possibly longer depending on the results of sperm counts. Arrangements were made for sperm counts to be made every 2 months. A week after the accident, the cytogenetics laboratory reported a whole-body dose of 120 rads. This lower dose was interpreted as possibly resulting from some shielding of the lower half of his body by laboratory equipment present in the vault. The patient was released for work in a nonradiation work area after the laboratory results showed no progressive adverse trends for 3 weeks after the accident. A follow-up program of weekly blood counts and examinations was made for up to 6 weeks after the exposure.

Case 3: Exposure to radioiodine

A nuclear reactor maintenance man was examining a pump during a refueling shutdown period. A radiation alarm suddenly rang and he evacuated the room as instructed. Health physicists determined from air monitors that a release of radioactive gas had occurred in the area. Gamma spectroscopy identified the radioactivity to be mixed fission products, but with a significant fraction of iodine-131. The health physicist made a gamma survey over the man's thyroid and found he had a slightly elevated thyroid count. Extrapolation from a 30-minute thyroid uptake to a 12-hour uptake suggests a probable ultimate iodine-131 deposition in the thyroid of 3 microcuries. One microcurie in the thyroid results is a dose of about 6.5 rem; three microcuries gives nearly a 20 rem dose to the thyroid. He was taken immediately next door to the medical department at the plant, where the nurse in accordance with her standing orders immediately gave him six drops of saturated solution of potassium iodide in a glass of water. This thyroid blocking agent given within 1 hour will reduce iodine-131 deposition in the gland by about 80%. The deposition is reduced less than 50% if treatment is given 6 hours after exposure and little effect can be achieved if the delay is 12 hours or more. The nurse instructs the man to take a

300 mg KI tablet daily for the next 7 days and possibly longer if necessary as determined by his counts. Additional thyroid counts made by the health physicist will determine the worker's thyroid dose from this exposure.

REFERENCES

1. American Medical Association Council on Scientific Affairs: Harmful effects of ultraviolet radiation, *JAMA* 262:380, 1989.
2. American Medical Association: *A guide to the hospital management of injuries arising from exposure to or involving ionizing radiation,* Chicago, 1984, American Medical Association.
3. Andrews GA: Medical management of accidental total-body irradiation, in Hubner KF, Fry SA, editors: *The medical basis for radiation accident preparedness,* New York, 1980, Elsevier North Holland, Inc.
4. Bickers, D: Sun-induced disorders, *Emerg Med Clin North Am* 3:659, 1985.
5. Bonde JP: Semen quality in welders exposed to radiant heat, *Br J Ind Med* 49/1:5, 1992.
6. Carpenter RL, Hagan GJ, Donovan GL: Are microwave cataracts thermally caused? in *Symposium on the biological effects and measurement of RF and microwaves,* HEW Publication FDA 77-8026, Rockville MD, 1977, Center for Devices and Radiological Health.
7. Cridland NA: Cellular and molecular approaches to assessing the carcinogenic potential of electromagnetic fields, *NRPB Rad Prot Bull* 138:13, 1993.
8. D'Andrea JA: Microwave radiation absorption: behavioral effects, *Health Phys* 61:29, 1991.
9. Drum DE, Rappeport JM: Treatment of whole-body radiation accident victims, in Mettler, Jr. FA, Kelsey CA, Ricks RC, editors: *Medical management of radiation accidents,* Boca Raton, 1990, CRC Press, Inc.
10. Fry SA, Sipe A: *DOE-REAC/TS radiation accident registries: serious radiation accidents worldwide,* unpublished report, Oak Ridge, Tn, 1992, Oak Ridge Associated Universities.
11. Hiller R, Sperduto RD, Ederer F: Epidemiologic associations with cataract in the 1971-1972 National Health and Nutrition Examination Survey, *Am J Epidemiol* 27:213, 1983.
12. Hocking B, Joyner KH, Fleming AHJ: Implanted medical devices in workers exposed to radio-frequency radiation, *Scand J Work Environ Health,* 17:1, 1991.
13. International Commission on Radiological Protection: 1990 recommendations of the International Commission on Radiological Protection, *Ann ICRP 21,* no 1-3. ICRP Publ 60, New York, 1991, Pergamon Press.
14. International Commission on Radiological Protection: Risks associated with ionizing radiations, *Ann ICRP 22,* no 1. New York, 1991, Pergamon Press.
15. Jauchem JR, Merritt JH: The epidemiology of exposure to electromagnetic fields: an overview of the recent literature, *J Clin Epidemiol* 44:895, 1991.
16. Kavet R, Tell, RA: VDTs: field levels, epidemiology, and laboratory studies, *Health Phys* 61:47, 1991.
17. Kligman LH, Atkin FJ, Kligman AM: Sunscreens promote repair of ultraviolet-induced dermal damage, *J Invest Dermatol* 81:98, 1983.
18. Lilienfeld AM et al.: *Foreign service health status study—evaluation of health status of foreign service and other employees from selected eastern European posts,* final report contract no 6025-619073, Washington, 1978, Department of State.
19. Marco D, Eisinger G, Hayes DL: Testing of work environ-

ments for electromagnetic interference, *PACE* 15:2016, 1992.

20. Mettler, Jr. FA, Kelsey CA, Ricks RC, editors: *Medical management of radiation accidents,* Boca Raton, 1990, CRC Press, Inc.

21. National Council on Radiation Protection and Measurements: *Ionizing radiation exposure of the population of the United States,* NCRP report 93, Bethesda, 1987, NCRP Publications.

22. National Council on Radiation Protection and Measurements: *Biological effects and exposure criteria for radiofrequency electromagnetic fields,* NCRP report 86, Bethesda, 1986, NCRP Publications.

23. National Council on Radiation Protection and Measurements: *Management of persons accidentally contaminated with radionuclides,* NCRP report 65, Bethesda, 1980, NCRP Publications.

24. National Council on Radiation Protection and Measurements: *Radiofrequency electromagnetic fields—properties, quantities and units, biophysical interaction, and measurements,* NCRP report 67, Bethesda, 1981, NCRP Publications.

25. National Council on Radiation Protection and Measurements: *Exposure criteria for medical diagnostic ultrasound: I. Criteria based on thermal mechanisms,* NCRP report 113, Bethesda, 1992, NCRP Publications.

26. National Council on Radiation Protection and Measurements: *Limitation of exposure to ionizing radiation,* NCRP report 116, Bethesda, 1993, NCRP Publications.

27. National Research Council, National Academy of Sciences: *Health effects of exposure to low levels of ionizing radiation,* BEIR V report of the Committee on the Biological Effects of Ionizing Radiation, Washington, DC, 1990, National Academy Press.

28. National Research Council, National Academy of Sciences: *Health risks of radon and other internally deposited alpha-emitters,* BEIR IV report of the Committee on the Biological Effects of Ionizing Radiation, Washington, DC, 1988, National Academy Press.

29. Robinette CD, Silverman C, Jablon S: Effects upon health of occupational exposure to microwave radiation (radar), *Amer J Epidemiol* 112:39, 1980.

30. Sahl JD, Kelsh MA, Greenland S: Cohort and nested case-control studies of hematopoietic cancers and brain cancer among electric utility workers, *Epidemiology* 4:104, 1993.

31. Schwartz G et al: Sun-induced disorders, in Schwartz G et al: *Principles and practice of emergency medicine,* Philadelphia, 1992, Lea & Febiger.

32. Theriault GP: Health effects of electromagnetic radiation on workers: epidemiologic studies, in Bierbaum PH, Peters, JM, editors: *Proceedings of the scientific workshop on the health effects of electric and magnetic fields on workers,* DHHS (NIOSH) publication no 91-111, Cincinnati, 1991, National Institute for Occupational Safety and Health.

33. Tornqvist S et al: Incidence of leukaemia and brain tumours in some 'electrical occupations,' *Br J Ind Med* 48:597, 1991.

34. United Nations Scientific Committee on the Effects of Atomic Radiation: *Ionizing radiation: sources and biological effects,* 1982 Report to the General Assembly, New York, 1982, United Nations.

35. Weiss JS et al: Topical tretinoin improves photodamaged skin: a double-blind vehicle-controlled study, *JAMA* 259:527, 1988.

SUGGESTED READINGS

American National Standards Institute: *Safety levels with respect to human exposure to radiofrequency electromagnetic fields, 300 kHz to 100 GHz,* report no ANSI C95.1-1982, New York, 1982, The Institute of Electrical and Electronics Engineers, Inc.

Lushbaugh CC, Comas F: Clinical studies of radiation effects in man, *Radiat Res* (suppl) 7:398, 1967.

31 Occupational Electrical and Lightning Injuries

Electrical hazards constitute a small but important class of occupational physical hazards. Since the first reported death in 1879 of a carpenter exposed to a 250-volt generator, electric current has been increasingly responsible for numerous accidents often resulting in severe injury or death.

There are about 1,500 cases of electrocution annually in the United States, including 100 to 300 cases of lightning deaths (Mellen, 1992). Approximately 400 electrocutions occur at work in the U.S. each year; the majority could be prevented if current safeguards are used and proper procedures followed. Although the number of accidents has not risen correspondingly with the increasing use of electric power, the accidents tend to be serious and often fatal when they occur. Despite the existence of a vast amount of experimental and technical knowledge concerning the hazardous nature of electricity and the measures required for electrical safety, electrical fatalities still account for a significant number of deaths in the workplace. The majority of injuries and deaths occur while workers are performing duties they normally undertake in the course of their job, suggesting inadequate preparedness and training in electrical hazards (Harvey-Sutton, 1992). It is important for the occupational specialist to understand the pathophysiology, clinical manifestations, and treatment of these often bizarre and devastating injuries. Knowledge of epidemiologic risk groups and high-risk settings is imperative, as most of these injuries are clearly preventable.

Electric current can cause a spectrum of acute and chronic health effects and often results in multi-organ system manifestations. Injury in electrical exposure is most often the result of a direct effect on the heart, nervous system, skin, and deep tissues. Ventricular fibrillation, respiratory arrest, or burns are the most common causes of immediate death. Burns can be minor, requiring minimal debridement, or cause devastating destruction requiring aggressive resuscitation and major limb amputation. Other health effects can include vascular damage such as thrombosis, rhabdomyolysis and subsequent renal failure, fractures due to high temperature or tetanic contractions, cataracts, neuropsychologic changes, degenerative neurologic syndromes, and associated trauma such as falls.

EPIDEMIOLOGY

Although the number of electrical accidents is usually a small proportion of the total number of work-related accidents, the percentage of electrical injuries that prove fatal is often much higher than the percentage of fatalities in accidents taken as a whole. Some injury registries have found the fatality ratio to be as high as 21% (Jones, 1991). Of the 7,000 to 11,500 work-related deaths occurring each year in the United States, approximately 5% result from electrical injury (Cone, 1991). According to the National Institute for Occupational Safety and Health (NIOSH) data on occupational deaths from 1980 to 1985, fatalities from electric current were the fifth leading cause of death on the job. Certain state occupational injury registries have found electricity-related deaths to rank even higher (Jones, 1991). While there is general agreement that occupational fatality data is incomplete and suffers from underreporting, data on the incidence of nonfatal electrical injuries are more sparse and many such injuries go undocumented. Somewhere between one half and two thirds of all electrical accidents are work-related. Electrical burns, a common sequelae of high-voltage injuries, result in numerous admissions to burn units. Lightning injuries differ in significant ways from other electrical injuries and will be discussed in a separate section.

OCCUPATIONAL SETTING

Occupational electrical injuries occur in many different workplace settings and through several mechanisms of injury. The most common scenarios resulting in electrical injury include (1) the use of portable power tools such as drills and saws; (2) the use of faulty power tools, electrical outlets, and connectors; (3) the use of portable arc-welding equipment (Suruda, 1992); and (4) contacting power lines with ladders (approximately 4% of yearly electrocutions), cranes, scaffolding, irrigation, or tree-trimming equipment.

Risk factors for injury include contact with moisture such as use of electric hand tools with wet or perspiration-covered hands that lower the resistance to electricity passing through the body, and wearing clothing inadequate to protect from electrical charges. Working on damp ground or where water is an integral part of the process, such as in irrigation, concrete work, and slaughtering, predisposes to electrical shock. Aerial powerlines are a well-known hazard in the vicinity of irrigation pipes. In some agricultural regions irrigation pipes have been the most common source of fatal human contact with electrical lines (Helgerson, 1985).

U.S. electric linemen suffer the highest rates of electrocutions, more than four times that of electricians, who suffer the second highest rate (MMWR, 1989). Utility workers appear to have a high fatality ratio, probably due to more frequent contact with high-voltage power sources. The hazard of this work greatly increases when repairs are conducted under conditions of widespread damaged electrical transmission and distribution systems, as in the aftermath of a natural disaster such as a hurricane (MMWR, 1989). Other occupational groups at high risk for electrical injury include the construction industry where electrocution is the second leading cause of death. Painters and roofers seem to be at particular risk most likely from working near overhead power lines with ladders and other equipment. Plumbers and other workers at temporary construction sites are at risk of electrocution. The constantly changing worksite exposes the worker to temporary wiring that may be substandard and to harsh conditions that damage tool power cords and plugs (Suruda, 1992). Portable arc-welding equipment is also responsible for numerous accidents, often resulting from improperly grounded equipment. The mining and agricultural industries have high rates of injury, and machinery operators have some of the highest fatality rates.

The greatest number of injuries occur in white males in the 20- to 29-year age group, predominantly during the summer months. This is most likely related to increased outdoor activity and the use of electrical equipment and machinery during this time of year. Increased sweating during the warmer months may also predispose to shock (Fatovich, 1992). Alcohol and drugs have not consistently been found to be significant contributing factors in most work-related cases, although widespread postaccident testing has not been routinely performed (Baker, 1982; Berkelman, 1985).

Persons exposed to electrical risk fall into two categories: those with training and experience in electrical work, such as electricians and linemen, and those untrained in electrical hazards but who use equipment with potential electrical risk. Avoidance of injury requires both education regarding hazards and attention to safe work practices.

ELECTRICAL ENERGY AND MECHANISMS OF INJURY

In order to understand the consequences of human exposure to electricity it is important to understand certain basic concepts of electrical energy. The tissue damage produced by electricity is proportional to the intensity of the current that passes through the body as stated in Ohm's law: resistance (ohms) = voltage/amperage. Voltage (tension or potential) is the electromotive force of the system; amperage (intensity) is a measure of current flow per unit time; and an ohm is a unit used to measure the resistance to conduction of electricity.

Two types of current are encountered in the workplace. Voltage is supplied either as a continuous source (direct current—DC) with electron flow moving in one direction, or as a cyclic source (alternating current—AC) with a cyclic reversal of electron flow. Nearly all injuries are the result of contact with the more common AC with the exception of lightning, which can be thought of as a high-voltage direct current shock. Alternating electric current (AC) is generated by large electromagnetic devices and generating stations and transmitted many miles at high tensions greater than 100,000 volts. Transformers reduce this voltage to 7,620 volts, the usual voltage in residential and industrial distribution lines. At residences, the voltage is again decreased to 110 to 220 volts for domestic use (Kobernick, 1982). The frequency of most commercial AC current in the U.S. is 60 cycles per second (Hz). This means the flow of electrons changes direction 60 times per second. The use of 60 Hz frequency has evolved because it is optimal for the transmission and utilization of electricity and it has advantages in terms of generation.

Whether or not death or injury occurs is directly related to several factors:

1. Type of current (AC or DC)
2. Frequency of current
3. Voltage
4. Amperage
5. Duration of exposure

6. Exposure pathway through the body
7. Area of contact, and
8. Resistance at points of electrical contact and in tissues.

AC vs DC

AC is significantly more dangerous than DC at similar voltages. AC can produce tetanic contractions that freeze the victim to the source of the current and interfere with the respiratory and cardiovascular centers. Victims do not freeze to DC current as with AC but can be injured when hurled from the point of electrical contact by the shock or when burned.

Frequency

The frequency of AC is of importance physiologically. The most critical frequencies are in the range of 20 to 150 cycles per second. Human muscular tissue responds well to frequencies between 40 and 150 Hz. Household current (60 cycle) lies directly within this range and may span the vulnerable period of the cardiac cycle causing ventricular fibrillation. As the frequency increases beyond 150 Hz, human tissue response is decreased and the current is generally less dangerous.

Voltage

Although somewhat arbitrary, harmful effects from electrical current can be subdivided into the effects of high voltage (current greater than 250 V) and the effects of low voltage (current less than 250 V). Although most recognize the danger of high voltage, such as a high-tension overhead powerline, low-voltage current can prove equally deadly. Occupational fatalities have been found to divide fairly equally between high- and low-voltage electrocutions, and ventricular fibrillation is the most common cause of immediate death. Severe burns are more common with high-voltage currents. Injury or death can occur by currents of very low voltage with instances of death with AC of 46 and 60 volts reported. It is claimed that any voltage over 25 should be considered potentially lethal.

Amperage

The amount of current flow, or amperes, is the single most important factor in injuries by electricity. Low-power alternating currents may be characterized by the thresholds of perception, by let-go, and by ventricular fibrillation. The threshold of perception is the minimum current to cause any sensation in the human body. The let-go current is the maximum level of current flowing through an electrode at which a person taking hold of the electrode is still able to release it. Currents greater than the threshold of let-go can be considered specially dangerous since the body receiving the shock is unable to respond to it and break away. General values for the thresholds of perception and let-go have been derived by the International Electrotechnical Commission (ICC). The threshold of perception is 0.5 mA and the threshold of let-go is 10 milliampere (mA) for signal frequencies in the range of 15 to 100 Hz.

Duration of exposure

The threshold for an adverse effect is clearly related to the duration of exposure to the electrical energy. The ICC has derived values for the threshold of ventricular fibrillation by adapting results from animal experiments. They consider that for a 50/60 Hz signal, a current of 500 mA may cause fibrillation for a shock duration of 10 ms; likewise 400 mA for 100 ms, 50 mA for 1 s, and 40 mA for greater than 3s. The likelihood of ventricular fibrillation increases if the shock continues for a complete cardiac cycle.

Tissue pathway

The pathway of the current is also important. Current passing the head or chest is more likely to produce immediate death by affecting the central respiratory center, respiratory muscles, or the heart. Arm-to-arm conduction can pass through the heart, and head-to-foot conduction may affect the central nervous system and the heart. A small current through the chest could be fatal, but a large current passing through a single extremity may have little effect. The above values for the threshold of ventricular fibrillation are for current paths through the whole body, but fibrillation is only triggered by that level of current directly affecting the heart (Robinson, 1990). Nonfatal tissue injury is also determined by the current path. Prediction of injuries from observation of the tissue path, however, can be unreliable. Burn injuries have been shown to be more severe when the electrical energy traverses the long axis of the body.

Tissue resistance

The effect of electrical current on the body depends on the resistance of the tissues involved. Intact dry skin has a relatively high resistance, but this falls dramatically with moisture or cuts or abrasions. A calloused palm may reach resistances of 1 million ohms, dry skin may have 5,000 ohms, and wet skin less than 1,000. The resistance of individual tissues is thought to differ considerably and play a role in differential injury to tissues. Resistance to current flow occurs in decreasing order through bone, fat, tendon, skin, muscle, blood vessels, and nerves. However the concept of electric current always passing through the body along lines of least resistance may not be true; the path may largely depend on the voltage (Hunt, 1976).

Tissue damage

Controversy exists over the exact mechanism of tissue damage in electrical injury. The most widely held theory is that electrical energy is converted to thermal energy in tissues and causes damage by heating. The release of heat is described by Joule's law: $P = I/RT$; where P = heat, I = current, R = resistance, and T = exposure time. The heat produced is a function of the current's strength and duration of contact and tissue resistance. It is possible, however, that tissue damage is also partially a result of other undiscovered electrical effects. Chronic neurological changes are difficult to explain simply from thermal damage to tissue.

CLINICAL EFFECTS AND TREATMENT

Electrical injury resembles a crush injury more than a thermal burn. The extent of internal damage is often more severe than the cutaneous wound makes it appear. The small entry and exit wounds give no accurate indication of the extent of tissue damage and may not be present in brief low-voltage injuries. In addition there can be a direct electrical effect on the heart, nervous system, and skeletal muscle. Immediate death results from ventricular fibrillation, with or without asphyxia, from paralysis of the respiratory centers, or from prolonged tetany of respiratory muscles. Low voltage injuries more commonly produce ventricular fibrillation than severe burns. Current passing through lower resistance tissues causes necrosis of muscles, vessels, nerves, and subcutaneous tissues and can cause thrombosis and vascular insufficiency.

Cutaneous and deep tissue. Cutaneous injuries result from thermal burns, flame burns, and arc burns, a type of burn specific to electrical injuries and more common with high-voltage accidents. Arc injuries result from current coursing external to the body, jumping from its source to the victim, or arcing between different sites on an extremity. The flexor surface of the forearm is a frequent site of arcing injury. Arcing may cause significant flame burns from ignition of clothing or other materials. Frequently an entrance and exit wound can be identified, but there may be severe deep tissue damage with minimal cutaneous involvement. In severe burns extensive limb damage can occur, requiring debridement, fasciotomy, and limb amputation.

Cardiac. The heart is susceptible to electrical injury, and a wide range of abnormalities from arrhythmias to structural damage may be seen (For-

rest, 1992). Ventricular fibrillation is a common cause of death in electric shocks. In nonfatal cases arrhythmias are an important complication. The most common electrocardiogram (ECG) abnormalities noted are sinus tachycardia and nonspecific ST-T wave changes. Ventricular and atrial ectopy, atrial fibrillation, bundle branch blocks, and ventricular tachycardia have all been reported. These abnormalities do not generally persist. Patients exposed to low voltages who are asymptomatic and initially have a normal ECG do not develop arrhythmias (Fatovich, 1991). High-voltage injury can cause myocardial necrosis, although the diagnosis can be difficult to make because of the absence of typical chest pain and ECG changes (Chandra, 1990). Evaluation of myocardial injury is based on measuring the cardiac fraction of the creatine kinase enzyme. Recent evidence suggests that a raised CK-MB level is not necessarily indicative of myocardial damage (McBride, 1986). Myocardial infarction has been reported as a rare complication of electrical injury and is possibly the result of electrically induced coronary vasospasm (Xenopoulos, 1991). It has been suggested that the presence of extensive burns and entrance and exit wounds present in the upper and lower parts of the body can predict patients at risk of myocardial involvement and warrant intensive monitoring (Chandra, 1990).

Neurologic. Acute central nervous system (CNS) complications include respiratory center arrest or depression, seizures, mental status changes, coma, localized paresis, and amnesia. In mild cases headaches, irritability, dizziness, and trouble concentrating appear. These usually resolve in a few days. Peripheral nerve injuries are seen most often with extensive limb burns. Spinal cord damage is the most common permanent neurologic problem. It may cause progressive muscular atrophy or illness simulating amyotrophic lateral sclerosis or tranverse myelitis. Symptoms characteristically appear after a latency period with no or minimal neurologic symptoms in the acute stage. Some reports describe a stereotyped generalized cerebral dysfunction resulting in depression, divorce, unemployment, and a high incidence of atypical seizures (Hooshmand, 1989).

Renal. Electrical injuries produce an increased incidence of renal damage as compared to other burns. Factors include shock, direct damage to the kidneys by high voltage current, and the release of toxic products from breakdown of damaged muscles. Myoglobinuria is commonly present and is proportional to the amount of muscle injury. Timely administration of fluids and diuretics is important in the prevention of pigment-induced acute renal failure (Gupta, 1991). The development of acute renal failure in electrical injury correlates poorly with the extent of surface burns since the volume of tissue destroyed is much greater than in a surface burn (DiVincenti, 1969). Applying the formula for estimating fluid replacement in surface burns may seriously underestimate the fluid required in patients with electrical burns.

Vascular. Vascular complications have included immediate and delayed major vessel hemorrhage, arterial thrombosis, abdominal aortic aneurysms, and deep vein thrombosis. This large and small tissue damage may be responsible for the tissue damage in electrical injury that is not immediately apparent (Kobernick, 1982).

Other. Musculoskeletal injuries are often initially overlooked and can include multiple fractures and dislocations. Shoulder and scapular fractures are frequently reported. Injury may result from falls or from being hurled from the electrical source. Cataracts and conjunctival or corneal burns can occur. Cataracts usually form 2 to 6 months after the shock, but they can appear immediately or many years later (Van Johnson, 1987).

Treatment in the field involves rapidly and safely removing the victim from the source of current, immediate and prolonged cardiopulmonary resuscitation (CPR), attention to other life-threatening injuries such as cervical spine injury, and initiation of advanced cardiac life support. A rescuer can easily become an electrical victim. Before touching the victim one should attempt to turn off the electrical source. The victim can be separated from the power by using nonconductive materials such as rubber, a wooden axe handle, a mat, or heavy blankets. If it is not known whether the victim fell or was thrown, a cervical collar should be applied. If there is more than one victim, efforts should be made to revive those who appear dead, as there is a good chance that some will survive after prolonged resuscitation attempts (Kobernick, 1982). Fluid resuscitation ideally should begin in the field, especially in high-voltage injuries that can result in significant volume depletion secondary to exudation and sequestration of fluids in burns and damaged areas. Fluid requirements frequently are much greater than those recommended by formulas predicting fluid needs from the area of cutaneous burns. Because deep tissue damage can exist with limited surface burns, fluid should be administered in sufficient volume to maintain a urine output of 50-100 cc/hr to prevent renal insufficiency from myoglobin deposition. Mannitol is recommended by some to assure an adequate urine flow (Artz, 1967). Tetanus immunization should be administered if indicated.

No clear-cut criteria guide the necessity of hos-pital admission of less severely injured patients. Inpatient observation is advisable for patients who may show evidence of cardiac dysfunction, symptoms of neurologic impairment, presence of significant surface burns, suspicion of deep tissue damage, or laboratory evidence of acidosis or myoglobinuria.

REGULATIONS

The Occupational Safety and Health Administration (OSHA) requires use of nonconductive ladders where the employee or the ladder could contact exposed electrical conductors and requires that all metal ladders be prominently marked with a warning label. OSHA does have regulations for the construction industry.

PREVENTION

Each injury or fatality should be viewed as a sentinel health event and prompt analysis of the worksite should be initiated with an eye toward preventive measures. Any injury suggests the need for a job-specific electrical safety analysis and provides an opportunity for preventive intervention in the workplace. Most of these injuries occur either from lack of education concerning the specific hazards of the work or from failure to follow safe work practices. Primary prevention of electrical injuries is the ultimate goal and can be accomplished through the use of administrative and engineering controls, personal protective equipment, and education and training.

Administrative controls require commitment from management and workers and should be part of a written safety program. Their effectiveness depends on rigorous implementation in the workplace. An example could be a scheduled preventive maintenance program for all power tools and cords to prevent mishaps due to damaged or frayed power cords.

Because many electrical injuries occur among nonutility workers, these employees should be specifically targeted for primary prevention activities. Worksite electrical safety education should focus on recognition of potential electrical hazards and practical training on active protection measures for the worker (Jones, 1991).

Power lines have been involved in numerous electrical fatalities and their hazards can be reduced through measures such as visual enhancement with markers, sleeving to insulate the line in high-risk areas, deenergizing lines in work areas when possible, use of ladders made of nonconducting materials, and the use of steering lines attached to the upper ends of ladders to stabilize and prevent tipping backward into power lines. Using a lookout worker to help guide aerial equipment is desirable. A minimum of 10 feet should be maintained for the safe operation of aerial parts of a machine near a power line.

Many accidents occur while using electric machinery or portable powered hand tools. Repair of damaged power cords, proper electrical grounding, and the use of ground fault circuit interrupters (GFCI) can prevent the majority of these injuries. A GFCI is a device designed to open the power source circuit quickly when a fault of a minimum amperage is detected. When the difference between the supply and return current exceeds 4 to 6 mA the power source is automatically disconnected. This is less than the estimated 50 to 100 mA of 60 Hz current needed to cause ventricular fibrillation. Consistent use of GFCI is an engineering control that could save dozens of lives each year.

Workers must be educated in the potential lethality of low-voltage and always ground hand tools properly, especially portable powered hand tools. Extension cords used to supply power need particular attention because the grounding pin (third prong) is often removed to accommodate a two-pronged receptacle. Use of two-conductor extension cords may encourage removal of the ground pin from the tool power cord. Using battery-powered hand tools in place of low-voltage, current-supplied tools and using double-insulated tools can help prevent electrical shock even under adverse conditions.

In Australia the electrical workers' union has attempted to address the problem by improving education. All apprentice electricians are now shown a documentary film that reviews the hazards of working with electricity. The film recommends that electrical workers never work "live" and never work alone.

LIGHTNING INJURIES

In the United States, lightning kills more people every year than any other natural disaster. Of the 100 to 300 deaths and 1,000 to 2,000 injuries per year caused by lightning, it is estimated that approximately 30% are occupationally related (Duclos, 1990). Many of these occur in the agricultural and construction industries and other jobs where people work outdoors. Job-related injuries are an important and frequent issue with respect to lightning strikes. Working may be an incentive to stay exposed or workers may be forced to continue working (Duclos, 1990).

Most injuries occur during the summer months when thunderstorms are most frequent. The areas of the U.S. with the greatest number of deaths include the Southern and Atlantic states, and states on the Ohio, Mississippi, and Hudson Rivers. The Gulf coast and Rocky Mountains also have a high incidence of lightning injuries, while California and the West Coast are almost devoid of thunderstorms and lightning strikes and thus of related injuries (Nelson, 1985).

Lightning kills 30% of its victims, and survivors experience a high morbidity rate. The most common cause of death is immediate cardiopulmonary arrest. Lightning is dangerous due to high voltage, heat generation, and explosive force. Lightning may also injure indirectly by starting forest and house fires, causing explosions, or by dropping objects such as trees on occupied buildings or cars.

The factor that seems to be most important in distinguishing lightning from electrical current injuries is the duration of exposure to the current. Exposure to lightning current is nearly instantaneous, so that prolonged contact is not made. The energy generally travels superficially, causing a flashover. Distinct entry and exit wounds are rare and deep burns are infrequent. The explosive force of the lightning strike may cause significant blunt trauma as the victim is thrown by a direct strike or by the shock wave created by the flash. Clothing and shoes may literally be blown from the body. Injuries vary and may be classified from minor to severe and, as with electrical injuries, several organ systems may be affected and acute and chronic effects are seen.

With minor injury, patients experience confusion and temporary amnesia. They rarely have significant burns but may complain of paresthesias and muscular pain. A ruptured tympanic membrane is a frequent finding due to the explosive force of the lightning shock wave. Patients usually recover completely. With moderate injury patients may be disoriented, combative, or unconscious. Motor paralysis, more often of the lower extremities, with mottling of the skin and diminished or absent pulses due to arterial spasm and sympathetic instability may be seen. Hypotension should be ruled out and, if found, should prompt a search for inapparent blunt trauma and fractures. Victims may have experienced temporary cardiopulmonary arrest at the time of the strike. Respiratory arrest may be prolonged and lead to cardiac arrest from hypoxia. Seizures may also occur. Ruptured tympanic membranes are commonly found and minor burns may become apparent after a few hours. Patients generally improve although they may experience chronic symptoms such as sleep disturbances, weakness, paresthesias, and psychomotor abnormalities. As with electrical injuries, rare cases of spinal paralysis have been reported. Severely injured patients may present cardiac arrest with either asystole or ventricular fibrillation. In fact, victims are unlikely to die unless cardiopulmonary arrest occurred at the time of the lightning strike (Cooper, 1980). Resuscitation may not be successful if there is a significant delay in initiating CPR. Direct brain damage may occur. Findings of blunt trauma suggest a direct strike.

In severe cases, initial treatment includes rapid attention to cardiopulmonary resuscitation and support if necessary. In general, fluids should be restricted unless there is evidence of hypotension. Although minor burns may be present, vigorous fluid therapy and mannitol diuresis are not indicated unless myoglobinuria is found. Overhydration with resultant cerebral edema has probably killed more lightning victims than pigment-induced renal failure (Cooper, 1983). Fasciotomy is rarely needed in lightning injuries, as most burns are superficial.

Long-term sequelae in survivors also include visual and hearing deficits due most often to damaged tympanic membranes and cataracts. Persons who work in areas where lightning strikes are possible should be familiar with the preventive measures recommended by the National Weather Service.

CASE STUDIES
Case 1

An 18-year-old construction worker wearing rubber-soled boots, shorts, and no gloves was using a portable electric saw on a hot and humid summer day. He was working on top of a corrugated metal roof cutting a groove for flashing in a concrete wall. The electrical source was a properly grounded electrical outlet within the building with residential current of 110/120V, 60 Hz. The saw was connected to this outlet by a 50-foot extension cord. The grounding pin was missing from the extension cord's plug.

A co-worker watched as the worker knelt on the roof, turned on the saw, and immediately started jerking and attempted to yell. After a short period of time the co-worker pulled the plug and the victim collapsed on the roof. The co-worker attempted mouth-to-mouth resuscitation as the victim had no spontaneous respirations. The victim was transported to a local hospital but was pronounced dead shortly after his arrival, having never regained any spontaneous respirations or cardiac rhythm. An autopsy showed no anatomical cause of death, burns, or evidence of significant trauma. The diagnosis was death by electrocution.

The saw and extension cord were examined by a electrical testing laboratory. The switch was found to contain a short circuit causing the metal handle to become energized. The groundwire in the saw's cord was broken, causing the short circuit current to flow into the worker's hand instead of harmlessly through the ground circuit. As noted above, the grounding pin on the extension cord was missing. The laboratory simulated conditions of temperature and humidity similar to the day of the accident and found a voltage of 105 V flowing from

the handle to ground. From this information the amount of current the victim was exposed to can be calculated (amperage = voltage/resistance). The average resistance of the human body is 1,000 ohms. When V = 105, amperage is 105 milliamps. This amperage, when of sufficient duration, is capable of inducing ventricular fibrillation.

The laboratory also noted that the saw's switch housing was not dust or water tight and a layer of cement dust and dirt was present around the switch. This probably permitted current to flow when moisture from the worker's hand was present.

In summary, this death was the result of a number of preventable defects. The ground circuit was disrupted, the switch produced a short to the saw's metal handle, and the worker's bare legs provided direct contact with the metal roofing. The electrical path was likely from the saw handle through the arm, chest, abdomen, and one or both legs to the roof to ground. The autopsy results are consistent with a low-amperage electrocution. This example clearly illustrates how low-voltage equipment can cause death.

Case 2

A 33-year-old Hispanic female stocking clerk for a large chain department store was referred to the clinic by her human resources (HR) manager.

Her chief complaint was pain in her right forearm, off and on for the past month. She stated that a significant part of her job involved touch-up ironing of clothes and other cloth items as she unpacked them for display. She had had three episodes of electrical shock from the iron, the most recent being that morning, and she was sure that the arm pain was from the shocks.

She described the sensation as a "buzzing, quivering feeling" in her hand and forearm when she lifted the iron. It did not happen all the time when she used the instrument, but had happened several weeks previously and then twice this week. She had told her supervisor about it, afraid that she would get a bad shock and "be electrocuted." (She was divorced from her husband and was a parent of two school-age children.) However her supervisor had done nothing about it.

On physical examination she was mildly tender to palpation over the right lateral epicondylar area. Resisted wrist extension test was negative. Other musculoskeletal and neurological examination of the right arm was normal.

She was diagnosed as having a mild lateral epicondylitis in her dominant right arm, from her work tasks of moving and opening big boxes, ironing with a heavy old iron, and so forth, but not from the electric shocks. However she was commended for bringing that problem to the attention of management. A call placed to the HR director resulted in immediate removal of the old iron and replacement with a new, lighter model. The patient was prescribed a forearm band, balm, and advised about icing. The case was resolved without further treatment.

Case 3

A 58-year-old farm laborer was reeling in an extension cord inside a barn. The cord connected a small mulching machine to an electrical outlet inside the farmhouse. The worker was standing on a damp earthen surface and did not notice a damaged area in the cord as he was coiling it up around his arm. He experienced a sudden shock as his hand grabbed the bare region of the cord and he was unable to release himself. Another worker witnessing the accident took a wooden-handled shovel and knocked the power cord out of his hand. The worker slumped to the ground, apparently not seriously injured and without loss of consciousness. He was taken to a small rural clinic for evaluation, as the nearest hospital was 30 miles away.

At the clinic he complained of arm and shoulder pain and numbness in his hand. On examination he was pleasant and cooperative and in moderate distress from arm pain. His vital signs showed a temperature of 98.2° F, regular pulse of 80, blood pressure of 150/92, and a respiratory rate of 14. His skin showed no evidence of a burn or entry or exit wounds. There was slight redness around his wrist where his watch had been worn. He also said his ring felt tight on his finger but there was no obvious edema of the hand or arm. The remainder of the examination was normal with the exception of moderate pain during palpation of the right forearm, upper arm and shoulder girdle, and anterior right chest wall. He had normal pulses in his arm and hand. There was full range of motion in the arm with moderate pain. The neurologic examination revealed normal mental status and cranial nerves, reflexes, and sensory response. An electrocardiogram was normal. The patient was discharged with a prescription for an antiinflammatory medication and was told to ice the arm and return to the clinic if his symptoms did not resolve.

Shortly after returning to the farm he began complaining of worsening pain and swelling in his hand, arm, and shoulder. On reexamination in the clinic he had evidence of increased swelling in his hand and arm with a diminished radial pulse. Arrangements were made for helicopter transport to the nearest hospital that was able to treat burns.

On arrival the patient was immediately assessed for a compartment syndrome. Shortly after admission he was taken to the operating room for fasciotomy and debridement of deep tissue injury. Laboratory studies revealed a CK of 3400. Urine myoglobin was present and the patient's initial creatinine was 1.4 mg/dl. Despite initial management with fluids, mannitol, and loop diuretics, the patient's course over the next 10 days was marked by oliguric renal failure with peak BUN of 182 mg/dl and peak creatinine of 9.3 mg/dl. Klebsiella sepsis occurred on the twelfth hospital day. The patient responded to antibiotic therapy but required a prolonged stay in the intensive care unit. The patient's renal functions returned to normal by the third week in the hospital. His arm required skin graftings but fortunately he retained full function of his hand.

SUGGESTED READINGS

Artz CP: Electrical injury simulates crush injury. *Surg Gynecol Obstet* 125:1316, 1967.

Baker SP, Samkoff JS, Fisher RS, Van Buren CB: Fatal occupational injuries. *JAMA* 248:692-697, 1982.

Berkelman RL, Herndon JL, Callaway JL, Stivers R, Howard LB, Bezjak A et al: Fatal injuries and alcohol. *Am J Prev Med* 1:21-28, 1985.

Branday JM et al: Visceral complications of electrical burn injury. A report of two cases and review of the literature. *West Indian Medical Journal* 38:110-113, 1989.

Brokenshire B: Deaths from electricity. *NZ Med J* 97:139-142, 1984.

Brokenshire B, Cairns FJ, Koelmeyer TD, Smeeton WM, Tie ABM: Deaths from electricity. *NZ Med J* 97:139-142, 1984.

CDC: Electrocutions in the construction industry involving portable metal ladders—United States, 1984-1988. *MMWR* 41:187-189, 1992.

CDC: NIOSH alert: preventing electrocutions during work with scaffolds near overhead power lines. *MMWR* 41:146-147, 1992.

CDC: Up-date: work-related electrocutions associated with Hurricane Hugo—Puerto Rico. *MMWR* 38:718-720, 1989. (Also Nov. 24, 1989.)

CDC: Occupational electrocutions in Texas 1981-1985. *MMWR* 36(4):26-28, 1987.

CDC: Fatal occupational injuries—Texas, 1982. *MMWR* 34:130-134, 139, 1985.

Chandra NC, Siu CO, Munster AM: Clinical predictors of myocardial damage after high voltage electrical injury. *Critical Care Med* 18:293-297, 1990.

Cone JE, Daponte A, Makofsky D et al: *J Occup Med* 33:813-817, 1991.

Cooper MA: Lightning injuries. In Auerbach PS and Geehr EC, editors: *Management of wilderness and environmental emergencies.* New York, 1983, Macmillan Publishing Co., Inc.

Cooper MA: Lightning injuries: prognostic signs for death. *Ann Emerg Med* 9:134, 1980.

Cooper MA, Rund D: Lightning injuries. In Nelson R, Rund D, Keller M, editors: *Environmental emergencies,* 1985, WB Saunders Co.

DiVincenti FC, Moncrief JA, Pruitt BA: Electrical injuries: a review of 65 cases. *J Trauma* 9:497-507, 1969.

Fatovich DM: Electrocution in Western Australia, 1976-1990. *Med J Aust* 157:762-764, 1992.

Fatovich DM, Lee KY: Household electric shocks: who should be monitored? *Med J Aust* 155:301-303, 1991.

Forrest FC, Saunders PR, McSwinney M, Tooley MA: Cardiac injury and electrocution. *J Royal Soc Med* 85:642-643, 1992.

Gallagher JP, Tabert OR: Motor neuron syndrome after electric shock. *Acta Neurologica Scandinavica* 83:79-82, 1991.

Gupta KL, Kumar R, Sekhar S, Sakhuja V, Chugh KS: Myoglobinuric acute renal failure following electrical injury. *Renal Failure* 13:23-25, 1991.

Harvey-Sutton PL, Driscoll TR, Frommer MS, Harrison JE: Work-related electrical fatalities in Australia, 1982-1984. *Scan J Work Environ Health* 18:293-297, 1992.

Helgerson SD: Farm workers electrocuted when irrigation pipes contact powerlines. *Public Health Rep* 100:325-328, 1985.

Hooshmand H, Radfar F, Beckner E: The neurophysiological aspects of electrical injuries. *Clin Electroencephal* 20:111-120, 1989.

Knight B: Injury and death from physical agents. In Knight B: *Legal aspects of medical practice.* Edinburgh, 1982, Churchill Livingstone, 144-153.

Kobernick M: Electrical injuries: pathophysiology and emergency management. *Ann Emerg Med* 11:633-638, 1982.

Kraus JF: Fatal and nonfatal injuries in occupational setting: a review. *Annu Rev Public Health.* 6:403-418, 1985.

Lee WR: Deaths from electric shock in 1962 and 1963. *Brit Med J* 2:616-619, 1965.

Lee WR: A clinical study of electrical accidents. *Br J Ind Med* 18:260-269, 1961.

McBride JW, Labrosse KR, McCoy HG et al: Is serum creatine kinase-MB in electrically injured patients predictive of myocardial injury? *JAMA* 255:764, 1986.

Mellen PF, Weedn VW, Kao G: Electrocution: a review of 155 cases with emphasis on human factors. *J Forensic Sci* 37:1016-1022, 1992.

Middleton D: The deadly current. *J Emerg Med Services* 12:341-343, 1987.

Murray R: Hazards to health—electric shock. *NEJM* 268:1127-1128, 1963.

Ng D, et al: Work-related burns: a 6 year retrospective study. *Burns* 17:151-154, 1991.

NIOSH: Preventing electrocutions of workers using portable metal ladders near overhead powerlines. Cincinnati, 1989. (DHHS publication 89-110.)

Robinson MN, Brooks CG, Renshaw GD: Electric shock devices and their effects on the human body. *Med Sci Law* 30:285-300, 1990.

Schein RM, Kett DH, De Marchena EJ, Sprung CL: Pulmonary edema associated with electrical injury. *Chest* 97:1248-1250, 1990.

Suruda AJ: Work-related deaths in construction painting. *Scan J Work* Environ Health 18:30-33, 1992.

Suruda A: Electrocution at work. *Prof Saf* 33:27-32, 1988.

Suruda A, Smith L: Work-related electrocutions involving portable power tools and appliances. *J Occup Med* 34:887-891, 1992.

Trent RB, Wyant WD: Fatal hand tool injuries in construction. *J Occup Med* 32:711-714, 1990.

VanJohnson E, Kline LB, Skalka HW: Electrical cataracts: a case report and review of the literature. *Ophthalmic Surgery* 18:283-285, 1987.

Wharton MD, Levine MS, Radford EP: A preventable death from an electrical hand tool malfunction. *J Occup Med* 9:589-591, 1975

Wright RK: Death or injury caused by electrocution. *Clinical Lab Med* 3(2):343-353, 1983.

Wright RK, Davis JH et al: The investigation of electrical deaths: a report of 220 fatalities. *J Forensic Sci* 25:514-521, 1980.

Xenopoulos N, Movahed A, Hudson P, Reeves WC: Myocardial injury in electrocution. *Am Heart J* 122:1481-1484, 1991.

32 Psychiatric Issues: Stress, Somatization, Violence, and Suicide

CONCEPT OF STRESS

Stress is ubiquitous, and occasionally deleterious in its effect. Most states have concluded that work function impairment and disability can be the result of psychiatric as well as physical factors. Stress injuries are difficult to quantify, often more multifactorial in etiology than the patient would prefer to believe, and costly to treat. In response, many states, such as California, are struggling with plans to revise the legal definition of compensable work-related stress. An understanding of the concept of stress and its varying clinical presentations will help the physician more effectively evaluate and treat the worker complaining directly of stress, or expressing psychologic and emotional difficulties in one of many displaced ways.

Cannon (1935) first used the term "stress" to indicate an individual's typical pattern of fight or flight reaction to noxious stimuli. He also used the term "homeostasis" to indicate the organism's wish to return to a steady state of functioning.

Selye (1956) described a nonspecific response on the part of the body to demands made on it. He conveyed that stress was the body's mental, emotional, and physical reaction to forces that impinge upon it. Certain forms of stress, or arousal and responsivity, are productive, helpful, and adaptive. As an example, physical, mental, and emotional arousal that occurs in the context of a major job opportunity will be channeled productively if expressed in the form of animation, focused thoughts, appropriate excitement, and other such overt responses. If it takes the form of tremulousness, vigilant apprehension, and stuttering, the result is likely to be less satisfactory. In general, stress theory would suggest that the stress response is most often idiosyncratic and related to a specific network of genetic, temperamental, developmental, general psychologic, situational, and prospective factors.

Caplan (1981) summarized 30 years of work studying responses to stressful life circumstances by describing the components of mastery, a process of effectively dealing with stress. This involved a pattern of responding to external, psychosocial, or intrapsychic stressors so that emotional arousal was reduced to tolerable physiologic and psychologic levels during and shortly after the stressful event occurred, and mobilizing internal, interpersonal, and environmental resources to develop "new capabilities in him that lead to his changing his environment or his relationship to it, so that he reduces the threat or finds alternate sources of satisfaction for what is lost" (p. 413). Caplan defined stress as a "condition in which there is a marked discrepancy between the demands made on an organism and the organism's capability to respond, the consequences of which will be detrimental to the organism's future in respect to conditions essential to its well-being" (p. 414). He described four phrases of response to stress: changing or escaping from the environment; acquiring new capacities for coping with circumstances; defending against negative effects; and a general process of internal readjustment.

An understanding of basic psychologic defenses is critical to respond to a patient's complaints of stress and its cause(s). Part of the homeostatic process initially defined by Cannon involves efforts at altering the external environment and/or the internal world and perspective. Psychologic defenses serve to organize, mediate, and moderate perceptions. Primitive defenses involve such behaviors as wholesale denial of discomfort, delusional rationalizations and explanations of experiences, and the polarization of feelings and perceptions into an all-good or all-bad framework. High-level defenses include appropriate suppression of certain perceptions and emotions on a temporary basis for adaptive reasons, sublimation, and altruism.

Vaillant (1977) defined a series of intermediate defenses that are moderately effective in managing aroused discomfort and distress. These include such internal actions as excessive repression (making conflicts unconscious), displacement (unconscious shifting of feelings from one thing or idea to another), rationalization (unconscious justification), reaction formation (manifesting feelings and/or behavior antithetical to internal urges), and

479

somatization (experiencing and expressing psychologic and emotional conflicts in physical terms). The individual using defenses at this level is often unaware of the primary or full set of factors potentiating the focus of his or her response. With this in mind, displacement, denial, rationalization, somatization, and other such defenses significantly influence a patient's internal representation of her experiences and their causality. For this reason, the comprehensive history to be described later should be undertaken to gather a full understanding of the potential sources of conflict and emotional stress with which an individual might be dealing. When these areas are not evaluated, the examiner is simply left to accept the patient's complaints at face value, or to find them unreasonable without having any idea why.

Psychosocial development

Among many clinicians who have written extensively on normal and pathologic development, Eric Erikson (1963) elaborated a particularly useful model of psychosocial development that viewed development as a lifelong process with important biologic, psychologic, and social tasks and demands. He concluded that life after birth confronts the individual with a series of adaptational tasks. These tasks can be intrapsychic, physical, environmental, or interpersonal. In normal development, they occur in a manner that is predictable, sequential, and hierarchical. Developmental demands occur and evolve throughout the life cycle. Metered frustration is an essential component for adaptation and psychologic, emotional, and intellectual growth. Success or failure at mastery of earlier adaptational tasks affects the capacity to cope with later developmental demands and life crises. Table 32-1 contains an overview of the effects of successful versus unsuccessful adaptation to the sequential and hierarchical series of adaptive demands on the organism that occur during a normal life span. These are listed in order from earliest to latest life demands.

Individuals respond to internal conflicts and interpersonal problems largely through the use of habituated coping mechanisms. These vary widely in efficiency, effectiveness, and adaptiveness. The specific choice and effectiveness of such mechanisms is determined by the interaction of:

- Inborn temperamental variables as described by Chess and Thomas (1986).
- Inborn ego (mediating) factors, such as intellectual capacity.
- Role modeling of primary identificatory figures.
- The nature, magnitude, phase appropriateness, and sequencing of adaptational demands.

Ideally, normal development proceeds by presenting the individual with graded, hierarchical demands that are mastered by using previously acquired resources and the internalization of coping skills modeled by parents, other significant adults, and peers.

Normal psychologic development includes the primary task in infancy of communicating needs experienced through bodily sensations. Infantile affects serve to cue parenting figures to respond to

Table 32-1 Sequelae of psychosocial development—Erikson's model

Successful adaptation	Compromised adaptation
Sense of basic, situationally-appropriate trust, reliance	Basic mistrust of the intentions of others
Capacity to rely on others in an interdependent way	Excessive dependence or pseudoindependence
Personal initiative without guilt; capacity for self-determining behavior and willing cooperation	Stubbornness, defiance, ambivalence, sadomasochism
Respect for the autonomy of others	Controlling behavior, fragile autonomy
Healthy, stable sense of self	Feelings of insecurity, inadequacy; narcissistic defenses
Conscience; sense of responsibility, dependability, self-discipline; appropriate independence	Chronic guilt or lack of appropriate internal prohibitions
Capacity for taking initiative	Inhibitions in facing new problems
Sense of pleasure in work, capacity for perseverance	Sense of incompetence in response to adversity
Positive sense of stability and continuity	Lack of a stable sense of identity and purpose
Capacity for mutually gratifying, mature, intimate relationships	Sense of personal isolation; strained, stiff relationships
Acceptance of limitations; sense of evolving fulfillment of one's potential	Self-absorption; self-indulgence
Capacity to place the needs of others before one's own	Lack of empathy; a geocentric world view

needs. A predominant mode of bipersonal communication develops and becomes a motif for the later expression of needs through symbolic language. Normal psychologic development includes parental facilitation of a differentiation within and between psychologic and somatic sensations. Families and cultures vary widely in the degree to which they encourage the ultimate primacy of language to communicate distress. The capacity to communicate disturbing emotions in verbal terms depends on a number of variables including:

• Patterns established early on with regard to the interplay between expressed sensations/needs and parental responsiveness.
• The degree of parental encouragement of verbal communication.
• Implications within the family and culture for expression.
• The capacity within the family to productively address conflict.

Within some families the form and type of communication is such that significant depression and/or aggressiveness results, or there is subtle encouragement of the use of physical symptoms to gratify needs for attention, love, and nurturance. Difficulties in learning to express feelings of distress verbally may prompt an individual to seek developmentally earlier modes of expression such as acting on impulses or somatization. Sifneos (1973) described alexithymia, a difficulty in expressing disturbing affects in verbal form and a consequent proclivity to use a somatic vocabulary rather than a psychologic/emotional one. This was deemed likely to result from a pattern of neglect or punishment for communicating about affects. Excessive childhood pain, trauma, neglect, and active or passive thwarting of normal developmental needs result in a heightened presence of neurotic-level defenses. A tendency to carry forward into adult life a broad array of conflicts about which the individual feels unconsciously resentful and paralyzed in terms of achieving an adaptive, productive solution is another result. Such individuals are highly prone to enact and play out their conflicts from childhood in current intimate and work relationships. They will be likely to have a history of extremely limited success in terms of mastering normal stressors, a proclivity to report accumulated stress for which they are bereft of adequate solutions, or a tendency to have a dramatic and untoward response to what most individuals would consider to be modest problems.

With these factors in mind, a comprehensive history is essential to facilitate an understanding of the patient's complaints. Only with such a history can one determine whether displacement and somatization are being used on an unconscious or preconscious basis to play out unresolved, preexisting conflicts, or if the current focus of concern should be the primary focus of attention. It should be noted that many individuals with considerable, unresolved conflicts from their formative years not only displace those conflicts onto their present environment, but also can unwittingly prompt others (on an unconscious basis) to enact and recapitulate unresolved past conflicts and traumas. With a basic understanding of the complexity of psychologic defenses and Erikson's model of life as epigenetic and involving a recurrent recapitulation of unresolved developmental problems, in part as a process of attempting to master them, the clinician should not simply take the patient's report of work-related stress at face value. A comprehensive evaluation should be taken to accurately understand the range and weight of factors causing current symptomatic complaints.

INDICES OF PSYCHOLOGIC FACTORS AT PLAY IN THE CLINICAL PRESENTATION

Symptoms that develop in response to perceived stressors are numerous and are related to developmental, intrapsychic, interpersonal, and situation variables. Symptoms can be viewed as the patient's unconscious effort to mediate or compromise between developmental, and current internal and external demands. Typical conflict expression might be manifested in alterations in consciousness, changes in general pattern of behavior, affective upheaval, use of more primitive defenses, thought content or process disturbances, and/or a generalized decreased level of adaptive flexibility.

Because of their mature personality structures, some people are resilient and appropriately flexible. People who are less well integrated in terms of their personality structure often have fragile and brittle defenses and may have difficulty accommodating relatively small changes in their normal and usual routines. A typical example is the patient with borderline personality disorder who functions well in a structured environment, but evidences a declining ability to adapt as boundaries become ill-defined.

Individuals with limited flexibility and coping resources are more prone to become symptomatic when confronted with stressors. This is due in part to the fact that they will regress to earlier defenses and coping strategies. Often the first complaints of such patients are physical. Lipowski (1988) and other authors have pointed out that the initial complaints of over 50% of patients who have depression are physical, not psychologic and emotional.

They come to the family practitioner or the internist complaining of physical disorders when an underlying, masked psychologic and emotional disorder is the problem. If this is not suspected or diagnosed, the patient can lead the physician astray. It is critical that psychologic and emotional disturbances and illnesses be considered as part of the differential diagnosis of many physical complaints, particularly when the physical complaint has no equally obvious physical explanation. This not to say that the emotional problem should become a diagnosis of exclusion, but one has to scrutinize carefully to be sure there is no psychologic or emotional diagnosis when one cannot make a physical diagnosis to fully explain the scope and depth of symptoms.

One of the most prominent psychologic defenses that emerges in the context of a perceived occupational problem or stressor is somatization. This psychologic defense can be defined as the proclivity to experience and express psychologic and emotional conflicts in physical terms. It is differentiated from psychophysiologic symptoms by the lack of adequate physical findings to explain the professed degree of functional impairment in somatization. In a psychophysiologic disorder, psychologic variables are deemed to be central to the initiation or aggravation of identifiable physical pathologic condition. One of the most common presentations of somatization is in the form of somatoform pain.

Patients who somatize are invariably convinced that their symptoms are largely, if not totally, of physical origin. This conviction often assumes delusional-like proportions, and they frequently convince their physicians to vigorously pursue physical diagnoses that often turn out to be red herrings (Becker and Smith, 1992). At the worst, patients are treated with unnecessary medications, treatments, or even operations, after which they invariably do have physical problems.

A number of clues should alert the clinician to the possibility, if not the probability, of functional overlay or somatization. Indices suggesting the presence of confounding, if not primary, psychological factors in the patient's clinical presentation, report of symptoms, and cooperation with treatment are include the following, which is not an all-inclusive list:

- A history that is vague or implausible, given the circumstances.
- The use of flowery and elaborate imagery to describe pain. Nonsomatizers are more likely to describe it as acute, blunt or throbbing, without highly emotionally colored adjectives.

- Narcotic overuse or other substance dependence, reflective of chronic, frustrated dependency needs.
- Complaints of total body pain, or a positive review of systems with complaints in many organ systems.
- Extreme patient protestation about past independent functioning. This patient may really be telling the physician that her symptoms are a thin mask or facade behind which she conceals her emotional neediness, and that allow her to be taken care of without losing face.
- A history of considerable attention derived during childhood for medical problems, or a family history of such behavior. Even in childhood, illness can become a way to avoid responsibilities and a vehicle for securing attention. This behavioral pattern, if reinforced, is frequently carried into adult life. The patient who expresses fears that she may never be able to work again is often revealing in the fear an unconscious wish, since fears and wishes are closely related outside of conscious awareness.
- Low job satisfaction. It is generally accepted that job dissatisfaction is an important variable predisposing patients to ongoing symptoms, particularly back and extremity pain on an industrial basis (Bigos et al, 1991, 1992).
- Noncompliance with treatment regimens may well reflect a conflict between what a patient consciously says is desirable (namely, to get better and to return to work) and what is unconsciously wanted (namely, to be taken care of). Patients are often not aware of this unconscious desire and are, therefore, in conflict. The clinician should remember that actions speak louder than words, and it is clear from some patients who have little in the way of positive physical findings to explain their ongoing symptoms, that there is little motivation to report subjective improvement.
- The presence of significant domestic problems.
- Unrecognized depressive spectrum problems that precede the onset of physical complaints.
- Waddell (1980) has noted the importance among orthopedic patients of a discrepancy between sitting and recumbent straight leg raising in the context of complaints of chronic back pain, give-way weakness on muscle testing, and glove or stocking hypesthesia.
- Atypical aroused resentment or irritability in the physician may be in response to passive-aggressive, passive-resistent, or overtly angry behavior on the part of the patient.
- The presence of litigation. Numerous articles have described the observed fact that, all things

being equal, patients who are in litigation tend to keep their disabling symptoms until the litigation is resolved. Patients not in litigation get better faster and return to work sooner. Litigation clearly has an adverse effect on symptoms when a patient understands that he or she may not win the litigation once normal physical health has been restored and normal activities have been resumed.

No single factor from this list is sufficient to draw firm conclusions with regard to somatization. Rather, any positive findings should be thoroughly assessed in the course of the clinical interview and psychologic testing described later.

INITIAL SCREENING
OF STRESS CLAIMS

The patient asserting a stress claim, professing to have psychologic and emotional problems, or whom the physician feels may be somatizing warrants a thorough examination. This is particularly the case when issues of causality and apportionment may become pertinent. Such an evaluation is best conducted by a qualified psychiatrist or psychologist who has developed an expertise in medical-legal matters. It is usually impractical in the occupational medicine clinic setting to have such a professional on staff; as such, referrals will most often have to be made for the specialized examination process that will be described later. As a rule of thumb, it is recommended that all claimants with a primary complaint of stress be seen by the clinic staff physician for a screening interview. This serves several purposes:

- The patient believes that her concerns are being responded to thoughtfully and with respect.
- Referrals for specialized evaluations often must be made through primary care physicians, particularly in the psychiatric arena where many claims examiners have an immediately negative response to the assertion of a stress claim.
- The primary care physician often has a working relationship with the employer and can be of considerable help in educating the mental health consultant to certain realities of the workplace.
- On some occasions complaints of stress emanating from work are relatively straightforward and can be addressed efficiently and effectively by the clinic physician. Wherever professed problems appear to be complex and/or longstanding, or where characterological difficulties seem to be present, a referral should be made.
- The screening interview provides an opportunity to evaluate for identifiable physical problems that might be significant; for example, mitral valve prolapse in the patient with a presenting complaint of anxiety.

Referrals to the mental health professional of patients complaining of stress usually are not met with resistance. On the other hand, referrals made to psychologists and psychiatrists of patients who are felt to be manifesting somatization or functional overlay must be handled tactfully. These patients often assume that they are being dumped or that the physician is indirectly asserting that the symptoms are only the result of a mental disorder. A referral should be introduced as part of a multidisciplinary evaluation to ensure that the patient will not feel fundamentally rejected or disbelieved. At the same time, the assertion that all psychological symptoms are in reaction to primary physical problems stemming solely from work should not be assaulted.

CLINICAL EVALUATION
OF PSYCHOLOGIC FUNCTIONING

When personal injury or workers' compensation issues are at play, the patient should be notified that there is likely to be no confidentiality with regard to the history obtained and other matters discussed. If the evaluation is conducted by a psychiatric or psychological consultant, that individual should clearly state that the gathered database and findings will be forwarded to the referring physician and the patient's disability carrier. If this is not done, there will be inevitable occurrences in which the patient divulges a great deal while believing that treatment has begun with a professional who will maintain strict confidence. Where the referral has been made for authorized treatment, the patient should still be informed that regular reports on the content and status of treatment will make this process different from normal psychotherapy.

Comprehensive history

For a thorough and competent evaluation of a claim of job stress, a comprehensive history must be taken. Data in many domains must be gathered, including the following:

Chief complaint A brief summary of the patient's current signs, symptoms and psychiatric problems should be offered. As much as possible, this should be done through direct quotes from the patient's comments. The patient's representation and understanding of the cause of any professed symptoms should be summarized.

History of presenting circumstances The patient's representation about his problems and their development should be reviewed in detail in chronologic order. In the case of an injury incurred in the work setting, a detailed history of the individual's employment should be derived, including the nature of working relationships, performance evaluation ratings, and the patient's representation as to whether other factors contributed to the development and/or aggravation of symptoms.

Whenever possible, is it helpful to distinguish the state of the individual's various symptoms at several points since the alleged date of injury. This should start with the perceived precursors of the symptoms, their development, and their consequent elaboration and ramifications. The patient's current array of symptoms should be enumerated. The clinician should distinguish between those symptoms openly offered by the patient and those derived from direct inquiry.

Within this section of the report, all treatment obtained by the patient since the onset of the problems should be detailed. The nature and type of treatment provided by any mental health professionals should be given particular attention.

Psychiatric and relevant medical history All history related to any personal or family contacts with mental health professionals should be reviewed. As well, any history of suicide attempts or impulsive, violent behavior by the patient or any member of her family should be noted. Any history of symptoms similar to those which the patient currently is professing should be discussed.

Personal and family history A detailed developmental history is in order. Particular attention should be given to the frequency of geographical changes; the number of siblings and the stability and effectiveness of their functioning; the status of the primary caregivers from the patient's childhood; a description of parental character styles; education, life satisfaction, employment, and disability; the nature of the parental relationship and how conflict was managed by them; any history of physical or sexual abuse of the patient as a child; and the general pattern of relationships with siblings and peers.

A full educational history should be obtained including grades during high school, disciplinary problems, extracurricular activities, learning disabilities, and graduation status. A history of subsequent college (if any) and work experiences should be obtained, including details of what prompted the changes between places of employment. An inquiry should be made into whether the patient was ever terminated from a job and why. A history of any reprimands, suspensions, or disciplinary actions at work should be obtained. Any prolonged periods out of work or history of absen-

teeism should be noted. The patient's long-range vocational plans are worth understanding.

In addition, the patient's history of intimate relationships should be reviewed. If there have been multiple marriages, these should be noted. The status of any children and the nature of their current functioning should be gathered. It is relevant to understand the individual's pattern of conflict management in intimate relationships as an adult. Gathering an understanding of how relationships are initiated and ended will help in understanding the patient's basic method of conflict management. Any history of sexual trauma is noteworthy.

Additional domains that should be looked into include any military history, a history of arrests (the patient or any member of her family), medical hospitalizations as a child or adult, current medical problems other than those under discussion, and medications currently used. The issue of menopause for women in late middle life, automobile accidents in the preceding 5 to 10 years, alcohol or drug abuse by the patient or family members, any history of disability claims or involvement in civil litigation, any recent history of being subjected to investigations, and the nature of current living circumstances and financial status are also areas of inquiry.

Mental status examination A comprehensive mental status examination is always important. A mental status examination should involve some basic description of the patient's physical status and behavior, the nature of speech processes, mood and affect, and cognitive coping resources. Many mental health professionals prefer not to take a patient through a formal mental status examination. This is a mistake. Conducting a routine, formal mental status examination is essential, particularly when medical-legal issues are at play. With regard to evaluating the patient's sensorium, clinical measurement in the following areas is deemed to be essential:

- Level of consciousness
- Orientation
- Memory functions
- Abstract reasoning skills
- Fund of knowledge
- Ability to attend and concentrate
- Comprehension and grasp
- General verbal skill level
- Visual-motor speed and coordination.

At this juncture in the examination it would be pertinent to take the patient through a list of general psychiatric problems and symptoms to elicit whether anything has been left unaddressed. By this method, one can often uncover the presence of some significant psychologic disturbance that had otherwise been undetected, for example, certain phobias or discrete obsessive-compulsive behaviors.

Psychologic testing Testing can most usefully be thought of as a thorough, normative-based, systematic adjunct to the clinical interview and mental status examination. Tests that have been standardized are most useful. They are defined as measures in which the method of administration, procedures for scoring, and interpretive schema have been fixed so that precisely the same tests can be given at different times and places by different professionals. Objective psychologic tests usually offer evidence in accompanying documentation of demonstrable validity and reliability. Additionally, many objective tests offer scores that can be standardized and plotted on a normal distribution. Behavioral observations made during test administration are an essential component in developing a clear understanding of the implication of the test data, particularly in a medical-legal context where secondary gain may be a prominent factor. For example, an acutely angry and dismissive patient who responds to test items in a cursory manner will not produce test scores that should be considered to represent a full effort.

Two basic testing formats are used by clinical psychologists: psychologic and neuropsychologic. Neuropsychologic testing is used to assess the effects of alleged closed-head injuries (with and without loss of consciousness), subdural hematomas, postconcussion syndromes, exposure to neurotoxic substances, and other such problems. General psychologic testing usually involves administering a battery of tests, the purpose of which is to understand an individual's general cognitive, psychologic, and emotional makeup, as well as the effects of any situational factors. At a minimum, such an examination should consist of some measure of cognitive/intellectual functioning, the use of selected measures to assess specific symptoms, an objective personality inventory such as the Minnesota Multiphasic Personality Inventory (MMPI) 2 or the Millon Clinical Multiaxial Inventory (MCMI)-II, self-report measures, and some form of projective testing such as the Rorschach or the Rotter Incomplete Sentences Blank.

The MMPI and MMPI-2 is the most thoroughly researched psychologic instrument available. Because there are a number of useful validity indices and the clinical scales were derived empirically, this test has persuasive clinical power. Extensive literature documents this test's basic effectiveness in evaluating general psychologic and emotional symptoms, as well as somatization and specific issues including the prognosis for a subjectively positive response to medical treatment such as or-

thopedic surgery. The validity indices are extremely useful in enabling the psychologist to detail the specific nature of the patient's response set. The issue of malingering and symptom misrepresentation can also be directly addressed. Scales pertinent to these issues on the MMPI include L, F, K, Ds-R, Sd, Ss, Mp, and the Weiner-Harmon Subtle-Obvious subscales. Validity scales pertinent to the issues on the MMPI-2 include L, F, K, VRIN, TRIN, Fb, and the Lees-Haley Fake Bad Scale (Lees-Haley et al, 1991) for personal injury and workers' compensation claimants. In another article, Lees-Haley (1991) suggested that unusually low ego strength (Es) scores in the context of an absence of severe functional impairment was potentially suggestive of malingering. He recommended a cutoff score of 31. It should be noted that the MMPI-2 has been normed on individuals representing a relatively balanced cross section of American culture. Spanish versions of the MMPI and the MMPI-2 are available. The interpretation of test scores of individuals with backgrounds different from those in the normative sample should be done with caution.

Psychologic testing is an invaluable asset for developing a comprehensive clinical impression of a patient's psychologic and emotional makeup. Testing is particularly useful in delineating a number of areas, including:

- Cognitive coping style and skills
- Characterological style
- Malingering
- Psychiatric diagnosis
- A description of the patient in comparison to the population at large
- Situational versus characterological issues
- Symptomatic and functional change between evaluations
- Permanent and stationary status
- Prognosis including such factors as general verbal skill level, intelligence, abstracting capacity, ability to maintain a task set, degree of impulsivity, frustration tolerance, and other signs of functional difficulties in dealing with problems through adaptive, interpersonal and intrapsychic means
- Ability to make use of rehabilitation.

Psychologic testing, and particularly the MMPI/MMPI-2, can be extremely useful in evaluating chronic pain problems. This is the case when findings are insufficient to support the patient's purported degree of pain and disability, or significant questions are raised as to the patient's ability to subjectively profit from contemplated treatment(s). Wiltse and Rocchio (1975) demonstrated the validity of the MMPI Conversion V for discriminating which patients would have a positive subjective outcome after lumbar surgery. Sorensen (1992) found that among a sample of patients undergoing first lumbar spine surgeries, a number of psychologic test factors were predictive of good or poor outcomes. Elevation on the K scale of the MMPI seemed to be a positive predictor, whereas heightened scores on Hs and Hy predicted poor outcome. The best predictor of poor outcome was an elevation on the admission of symptoms (Ad) scale. This is a subscale of hysteria (scale 3) and has many items in common with the Harris-Lingoes subscales of lassitude-malaise (Hy3) and somatic complaints (Hy4). Sorensen, like many others, found that a conversion V was related to a poor subjective response to surgery. Tollison and Satterthwaite (1990) found that the MMPI aided in determining which patients would be likely to report a positive outcome from lumbar spine surgery. They indicated that the MMPI aided in determining which patients would be helped most by treatment other than surgery, or who would probably best benefit if provided perioperative psychotherapeutic and/or psychopharmacologic services.

Thorveldsen and Sorensen (1990) found that psychologic problems as indicated by the MMPI boded poorly for a positive subjective response to lumbar spine surgery regardless of surgical findings, preoperative general health, age, and gender. Gallagher et al (1989) found that when age and time out of work were controlled variables, physiological status alone was not an adequate predictor of the likelihood that an individual would return to work after developing lumbar pain. They found that psychosocial risk factors, in part evidenced through differential MMPI profiles, were central factors in understanding whether an individual would return to gainful employment. They specifically found that elevation on the MMPI Hy scale, perceived health locus of control, and ability to function in the course of doing daily activities were all important predictive variables for return to work within 6 months. In partial response to the issue of whether elevated MMPI scores reflect cause or effect in chronic pain evaluations, Leavitt and Katz (1989) found that identified positive physical findings alone were insufficient to result in the elevated neurotic scale scores among patients with a diagnosis of fibromyalgia. Milhous et al (1989) found that psychosocial and MMPI factors probably provided a better basis for predicting vocational potential for low back pain patients than did physical findings. They summarized, "Demographic, job-related, compensation and psychologic factors were found to be more impor-

tant than physical factors in predicting ability to return to work" (p. 593).

In a persuasive and comprehensive longitudinal study, Bigos et al (1992) followed 3,020 volunteers at Boeing's Everett, Wa., plant. The purpose was to assess factors that might predispose employees to file a workers' compensation claim alleging lumbar pain. It is noteworthy that the factors with the greatest predictive utility were dissatisfaction with job duties and distress as evidenced by an elevation on scale 3 of the MMPI. Bigos et al reiterated a common assumption that attention to physical factors alone in evaluating a patient with back complaints is not sufficient. The factors that might prompt a patient to report physical complaints might also prompt her to have potential problems in making effective use of provided treatment. The authors concluded that "60-65% of statistically significant factors for predicting acute back injury claims were nonphysical factors" (p. 26). Beyond immediate back pain complaints, the factors that carried the greatest weight for whether an individual would submit a complaint of back injury were job dissatisfaction and "certain psychosocial responses identified on the MMPI" (p. 27).

A number of cautionary comments regarding the use of psychologic tests are germane. Tests should only be used under circumstances that are consonant with standard test administration. A reasonable array of tests should be administered. Testing should be used in the context of a comprehensive clinical interview and mental status examination. Self-report measures should only be used and interpreted with the caution appropriate to the context of the examination. For example, self-report measures such as the Beck Depression Inventory are likely to yield data of limited utility in a medical-legal context. The test was neither developed nor normed with the intent to provide objective, legally unassailable information. Given the nature of the items and the obvious implications of answering in certain directions, measures such as this should only be viewed as reflecting how the patient wishes to be seen, rather than as indicative of actual functional state.

There are a number of common misuses of psychologic tests, particularly in workers' compensation and personal injury settings. It is generally deemed to be inappropriate for psychologists to administer and interpret tests for which they have had limited training. In such a circumstance, the psychologist is vulnerable to overinterpreting or misinterpreting the test results. Occasionally tests are used that are not suited for the context or questions at hand or do not have appropriate validity and reliability for the context in which they are administered.

Psychologists will occasionally fail to account for the context in which the test is administered, or will interpret tests without regard to available norms. For example, a relatively high elevation in one of the validity indices on the MMPI that would suggest significant defensiveness in a general population, has a different meaning in the context of a preemployment evaluation of a relatively educated job applicant. Psychologists will sometimes fail to use an appropriate array of tests or will not reconcile conflicting data. Of particular significance is the fact that the evaluating professional will often fail to evaluate and discuss potential motivational factors that might influence the patient's performance. Psychologists with limited testing experience will often rely on computer-generated interpretive reports of MMPI profiles. This practice is inappropriate, as these reports cannot account for critical contextual variables such as intelligence, implications of the test findings for secondary gain, social and ethnic factors, and immediate adaptational variables such as drug and alcohol usage.

Review of medical records

The evaluating professional should review all pertinent records available for material that clarifies the patient's current functioning and allegations. While these records may not provide telling material, they occasionally enable a clinician to discern a pattern of drug-seeking behavior and other problems that have previously gone unacknowledged and unnoticed. For example, in one legal evaluation, the female patient denied a history of substance abuse. It became apparent by carefully reviewing the records, however, that she was simultaneously receiving substantial prescriptions for vicodin from multiple physicians. In another case, a relatively obscure legal document pointed to the fact that an individual who claimed he was under no duress other than at work was actually under investigation for sexually abusing his child and for becoming involved in long-standing, mounting conflicts with a neighbor, resulting in legal action.

Diagnosis

Clear diagnostic conclusions should be made using Diagnostic and Statistical Manual (DSM) III-R, the current psychiatric diagnostic nomenclature.

Discussion and conclusions

This section of the report should bring together the material from all sources and specifically address the questions raised by the referral source. Where

pertinent, the issues of impairment, causality, disability status, apportionment, and vocational rehabilitation needs should be addressed. Additionally, recommendations with regard to psychiatric treatment should also be detailed.

Only with the extensive database described previously can the process of gathering an understanding of the patient's assets, liabilities, and vulnerabilities be done in a discriminating manner. Consistent with this conclusion are the findings of Schofferman et al (1992). They identified developmental factors that boded poorly for a positive subjective outcome to lumbar spine surgery. These included physical or sexual abuse by a caregiver, alcohol or drug abuse by a primary caregiver, perceived active abandonment by a primary caretaker, and a pattern of emotional neglect and abuse during the patient's formative years. Indices of surgical failure included repeat surgeries except for debridement related to infection; a failure to return to gainful employment within 6 months after laminectomy or 1 year after fusion; magnetic resonance imaging (MRI) or computerized tomography (CT) scans obtained 6 or more months after surgery; epidural steroid or nerve-root injection 6 or more months after surgery; and continued use of opioids 6 or more months after surgery. When only one risk factor was present, 75% of the patients subsequently had none of the described outcome indices. When three of the risk factors were present, only 20% of the patients were deemed to have had a successful outcome. This study provides persuasive evidence that developmental experiences have a substantive impact on an individual's subsequent ability to effectively master physical and psychologic crises.

MALINGERING

Malingering is a term colored by many negative connotations and is often thought of in a simplistic, binary manner. That is, it is often assumed that misrepresentation by a patient of basic history, current functioning, and circumstances is either present or not. In fact, symptom misrepresentation is often complex and can occur at conscious, preconscious, and/or unconscious levels. Additionally, Rogers (1990) has indicated that malingering is a contextual phenomenon and that simple models such as viewing the behavior as being an indication of a criminal background or severe psychopathology are inadequate. He suggested that indices of malingering are developed contextually and empirically.

The form malingering might take can vary depending on a variety of factors. For example, at a pain treatment program in Georgia, Chapman and Brena (1990) compared 17 subjects who had chronic low back pain and demonstrated at least one significant inconsistency in terms of their clinical presentation with 143 other patients who demonstrated no inconsistencies. They found that subjects with inconsistencies had much greater likelihood of being involved in civil litigation, a greater degree of professed pain symptoms and more dramatic complaints, poor compliance with proffered treatment, and lower overall levels of medical findings. These 17 subjects also reported a much lower level of general physical activity and did not profit as well from treatments offered. Chapman and Brenna noted that many of these patients' characteristics were consistent with those often described among individuals who are believed to be malingering, but the form was subtly different. They suggested that particularly careful assessment of self-report data and measures from patients with such characteristics was indicated.

It is our impression that pure form conscious symptom fabrication and misrepresentation in the context of a workers' compensation examination is relatively rare since the potential rewards are not particularly high. It is much more common to see such a process in a personal injury case. Most often, misrepresentation in a workers' compensation case is based on preconscious factors; that is, the patient convinces herself in the moment that what is being said is the truth, but on some level the claimant is aware that there is some degree of distortion at play. It should be noted that many individuals with pure form conscious misrepresentation are intelligent and extremely difficult to detect. Most other individuals who amplify, dramatize, and exaggerate their symptoms to some degree are often less sophisticated and make errors in their presentation that reveal the preconscious distortion factor.

Misrepresentation of clinical material often seems to involve the equivalent of the Catholic sins of commission and omission. Distortion involving commission includes the conscious reporting of problems, events, symptoms, and other such things that have not occurred or are functionally of less significance than the patient has portrayed. Distortions of omission involve withholding of important material despite direct inquiry into an area by the examiner or failing to offer salient information when it has not been specifically requested but would be clearly germane to the issues at hand. An example of the former of these two omission possibilities is the adamant denial of a history of arrests, when in fact there is a record of detainment, conviction, and jail time. An example of the latter of these two possibilities involves not mentioning that one is under investigation for sexual abuse of one's child when this is clearly a non-

industrial source of stress, but the examiner did not specifically ask about such matters. It is probably most commonly the case that where misrepresentation of clinical material occurs, it represents a partial, rather than full, explanatory basis for the claimant's current presentation. The physician should still attempt to rule out any medical pathologic condition or disease.

A number of data sources are useful in making a determination about the issues of conscious misrepresentation or embellishment. These include discrepancies within the clinical data obtained from a claimant; discrepancies between clinical data and material obtained from behavioral observation on mental status examination; and discrepancies between clinical data and the material in the medical and other records. Additionally, of particular utility in evaluating the issue of malingering or symptom embellishment is the MMPI/MMPI-2. These tests have a wealth of what have been termed validity scales that enable the examiner in a statistically based manner to describe the response set of the claimant. If the patient's MMPI profile is deemed to be internally consistent and reflective of a systematic style of responding, the other validity indices can be of great utility. These scales have been described previously. They offer substantial, objective data and will moderate or reinforce the health professional's clinical impressions.

Test data and clinical material can conversely be used to help buttress a conclusion that a patient's representation of work-related stress is valid. When an individual's stated symptoms are consistent with demonstrable stressors, her character structure, and the normal course of the identified disorder(s), test data suggesting a lack of preconscious and/or conscious embellishment and misrepresentation can be assuring.

EVALUATION OF SUICIDE AND VIOLENCE POTENTIAL
Homicide evaluation

In the midst of a seemingly routine evaluation of a patient complaining of harassment on the job, a medical colleague became increasingly concerned and distressed as the patient's level of anger and agitation escalated, and vague allusions were made to "shutting up" his supervisor "for good." Not knowing how to assess the patient's vulnerability to violent action, the physician began to believe that he was losing control of the evaluation.

Patients seen in a clinical setting for medical and/or psychiatric evaluation of complaints of occupational injury at times present with an appearance of potential precarious impulse control. Although violent impulses, whether expressed toward others or oneself, are infrequently carried over into direct action, homicide is one of the leading causes of death in the workplace. The expression, or appearance, of impending dyscontrol must be taken seriously and evaluated carefully. Listed below are the most salient factors in evaluating an individual's potential to act violently toward others. It is readily apparent that such an evaluation requires taking an in-depth history as described previously. The factors are as follows:

1. History of violent or impulsive behavior. Note the type and nature of impulsive aggression, the age of onset and last episode, and the objects of the aggressive impulses. This is generally considered the best predictive variable.
2. Life experiences that have created considerable resentment and bitterness.
3. Frequent quarrels with family members or other significant individuals in the patient's life.
4. Association with significant figures who have a history of violent behavior, particularly if these individuals are viewed positively.
5. An absence of gratifying, culturally-acceptable sources of self-esteem. This can result in a negative self-image and increases the likelihood of feelings of futility and lessened consequences to violent actions.
6. An interest in, and possession of, weapons.
7. Violent fantasies and daydreams, particularly ones that contain intense, negative affects.
8. A history of drug or alcohol abuse, particularly if it is recent. Substances promote disinhibition.
9. The degree of agitation.
10. Concreteness of plan.
11. A family pattern of substantial parental hostility, overt violence, and/or sexual provocativeness.
12. A constellation of childhood behaviors and symptoms that have been correlated with violence and include temper tantrums, hyperactivity, persisting stuttering, holding of breath, and other such behaviors.
13. A childhood history of pyromania, cruelty to animals, and enuresis.
14. Noteworthy findings on the mental status examination such as acute anxiety; expressed fear of loss of control; markedly ambivalent feelings toward people in the patient's environment; and undisguised, straightforward hatred and anger.
15. Impaired reality testing.

16. The quality of the patient's overall life circumstances including the availability of realistic avenues and methods for addressing perceived problems.

In general, the assessment of the violence potential of a patient depends on the history of violent behavior, the type of violent behavior contemplated or enacted, and the degree of control that the patient manifests, verbally and physically, during the interview. As well, the clinician should be attentive to the presence of psychiatric conditions that may serve to potentiate the vulnerability to aggressive impulse dyscontrol. A brief list of such conditions would include the following:

1. Schizophrenia, especially paranoid type.
2. Delusional disorders.
3. Acute delirium resulting from psychotomimetic or alcohol abuse.
4. Intermittent explosive disorder.
5. Temporal lobe epilepsy.
6. Antisocial personality disorder.
7. Bipolar disorder, manic type.
8. Organic states involving lesions to the limbic system or frontal lobes.
9. Socially maladjusted individuals without manifest, Axis I psychiatric disorders, but who evidence a history of recurrent impulsive, aggressive solutions to emotional conflicts.

A number of factors are considered to increase the likelihood of triggering an aggressive outburst by an agitated, threatening patient. These include bluntly refusing a patient's demands, attempting to force things on the patient, and setting either too many or too few limits. Handling the threatening patient requires a relative comfort with the climate of aroused aggressiveness and fluid responsiveness to the patient's immediate circumstances and demands. With regard to the management of the potentially violent patient in an office setting, a number of recommendations can be made. These include the following:

1. Do not make the patient wait. Even though the individual may have been preceded by several other patients, he or she should be seen quickly if there appears to be only precarious control over threatened aggressive impulses. Occasionally only a brief, preliminary meeting is required before the patient is able to wait for her appropriate turn. At other times the realities of the circumstance require that the evaluation and possible treatment of such an individual take priority over others in the waiting room. Forcing such an individual to wait without acknowl-

edgment and contact can often result in mounting anxiety, irritation, and agitation. It can unwittingly convey a message of disregard and seemingly recapitulate a general feeling that her concerns are not being heard.

2. Avoid responding to irritation or threatened aggressiveness with aggression of one's own, verbally or physically. Provocativeness significantly increases the likelihood that such individuals will express their aggression openly. Similarly, overtly expressed fear, anxiety, apprehensiveness, or other such emotions can also trigger an aggressive response in an individual who feels that she has gained the upper hand. As much as possible, the clinician needs to manifest a calm, benignly confident and nonadversarial exterior.

3. Efforts at controlling the patient and the behavior must be neutral and require acknowledging that the patient is clearly upset, irritated, and, if true, concerned about a loss of control.

4. Security personnel, whether private security officers or local peace officers, should be alerted by office staff as soon as possible with regard to the possibility of violence in the office. It is recommended that the involvement of such individuals be titrated to meet the needs of the circumstances. For example, when faced with an individual who may potentially lose control of aggressive impulses, but who does not appear to be in necessarily imminent danger of doing so, security or law enforcement officers might be asked to wait in a room off the waiting room while the evaluation continues. It is rarely helpful or useful for security personnel to burst into the office. Such behavior is most likely to potentiate a frightened, aggressive response on the part of the patient.

5. Where the interview of the patient is conducted depends on the assessment of the immediate vulnerability to a loss of control. If such a loss of control appears to be potentially imminent, coordinated activity on the part of staff can be helpful. While one member of the staff quietly ushers other people in the waiting room outside, the physician should engage the patient in preliminary discussion. Whether that takes place in the waiting room or in the office is dependent on the physician's basic sense of the patient's degree of impulse control and on concerns about safety issues.

6. In general, it is best if the individual evaluating the patient does not position himself or herself between the patient and an exit from the interview room. Many patients in such circumstances can feel increasingly agitated and apprehensive if they sense they cannot readily leave should they wish to do so.

7. It is occasionally appropriate to acknowledge, while managing, one's anxiety and provoked irritation if it is under reasonable control. This should be done in a neutral manner and not impulsively in response to aroused internal feelings. The effective management of one's own aroused emotions serves as a model that the patient can potentially use to help moderate her own internal feelings.

8. It is usually inappropriate to actively oppose or confront a patient's paranoid or angry beliefs. Usually the clinician does not have sufficient information to accurately contest such assertions.

9. In general, it is useful to encourage verbalization. It is always preferable for the patient to express violent fantasies verbally rather than act on them physically. In talking with the patient, it is important to convey a continuing professional interest in understanding the patient's concerns and a willingness to help address them in a reasonable manner. One can acknowledge the feelings evidenced by the patient without necessarily rebutting or concurring with their perceived causal basis. For example, one could state to an employee who is expressing violent fantasies about harming a manager, "I can see that you are extremely angry by what seems like very prejudicial behavior by Mr. North. If you will tell me all about what has gone on at work, perhaps we can find a way to help you effectively deal with the difficulties you have been having." Through the embedded use of the phrase "seems like," the physician acknowledges the patient's experience while keeping his own assessment in what we would call the "tentative mode." The physician is neither refuting nor accepting the patient's perspective but remains interested in gathering more information to generate an accurate understanding of the perceived problem.

10. When control of impulses appears precarious, a patient should be offered medications and told that they will help her control herself. The implicit message is that the patient is expected to control her own behavior with your help. Medications that potentially

could be of help under such circumstances include anxiolytics such as diazpam, chlordiazepoxide, or Restoril, as well as high-potency neuroleptics such as haloperidol. The specifics of the acute pharmacologic management of the potentially violent patient are beyond the scope of this chapter. The interested reader should consult knowledgeable colleagues or any of the numerous texts on managing psychiatric emergencies.

Although being confronted with the potentially explosive, aggressive patient is not a common part of office practice, nonetheless, it is worthwhile for the physician to have a plan for the management of such circumstances laid out in some detail with staff. For example, one or more individuals should be designated as the primary person(s) to intervene with the patient, another person should be designated to contact security or law enforcement officers as needed, and other staff members should be prepared to manage and provide for the safety of other patients currently in the facility. As indicated previously, most patients who present with threatened aggressive impulse dyscontrol rarely go on to act violently. The majority of them gain sufficient gratification from the verbal expression of their violent fantasies and the perceived, often pronounced upheaval that it causes in others. The direct expression of violent behavior, with all of the attendant consequences, does not occur.

When the risk of impulse dyscontrol is acute, most offices are ill-equipped to handle the problem effectively, and security or law enforcement officers should be involved immediately. Again, if procedures are in place for invoking the use of such professionals, the intervention will occur more smoothly.

Suicide evaluation

Evaluation of the potentially suicidal patient involves a somewhat similar set of criteria. The evaluation should include gathering data in the following domains, all of which affect the assessment of the probability of suicidal behavior:

1. A history of prior attempts, including their number and lethality. Hospitalizations in the past in an intensive care unit setting because of suicide attempts have ominous implications. On the other hand, many individuals with borderline personality disorders make repeated suicide gestures as a relatively routinized manner of engaging with their environment. Nonetheless, a history of gestures should not be trivialized or taken lightly. Weisman and Worden (1972) developed a model in which they rated suicidal behavior in terms of risk and rescue factors. Risk factors include the type of agent used, degree of resulting impairment of consciousness, degree of lesions and toxicity, reversibility of effects, and treatment required. Rescue factors include the location of the suicide attempt (familiar or remote), the person who initiated the rescue (a key person or a passer-by), the probability of discovery by any rescuer, the accessibility to rescue (ranging from actively asking for help before the attempt to not leaving any clue), and the duration of delay until discovery. Obviously, individuals with attempts that have involved a high degree of risk and a low degree of probability of rescue warrant careful, further evaluation.

2. Presence and extent of current ideation.

3. Concreteness of plan.

4. Availability of professed means.

5. Degree of depression. The presence of symptoms of major depression with associated anhedonia worsen the prognosis. The individual's pattern of sleep should be assessed. Significant sleep deprivation adversely affects a great array of general psychologic and cognitive coping resources, and heightens the likelihood of impulsive behavior.

6. Degree of impulsivity, both at the present time and by history.

7. Degree of current agitation.

8. Abuse of alcohol and other drugs.

9. Reality situation—the viability of current or prospective life circumstances.

10. Adequacy of the patient's social network.

11. Medical status. The presence of life-threatening illnesses can increase the suicide risk among individuals with a number of other critical factors.

12. Family history of suicide, and particularly the approaching anniversaries of any suicidal acts by such others.

13. Degree of involvement with friends, spouse (if any), and family. The presence of dependent children towards whom the patient experiences a significant sense of responsibility and meaning lessens the likelihood of suicidal behavior.

14. The particular meaning of death to the individual. Those who view death as endless sleep have a higher greater potential risk factor than those who view themselves as likely to be consigned to hell for taking their own lives.

15. The availability of significant others to observe the patient before the next planned visit.

16. Reality testing. Individuals who are delusionally depressed or who are experiencing command hallucinations to commit suicide represent a significantly heightened risk.

A number of demographic variables are considered to be important in the evaluation of suicide risk. These include the following:

1. Age. Suicide risk increases as people enter middle and later life.
2. Gender. Males are at higher risk than females.
3. Family status. Individuals who are separated, divorced, widowed, or isolated from family have an increased risk.
4. Race. Caucasians and Native Americans have a higher risk of suicide.
5. Profession. Individuals in competitive or highly personally demanding jobs have a somewhat increased risk.
6. Employment. Lack of employment results in increased risk.
7. Health. Poor health, chronic depression, or substance abuse increase the risk level.
8. Living arrangements. Individuals on the West Coast and who are transient have an increased risk. Living alone increases the level of risk.

Additional potentiating variables for the risk of suicidal behavior include a history of negative therapeutic relationships, recent or threatened loss, social disgrace, or loss of existing reasons to live. The presence of hopeless resignation, anhedonia, a history of high-in-risk and low-in-rescue factors, and an absence of any developed rapport across the course of the interview, bode ominously. Particularly noteworthy in the examination is whether an individual has undertaken a process of giving away personal possessions. This is often an ominous sign.

In general, the assessment of both suicide and violence potential is a complex, multifactorial process. Ultimate prognostic conclusions must be drawn by weighting the various factors. In general, the clinician should opt to take a conservative impression with regard to conclusions drawn.

The effective evaluation of suicide risk is contingent on conducting a thorough clinical examination of the patient. The prognostic factors described previously, as well as the broader backdrop of the patient's life, warrant exploration. At some point in the interview, it is worth asking the patient, "What makes your life worth living?" Any fantasies about death should be inquired into in some detail. Factors that might worry the physician would be descriptions of death as rest and sleep, peace at last, or a reunion with lost loved ones. The physician should function as an empathetic listener. The aim is not to specifically instill some reason for living, or hope, but rather to hear out the patient's feelings and beliefs and to make a professional judgment as to whether other professional resources, such as a psychiatrist or psychologist, or inpatient psychiatric hospitalization, are required.

With regard to the evaluation of violence or suicide potential in the office setting, it is important that the physician obtain consultation from a knowledgeable psychiatrist or psychologist once an initial impression has been developed. To minimize the likelihood that the referral process will fail, it would be important for the physician to indicate that she intends to remain involved but wishes to get outside expertise to augment her understanding of the patient's concerns and fears. If both suicidal and homicidal impulses represent a form of psychiatric emergency, the physician should have available the names of a number of professionals who could see the patient on relatively short notice. If an early appointment cannot be arranged, the patient should be referred to available psychiatric emergency services. Such services should be routinely used when the patient requires involuntary detainment and a direct admission to a psychiatric unit cannot be arranged, either for logistic or insurance reasons. Although procedures vary by city, county, and state, in most instances law enforcement officers are authorized to involuntarily detain an individual and take him to a psychiatric emergency service. Such a solution is a measure of last resort as it usually has a significantly damaging effect on the working relationship between the patient and physician.

SUMMARY

The evaluation of the injured worker is often an extremely difficult and complex matter given the numerous factors that are usually at play including the specific physical or psychologic injury, the contextual meaning of the injury in terms of the patient's job satisfaction and formative experiences, and the presence of primary and secondary gain variables. Only through a comprehensive evaluation as has been described previously can the clinician adequately respond to issues regarding differential diagnosis, causality, the possibility of malingering, apportionment, capacity to make use of any offered vocational rehabilitation, and long-term prognosis. When the initial presenting complaint is strictly physical and the patient does not respond to proffered treatments in a clinically reasonable timeframe, more careful screening for somatization and/or malingering is recommended. Toward this end, the treating physician should develop working consultative relationships with psychologists and psychiatrists who are knowledgeable about the special issues raised in medical-legal evaluations and treatment.

REFERENCES

Barnes D et al: Psychosocioeconomic predictors of treatment success/failure in chronic low back pain patients, *Spine* 14(4):427-30, 1989.

Becker GE and Smith RB: Psychological factors in back pain, In Kirkaldy-Willis WH and Burton CV, editors: *Managing low back pain,* New York, 1992, Churchill Livingstone.

Bigos SJ et al: A longitudinal, prospective study of industrial back injury reporting, *Clinical Orthopedics* 279:21-34, 1992.

Bigos SJ et al: A prospective study of work perceptions and psychosocial factors affecting the report of back injury, *Spine* 16(1):1-6, 1991.

Cannon WB: *The wisdom of the body,* New York, 1936, Norton.

Caplan G: Mastery of stress: psychosocial aspects, *The American Journal of Psychiatry* 138(4):413-420, 1981.

Chapman SL and Brena SF: Patterns of conscious failure to provide accurate self-report data in patients with low back pain, Clin J Pain 6(3):178-90, 1990.

Chess S and Thomas A: *Temperament in clinical practice,* New York, 1986, The Guilford Press.

Erikson E: *Childhood and society.* New York, 1963, Norton.

Gallagher RM et al: Determinants of return-to-work among low back pain patients, *Pain* 39:55-67, 1989.

Karasu TB and Bellak L: *Specialized techniques in individual psychotherapy,* New York, 1980, Brunner/Mazel.

Kinder BN and Curtiss G: Alexithymia among empirically derived subgroups of chronic back pain patients, *Journal of personality assessment* 54(1&2):351-362, 1990.

Leavitt F and Katz RS: Is the MMPI invalid for assessing psychological disturbance in pain-related organic conditions? *Journal of Rheumatology* 16(4):521-26, 1989.

Lees-Haley PR: Ego strength denial on the MMPI-2 as a clue to the simulation of personal injury and vocational neuropsychological and emotional distress evaluations, *Perceptual Motor Skills* 72(3):815-9, 1991.

Lees-Haley PR et al: A fake bad scale on the MMPI-2 for personal injury claimants, *Psychological Reports* 68, 203-210, 1991.

Lipowski ZJ: Somatization: the concept and its clinical application, *Am. J. Psychiatry,* 145(11):1358-1368, 1988.

MacKinnon RA and Michels R: *The psychiatric interview in clinical practice,* Philadelphia, 1971, WB Saunders Company.

Milhous RL et al: Determinants of vocational disability in patients with low back pain, *Arc Phys Med Rehabil* 70:589-93, 1989.

Rogers R: Development of a new classificatory model of malingering, *Bulletin, American Academy of Psychiatry and the Law* 18(3):323-33, 1990.

Rosenbaum CP and Beebe JE: *Psychiatric treatment: crisis/clinic/consultation,* New York, 1975, McGraw-Hill Book Company.

Schofferman J et al: Childhood psychological trauma correlates with unsuccessful lumbar spine surgery, *Spine* 17(6 Suppl):S138-44, 1992.

Selye H: *The stress of life,* McGraw-Hill, 1956, New York.

Sifneos P: The prevalence of alexithymic characteristics in psychosomatic patients, *Psychother Psychosom* 22:255, 1973.

Sorensen LV: Pre-operative psychological testing with the MMPI at first operation for prolapsed lumbar disk, *Danish Medical Bulletin* 39(2):186-190, 1992.

Thorveldsen P and Srensen EB: Psychological vulnerability as a predictor for short-term outcome in lumbar spine surgery. a prospective study, *Acta Neurochir* 102(1-2):58-61, 1990.

Tollison CD and Satterthwaite JR: Multiple spine surgical failures. The value of adjunctive psychological assessment, *Orthopedic Review* 19(12):1073-7, 1990.

Vaillant GE: *Adaptation to life,* Boston, 1977, Little, Brown & Company.

Waddell G et al: Non-organic physical signs in low back pain, *Spine* 5:117-X, 1980.

Wiltse L and Rocchio P: Pre-operative psychological tests as predictors of success of chemonucleolysis in the treatment of low back syndrome, *Journal of Bone and Joint Surgery* 57:478, 1975.

SECTION IV

PREVENTION AND CONTROL

33 Medicine and Safety Resources for the Physician Treating Occupationally Injured Workers

The proper treatment and care of an injured worker often requires the physician to obtain information about how and what caused the injury. Usually this information is obtained directly from the injured worker. If the worker has been exposed to some unknown chemical or physical agent, however, an industrial hygienist or safety professional should be consulted. These professionals can also measure exposure levels, evaluate routes of exposure, implement personal protective equipment programs, and design engineering controls.

The purpose of this chapter is to give the physician who evaluates and treats an occupationally exposed worker resources that will provide valuable information to use in managing the patient's exposure.

OCCUPATIONAL INJURIES

Today's workplace contains a wide range of potentially dangerous physical and chemical agents. As industry has grown in size and complexity so have the number and types of chemical, biological, and physical agents that can cause injury. Chemical agents include literally thousands of compounds. The toxicity of some of these chemicals and the levels of exposure that affect workers' health are relatively well known. But the toxicity of numerous other chemicals used in industry is not well understood. In the last 15 years the use and development of biologic agents has presented an even wider opportunity for adverse effect on a worker's health.

Along with chemical hazards, physical agents including noise, lasers, and ionizing and nonionizing radiation can injure workers. Finally, mechanical hazards such as rotating equipment and fire hazards can also cause injury.

Diagnosis and treatment

With this assortment of potential injury-causing agents, the attending physician may need additional technical and environmental information to diagnose and treat the injured worker. Two main groups of nonmedical professionals can aid the physician with occupational injuries: safety professionals and industrial hygienists. The safety professional (the historical term is safety engineer) is trained in a range of disciplines that deal with accident prevention and loss control. The industrial hygienist focuses on health protection by identifying agents in the workplace that are harmful to health, measuring exposures, and preventing and controlling exposure to these agents.

The physician can use a safety professional or industrial hygienist to evaluate the workplace to provide information necessary for diagnosis and treatment, and to prevent injuries from recurring. The safety professional or industrial hygienist can evaluate complicated mechanical and chemical manufacturing processes, obtain environmental samples, and interpret results, thereby supplying the physician with important information.

In the following types of injuries the physician often works with a safety/industrial hygiene professional.

Chemical exposures. The physician needs to know what chemical(s) the worker was exposed to and an estimate of the amount of exposure. It is critical to the treatment of the worker that this information be obtained quickly. Follow-up work should include recommendations for preventing future exposures by engineering controls and the use of proper personal protective equipment (see Chapter 25).

Indoor air quality. The recent increase in health problems related to indoor air quality (sick building syndrome) has presented the physician with cases that are difficult to diagnose and treat. An experienced safety/industrial hygiene professional can help identify possible causes and solutions for indoor air quality problems (see Chapter 23).

Musculoskeletal complaints. A safety or industrial hygiene professional can analyze worksites and make recommendations about work habits and conditions to prevent repetitive trauma cases such as carpal tunnel syndrome (see Chapter 22).

Hearing loss. The diagnosis of hearing loss caused by high noise levels requires the involvement of a safety or industrial hygiene professional to measure exposure levels and recommend engineering control or personal protective equipment to reduce noise exposure (see Chapter 27).

If the physician treating an occupational injury does not have adequate information for diagnosis and treatment, the physician should contact the employer of the injured worker and ask for the safety officer. The Occupational Safety and Health Administration (OSHA) safety regulations require most companies to have a safety officer who is responsible for the safety program. This officer is required to have information on the chemicals used in each department.

It is important to note that safety officers for small and medium-sized companies are often not trained safety or health professionals. The safety officer in these companies is often a production or staff supervisor/manager who has been given the safety officer responsibility as an addition to his other job. The level of technical information available will vary from company to company. In larger companies, the safety officer is often a trained safety or industrial hygiene professional and should be qualified to provide valuable and accurate information about how a worker was injured. If the safety officer is unable to provide the needed information and support, a number of other resources are available to the physician.

SAFETY AND INDUSTRIAL HYGIENE RESOURCES

Both the safety professional and the industrial hygienist have national organizations with local chapters. The American Society of Safety Engineers* is the largest national safety organization. The American Industrial Hygiene Association* and the American Conference of Governmental Industrial Hygienists* are the two established industrial hygiene organizations.

The safety professional and the industrial hygienist often have a good understanding of industrial manufacturing and research processes and procedures. They are familiar with how to investigate accidents and identify what caused the injury. Industrial hygienists have the equipment and knowledge to measure exposures to chemical and physical hazards and can make recommendations on how to prevent future exposures.

---

*See Appendix A.

Certified safety professional (CSP)

The Board of Certified Safety Professionals* defines a Certified Safety Professional (CSP) as

someone who has met the academic, experience and examination requirements for certification established by the Board of Certified Safety Professionals, as they apply to the prevention or mitigation of accidents and other harmful exposures and personal injury/disease, property damage, and economic loss that may ensue. The CSP uses a knowledge of engineering and the various human and physical sciences in the development of procedures, processes, specifications, and systems to achieve optimal control and reduction of hazards and exposures detrimental to life, health and property.

Under current requirements for the CSP certification an applicant must have:

1. Graduated from college or university with an accredited baccalaureate degree in safety
2. Four or more years of professional safety experience acceptable to the Board of Certified Safety Professionals
3. Achievement of passing scores on each of the two written examinations

Certified industrial hygienist (CIH)

The American Board of Industrial Hygiene defines industrial hygiene as follows:

Industrial hygiene primarily involves: (1) the recognition of environmental factors and stresses associated with work and work operations and the understanding of their effects on man and his well-being in the workplace and the community; (2) the evaluation, through training and experience, and with the aid of quantitative measurement techniques, of the magnitude of these factors and stresses in terms of ability to impair man's health and well-being; and (3) the prescription of methods to control or reduce such factors and stresses when necessary to alleviate their effects.

Under current requirements the American Board of Industrial Hygiene* requires that an applicant for CIH certification must have:

1. Graduation from college or university with a bachelors degree in industrial hygiene, chemistry, physics, chemical, mechanical or sanitary engineering or biology
2. Five years of full-time employment in the professional practice of industrial hygiene
3. Achievement of passing scores on each of the two written examinations

Toxicologist and health physicist

In addition to safety professionals and industrial hygienists, two other professional groups may be of assistance to a physician treating an injured worker. The toxicologist can provide valuable assistance in cases of exposure to a toxic chemical, and the health physicist can be of assistance when dealing with ionizing and nonionizing radiation exposures. The Society of Toxicology* and the Health Physics Society* are the organizations to be contacted if the assistance of these two disciplines are required.

GOVERNMENT RESOURCES

Several government agencies can help when dealing with occupational injuries. The Occupational Safety and Health Administration (OSHA) is the main government agency responsible for safety and occupational health protection in the workplace. About half of the states have their own OSHA programs. These agencies can answer questions about compliance with regulations.

The National Institute for Safety and Health (NIOSH) carries out field investigations, conducts safety and health research, and develops new safety and health standards.

Federal OSHA programs

There are 10 federal OSHA regional offices* that can provide assistance and information. OSHA responds to complaints and will carry out site inspections and investigations. Citations can be issued when violations are found. The OSHA regional and area offices can provide a wide range of technical information about specific safety and health topics. Copies of individual OSHA regulations can also be obtained from these offices. A list of the regional offices including addresses and telephone numbers can be found in Appendix A.

State OSHA programs

About half of the states have their own OSHA programs that have been approved and are monitored by the federal OSHA. The state programs publish their own safety and health standards and have their own enforcement staff. State programs must have standards that are identical to, or at least are as effective as, the federal standards. Some state programs include a consultation branch that answers questions and will make site inspections without involvement of the enforcement branches. The location of the state OSHA programs can be found by calling the nearest federal regional office.

National Institute for Safety and Health

The National Institute For Safety and Health (NIOSH) is the federal government's research and standards development organization. This organization completes field studies and research in support of proposed safety and health regulations and publishes a wide range of health and safety information. Lists of NIOSH publications can be obtained by calling (800) 35-NIOSH.

OTHER RESOURCES FOR THE PHYSICIAN

If the physician is not able to obtain the safety and industrial hygiene support needed from the company safety officer, there are at least two other sources: workers' compensation insurance carriers and consultants.

Most workers' compensation insurance carriers have safety and industrial hygiene departments. The physician can contact the injured employee's workers' compensation insurance carrier and have an appropriate safety or industrial hygiene person investigate the injury.

Consultants are often called to investigate accidents that involve worker injuries and illnesses. Companies as well as insurance carriers call on outside consultants to evaluate worker injuries both to determine compensation and to prevent future accidents. Physicians can also request that a safety or industrial hygiene consultant be brought in by the company or by the insurance carrier to assist the treating physician.

The American Industrial Hygiene Association publishes semiannually a list of industrial hygiene consultants. A copy of the current list can be obtained by contacting the AIHA (see Appendix A). The American Society of Safety Engineers also publishes a list of safety consultants. A copy of this list can be obtained by contacting the ASSE (see Appendix A). There is a charge for the ASSE list.

PRODUCT HEALTH AND SAFETY INFORMATION AND DOCUMENTATION

A number of sources for information about specific products are helpful to a physician managing an occupational injury.

Material safety data sheets (MSDS)

Several questions face a physician treating a patient exposed to a chemical substance. The physician must identify the specific chemical(s), know the toxicity, and assess how much exposure the worker received.

Brand names and labels often do not provide enough information. When a worker is admitted to the emergency room with serious respiratory problems from exposure to a paint remover, for example, the brand name of the remover should be

---

*See Appendix A.

MATERIAL SAFETY DATA SHEET

I PRODUCT IDENTIFICATION

MANUFACTURER'S NAME	REGULAR TELEPHONE NO. EMERGENCY TELELPHONE NO.
ADDRESS	
TRADE NAME	
SYNONYMS	

II HAZARDOUS INGREDIENTS

MATERIAL OR COMPONENT	%	HAZARD DATA

III PHYSICAL DATA

BOILING POINT, 760 MM HG		MELTING POINT
SPECIFIC GRAVITY (H_2O = 1)		VAPOR PRESSURE
VAPOR DENSITY (AIR = 1)		SOLUBILITY IN H_2O, % BY WT
% VOLATILES BY VOL		EVAPORATION RATE (BUTYL ACETATE = 1)
APPEARANCE AND ODOR		

Fig. 33-1 Sample material safety data sheet form.

identified. The worker's company should be contacted for the material safety data sheet (MSDS) for the specific brand of paint remover. Ideally the MSDS accompanies the worker to the physician's office or emergency room at the time of injury.

Under OSHA regulations all manufacturers of chemical products are required to supply an MSDS to all purchasers of their products. The sheets are required to cover the following topics:

Section 1. Product identification
The trade name, common name, and scientific name including CAS number as well as the manufacturer's name, address, and telephone number.

Section 2. Hazardous ingredients
The chemicals present in the product and the concentration of each chemical is required. Information about the toxicity and other hazards should be identified. If a permissible exposure level (PEL) has been established, it is to be identified.

Section 3. Physical data
Data, including boiling point, vapor density, pH, percentage volatility, and other physical data are listed.

Section 4. Fire and explosion data
The flammability and the conditions under which the substance will explode are included.

Section 5. Health hazard information
Overexposure symptoms, first aid, and additional treatment procedures are to be presented.

IV FIRE AND EXPLOSION DATA					
FLASH POINT (TEST METHOD)			AUTOIGNITION TEMPERATURE		
FLAMMABLE LIMITS IN AIR, % BY VOL		LOWER		UPPER	
EXTINGUISHING MEDIA					
SPECIAL FIRE FIGHTING PROCEDURES					
UNUSUAL FIRE AND EXPLOSION HAZARD					

V HEALTH HAZARD INFORMATION
HEALTH HAZARD DATA
ROUTES OF EXPOSURE
INHALATION
SKIN CONTACT
SKIN ABSORPTION
EYE CONTACT
INGESTION
EFFECTS OF OVEREXPOSURE
ACUTE OVEREXPOSURE
CHRONIC OVEREXPOSURE
EMERGENCY AND FIRST AID PROCEDURES
EYES:
SKIN:
INHALATION:
INGESTION:
NOTES TO PHYSICIAN

Continued

Section 6. Reactivity data

Chemicals that react adversely with the product are listed.

Section 7. Spill, leak and disposal procedures

Environmental protection procedures are identified.

Section 8. Special protection information

Personal protective equipment including the proper respirators, gloves, and appropriate body protection are listed. Engineering controls, such as local exhaust ventilation systems, are recommended.

Section 9. Special precautions

Special labeling requirements or additional health and safety information can be listed.

The most important information to the physician treating a worker exposed to a chemical is found in sections I, II, and V. An example MSDS can be found in Figure 33-1.

The amount and accuracy of information on a data sheet varies considerably depending on the manufacturer. A great deal of information is known about large-volume commodity chemicals, for example, although little is often known about small-volume research chemicals. MSDSs for these compounds often provide minimal information.

The regional Poison Control Centers or Chemtrex (800) 424-9300 can provide toxicology information if the MSDS is not available or is inadequate. Both are available 24 hours a day.

VI REACTIVITY DATA
CONDITIONS CONTRIBUTING TO INSTABILITY
INCOMPATIBILITY
HAZARDOUS DECOMPOSITION PRODUCTS
CONDITIONS CONTRIBUTING TO HAZARDOUS POLYMERIZATION

VII SPILL OR LEAK PROCEDURES
STEPS TO BE TAKEN IF MATERIAL IS RELEASED OR SPILLED
NEUTRALIZING CHEMICALS
WASTE DISPOSAL METHOD

VIII SPECIAL PROTECTION INFORMATION
VENTILATION REQUIREMENTS
SPECIFIC PERSONAL PROTECTIVE EQUIPMENT   RESPIRATORY (SPECIFY IN DETAIL)
EYE
GLOVES
OTHER CLOTHING AND EQUIPMENT

Chemical exposure limits

The physician needs to know the extent to which the patient was exposed to a toxic chemical, particularly when exposure has been chronic. The industrial hygienist can measure worker exposure and report the levels to the physician.

Different chemicals require different air-sampling techniques. Absorption tubes, filter cassettes, and impingers are examples of collection media used for air sampling. The collection media is attached by a plastic tube to small battery-operated pumps attached to the worker's belt. The sample is collected in the worker's breathing zone to obtain a representative sample. The collection medium is then sent to a laboratory for analysis. The laboratory results are used to calculate exposure levels. The exposure levels can then be compared with OSHA's permissible exposure limits (PEL). The correct sampling method for a given chemical should be selected by an experienced industrial hygienist.

The PELs have been established by OSHA as safe levels of exposure for an 8-hour workday. The limits are usually listed in parts per million of the chemical in air or milligrams per cubic meter of air. The physician should use these numbers as guides in assessing health protection. It is important for the physician to keep updated on exposure

```
┌─────────────────────────────────────────────────────────────┐
│                    IX SPECIAL PRECAUTIONS                     │
├─────────────────────────────────────────────────────────────┤
│ PRECAUTIONARY                                                 │
│ STATEMENTS                                                    │
│                                                               │
│                                                               │
│                                                               │
│                                                               │
│                                                               │
│                                                               │
│                                                               │
├─────────────────────────────────────────────────────────────┤
│ OTHER HANDLING AND                                            │
│ STORAGE REQUIREMENTS                                          │
│                                                               │
│                                                               │
│                                                               │
│                                                               │
│                                                               │
├─────────────────────────────────────────────────────────────┤
│ PREPARED BY:                                                  │
├─────────────────────────────────────────────────────────────┤
│ ADDRESS:                                                      │
├─────────────────────────────────────────────────────────────┤
│ DATE:                                                         │
└─────────────────────────────────────────────────────────────┘
```

levels because the numbers are continually being lowered as more information is learned about the toxicity of individual chemicals. Presently, there is much debate as to whether these numbers are too high for long-term protection of all workers.

A list of PELs can be found in federal and state OSHA regulations. Copies can be obtained by contacting the nearest Federal or State OSHA office (see Appendix A).

The present OSHA PELs are copied from the threshold limit values (TLV) published by the American Conference of Governmental Industrial Hygienists. This group is careful to point out that the threshold limit values are only guidelines and a complete understanding of the limits is necessary before using the numbers to protect workers' health. For this reason it is important that the physician have a thorough understanding of the limitations of these chemical exposure limits. An experienced industrial hygienist can aid the physician in the interpretation and use of the exposure limit guidelines.

The TLV book also includes exposure guidelines for physical agents such as noise, vibration, lasers, heat, cold, and radiation (ionizing and nonionizing). Biological exposure indices for assessing exposure to certain chemicals are also included. Copies of the book can be obtained by contacting the American Conference of Governmental Industrial Hygienist (see Appendix A).

PREVENTION

One of the most important aspects of treating an occupationally injured worker is learning how the injury occurred so that steps can be taken to prevent it from recurring. The physician working with a safety professional or industrial hygienist can analyze the work environment to identify the dangerous agents or operations that caused the injury and take actions to prevent future injury.

The safety professional and the industrial hygienist are important assets to the physician when developing and implementing an effective program to prevent a future worker injury.

The following are case studies in which physicians have worked with industrial hygienists to successfully manage a worker's injury.

CASE STUDIES
Case 1

A physician was called in to evaluate the health problems being experienced by a number of hotel employees working at the reception desk. They all reported significant respiratory problems. The physician requested that the hotel hire an industrial hygienist to evaluate the work area. Appropriate medical evaluations and lab testing were done by the physician. The industrial hygienist interviewed the affected employees, inspected the work area, collected air samples, and measured the performance of the hotel's ventilation system.

The work revealed that two separate operations were contributing to the problem. The first was the use of a highly irritating oxalic acid-base marble cleaner by the janitorial staff at night. The second environmental problem was an upset in the chlorination system for the water in a decorative fountain/waterfall in the reception area. The oxalic acid marble cleaner was discontinued and a different biological control system was used for the fountain/waterfall. These simple changes solved the employees' problems without further medical intervention.

Case 2

An occupational physician was asked to investigate a sick building where employees were experiencing a wide range of health problems that they attributed to the air in the building. The symptoms included headaches, dizziness, cold symptoms, and fatigue.

After the physician's medical examination proved unremarkable, an industrial hygienist was brought in to evaluate the building's ventilation system, measure levels of pollutants, and interview the building's occupants. As a result of the work by the industrial hygienist it was discovered that the building's ventilation system was not supplying adequate air and that a water spill had resulted in high levels of fungal spores in the carpet for part of the building. An increased amount of fresh air was introduced into the building and the damaged carpet as well as the backing pad were removed. No further indoor air quality problems were experienced.

Case 3

A physician was retained by a workers' compensation insurance carrier to evaluate a claim for permanent disability. The injured worker claimed that the workplace caused permanent difficulty in breathing. A complete physical examination of the worker, including pulmonary function studies, did not indicate a cause for the respiratory problems. The physician requested that an industrial hygienist inspect the worksite and complete air sampling to determine whether there were workplace environmental factors causing or contributing to the patient's respiratory problem.

The industrial hygienist completed a detailed review of all work activities, inspected the building ventilation system, collected air samples, and reviewed the material safety data sheets for the limited number of chemicals in the workplace. The industrial hygienist determined that there was no evidence of any agent present to account for the respiratory problems being experienced by the worker. The workers' compensation claim was closed, and the patient, relieved that no significant medical problem was present, continued follow-up care with her personal physician as needed.

SUMMARY

The safety professional and the industrial hygienist are valuable resources for the physician responsible for managing an occupationally injured worker. When the treating physician needs additional information about the workplace and when the agents that caused the injury need to be identified, these professionals have the knowledge and resources to investigate accidents, provide valuable information for treatment, and make recommendations to prevent future injuries.

34 Personal Protective Equipment

Protection against hazards at work can be provided in three primary ways: engineering controls, administrative controls, and personal protective equipment (PPE). Engineering controls generally are the best choice, because a better ventilation system, sound baffling to reduce noise, and other changes that reduce the exposure at the source require no effort on the part of the employee. Administrative controls, such as rotating tasks to reduce exposure levels, are a good option and usually require much less money than engineering controls, although they are less adaptable for small businesses with relatively fixed tasks and limited staff.

Personal protective equipment therefore, although the least desirable method as far as the Occupational Safety Health Act (OSHA) is concerned, is frequently the option used most in small and medium-sized industries. This method of protecting employees, however, is not perfect. Many medical concerns may still be brought to the attention of the local occupational or primary care physician. The purpose of this chapter is to give the local clinician an overview of the types of PPE, the problems likely to be encountered, and resources for further information.

A logical approach to the problem of personal protective equipment requires that the treating physician understand what kind of work is performed by the patient. Many forms exist to obtain a self-report occupational history. Choose one that allows the patient to identify PPE worn as well as types of hazards faced. The clinician, faced with a patient possibly exposed to toxins, should obtain further information using the approach and resources identified in Chapter 25, on chemical hazards. Specific information about the types of PPE (brand name, model number, size, source, as well as the patient's opinion of fit, comfort, effectiveness, and how much of the time the item is actually worn) should be sought. Finally, inquiry should be made into how and how often the item is cleaned and what solution is used. It is helpful to have on file for each client company of the clinic a list of PPE, with all the information described previously for each item.

PPE: RESOURCES FOR THE CLINICIAN

Most clinicians do not feel intellectually or legally comfortable recommending specific kinds of personal protective equipment for their patients. Unfortunately, most workers and employers also lack this information, with the result that employees too often are handed masks and gloves purchased from a local hardware store. Such makeshift equipment may be hopelessly inadequate for the task. Worse, it can result in a false sense of security, leading to dangerous or toxic exposures.

In cases of possible toxic exposure, review of PPE can often identify the reason for the exposure and guide the clinician toward a solution. In addition, the local clinician can send employers copies of appropriate pages from safety catalogues with the suggestion to explore these alternatives, because "the current equipment does not appear protective." A referral to a local OSHA consultation service or to several local industrial hygiene firms for follow-up can also be most helpful for employers who may not know that these resources exist.

A key resource that merits mention in the beginning of this chapter is *Best's Safety Directory* (1994, approximately $50 annually). This two-volume set lists, by type of equipment, most models of all safety equipment produced by United States safety supply manufacturers. It is divided into sections (e.g., respiratory protection, hand protection, and so forth) and each section is preceded by a concise overview of the latest legal statutes and the field's developments. Particularly useful is a review of all current OSHA standards related to the topic. For example, the section on hand protection includes an overview and a separate list and summary of each OSHA standard that specifically mentions gloves.

Because there are actually few safety supply stores in any given geographic area, it is helpful to supplement the information in the annual *Best's* with supply store catalogues and some samples from local vendors. If an employer's equipment is not appropriate, either discuss recommended changes or refer the employer to a resource for help. Contacting the local safety supply company's sales office can lead to an unsolicited call by the representative who can recommend to the employer the particular types of items identified as needed.

If the employer is recalcitrant and the clinician is certain of a hazard to patients from poor or inappropriate protective equipment, a call to OSHA should be considered. This action clearly has major implications, but the health of the patient who faces a serious hazard is the most important issue and the clinician's biggest liability.

PROTECTING THE HANDS
Gloves

Gloves are the most common type of protective equipment worn in industrial operations. Dozens of companies produce a wide variety of gloves designed to protect the employee against diverse biological, chemical, and physical (heat, cold, vibration) hazards. Two major questions must be asked by the clinician caring for a worker whose work requires glove use:

1. Is the type of glove provided actually appropriate for the hazard?
2. Is the glove material likely to cause harm to this employee?

Biologic hazards. Gloves to protect workers against biological exposures are usually made of latex or polyvinyl. They are frequently boxed in 100s and in sizes small, medium, and large. They are meant for single use and are disposable. The OSHA blood and body fluid standard mandates provision of gloves for any employee potentially exposed more than once a month.

There is good documentation now that these gloves even provide some protection against needlesticks that penetrate the skin through the glove. The glove layer itself significantly reduces the number of infectious particles that are transmitted. Problems arise most often in the uncontrolled settings of emergency care, where firefighters handling a rescue at an auto crash or where emergency room (ER) personnel dealing with a cardiac arrest find the gloves too loose and flimsy, easily ripping or allowing blood to slip inside to contact the wearer's skin. Another major problem is allergic reaction to the rubber or extreme drying or maceration of the skin from a combination of frequent hand washing and talc powder inside the gloves.

A number of industrial gloves are disposable but are longer and fit better than the latex ones usually provided. These should be considered for firefighters and other emergency rescue personnel. For those with allergic reactions, hypoallergenic gloves may be purchased through hospital and medical supply companies, and nonlatex gloves such as those made with disposable polyvinyl chloride (PVC) are now available. Gloves without talc can be suggested along with appropriate skin care techniques described in Chapter 16, dermatologic injuries. Excellent care of the skin must be emphasized to the patient potentially exposed to biologic hazards. Intact skin is an excellent barrier against germs, whereas damaged skin, even somewhat defatted, can provide an entry for these agents into the body. (Several of the health care workers whose human immunodeficiency virus (HIV) infections are deemed occupational were exposed through blood contact with damaged skin).

Chemicals. Dozens of manufacturers produce literally hundreds of models of gloves for protection against chemical exposures. Originally only natural rubber was available, but new synthetic rubbers (nitrile, butyl, or neoprene rubber) and increasing numbers of other synthetic materials (viton, polyvinyl chloride, polyvinyl alcohol, polyethylene) allow the purchaser to select appropriate materials based on chemical interaction features and type of use expected.

Permeability is a key consideration. Gloves that fully protect against one type of exposure may dissolve on contact with other chemicals. Degradation, or the ability of the material to withstand rough handling, is another important feature. Length, thickness, amount of use, exposure to temperature extremes and to sharp edges are also features that must be considered. Most safety catalogues have tables that cross-reference glove features with type of exposure so that the clinician can easily determine whether appropriate protective equipment has been issued in cases of possible chemical exposure. For example, natural rubber (latex) is usually resistant to acids, bases, aldehydes, and ketones but dissolves on contact with solvent. Neoprene is good protection against phenols and glycol ethers, whereas nitrile rubber can provide protection from some but not all solvents, oils, esters, and glycols but not ketones. PVC is tough and effective against many alkalis, acids bases, and alcohols, but it is not good for solvents and ketones. (Note that these cover general classes of chemicals only and may well not include many of the over 100,000 chemicals used in U.S. industrial operations today. If the appropriate choice is unclear, the employer should be referred to an industrial hygienist or OSHA for further advice.)

Physical hazards. Extreme heat or cold, sharp edges, vibration, slippery surfaces, and other physical hazards make additional demands on worker's hands, and there are gloves designed to meet all of these needs. Many combine several features. For example, a meat-packing worker needs hand protection to provide warmth, a good gripping surface for slippery knife handles, and protection against sharp edges, both bone and knife. A safety supply catalogue can provide the clinician with ideas to give to the employer or the patient.

PROTECTING THE LUNGS
Respirators

Respirators are probably the next most frequently used piece of equipment and the most problematic for the industrial clinician. Most physicians, when asked about respirators, think of the intensive care unit. In fact, industrial respiratory protection has been documented as early as the Roman era, when pig bladders were used to protect slaves against dust in mining operations.

Current respiratory protection falls into two categories: supplied air (positive pressure) and filtering devices (negative pressure). Supplied air respirators are used in the most dangerous work situations, such as fighting fires, working in low-oxygen atmospheres, or working with toxic chemicals. These work atmospheres are called IDLH or immediately dangerous to life and health. In these work settings, being without the respiratory protection for even a few seconds or minutes may result in serious illness or death.

Supplied air respirators provide a source of clean air and prevent pulmonary exposure to toxins. The most familiar version is the SCBA or self-contained breathing apparatus used for firefighting and deep sea diving operations. Air is provided through tanks carried on the worker's back and supplied to the face through a short hose attached to a face mask. The unit is good only while the compressed air lasts, and the usual range is 20 to 60 minutes. In heavy work such as firefighting, however, the increased respiratory rate and tidal volume decrease effective air time. The major problem unique to this type of respirator is the unit's weight, approximately 20 to 30 pounds.

Air line respirators, a mask attached to a hose leading to an air compressor, are the second type of supplied air respirator. The unique hazard with this type is contamination of the air at the source (the compressor) with oil, carbon monoxide, or other toxins. An additional problem is the vulnerability of the air hose and the wearer's limitation in range and movement.

Air-purifying respirators filter air through a cartridge (usually replaceable) designed to remove specific hazardous substances from the inspired air. Most frequently these are attached to the face-piece, which can be half-face (covering nose and mouth) or full-face (covering eyes as well). This is the most common type of respirator, costing between $20 for average half-face to $100 for a full-face respirator. The cartridges are specific to the hazard, so knowledge of the type of hazard is critical to effectiveness. A filter for dusts will not protect against solvent vapors or acid gases. Over 20 different cartridges or combinations have been approved by the National Institute for Occupational Safety Health (NIOSH) for industrial use. Industrial supply catalogues also have lists of approved cartridges.

A modification of the negative pressure or cartridge respirator is the powered air-purifying respirator (PAPR). The face mask is attached by a hose to a battery pack with a filter at the waist. Air is drawn in through the filter at the waist and then sent up to the face mask. Although the work of breathing is less and the air is cooler, the mask is still considered negative pressure because the air is filtered and not supplied at high enough velocity to provide the protection level of supplied air respirators. The units are also much more expensive, approximately $500, although one battery pack can be purchased for use by multiple employees each with their own masks.

All respirators have certain common problems. Allergies can develop to the mask components, particularly rubber. Persons with severe acne or other types of dermatologic conditions may find that wearing a respirator makes their skin condition worse, and, conversely, skin conditions or facial hair may cause a bad facepiece seal.[7] A small percentage of the population is genuinely claustrophobic and unable to tolerate something covering the face. All respirators increase the physiologic dead space of breathing, and adversely affect breathing effectiveness by decreasing effective tidal volume.[5,7] Peripheral vision is decreased in any full-face model, and the masks are hot and sweaty. If not issued to a single individual, assorted infectious diseases are transmissible, and inappropriate storage methods can lead to microbial growth on the filters unless rigorous cleaning protocols are followed.[12]

In addition to the above drawbacks, individual types of respirators have other specific health effects. SCBAs are heavy and increase cardiopulmonary and musculoskeletal strain because of the extra weight. Air line respirators depend on uncontaminated air and integrity of the air hose. Air-filtering devices increase the work of breathing because of increased inspiratory resistance through the filter and increased expiratory resistance through the exhalation valve.[1,5,6]

Physicians are frequently asked to medically clear an employee to wear a respirator. Knowledge of these hazards leads to a simple but effective medical protocol that can be used to screen employees who will be assigned to duty requiring respirators. Key to this protocol is understanding the increased cardiopulmonary strain (as a result of the increased inspiratory and expiratory resistance and dead space described previously) caused by wearing respiratory protection. Studies have shown that some individuals develop a paradoxical decreased respiratory or cardiac rate, particularly at maximal exercise.[9] Normal individuals can tolerate this, but those with preexisting disease may not. Questions to screen for cardiac and/or pulmonary disease and risk factors are the major focus. Additional questions cover skin problems, claustrophobia, and musculoskeletal problems. Specific information about the type of respirator to be worn, frequency and duration of wear, and heaviness of the work to be performed should also be obtained.

The physical evaluation emphasizes heart, lung, pulse rate, and blood pressure evaluation for non-IDLH users. Spirometry should be performed by someone certified through a NIOSH course or pulmonary function technician training. This simple evaluation, including review of the history and physical examination, can be performed by a registered nurse under the protocol for non–IDLH air-filtered respirators. A physician should sign off all charts and medical clearances.

Those wearing SCBAs for emergency response work or other IDLH work should be evaluated by a nurse practitioner or physician, with additional attention paid to cardiac risk factors, exercise patterns, and actual level of functioning. If questions exist in clearance for IDLH cases, a pulmonary exercise treadmill test should be performed for nonsymptomatic individuals. Those subjects with high-risk profiles and symptoms suspicious for angina should be referred through their own private insurance plans for cardiac evaluation including a treadmill stress test (TMST).[4,11,14]

OSHA regulations suggest periodic reevaluation. Usually this is done each year, although annual frequency is not required by law. All records of medical evaluation and testing must be kept in the clinician's office, accessible if proof is required by OSHA of an employer's compliance with the law. Employers are not legally privy to the medical records but should receive a copy of the medical clearance form for the personnel records. The employee should be given a wallet card to keep a record of both the medical examination and the types of approved respirators when later fit-tested.

PROTECTING THE BODY
Chemical-resistant suits

Workers are increasingly assigned to tasks requiring the use of occlusive full-body suits in addition to gloves and respirators. Federal regulatory agencies including the Environmental Protection Agency (EPA), OSHA, and the National Fire Protection Association (NFPA) involved in hazardous materials work have developed a grading system for this clothing, with Level A protection being the most protective—fully occlusive suits used with an SCBA.

Medical concerns associated with this clothing relate to its actual effectiveness for the hazard under consideration and the medical effects from wearing the clothing. Research shows that wearing fully occlusive clothing will raise core body temperature at moderately strenuous workloads within 15 minutes, leading to risks of heat stress and cardiopulmonary strain. (See Chapter 26 on temperature-related injuries for further discussion of this problem.) All employees who are asked to perform work in this type of clothing should be evaluated by a clinician for preexisting problems such as heart disease, diabetes, or pulmonary disease. Most job classifications requiring use of this clothing fall under the OSHA hazardous waste work standard that mandates medical evaluation.

PROTECTING THE FEET
Shoes and boots

Foot protection is provided for reasons similar to those for providing gloves: to protect against chemicals, wet environments, heat and cold, electrical shock, injury from sharp or blunt objects, or trauma. Concerns about the material's resistance, longevity, degradation potential, and the like, apply to foot protection just as to glove protection.

The major medical effects of foot protection are fungal infections from occlusive boots and cumulative trauma to the foot from poorly fitting footwear. Fungal infections of the feet can be common and resistant to treatment. The mainstay of treatment involves the use of cotton socks; footwear that allows air circulation as much as possible while not at work; provision of several pairs of boots so that they can air out between wearings; and the use of topical antifungal preparations. Referral to a podiatrist for ongoing care may be needed in resistant cases.

Poorly fitting boots can also result in injuries (such as plantar fasciitis) that are difficult to treat and potentially can result in temporary disability. If appropriate fitting footwear does not rapidly correct the problem, a referral to a foot specialist may be needed.

PROTECTING THE EYES*
Safety glasses

It is important to remember that the worker as well as anyone who enters the work area must be adequately protected. To be effective, eye protection must be required for everyone entering a hazardous area, including the supervisor, shop steward, visitor, or the employer. The American National Standards Institute (ANSI) standard practice for occupational and educational eye and face protection (287.1-1979), describes three types of basic safety spectacles:

1. Spectacles with no side shields
2. Spectacles with orbital-fitting, cup-type side shields made of wire mesh or perforated/nonperforated plastic
3. Spectacles with semi- or flat-fold side shields.

Safety spectacles that meet these standards are clearly marked with the manufacturer's hallmark etched on the lenses and the trademark indicated on the frame. In addition, the designation "Z87" appears on all major component replacement parts. It is important to note that safety lenses of Z87.1 quality mounted in streetwear frames instead of industrial safety frames do not provide adequate protection. Similarly, scratched or pitted safety lenses frequently lose their impact resistance and should be replaced.

Each of the three styles of safety spectacles is designed to protect against different types of environmental hazards. Spectacles that have no side shields protect against missiles or impact from in front of the worker but offer little or no protection from harmful missiles from above, beside, or below. Side shield safety spectacles provide important additional protection from hazardous material from the side, below, above, and behind. Spectacles with semi- or flat-fold side shields provide an intermediate level of protection. With these spectacles, a portion of the eyes and orbit remain vulnerable to harmful agents from above and to the side and from below and to the side. The selection of an appropriate eye protection device depends on the environmental hazards involved. The experience of many industries, however, has shown that wire mesh side shield safety spectacles are the most effective, except in work involving splatter risks, such as health care.[2]

Depending on a worker's visual needs, safety glasses may be either corrective or noncorrective. Workers who normally require corrective lenses to see clearly must use corrective safety eyewear on the job as well. If glasses are typically not required for good vision, clear lenses without correction (plain safety glasses) are all that is necessary.

Goggles

Some jobs require that basic eye protection be supplemented by an additional protection device. One example is a pair of eyecups or rigid cover goggles used for protection against chipping, dust, or splashes. Another example is a set of welding or cutting goggles.[11]

A useful device for the protection of visitors and new employees is a coverall goggle that may be worn as basic eye protection over streetwear glasses. This type of goggle may be used as supplementary protection when worn over the basic safety eyewear required for some jobs. Coverall protectors of this type are useful and inexpensive. They should be worn, for example, while hammering, making auto repairs, and working with power tools, a power mower, or auto batteries.

Use of contact lenses in the workplace

The use of contact lenses while at work has been somewhat controversial.[13] Contact lenses do not provide barrier protection for the eye or orbit. Furthermore, soft lenses may absorb small amounts of chemical solvents, potentially allowing prolonged exposure of the cornea to these chemicals. Some studies suggest, however, that hard lenses may actually seal off the cornea, providing protection from chemical irritants.[3]

With the few exceptions noted here, the use of contact lenses in industry is permitted. The American Academy of Ophthalmology in 1980 issued a policy statement endorsing contact lens wear at work in conjunction with appropriate safety eyewear, except in harsh environments. The general prohibition against wearing contact lenses is in the process of being removed from industrial regulations. For the most part, any prohibitions against the use of gas-permeable and soft lenses are not being enforced pending reevaluation of the standards. The wearer, of course, must be appropriately protected from hazards to eye injury whether or not lenses are worn.

In general, contact lenses are allowed in any work area where eyeglasses and the naked eye are permitted. Contact lenses may be worn under safety goggles and may well increase worker compliance with wearing safety eyewear. Where not prohibited by regulation, contact lenses may also be worn under a respirator without problem, although the circulating air in some respirators may have a drying effect on the lenses. The use of contact lenses with safety goggles or respirators is

* This section was written by T. Otis Paul, MD, of the Department of Ophthalmology at California Pacific Medical Center, and Thomas Herington, MD.

much less expensive than purchasing prescription safety eyewear or attaching prescription lenses inside respirator facepieces.

Federal regulation prohibits the wearing of contact lenses when working with the following chemicals:

1. 1,2-dibromo-3-chloropropane (DBCP) *(Code 1910.1044)*
2. Acrylonitrile *(Code 1910.1045)*
3. Ethylene oxide *(Code 1910.1047)*
4. Methylenedianaline (MDA) *(Code 1910.1050)*

OSHA also recommends against the use of contact lenses in the laboratory unless necessary, and prohibits their use by welders. Finally, OSHA prohibits wearing contact lenses with a respirator in contaminated atmospheres, although this ruling is changing with new evidence. The use of eyeglasses inside a respirator is also problematic because the temple bars extend through and break the seal of the facepiece. This is illegal. Glasses with short temple bars taped to the head inside the facepiece or prescription lenses, professionally mounted inside the facepiece, are recommended.

Companies should develop policies around the use of contact lenses at work and should identify all those who wear contact lenses in the workplace. Workers and safety or medical personnel should be familiar with proper lens care, with company policy around the use of contact lenses, and with first aid procedures for lens wearers who sustain eye injuries. In particular, safety personnel should be trained in procedures for removing hard and soft lenses.

PROTECTING THE EARS*

The physician needs to educate all employees who are at risk for NIHL (noise-induced hearing loss) about hearing protectors. There are basically two types, and each has its own advantages and disadvantages.

Hearing protection reduces noise levels so the intensity reaching the ear will be at safe levels. First and foremost, hearing protection must provide adequate attenuation. If adequate attenuation cannot be achieved by one type of device, two different types of devices (such as earplugs and muffs), may be necessary to protect the ear from hearing loss.

Many non–hearing-impaired workers also do not accept the concept that with hearing protec-

tion, speech discrimination actually improves in a noisy environment. This is because speech-to-noise ratios are kept constant, and the protected inner ear hair cells do not fatigue. With lower overall noise levels, the ear will not distort the speech perceived.

Hearing protectors reduce both the noise and voice levels so the ear can operate more efficiently. Speech is dulled in a quiet environment with hearing protection but not in noisy environments. The physician needs to convince the employee that one's speech discrimination will be more acute with hearing protection than without.

Ear plugs

Insert-type hearing protectors (earplugs) are easily portable and do not interfere with eyeglasses, safety helmets, and so on. Most people find them comfortable to wear, and they are ideal for work in confined spaces. The disadvantages, however, are that they need to be inserted properly for maximum attenuation and that they can only be inserted in a healthy ear canal (canals that are free of eczema and infection). Because they are not readily visible when worn, it is difficult for the supervisor to monitor compliance.

Ear muffs

Ear muffs can be worn even if the employee has otitis media. Muffs are easier to put on correctly. They can be seen at a distance so compliance can be monitored by the supervisor. Ear muffs are bulky and hot, however, and cost more than most earplugs. The attenuation factor is reduced by wear and tear and deliberate bending of the frame. They can also become loose when someone is either talking or chewing.

Fitting hearing protection devices

Every worker's ear should be visually inspected before hearing protective devices are issued. Medical problems that may preclude a worker from wearing hearing protection include ear tenderness or inflammation, sores externally or in the ear canal, eczema of the pinna or of the canal, and any congenital or surgical malformations of the external ear. The physician or other health professional should note cerumen impaction and/or excessive cerumen. It is widely believed that earplugs increase cerumen production and the possibility of impaction, but few studies have been done on the effects of earplugs on cerumen formation.

Although good hygiene and routine cleaning of ear protection to prevent ear infection is a good general policy, no good epidemiologic data link the use of hearing protective devices and otitis externa or infections of the ear.

---

* This section was written by Susan Tierman, MD, of the Department of Occupational Medicine at Palo Alto Medical Foundation, Palo Alto, Calif.

The physician or other health professional should never assume that an ear irritation or infection is caused by the patient wearing hearing protective devices. A good history is essential. There are other causes of ear infections such as swimming, hot tub use, water skiing, excessive scratching or picking at the ear with cotton applicators or bobby pins, and various causes of dermatitis unrelated to hearing protection use.

When hearing protection is implicated, caustic or irritative materials contaminating the muffs or earplugs are often the problem. Foreign material from the workplace can get caught in the hearing protective device. It is the irritation from concrete, fiberglass, acid, coolants, and the like that is the primary problem, not the actual hearing protective device itself. When examining a patient whose chief complaint is irritation of the ear as a result of wearing hearing protective devices, the employee should always bring in the device so it can be visually inspected.

There is little likelihood of an inserted earplug doing damage to the tympanic membrane. The ear canal becomes increasingly sensitive the closer it is to the tympanic membrane. At the first sensation of pain the worker will be alerted to stop pushing the plug further in, before any damage can occur. There can be a problem, however, with earplugs that form an airtight seal. These earplugs are usually premoulded and are manufactured out of vinyl or cured silicones. The worker must be instructed to withdraw the plugs slowly with a twisting motion to break the seal. Rapid removal of the earplug may build up pressures so high that the tympanic membrane can be managed. Foam and fibrous earplugs do not form a pneumatic seal.

OTHER PROTECTIVE EQUIPMENT

No major issues are associated with the use of other types of protective equipment such as faceshields, hard hats, aprons, and the like, except when injury occurs because they are not used. This simple equipment can be suggested, prescribed, or required for treatment or prevention of injury when needed.

The following case studies underscore the importance of understanding the relationship between the worker's health and the entire work environment.

CASE STUDIES
Case 1

A 43-year-old man came to the occupational medicine clinic with painful, cracked, and bleeding dermatitis of the hand, frequent sore throats, and frequent coughing. He worked in a plating shop that had open tanks of a variety of acids, caustics, and solvents. Ventilation was provided through a ceiling fan, one window, *and large doors that were left open during the day. Protective equipment included a cloth mask, disposable gloves, a rubber apron, and boots. The patient mentioned that a "haze" was present in the shop on most days and, when questioned by the physician, he reported that he had to change gloves every few hours because they got sticky and dissolved.*

Treatment focused not only on the hand and respiratory problems but also on getting the worker better protective equipment. The man was an illegal immigrant and thus afraid of being fired or deported. The physician called a local safety supply store that had an industrial hygienist as a sales representative. The representative visited a number of facilities in the area, including the patient's small plant. The employer was receptive to his suggestions, ordered more appropriate gloves and respirators, and installed additional fans for dilution ventilation.

Case 2

A wastewater treatment plant contracted with a local occupational health clinic to screen employees for medical clearance to be assigned to the emergency response team (ERT) in the event of a chlorine leak. The facility covered several square blocks, and ERT members would be required to run to the site of the stored SCBAs and chemical suits, don them, run to the site of the leak to rescue anyone overcome, and then contain the leak.

Screening proceeded, using the protocol for use of air-filtered respirators. One 41-year-old supervisor, whose continued shift assignment depended on his clearance for the ERT, was found to have a history of a sedentary lifestyle. He had smoked one and one half packs of cigarettes a day for 22 years (recently reduced to less than 1 pack per day) and had a history of elevated cholesterol. His examination was significant for an FEV_1 of 79% predicted, occasional rhonchi on auscultation, and repeated blood pressure in the 160/96 range. He also was obese.

The employee was strongly counseled about weight loss, exercise, a low-fat diet, and quitting smoking, but initially he was unresponsive to these recommendations. Per protocol, he was referred for a screening pulmonary treadmill test, which had to be deferred three times because his initial blood pressures were too high. Weight loss, quitting smoking, and exercise were reinforced each time, and finally the patient took it seriously. He lost 24 pounds, stopped smoking, brought his cholesterol under control, and began a walking program. He passed his evaluation 6 months later.

SUMMARY

By familiarizing himself with the basic types and correct use of protective equipment, a local practitioner who treats occupational injuries can serve as a valuable resource for both employer and employee. The creative techniques identified in this chapter and illustrated in the case studies are approaches that have proved effective in difficult cases.

REFERENCES

1. Bentley G et al: Acceptable levels for breathing resistance of respiratory apparatus, *Arch Environ Health* 27:273-280, 1983.
2. Garrett SJ, Robinson JK: Disposable protective eyewear devices for health care providers: how important are they, and will available designs be used? *J Occup Med* 17:163-165, 1975.
3. Guthrie JW, Seitz GF: An investigation of the chemical contact lens problem, *J Occup Med* 35:1043-1047, 1993.
4. Harber P: Medical certification for respirator use, *J Med* 26:496-503, 1984.
5. Harber P et al: Determinants of breathing during respirator use, *Am J Ind Med* 13:253-262, 1988.
6. Harber P et al: Effects of respirator dead space, inspiratory resistance and expiratory resistance ventilatory loads, *Am J Ind Med* 16:189-198, 1989.
7. Hyatt EC, et al: Effect of facial hair on respirator performance, *Am Ind Hyg Assoc J* 34:135-142, 1973.
8. James: Breathing resistance and dead space in respiratory protection devices, pub no 77-166, 1976, National Institute of Occupational Safety and Health, Department of Health and Human Services.
9. Lohevarra VA: Physiological effects associated with the use of respiratory protective devices, *Scand J Work Environ Health* 10:275-281, 1984.
10. Mahoney WP: No contacts for welders using respirators, *J Occup Med* (letters).
11. Morgan WP, Raven PB: Prediction of distress for individuals wearing industrial respirators, *Am Ind Hyg Assoc J* 46:363-368, 1985.
12. Pasanen AL et al: Microbial growth on respirators from improper storage, *Scand J Work Environ Health* 19:421-425, 1993.
13. Perry GF, editor: What are the current recommended guidelines concerning the use of contact lenses in industry? Occupational Medicine Forum, *J Occup Med* 35:650-652, 1993.
14. Raven PB et al: Clinical pulmonary function and industrial respirator use, *Am Ind Hyg Assoc J* 42:897-903, 1981.

SUGGESTED READINGS

Best's safety directory, vols 1 and 2, Oldwick, NJ, published annually, AM Best.
Rajhans, Blackwell: *Practical guide to respirator usage in industry,* Boston, 1985, Butterworth.

35 Ergonomics and Occupational Disorders

Ergonomics is the interdisciplinary approach to the interface between the worker and the worksite, work tools, and work tasks. The major United States texts on the subject all relate the beginning of serious research to World War II.[1,3,11] Work in the past has focused on job skills acquisition and error avoidance. The current focus is on prevention of chronic musculoskeletal or cumulative trauma disorders. Ergonomic hazards are not only a major focus of the Occupational Safety and Health Act (OSHA) but also a rising liability in terms of workers' compensation claims.

Since ergonomics involves the fit of the worker to the job, the study of anthropometrics—understanding human anatomy and average/range of sizes within a group—is important. The earliest United States study, published in 1953, was conducted on over 3,000 male Army inductees.[2] Most were healthy caucasians between the ages of 17 and 24. Even though the data collected consisted of the measures that a tailor would require, such as sleeve length or head circumference, the information was also used to design equipment for use by the general population. Later applications included the design of aircraft controls and equipment for ease of use and reduction of error. Since the Armed Forces were primarily male and the discipline of ergonomics in the United States relied heavily on military resources, the focus has been on males.

Current anthropometric tables are commonly based on Air Force data, first of the males, gathered in the 1950s, and later of Air Force females, published in 1983.[12] In addition to the racial and physical conditioning biases, the female data were also limited to women up to age 45. Rogers and Salvendy both point to its limitations in their texts. Few additional studies have been published in the English language literature that supplement these databases with information about different ethnic or age groups.[4,7,8,10] This chapter takes into account the increasing numbers of women in the workplace and draws from previously published material on the subject in Morse and Hinds (1993).[9]

THE CHANGING WORKFORCE

Women are entering the workforce in increasing numbers and remaining in it longer. Statistics show that while only 37.7% of American women worked in 1960, that figure had risen to 56.5% in 1988, with further increases projected for the future.[5,6] The increasing rate of minority immigration into this country adds an additional problem to the use of design criteria based on military data—the issue of physical differences due to genetic and/or nutritional backgrounds. By 2050 nonHispanic whites are projected to be only 53% of the U.S. population, with Hispanics projected at 21%, African-Americans 16%, Asians 11%, and Native Americans 2%. Finally, many U.S. corporations are moving parts of their operations to other countries (Mexico and Asia, in particular). Questions are being raised about the appropriateness of equipment developed for a U.S. workforce when this equipment is installed in another country.[7,10]

Approach to human factors in the workplace

The significant rise in the number of women and minorities in the workforce combined with America's economic importance necessitates a different approach to human factors and ergonomics. This approach requires research focused on developing anthropometric and biomechanical data describing the reality of our current and projected workforce. That information then needs to be applied to all aspects of the field, from tool and furniture design to sophisticated information-processing equipment such as voice-activated computers. Failure to do so will perpetuate our rising injury rate due to ergonomic hazards.

As Salvendy eloquently states: "The country is gradually becoming aware of the enormous human resources that have been wasted because of prejudice against women, minority races, the handicapped, and older citizens. The opportunity to work and serve in some useful capacity must be made available to the broadest possible spectrum of individuals."[10] Occupational health professionals, including ergonomists and human factors spe-

513

cialists, have a major contribution to make in aiding the development of safe and healthy workplaces that include all individuals.

Much of the work available to women as they have entered the workforce in recent decades has been in light assembly production operations or in information processing. Most of these jobs are seated, and most of the women have been seated at workstations with designs that are based on anthropometric measurements of men in the Air Force, as previously mentioned. The more recent addition of women from minority groups, especially from Puerto Rico, Mexico, Central America, (and other Latin American Countries), and those from Southeast Asia and China further decreases the appropriateness of these data for the fit of the furniture and tools.

Traditionally, a work surface in the United States is 29 to 31 inches high, excellent for a 5'10" male but totally inappropriate for a 5'1" female, who requires a work surface height of approximately 23 to 25 inches. Similarly, chairs are built with deep seat pans, fine for long-legged employees but forcing those who are smaller to sit forward with no lumbar support because if they sit against the back of the chair their legs extend out. Providing chairs with arms is often useless because the armrests are too far away from the body.

Hand tools are also poorly designed for this segment of the workforce. Grips are too thick, and tools such as pliers require an overwide grasp (or even two-handed grasp) resulting in inappropriate pressures on the palm and loss of functional efficiency.

Even when consideration is given to the growing female participation in the labor force, the measurements used are still based on a selected segment of the population, the white Air Force women. In a 1984 workshop on ergonomics, Chaffin said, "It was not long ago that a job designer would assume that if an overhead reach was required, a male would be given such a job. Today that is not the case with over 43% of the labor market composed of women in the U.S. . . . Where an easy overhead grasp reach of about 77 inches (195 cm) was given in design books in reference to men, now approximately 73 inches (185 cm) is recommended to accommodate 95% of women," he continued, and referenced the NASA data.

Finally the issue of the older female worker must be addressed. Women live longer than men, and older women often must work to avoid impoverished existences. Loss of lean muscle mass begins in the early 30s in both males and females, and in women the loss of strength is combined with a loss of bone mass after menopause. This is the most likely explanation for women's noted decrease in height as they get older. The aging population, and in particular the female aging population, brings certain special issues to the workplace that we must address ergonomically to prevent injury.[4]

THE ROLE OF THE OCCUPATIONAL HEALTH PROFESSIONAL

Occupational health professionals can do much to correct poor ergonomic conditions in the workplace. Attention should be paid to three factors: the worksite and work tools, the work tasks, and the individual employee's work practices. In considering these three factors, one must remember the three types of controls of occupational hazards: engineering, administrative, and personal protection. Finally, it is very important to recognize that the ideal musculoskeletal position for any job is rarely held for more than a few minutes. Human beings evolved to move, not to sit in one spot all day in a perfect 90-degree position with feet flat on the floor, spine straight, and elbows locked at right angles. Many training courses focus on this as the ideal position, but an honest self-assessment and review of groups of employees doing seated work reveal that most people shift around in their chairs frequently.

Most individuals develop certain position behaviors to ease the load on various parts of the body. A chair may look properly adjusted, but the individual may slump forward or push back with thigh pressure in order to find a mid-range comfortable position for the lumbar spine that may be quite lordotic in one person and quite flat in another. Varying degrees of body fat and muscle mass also result in varying perception of direct pressure on buttocks, thighs, back, and arms. People may shift about frequently in order to alleviate soft tissue pressure. The seated workstation should be set up to recognize this fact and should support the worker's body as she moves through a variety of positions during the day.

Engineering controls

Intervention in the worksite and work tools ideally begins with ordering appropriate equipment. Manufacturers are quick now to stamp the words "ergonomically designed" on their products. Occupational health professionals can be of significant service to their companies and/or consult clients by reviewing the features of the equipment, especially focusing on range of adjustability and/or sizes offered, the database on which these were predicated, and the designer's credentials. (For example, one "state of the art" piece of computerized information processing equipment, believed to be responsible for many injuries, had been designed by someone educated in ceramics.)

Furniture. Multifaceted, multiuse furniture is the wisest purchase. Even executives and judges use computers and need multitask chairs and workstations. Those performing light assembly jobs or information processing require workstations that provide support through a range of positions. Fully adjustable work surfaces and similarly adjustable chairs that provide support for the upper back and/or neck and arms are the ideal.

Most manufacturers have a number of products in various phases of design and prototype production. Large corporations with significant problems may want to meet with the manufacturer to discuss their particular needs and may even delay an order in anticipation of an ergonomically superior product in the near future.

Companies with specific needs also can make specific demands. One large electronics manufacturing company was able to insist on lower chairs after the nurse practitioners measured all 246 workers (largely female and foreign-born) and found the average worker to be below the 5th percentile in size on the National Aeronautics and Space Administration (NASA) tables.

Deleting a bad ergonomic problem through automation is also an excellent solution. Biotechnology firms frequently use this option, identifying high-risk tasks early, and rotating employees through these until the company is large enough to justify automation. Since biotechnology involves not only new drug production but also development of new high technology equipment for gene-splicing and so forth, there are resources within the industry for development and production of completely new pieces of equipment to automate a repetitious task.

Many industries will not have those same resources at hand, but the problem frequently has been solved already with available equipment. A State of California insurance commissioner's study on workers' compensation illustrates the types of savings, in both human and monetary terms, that can be accrued by using engineering controls in materials handling and other high-risk jobs. If specific equipment does not exist, companies should discuss the issue with an industrial engineer, a specialist with the training to create new machinery and tools.

Many companies cannot afford huge furniture or equipment purchases, however, and must seek less expensive interventions. Workstations that are too high can be adjusted by elevating the chair and providing a footstool. For some employees who are very short, the commercially available footrests will need to be attached to a block of

wood for further elevation. If the work surface is too low, the desk or table can be elevated on blocks or newly available risers.

Chairs that are too deep can be corrected by inserting a pillow behind the employee. A variety of lumbar support cushions are available, with velcro attachments for cloth chairs and elastic straps for vinyl ones. They come in varying sizes and depths for different preferences. A quick fix is the temporary use of a bed pillow or couch cushion. If the arm rests are too short or too widely separated, wrapping them with foam or cervical collars (which are made of 1-inch thick foam with a velcro strap) will frequently be helpful.

Employees with very high work surfaces frequently stand or are required to sit on high stools with small backs and a ring at the base for foot support. An alternative is the sit-stand stool, where the employee leans back against a semi-sit surface. This is much easier if frequent moves into and out of the standing position are required.

Computer workstations. The computerized workstation must be evaluated to ensure that the monitor screen is at the appropriate height (placed so that the top of the screen is at or slightly above eye level). Employees with glasses should have the screen set at their focal distance or they will lean forward in order to see, straining the neck and back. Those with bifocals will frequently tilt the head back in order to see out of the lower reading section of the glasses, and they are at risk of neck injury unless the screen is lowered. Employees who have reached the age (40) where they are developing presbyopia may benefit from an adjustable computer monitor arm that can be moved easily to accommodate vision changes. Glasses with specific correction for the focal distance of computer use, with biannual replacement, can be provided.

Keyboards and peripherals (such as mouse and trackball) should ideally be placed on a work surface so that the employee can type with shoulders relaxed, elbows comfortably at the side of the body, and bent at a 90-degree angle or slightly more open. This usually requires some type of adjustable work surface or keyboard tray, drawer, or table. In addition, the employee should be provided with a wrist rest for the keyboard and another one for the mouse or trackball. Dozens of wrist rests are commercially available, and attention should be paid to their features as well as their cost. An ideal wrist rest should have a foam core, a smooth surface (preferably felt, or vinyl if it will have multiusers) and rounded edges. Ideally it should extend under the keyboard so that it is weighted down, and it should be high enough so that the wrist of the user is not extended or flexed in use. It must be deep enough to comfortably support the wrist during use of all keys including the space bar (approximately 4 inches deep by 1 to $1\frac{1}{2}$ inches thick). Placing the wrist rest at the edge of the work surface also eliminates the sharp edge that can place undue pressure on the ulnar nerve. Special foam wrist rests are commercially available for keyboard trays, cut so as to fit over the plastic or metal lip of the tray.

For many information processors and some assembly workers, adjustable forearm supports may prove useful. These clamp on the work surface edge and are articulated for full movement of the forearms. Key features include sturdy construction, smooth joints, and a soft cup surface for the forearms, as well as some adjustability in height of use. Just as with wrist rests, careful attention should be paid to construction and ease of use. There are excellent products on the market and, conversely, forearm supports that are poorly made do not provide firm secure support.

Phone adaptations. Those involved in heavy telephone work should use a headset. Headsets have long been provided to directory assistance operators and telephone sales solicitors. Increasing numbers of workers, including management executives, reporters, software support engineers, financial advisors, advice nurses, and the like, are required to use the telephone 2 to 6 hours a day, often while simultaneously typing on a computer or researching information. A headset will prevent the neck and upper back problems associated with trying to hold the phone between the neck and shoulder while using the hands for a different task.

Tools. Work tools are often a source of significant problems. Fortunately, ergonomic tools not easily found 10 years ago are now available. In situations where purchase of ergonomically designed screwdrivers, pliers, scissors, and other tools is cost-prohibitive, modifications that will make a dramatic difference can be made with inexpensive material. Caulking material can be used to build up the handles of many tools, turning a hard slippery plastic surface that required a forceful grip into a larger, soft, roughened grip customized to the user's hand size. Newer thermophilic plastic materials with the same abilities are now available, can be more easily cleaned, and can tolerate some chemical and temperature exposures. Even taping the handle or slipping foam rubber sleeves over the handles makes a big difference.

Administrative controls

Work task interventions can be accomplished through several means. Evidence exists to show that work performance will increase and visual complaints from close work decrease if the work activity is rotated or interrupted by rest breaks. One simple intervention is to teach employees to do a stand-and-stretch moment every 20 to 30 minutes. This is not a break or rest period; it simply means getting up out of the chair to perform 60 to 120 seconds of gentle movements designed to loosen the muscles, break up the constrained posture, and improve bloodflow and tendon lubrication in the affected areas.

This maneuver is most successful when supervisors are responsible for its performance and the whole work unit does it simultaneously. In addition to stand-and-stretch, employees should be taught to vary tasks within their workday as much as possible. If a worker performs 4 hours of typing and 4 hours of telephone work, the tasks should be interwoven throughout the day rather than one task all morning and the other all afternoon.

Within employee groups, the same principle also is relevant. Employees should be cross-trained and job tasks rotated so that different muscles are used. High-risk jobs, with significant repetitive work, should be periodically analyzed for new interventions. In the interim, these jobs should be rotated among as wide a group of employees as possible, for as brief a period of exposure as possible. These are also the jobs that should be considered for automation.

Evaluating production standards. Finally, the most basic work task intervention is periodic reevaluation of production standards. Economic solutions have resulted in significant lay-offs and consolidation of many jobs without reducing required output. At the same time, particularly in computerized information processing operations, equipment developments allow work to be performed much faster than before. The result may be that employees are expected to do too much. Management, in conjunction with health and safety personnel, should periodically review this issue and, particularly when layoffs are needed, consider what job tasks are noncritical and can be cut.

When new equipment that increases efficiency is purchased, careful consideration should be given to defining appropriate production standards, including a graduated increase in output during a learning period. Employees who have been off on long-term leave, such as for childbirth or heart attack, should return to full production gradually. One large corporation routinely required returning employees to start back to work at 50% of production, and to increase over several weeks in a clearly defined pattern to avoid development of cumulative trauma disorders (CTDs) due to deconditioning. Encouraging return to work in mid-week is another practice that eases the transition period for many employees.

Personal protection

Work practices or an individual's work style are also key areas for intervention. If a group of employees who perform the same job on the same equipment is evaluated, a significant difference in how the employees do their work will be noted. Some will move with high force, velocity, and extreme ranges of motion. Others will be gentle and graceful, with minimal movements. The former group is at higher risk, based on clinical experience and results of research studies. Supervisors, safety personnel, or health care professionals can teach employees to alter their work style by pointing out the differences between their movements and those of others. In addition, encouraging frequent stand-and-stretch moments allows employees to think about their work style.

Finally, in our experience, the workers most frequently injured are those who do not take coffee or lunch breaks and often work overtime. While management, particularly in this economic era, may encourage these practices, the result is too often an injury to the most valuable and dedicated employees. Workers should be encouraged to take lunch away from their work areas and to take coffee breaks. This allows bodies and minds a needed respite.

ERGONOMIC STANDARDS

Currently there are no comprehensive ergonomic standards in force in the United States. Industries are subject to citation under the General Duty Clause that requires employers to provide a safe and healthy workplace. The past five years have seen major fines and the attention of the Occupational Safety and Health Act (OSHA) to cumulative trauma disorders in the meat-packing and other industries. However, challenges are being made to the use of this clause for CTDs in the absence of an ergonomic standard.

Both federal and some state plans are currently considering ergonomic standards. Federal OSHA's draft plan and California's draft plan are similar in that they are performance standards. They both require employers to evaluate their injury and illness statistics or perform a survey to see if a problem exists; to develop an approach for correcting the problem, including medical intervention; to institute corrective action; and to reevaluate the situation to see if the intervention was successful.

Major political issues surround the debate over these proposed standards, and the drafts are changing constantly. It is clear, however, that ergonomic hazards are now and will be in the future a major focus of OSHA action and a rising liability in terms of workers' compensation costs. The wise employer and occupational health professional will develop a formal plan for dealing with this issue and work on its implementation. This will both prevent or reduce costs and place the company or institution in a much better position if inspected by OSHA.

REFERENCES

1. Chaffin DB, Anderson G: *Occupational biomechanics,* New York, 1984, Wiley & Sons.
2. Daniels GS, Meyers HC: *Anthropometry of male basic trainees,* Dayton, Ohio, 1953, McGregor & Werner.
3. Human factors section: *ergonomic design for people at work,* vols 1 and 2, New York, 1983, Van Nostrand Reinhold.
4. Kelly PL, Kroemer KHE: Anthropometry of the elderly: status and recommendations, *Hum Factors* 32:571-595, 1990.
5. Lewis M: Surprising growth in US forecast by Census data: the population explosion is hitting closer to home, *San Jose Mercury News,* p 1A, December 4, 1992.
6. Lewis M: Labor force transformed by women's growing needs, *San Jose Mercury News,* p 1A, May 17, 1992.
7. Li S, Xi Z: The measurement of functional arm reach envelopes for young Chinese males, *Ergonomics* 33:967-978, 1990.
8. Mebarki B, Davis BT: Anthropometry of Algerian women, *Ergonomics* 33:1537-1547, 1990.
9. Morse L, Hinds LJ: Women and ergonomics, *Occupational medicine state of the art reviews* 8(4): 721-732, 1993.
10. Ong CH et al: Anthropometrics and display station preferences of VDU operators, *Ergonomics* 31:337-347, 1988.
11. Salvendy E: *Handbook of human factors,* New York, 1987, Wiley & Sons.
12. Young JW et al: Anthropometric and mass distribution characteristics of the adult female, Georgia Air Force Base, Calif, 1983.

36 Vocational Rehabilitation and the Injured Worker

Work is more than a means for earning a salary. Injured workers, separated from the workplace for physical or cognitive impairment, must adjust not only to financial obligations but also to fears of dependency, medical procedures, hospitalization, and family difficulties. Through impairment, workers fear losing not only a job but also a part of themselves as they believe their family, friends, and society define them. (Demore-Taber and Cohen-Siskind, 1990.)

OVERVIEW

An employee injured on the job and placed on workers' compensation disability leave may face with her family an immediate loss of income and disrupting changes in routine, in addition to the possibility of long-term losses. For the first time, the worker may have to deal with an insurance company, lawyers, doctors, and situations about which she may know nothing and over which she seems to have little control. For some people, being injured will become a central issue in life; for some, injury will involve only medical treatment; for others it will require adjusting to a new way of working.

In the first few days and weeks after the injury, it makes sense that everyone—the insurance carrier, the doctor, the worker, and the family—will be preoccupied with the medical treatment. The issue of return to work may not even surface until the medical condition has stabilized. At that time, the doctor is expected to state when, or even whether, the person will be able to return to work. When it seems clear that the only option open is a new job, the worker may be referred for vocational rehabilitation counseling. By then, it may be too late.

If we are to reduce the number of persons whose work-connected injuries become lifetime handicaps, return to work must become a central part of the medical treatment plan, and vocational counseling must address return to work issues early in the course.

Otis Byrd, a California rehabilitation consultant for the rehabilitation unit of the Division of Work-

ers' Compensation Office of Benefits Determination states that physicians have a critical, clear role in determining and documenting the medical restrictions of the worker's injury. The doctor's responsibility is to describe precisely how the worker's injury precludes her from previous duties; this is the keystone to legal eligibility for vocational rehabilitation counseling. The doctor can also be the linchpin in early assessment, creative planning, and effective mobilization of resources. Mr. Byrd also stated that doctors who include specific ideas for accommodations give his office the leverage to approach employers. This chapter is intended to provide some of the practical skills required to fulfill these responsibilities.

This chapter begins by defining vocational rehabilitation in the context of the workers' compensation system—its history and basic services. Next, the chapter describes the vocational rehabilitation counseling process from referral through placement. Two ideas are stressed: vocational rehabilitation is not solely an issue of retraining; and successful vocational rehabilitation requires a variety of professional services aimed at understanding the job and at delineating the worker's assets, liabilities, and the vocational alternatives. The chapter then concludes with case studies that will illustrate these ideas.

Vocational rehabilitation counseling is an important adjunct to the treatment of injured workers. Occupational medicine emphasizes the provision of service designed to prevent work hazards and maintain the health of the worker at work. Occupational health is really about maximizing worker safety and minimizing work injury/illness. Practitioners will find that an understanding of vocational rehabilitation can be useful to the reinstatement of any injured worker, not just to those covered by workers' compensation benefits. Because 1992 legislation (the American Disabilities Act, or ADA) has added new employer responsibilities in the accommodation of the disabled and because non–work-related medical conditions can

519

also disable workers, return-to-work planning and assessment measures may soon be essential features of any comprehensive employee health care service.

VOCATIONAL REHABILITATION COUNSELING AND WORKERS' COMPENSATION

Society's willingness at any point in time to attend to the needs of the disabled was greatly determined by the perceived cause of the disability, the prevailing economic conditions, and the existing medical knowledge (Rubin and Roessler, 1978).

The history of vocational rehabilitation services

As has been true in other medical specialties, rehabilitation services have usually experienced the greatest periods of growth and innovation after a major war. After World War I, for example, technology and interest combined with the advent of the federal income tax to create the funding for vocational rehabilitation services, first to veterans and later to civilians (Rubin and Roessler, 1978; Levitan and Taggart, 1982). By 1929, all but four states had established vocational rehabilitation services (Rubin and Roessler); by 1954, state vocational rehabilitation agencies had been established in their present form. For the next 20 years, an expanding network of similar-appearing agencies with national eligibility and service standards provided for the employment needs of congenitally and adventitiously disabled adults (Rubin and Roessler, 1978; Bitter, 1979).

In the 1970s, a combination of large numbers of returning disabled Vietnam veterans and a new self-advocacy movement among people with severe disabilities helped create a shift toward serving a more severely disabled population. Legislation was introduced mandating wheelchair accessibility to public buildings (Bitter, 1979). The concept of "reasonable accommodation," the idea that people with physical and mental disabilities must have equal access to the employment mainstream, became part of the national vocabulary and part of advocates' demands. The first Center for Independent Living was organized in California by Ed Roberts, who is severely disabled himself. This self-advocacy group worked to secure the same civil rights protection for people with disabilities that other minorities were demanding. For the first time, disabled people became actively involved in setting their own service needs. Centers staffed by and for disabled people appeared all over the country. Whatever changes took place in the grassroots movement, the legacy of self-advocacy remains. What began as a "field . . . created, shaped, and subsidized primarily by federal mandates and appropriations designed to assist handicapped Americans to return to work," (Matkin, 1985) had been expanded by the demands of people with disabilities to include equal participation in the planning and provision of services.

The history of workers' compensation

Western industrialization developed in an atmosphere of laissez-faire government that did not believe in interfering in worksite safety, protection, medical remediation, or compensation for injuries. Evidence of the extremely dangerous conditions in the coal mines and on the railroads prompted the first federal standards for industrial safety (Nagi, 1970; Weeks, 1991; Corn, 1989; President's Commission on Coal, 1980).

The notion that injured workers should receive financial reimbursement or rehabilitation is entirely modern. Rubin and Roessler noted that the first "workmen's" compensation law in the United States was passed in New York in 1910; these early laws made no provision for vocational rehabilitation services. Initially, compensation for job-connected injuries and salary loss required proof of employer negligence, but this soon changed. "Some identify the deep concern felt by liberals who saw bodies maimed and deaths occurring with no income replacement while the tort process worked its way through the courts, as the significant impetus to passage of the first 'no fault' legislation," (Akabas, 1987). At present, workers' compensation insurance is a no-fault program: neither the injured worker nor the employer is required to prove that the injury occurred because of the fault of one of the parties. (Refer to Chapter 2 for further discussion of workers' compensation.)

In 1975, California enacted the first mandatory vocational rehabilitation counseling service in the United States for injured workers (Deneen and Hessellund, 1986). All states continue to provide vocational rehabilitation counseling services through public agencies, but each state has defined its own workers' compensation practices. Therefore, the benefit amounts, claims procedures, and the eligibility or provisions for vocational rehabilitation will vary (Rothstein, 1990). The New York state statute mandates only medical rehabilitation and, in the opinion of one commentator, contains "no incentives, but numerous disincentives, to undertake or provide rehabilitation," (Freireich, 1987).

Workers' compensation and vocational rehabilitation counseling

The role of the rehabilitation counselor, in the context of the workers' compensation system includes all the basic duties described by Rubin and Roessler: "(1) case finding, (2) intake, (3) diagnosis, (4) eligibility determination, (5) plan development and completion, (6) service provision, (7) placement and follow-up, and (8) post-employment services . . . [which] require the rehabilitation counselor to have a knowledge of the rehabilitation process, as well as counseling, evaluation, decision making, service provision, monitoring, and placement skills."

For the purpose of this discussion, vocational rehabilitation counseling may be defined as "the coordinated activity that is (1) directed toward an individual with a chronic or permanent functional limitation or disability, (2) intended to restore an individual's working or functional capacity to its maximum, and (3) includes measures aimed at developing an individual's own resources or removing obstacles imposed by the environment," (Javikoski and Lahelma, 1980). Counseling concentrates on identifying and supporting individual strengths and on preparing the individual for active participation in the recovery process; both activities are required for successful rehabilitation.

In this kind of counseling, as in other professional relationships concerned with change, success depends on the trust and confidence established between the parties. But during rehabilitation problems occur that may have nothing directly to do with the counseling relationship. It is important to remember that the worker comes to her injury status with a fully developed extra-employment life that can complicate and obfuscate recovery. "Unfortunately, it is becoming increasingly more common for the worker's recovery from a seemingly uncomplicated condition to be inexplicably lengthy. The evaluating physician (and the counselor) may be stymied, unable to apply medical explanations to psychosocial vocational problems. Marital difficulties, drug dependency, job dissatisfaction, and other matters can masquerade as medical problems that do not improve," (Scheer, 1990). Further complications can arise from the workers' compensation process in the form of questions about the legitimacy of the claim or the injuries. The injured worker functions in an ironic legal and social bind. "On the one hand [disabled workers] need to believe in the seriousness of their limitations in order to maximize chances and amount of benefits, while on the other hand they are expected to focus more on their residual capacities and cooperate with rehabilitation efforts," (Nagi, 1970). The workers' compensation system, because of its antagonistic nature, often makes unnecessary adversaries of management and employee. The injury claim can become both a symbol and a red flag for other problems. It is often necessary to separate some of these issues and deal with them before the employee can make any progress toward returning to work.

There are many important issues in vocational rehabilitation counseling, but the two basic principles are as follows: (1) successful rehabilitation requires the active participation of the injured worker, and (2) the timing of the return to work is critical. The first principle is a basic tenet of any counseling: no counselor can make any client successful. The skills of the most competent counselor can not counterbalance the lack of commitment from a disheartened, alienated, or disinterested client. No rehabilitation plan, no matter how logical or well-considered, will succeed if the client is not involved in the selection of the vocational goal and in the negotiation of the plan's details. There is no quicker way to infantilize an adult than to exclude her from decision-making; there is no surer way to guarantee that the plan will be sabotaged than to have the counselor plan everything for the client.

This is a deceptively simple principle: everyone—the worker, the doctor, the family, the insurance company, even the counselor—will tend to defer to the professional. But under no circumstances should vocational planning be something that happens to a client. Even if the counselor is capable of making a quicker, more efficient decision, the client must make her own choices to acquire the problem-solving skills that can serve future job-seeking needs. The client's task is to remain active—to visit schools, talk to people, take in and evaluate information, read, or, if necessary, be read to. The greater the client's active involvement in the plan's development, the greater the commitment to making the plan work.

The second principle is just as simple—the sooner an individual returns to work, the greater the likelihood of successful rehabilitation. Those workers who are less seriously injured and/or can be accommodated by their previous employers will have the fewest problems resuming their normal routine. It is important, however, for every injured person to be out of work for as short a time as possible. As will be discussed later, a lengthy hiatus can be associated with depression, loss of role status, a troubling preoccupation with the medical condition, and an alienation from the world of work.

Timing and involvement of the client are related to successful outcomes because of the social context in which the constructs of work and disability are embedded. In a country that places considerable emphasis on the achievement of the individual, irrespective of background or circumstance, being out of work means that something is wrong with you. Income is only part of the motivation to work (Rusk, 1971); occupation defines socioeconomic status for researchers (Kitagawa and Hauser, 1973; Hay, 1988; Winkleby et al, 1992) as well as for the lay public. When work is a critical part of one's identity, loss of work becomes synonymous with loss of self. This loss may be particularly marked in families that assign work and status along traditional gender lines. Able-bodied people who lose their jobs because they are laid off or fired can become depressed when they remain unemployed for an extended time. As their time away from work extends, they may delay seeking work. People injured on the job can have the same problems, but situations are more complicated: there is a medical problem, a legitimate reason for not seeking work.

The maintenance of the disability can become a separate barrier to returning to work. Having the outward signs of a medical condition—a cast, a neckbrace, a wheelchair, or a surgical scar—can legitimize the disabled worker's complaints. But the injured worker who has no such visible evidence, or whose disability becomes protracted, may find it difficult to continue convincing others of a legitimate basis for pain and inactivity. In some cases, the lack of support from family and friends will persuade the injured worker to return to work. In some instances, the worker's symptoms will become more intractable the less she is believed.

The danger in attempting to legitimize the injury is that the harder the injured person works to prove she is disabled, the less she will try to do; the lower the activity level, the longer the person will be out of work; the longer the time the person is away from work, the less the chance she has of ever returning. The physician's assertions that the injured worker is ready to return to work may be greeted with reluctant compliance: "I'll go back . . . I'm not sure I'll be able to do it, but I'll try." This kind of statement must be taken seriously and regarded as an early warning that the person is in need of thoughtful intervention.

There are several other early warning signs that problems may be developing. One is decreased contact with the former job site or the supervisor. Other early indicators are an absence of any activities that might be a precursor to work—volunteer work, informational job interviews, visiting schools, library research, reading the want ads, networking with friends and relatives, or even talking about ideas for future job possibilities. People may make the medical condition their career. Days are recalled in terms of doctors' appointments. Responses to questions about returning to work are characterized by phrases such as, "I've decided not to think about that until I am well," or "I won't know what I can do until you tell me," or "I haven't thought about that," or "I'll

wait until the doctor tells me I can work." In our experience, these comments should indicate to the practitioner that the injured person is seriously distant from her own recovery process.

The most serious problems occur when an injured worker and her friends and family begin to show inappropriate signs of accommodating the disabled status. The accommodation may be displayed in new habits formed around the medical condition, such as changes in the assignment of chores. The change will be most striking when the person's role in the family becomes significantly altered—when activities such as discipline or decision-making are reassigned to other family members.

These changes can be accompanied by the uninjured spouse's enabling behavior that can compromise any plan for rehabilitation. A special bed or chair may be purchased, excessive medication or alcohol use may be justified. Structural changes in the family system, such as a spouse assuming new responsibilities for providing and managing the family's income, can be a sign that the disabled behavior is becoming entrenched. If the new accommodations also help the injured worker avoid uncomfortable situations or provide a source of special attention or sympathy, the medical condition is supplying a secondary gain. If that happens, rehabilitation becomes extremely difficult, if not impossible.

In considering the social context of rehabilitation and recovery, it is important to note that the relationship between the worker and the supervisor plays a critical role. Often the behavior that follows the on-the-job injury reflects and summarizes the dynamics already present in that relationship. The injury may be just the tip of unresolved work-connected issues: the worker and her supervisor may have been having difficulties for some time, and the injury may be a way out for both of them. The injury may even be the result of that conflict. It is interesting to note that some of the most complicated recoveries have occurred for employees with histories of excessive absenteeism and/or job performance problems at the time of the injury. Their difficulties may not become clear until the supervisor refuses to have the employee return to work, or until the employee's protracted disability continues beyond the expected time frame. This is not to imply that the relationship between employer and employee is always a causal factor. The problems present may be associated with other work issues, such as the worker's difficulty with authority, a specific employment practice, inappropriate company policy, or an unsafe or frustrating working situation. Nevertheless, this relationship is a rich source of explanatory material and must be examined for sources of conflict or facilitation.

The earlier the physician poses questions about the injured worker's job, relationships with family and employer, typical day, or about future vocational plans, the sooner problems can be identified. The sooner these issues are clarified, the sooner problems can be dealt with. Typically, the patient will turn to the physician for guidance and reassurance. In the context of their relationship, the doctor may find that the injured worker will be willing to discuss these potential problems. But it is also important for the treating doctor to know she need not be alone in dealing with these problems. Rehabilitation is, by definition, the sum effort of many different health professionals.

Vocational rehabilitation counseling of injured workers

Step 1: Referral to the vocational rehabilitation counselor

Once the worker has been injured how does she usually get referred to a counselor? Unfortunately, there is a paucity of written literature on the procedures used by various state workers' compensations systems (Byrd, 1993). According to Deneen and Hessellund, most vocational rehabilitation referrals are made by the insurance carrier working in concert with the injured worker's attorney, if the worker is represented. In some states, legal regulations cover the timeframe for notifying the injured worker of the vocational rehabilitation benefit. Furthermore, regulations may set similar time guidelines for the physician who is being asked to determine, on the basis of a description of the job duties, whether the injured worker qualifies for vocational rehabilitation services. The specific time standards may vary by state, but the physician's written judgement of the worker's functional abilities and limitations remains key to initiating the referral process.

Step 2: Evaluating the injured worker

A. Establishing eligibility. As the first state to mandate vocational rehabilitation services, California uses the following criteria to determine eligibility for vocational rehabilitation: "(1) When the effects of the injury, whether or not combined with the effects of a prior injury or disability, permanently prevent the worker from engaging in either a usual and customary occupation, or in engaging in the position in which he/she was employed at the time of the injury, and (2) if the injured worker can be reasonably expected to benefit from a rehabilitation program," (Deneen and Hessellund, 1986). These are general criteria, however, drawn from the federal requirements for state vocational rehabilitation agencies. Any practitioner whose patients are referred directly to the state agency will encounter these same eligibility criteria.

In addition to documenting the client's medical condition and describing the ways in which the condition is a barrier to returning to work, rehabilitation counselors have a primary responsibility for determining whether the disabled person is capable of using services to return to work. This last factor, sometimes referred to as feasibility, may be the most important part of determining eligibility. This is also the criterion for which it is most difficult to establish clear-cut, objective standards. Sometimes when counselors refer to a person as "feasible" or "nonfeasible," they are giving an opinion about the client's readiness to accept counseling. The term is sometimes used to justify the decision not to work with a difficult or complicated client. In general, this term is used to cover issues connected with motivation to return to work (Deneen and Hessellund, 1986). Even though feasibility is an elusive term to define, a competent counselor will be able to explain the basis for the decision regarding a client's eligibility.

B. Evaluating background. Just as the social worker is concerned with the social systems in which the clients function, the rehabilitation counselor's concern is to examine the vocational systems in which the clients have participated and the roles the clients have assumed in those systems. The educational and employment history provides an information-rich context and the most accurate source for predicting future behavior (McGowan and Porter, 1967; Scheer, 1990). The goal of the initial evaluative sessions is to provide a personal profile of assets, skills, and liabilities. In addition to collecting the details about job titles, dates of employment, employers' names, skills learned, and training experiences, the counselor is concerned with the implications of the history. What does the overall work-seeking pattern reveal about the client: has she proactively sought out new jobs that were increasingly demanding, as opposed to taking whatever has come along? What does the length and breadth of past job situations tell about the client's stability, ability to get along with others, ability to learn on the job, and so on? What was the client's experience with education and training? Will this client expect to be challenged or intimidated by a training program? What evidence does the employment and educational history provide of transferrable skills? Responsibility taking? Supervising others? What does the history suggest about problem-solving experiences and/or predict for the present set of problems? What other personal assets—family support, personal strengths, interests, hobbies—does the person bring to a process aimed at returning to work?

C. Evaluation of capacities. The timing of the evaluation of an injured worker's capacity is often linked to the stability of the medical condition (Thomas, 1990). Although medical stability can help guide the timing of a referral, it cannot be the only criterion used. Even if an evaluation does not indicate the client's full functional potential, it may provide necessary encouragement and confidence; in some cases, evaluation may be used to "establish the need for rehabilitation, training or reasonable accommodations," (Wickstrom, 1990).

Evaluation can, certainly, occur prematurely and, with some clients, contribute to the perception that return to work is impossible. This may be avoided by discussing plans with the worker before the referral is made. The discussion should include a full description of what will occur, including the action that will be taken if some part of the evaluation proves too difficult for the worker to complete. The worker must have a clear understanding of the purpose and content of the evaluation, and of the options and control she can expect. As in other parts of the return-to-work process, the client can either facilitate or sabotage the objectives. Adults are less likely to sabotage plans when they understand the purpose and have agreed to participate.

The goal of any vocational evaluation is to collect information that will allow the development of an appropriate rehabilitation plan. The information can be general: profiling overall vocational interests and aptitudes, determining functional capacities including physical issues such as sitting, standing, weight-handling, body mechanics, and cognitive skills such as concentration, interpersonal skills, ability to take directions, and so on. It can also be used to assess the physical and mental requirements of a particular job choice.

Evaluations are usually performed by trained experts—occupational/physical therapists, ergonomists, and certified vocational evaluators—with highly sophisticated equipment. Depending on the practitioner's proximity to a major market center, these services may be provided in a hospital, at a site such as a Salvation Army or Easter Seal center, or in a private clinic. Depending on the practitioner's setting and resources, it may be appropriate to organize one's own evaluation service. The equipment and materials to be described can be purchased and/or developed by most rehabilitation teams. An evaluator must be capable of safely and formally addressing the questions formulated by the doctor, the worker, the insurance company, and/or worker's representative regarding the capabilities and limitations of the injured worker. Such questions could include the following:

- Can the worker perform all the specified physical demands of the former position? Which tasks continue to present problems? Can this performance be improved? What kinds of assistive device or work reorganization would make it possible for the worker to return to that job?
- Does the worker have the specific aptitudes and/or abilities to pursue a selected vocational direction? What about the physical endurance to tolerate a training situation? What accommodations would make it possible for the worker to succeed in such an employment situation?

The following are brief descriptions of vocational evaluation methods that practitioners have found useful. These evaluations can be brief (hours) or lengthy (days) depending on the complexity of the case and the questions that need to be answered.

Job analysis. A well-done job analysis can be used as an evaluative tool (see Figure 36-1). If done correctly, a job analysis provides a detailed description of the physical and mental demands of a specific position. It would also provide a description of the work setting and of any equipment that is customarily used to perform the job. The job analysis should permit the physician to decide whether the worker will be able to return to a specific job; and it should permit the worker, doctor, attorney, insurance company, rehabilitation therapist, and the employer to consider the options for work hardening and/or accommodation.

A job analysis can be adequately completed by a variety of trained rehabilitation professionals, including rehabilitation counselors. In our experience, occupational therapists, by training and perspective, are well equipped to look at the present job situation, collect accurate information, and plan appropriate reorganization and/or accommodation measures. A well-trained ergonomist may have similar skills.

Functional capacity evaluation: This evaluation is generally used to provide details about the physical activities the injured worker can safely tolerate. Because of the potential danger to the worker, this evaluation should only be done under the close supervision of a trained medical professional. This professional should discuss the nature of the injury with the treating doctor and preclude the client from activities that would exacerbate the injury. A rehabilitation counselor may be a useful consultant, particularly in framing the questions to be addressed during the evaluation. In our experience, occupational therapists, especially those who have received specialized work evaluation training, bring highly appropriate professional backgrounds and skills to these assessments. Their awareness of the world of work combined with their training in the physical and mental dimensions of disability make them qualified to evaluate and teach injured workers.

Work-hardening. When an evaluation must be more than a snapshot of current competencies, and when the purpose is to assess whether current levels of functioning can be improved over time, work-hardening may be implemented. Like the functional capacity evaluation, work-hardening requires close careful supervision by a trained health professional. In our experience, both occupational and physical therapists are skilled at using medical information to break down a goal into appropriate, progressively more demanding steps aimed at increasing strength and endurance. Work-hardening activities present the perfect opportunity to correct the worker's body mechanics and decrease the chances of reinjury.

Situational assessments. A more specific use of ongoing evaluation is the situational assessment. These assessments involve placing the injured worker on an actual job assignment or in a structured testing situation set up to closely resemble the actual job, or in some combination of these two situations. This kind of assessment can offer a low-risk way to evaluate the worker's ability to handle a particular job, job setting, or family of job skills. Again, it should be closely supervised by a health professional who can set appropriate limits. The realistic aspects of the situation can provide the worker with an opportunity to try out a job without prejudicing a future employer with trial-and-error learning.

Work sample testing. Another example of this approach to work-oriented evaluation involves isolating and reproducing job tasks. Work sample tests may require the individual to assemble small objects, add columns of numbers, categorize or organize materials. The tests may be normed to permit comparisons of the injured worker's performance. Caution should be exercised in studying these scores, however, and it is reasonable to ask for information on the population with whom the injured worker is being compared. This kind of evaluation may be effectively performed by a certified evaluator or by an occupational therapist. It is possible to set up work samples and use local groups and one's own experience to evaluate individual scores. Work sample testing can provide a broad-spectrum evaluation of the injured worker's skills and abilities.

Ability, aptitude, and interest training. Another approach to skills assessment comes from paper and pencil tests: ability testing defines the client's present skills levels; aptitude testing describes special and/or potential skills that can be developed with further training; and interest testing helps to describe the patterns of vocational preferences. Testing can provide suggestions for further vocational exploration. The advantages of the use of standardized tests are obvious: the tests provide an objective means of measuring the client's competence, as well as placing the score in an appropriate comparative context. Some tests, for example, have norms that allow the counselor to compare the client's performance with people already successfully employed in the occupation under consideration. Because of the reliability and validity of some tests, scores can be used to justify a specific vocational plan. The decision to use paper and pencil tests should be based on a number of factors, including the client's reading level, the vocational goals being considered, the client's past educational attainments, and the client's interests and informational needs. A client with a junior high school education and a manual work history, for example, may do better in a work sample or situational assessment situation. A client with a high school education, demonstrated skills in supervision, and an interest in further training may make effective use of paper and pencil tests.

All tests have limitations. Even when a test is standardized, the norms may provide an inappropriate comparison group. Tests can be culture-bound depending on how the tests were standardized, and the norms can give an inaccurate picture — either inflated or unnecessarily pessimistic — of the client's potential. It is critical, therefore, that the population norms be explicated and that their applicability in the specific case be justified. In addition, some injured workers will perform poorly in this kind of testing situation, no matter how well prepared or skilled, because of previous bad testing experiences or nervousness. For these workers, paper and pencil testing raises unnecessary anxiety and provides an inadequate picture of capacity. Furthermore, paper and pencil testing rarely shows a totally unexpected skill; clients (and sometimes their attorneys, families, or physicians) may hold the unrealistic expectation that these tests will supply the best answer. Tests are tools to be used judiciously and only in conjunction with ongoing counseling, triangulated with other information. A good rehabilitation plan includes *all* the data that support a vocational decision, not just the paper and pencil testing results. Tests are static instruments; although some are much better than others, they can become outdated. Even at best, tests have the disadvantage of providing a one-shot, laboratory assessment.

INSTRUCTIONS: Accurate information regarding job requirements is necessary to provide safe work assignments for employees. Please complete this form, consulting with employees if necessary, and return to Human Resources, 0000 Main Street, Attn: Mary Jones. Your additional comments will be helpful.

Department/Location/Cost Center/Employee Name	Direct Supervisor

Job Title and Code	I Full-time [ ] Part-time [ ] Per Diem [ ] Temp [ ]

Status Exempt [ ] Non-Exempt [ ]	Shift: Days [ ] Eve [ ] Night [ ] Rotating [ ]

Overtime /wk (hours):
0–5 [ ]   5–10 [ ]   10–20 [ ]   20+ [ ]   Scheduled Hours _____

Description of essential functions:

Check the appropriate entry for each of the following items to describe the extent of the specific activities performed by this position:

N = Never   R = Rarely (1–2 hours/day)   O = Occasionally (3–4 hours/day)
F = Frequently (5–6 hours/day)   A = Always (7–8 hours/day)

	N	R	O	F	A		N	R	O	F	A
1. Sitting	[ ]	[ ]	[ ]	[ ]	[ ]	15. Grasping:					
2. Standing	[ ]	[ ]	[ ]	[ ]	[ ]						
3. Walking	[ ]	[ ]	[ ]	[ ]	[ ]	A. Simple/Light					
4. Bending over	[ ]	[ ]	[ ]	[ ]	[ ]						
5. Crawling	[ ]	[ ]	[ ]	[ ]	[ ]	1. Right only	[ ]	[ ]	[ ]	[ ]	[ ]
6. Climbing	[ ]	[ ]	[ ]	[ ]	[ ]	2. Left only	[ ]	[ ]	[ ]	[ ]	[ ]
7. Reaching overhead	[ ]	[ ]	[ ]	[ ]	[ ]	3. Both	[ ]	[ ]	[ ]	[ ]	[ ]
8. Crouching	[ ]	[ ]	[ ]	[ ]	[ ]						
9. Kneeling	[ ]	[ ]	[ ]	[ ]	[ ]	B. Firm/Strong					
10. Balancing	[ ]	[ ]	[ ]	[ ]	[ ]						
11. Pushing or pulling:						1. Right only	[ ]	[ ]	[ ]	[ ]	[ ]
a) 10 lbs or less	[ ]	[ ]	[ ]	[ ]	[ ]	2. Left only	[ ]	[ ]	[ ]	[ ]	[ ]
b) 11–25 lbs	[ ]	[ ]	[ ]	[ ]	[ ]	3. Both	[ ]	[ ]	[ ]	[ ]	[ ]
c) 26–50 lbs	[ ]	[ ]	[ ]	[ ]	[ ]						
d) 51–75 lbs*	[ ]	[ ]	[ ]	[ ]	[ ]	16. Fine Dexterity:					
e) 76–100 lbs*	[ ]	[ ]	[ ]	[ ]	[ ]						
f) Over 100 lbs*	[ ]	[ ]	[ ]	[ ]	[ ]	A. Right only	[ ]	[ ]	[ ]	[ ]	[ ]
12. Lifting or carrying:						B. Left only	[ ]	[ ]	[ ]	[ ]	[ ]
a) 10 lbs or less	[ ]	[ ]	[ ]	[ ]	[ ]	C. Both	[ ]	[ ]	[ ]	[ ]	[ ]
b) 11–25 lbs	[ ]	[ ]	[ ]	[ ]	[ ]						
c) 26–50 lbs	[ ]	[ ]	[ ]	[ ]	[ ]	17. Other:					
d) 51–75 lbs*	[ ]	[ ]	[ ]	[ ]	[ ]						
e) 76–100 lbs*	[ ]	[ ]	[ ]	[ ]	[ ]	A. Work 3' above					
f) Over 100 lbs*	[ ]	[ ]	[ ]	[ ]	[ ]	the floor	[ ]	[ ]	[ ]	[ ]	[ ]
13. Repetitive use of foot control:						B. Drives:					
a) Right only	[ ]	[ ]	[ ]	[ ]	[ ]	1. Van	[ ]	[ ]	[ ]	[ ]	[ ]
b) Left only	[ ]	[ ]	[ ]	[ ]	[ ]	2. Truck	[ ]	[ ]	[ ]	[ ]	[ ]
14. Repetitive use of hands:						3. Car	[ ]	[ ]	[ ]	[ ]	[ ]
a) Right only	[ ]	[ ]	[ ]	[ ]	[ ]	* Please use comment section if over 50					
b) Left only	[ ]	[ ]	[ ]	[ ]	[ ]	pounds; specify frequency and objects					
c) Both	[ ]	[ ]	[ ]	[ ]	[ ]	lifted					

Fig. 36-1 The job analysis form is intended to be used as a guide to collect and analyze information relating to job demands.

Visual Requirements	Yes	No		Yes	No
20/50 or better	[ ]	[ ]	Both eyes needed	[ ]	[ ]
Depth perception	[ ]	[ ]	Dept. of Transportation	[ ]	[ ]
Full field of vision	[ ]	[ ]	Shades of colors	[ ]	[ ]

Hearing Requirements	Yes	No		Yes	No
Quiet conversations	[ ]	[ ]	Hearing aid permitted	[ ]	[ ]
Hearing without aid	[ ]	[ ]			

Environmental Factors	Yes	No
Exposure to infectious diseases	[ ]	[ ]
If yes, list mode of exposure: _____		

Medications	Yes	No		Yes	No
Cytotoxins	[ ]	[ ]	Ribavirin	[ ]	[ ]
Pentamidine	[ ]	[ ]	Other: (List)	[ ]	[ ]

Environmental Exposures	Yes	No		Yes	No
Outside	[ ]	[ ]	Radiation	[ ]	[ ]
Outside & inside	[ ]	[ ]	Electricity	[ ]	[ ]
Extreme heat	[ ]	[ ]	Slippery/uneven walking	[ ]	[ ]
Extreme cold	[ ]	[ ]	Moving machinery parts	[ ]	[ ]
Humidity	[ ]	[ ]	Moving vehicles/objects	[ ]	[ ]
Dampness & chilling	[ ]	[ ]	Ladders/scaffolding	[ ]	[ ]
Intermittent noise	[ ]	[ ]	Working below ground	[ ]	[ ]
Constant noise	[ ]	[ ]	Hands in constant water	[ ]	[ ]
Vibrations	[ ]	[ ]	Lasers	[ ]	[ ]
Working alone	[ ]	[ ]			

Substance Exposures	Yes	No		Yes	No
Paints	[ ]	[ ]	Strong acids/alkalines	[ ]	[ ]
Thinners	[ ]	[ ]	Formaldehyde	[ ]	[ ]
Solvents	[ ]	[ ]	Carbon monoxide	[ ]	[ ]
Epoxy	[ ]	[ ]	Cutting oils	[ ]	[ ]
Sand	[ ]	[ ]	Sewage/waste	[ ]	[ ]
Lead	[ ]	[ ]	Dusts	[ ]	[ ]
Asbestos	[ ]	[ ]	Gases/fumes (e.g. ETO)	[ ]	[ ]
Others (List)	[ ]	[ ]	Waste anesthetic, etc.	[ ]	[ ]

Works with VDTs (Video Display Terminals)	Yes	No		Yes	No
Occasionally	[ ]	[ ]	4+ hours/shift	[ ]	[ ]
< 4 hours/shift	[ ]	[ ]	30 hours/week	[ ]	[ ]

Safety Equipment Used	Yes	No	hr/dy		Yes	No	hr/dy
Lead apron	[ ]	[ ]	____	Chemical apron	[ ]	[ ]	____
Surgical mask	[ ]	[ ]	____	Safety glasses/goggles	[ ]	[ ]	____
Hearing	[ ]	[ ]	____	Gloves (type)	[ ]	[ ]	____
Respirator (type)	[ ]	[ ]	____	Other (list)	[ ]	[ ]	____

Comments:

_____

_____

_____

Prepared by: _____   Date: _____

_____   _____
      Department Manager   Telephone #

When a dynamic, interactive evaluation is more appropriate, a situational assessment will supply much of the same information in a more useful form. A standardized test can indicate whether one has the math skills to handle a cash register; a situational assessment can reveal how well the client interacts with customers.

Safety engineer's ergonomic site analysis. Finally, it is important to be able to think about evaluation as a process that exceeds the bounds of a single injury. In instances of repeated injuries, such as multiple cases of cumulative trauma disorders, it may be wiser to look at the safety and engineering aspects of the work than at the rehabilitation of individual workers. A safety engineer's or ergonomist's analysis may permit the prevention of future injuries by identifying the structural sources of unsafe working conditions. Ergonomic changes have been responsible for reducing work-connected injuries in even the most dangerous industries (Robertson, 1975; Weeks et al, 1991; USDHHS, 1992).

In summary, the evaluation phase has two objectives. The first to establish legal eligibility, which requires collecting data from medical records and documenting specific ways in which the medical condition constitutes a barrier to employment. The second objective is to define the client's assets and liabilities, which requires careful assessment of the individual. This includes vocational/educational background; full and objective analysis of the previous job, assessment of the present level of functioning, and assessment of the potential for change. Part of the second objective is to prescribe the appropriate assistive devices or accommodation required to get the person back to work.

Step 3: Developing and writing the rehabilitation plan

Once the evaluative phase of counseling is completed, the counselor and the client work to define the vocational goal and formally delineate the service required to reach that goal. The best rehabilitation plans are often the simplest ones. It is generally believed that the most effective rehabilitation plans involve returning injured workers to jobs that are close to or the same as their preinjury positions (Matkin, 1985). This kind of plan promises the advantages of minimal adjustment and maximum reuse of the client's experience. The second best plan involves the next least level of personal disruption: the worker returns to the same employer but in a different capacity. The third choice retains some stability by transferring a portion of the individual's skills and experience to a new position, with a new employer. The fourth, and least satisfactory choice is retraining. Even with the final and most extreme alternative, the

personal disruption can be minimized by selecting a new occupation that builds on previous skills.

Each plan will have unique aspects because it must reflect the special combination of restrictions, interests, and experiences of each client. Most plans include these common elements:

Modified work/accommodation. The physician may be the key to considering this alternative to retraining, which may be accomplished either as an interim measure (even before the decision must be made to refer the worker for rehabilitation counseling) or as a permanent alteration in the job description. Temporary placements in a modified job can make immediate return to work possible even before full recovery occurs or when immediate accommodations are not possible. Modified work can involve placement in a less physically or mentally demanding job or the temporary elimination of duties from the preinjury job the injured worker cannot perform. Another similar approach, the graded return to work, allows the injured person to begin with a shortened day or work week, building by appropriate increments to full-time employment. Both approaches can make use of the worker's skills while keeping the time out of work to a minimum. More permanent changes in the job structure may require more negotiation. If such permanent changes are necessary, the rehabilitation plan can include the purchase of assistive equipment, special furniture, or even the reorganization of a job that permits the employment or reemployment of the injured worker. These plans work best when a multidisciplinary team, consisting of the doctor, the rehabilitation counselor, occupational and physical therapists, psychologists, and other rehabilitation professionals, work with the employer and the employee.

On-the-job training. On-the-job training (or OJT) has the advantage of allowing the client to demonstrate competency while learning a new skill or expanding existing skills. It also permits work-hardening. It may be organized so that the worker moves through training states completing the apprenticeship by becoming a full-fledged employee of the training employer. This kind of plan has advantages for the worker and the potential employer: both are allowed to evaluate the other in a situation with prestructured performance standards. A plan that uses this training method would need to delineate the fees and salaries (specifically dealing with how the worker's benefits will be affected, if at all), external/adjunctive training, the amount of supervision that will be provided, and the timeframe for the OJT. As much as possible, expectations about what will follow the OJT should be directly addressed in the plan. Any mix-up on this issue could significantly undermine the counseling, as well as the employee/employer, relationship.

Direct job placement. In the case of an injured worker whose skills remain largely intact after the injury, direct job development/placement may be the best plan. The services will include all the elements that are essential to any appropriate plan: justification of the specific vocational goal (in this case, minimally supported by a labor market survey that defines the local potential for successful placement) and detailed descriptions of the kinds of support services that will be provided to ensure a positive outcome. In a direct job placement plan, such services could include training in job-seeking skills, resume writing, job interviewing techniques, and the provision of a job-seeking support group and/or supportive counseling.

Formal training programs. In the event that training will occur in a formal educational setting, whether a vocational school, junior college, university, or private school, the plan is usually justified by a combination of information from testing, a labor market survey, and data from the worker's background. In addition, the plan should discuss why this particular school was chosen, including the background of school and faculty, placement rate and/or school reputation. Availability of training programs will influence the choices, but counselors may also find that a combination of formal training and OJT can overcome local curricula limitations.

Decisions about plans are generally based on the individual client's needs and interests balanced against the local employment situation. For some clients the best choice will be retraining for an entirely new career, even though that alternative can be the most disruptive. Disruption may be a minor issue compared with the drawbacks of returning the employee to a work situation that is intolerable. In short, there are many different options to consider and no preordained rules should be applied to injured people in a wholesale fashion. The rehabilitation plan must make sense in the context of the specific skills, background, and medical condition of the injured worker.

According to the California regulations governing workers' compensation, a vocational rehabilitation plan is the "written description of and rationale for the manner and means by which it is proposed a[n] . . . injured worker may be provided the opportunity to return to suitable employment. The plan may contemplate modification of the employee's occupation at the time of injury, provision for alternative work with the same employer, direct job placement assistance, on-the-job training, retraining, job placement assistance or self-employment," (Workers' Compensation Laws of California, 1993). But the plan is not only a summary of services; it is a written agreement of the goals set in counseling:

> In many ways analogous to a business contract, the rehabilitation plan identifies the vocational goals, the vocational specialist's responsibility in achieving those goals, and the roles of the client and outside providers (e.g., private rehabilitation nurse, attorney, other vocational counselor), and the treatment team. Furthermore, the rehabilitation plan outlines the rehabilitation process with objectives and time frames. . . . The counselor . . . reviews the plan with the client, giving the client an opportunity to question the plan, to assess what it requires, and to modify the overall vocational plan if the client is uncomfortable with it" (Demore-Taber and Cohen-Siskind, 1990).

The resemblance of the rehabilitation plan to a business contract ends at its inability to legally bind the signing parties. Rather, it is an effort to spell out services and responsibilities of all parties to minimize miscommunications, assumptions, and unrealistic expectations. Such difficulties can arise in any interaction. In a counseling process securely tied to legal, financial, and medical benefits, it is essential that the process be as explicit and agreed on as possible. If misunderstandings should develop, the rehabilitation plan can be consulted. It should contain sufficient detail to permit resolution of these misunderstandings. It must be a collaborative effort to accomplish this purpose. The client should be given time to read and consider the plan fully, to consult with her attorney if the client is so represented, and to consult with a spouse or other family members/partners, or friends, if so desired. The rehabilitation plan is, finally, a working compromise that must represent the best, real chance of helping the injured worker return to work.

Step 4: Placement and follow-up

In workers' compensation, as in any rehabilitation counseling process, the overall goal of the plan is "always to return the injured worker to a level of functioning that is as close as possible to his or her previous level of functioning, as well as to jobs that will yield the workers' pre-injury income," (Demore-Taber and Cohen-Siskind, 1990). As noted previously, a rehabilitation plan can focus exclusively on direct placement, or placement services may be part of a more elaborate rehabilitation plan. Within the workers' compensation system, it is not unusual for placement activities to be the responsibility of a specialist. Sometimes this individual will provide the same services as an employment agency—lining up job interviews, following up to see how the client fared, using contacts to secure positions for clients. It bears repeating that this is an efficient method of securing a job; but to the greatest degree possible, the client must be involved in direct job-seeking activities in the same way, and with the same benefits, as in other aspects of the counseling process. Placement is not the last step:

Follow-up, our final classification of the services in the vocational rehabilitation process, refers to the counselor's activity in assisting the client to deal successfully with job problems. This may require counseling sessions with the client concerning relationships with supervisors and fellow employees, job performance and job satisfaction, need for further training, social and recreational needs, housing and transportation. Follow-up may also include contact with employers, a service that can be effective in clarifying and resolving job problems" (Rusk, 1971).

Timeframes for follow-up will vary by state, but, in general, follow-up will represent the completion of services provided for the injured worker. The final success of the entire plan may depend on how thoughtfully this final step is executed.

CONCLUSION

The basic purpose of this chapter is to provide the practitioner with information about rehabilitation services that can be used to assist injured workers in a sensible return to work. The doctor, who has a critical role in this process, can draw on the expertise of a variety of other resources, including the injured worker, to fulfill the legal and medical responsibilities. The services described here should prompt the practitioner to two actions: early questioning and early referral.

CASE STUDIES
Case 1

A 58-year-old man, whose job involved shaving and weighing patients before surgery, had worked for his employer for over 28 years when he sustained a back injury. Proud of his past job performance, he was afraid he was no longer capable of the same work standards. He had several significant vocational handicaps that complicated his rehabilitation: limited educational background (sixth grade in his native country of Nicaragua), limited English language skills (his reading and writing skills were only rudimentary in both English and Spanish), and limited employment experience. He had no real interest in working anywhere else; with his length of service and expectation of retirement in the near future, it made little sense to consider retraining or direct placement with another employer. On the positive side, he had an excellent relationship with his employer: he had been a highly dependable employee, and his employer was willing to retain him in his position if assured it would be safe to do so.

Once his condition stabilized, his physician had questions about whether he could continue in the same job. First, the physician requested the occupational therapist to do a job analysis. This analysis showed that the most serious preclusion was pushing and pulling an antiquated, heavy bedside scale that was difficult to maneuver. As part of the job analysis, the occupational thera-

pist investigated alternative equipment; newer, lighter, and more manageable versions of the bedside scale proved to be readily available. The physician then determined that only with new equipment could he continue in his present job. This information was communicated to the insurance carrier, who assigned a rehabilitation counselor. The rehabilitation counselor worked with the employer and the carrier to purchase the necessary equipment. The patient was then taught how to use the new equipment and how to avoid further injury. In the end, his rehabilitation plan involved a simple accommodation—the purchase of a modern piece of equipment. This purchase allowed him to continue working uninjured until retirement and allowed the hospital to gain and use equipment that would not endanger another employee.

Case 2

A 40-year-old woman had an AA degree in nursing and a disabling back injury that her physician had determined would preclude her from doing heavy lifting, thereby preventing her return to bedside nursing. Although she had advanced educational training, her experiences in school had not been positive, and she was not interested in further formal training. She had, however, a stable and diverse nursing background. Early in her medical treatment, her physician was fairly certain she would be precluded from returning to bedside nursing but was not sure what kind of work would be more appropriate. Because of her similar concern, the patient expressed interest in transferring to another position that would use her medical expertise. She investigated several work areas at her employment site and finally decided she was interested in the work of the quality assurance unit. Her physician was impressed by her initiative. He ordered a functional capacity evaluation that revealed that it was unsafe for her to handle more than 25 pounds of weight, but that her general endurance, sitting, standing, walking, and handling capacities were all within normal limits. She tolerated the evaluation well and was described by the occupational therapist as well organized, calm, dependable, and cooperative.

By this time, her medical condition had stabilized and her physician made the determination that she was unable to return to her usual and customary job. He communicated this information to her insurance carrier, who assigned a rehabilitation counselor to work with her. The counselor completed and returned a detailed job analysis for a position in the quality assurance section. Based on the job analysis, the physician was able to give his opinion that this new work area was well within the patient's functional capacities.

She and her counselor designed an OJT situation. The plan formally required that she return to her previous employer as a trainee for 6 months, during which time it was expected that she would receive direct, supervised experience in all the aspects of quality assurance. It was understood that the hospital could offer her a job at the end of training, but no specific commitments were made by either party.

The patient was successful in her OJT. At the end of the 6 months, she found a position at another local *hospital. She continued to meet with the counselor until it was clear that she had made a successful transition into her new occupation.*

Case 3

A 35 year-old janitor complained to his personal physician that he was having problems physically performing his job duties. He specifically cited difficulties using heavy, unwieldy equipment to strip the wax from floors. He requested that the doctor take him off this job and help him find something less physically demanding.

Initially, the doctor was understandably concerned about the patient's ability to perform his regular job duties. From the description, it appeared that these duties could cause future difficulties even if he was capable of performing them for the present. Before making her recommendations, however, the doctor sought additional information. She requested a job analysis, which revealed two important, additional facts: first, the janitor had been performing a job task outside his customary duties when his problems occurred; second, it became clear from the occupational therapist's job analysis that the equipment was not as cumbersome as had been described. The occupational therapist had been informed that the janitor had been asked to strip the wax because the person who usually did this job was ill. The employer was willing to assign this task to someone else if the need should again arise. After reviewing the job analysis, the doctor met again with the janitor. This discussion revealed that he did not like the task of stripping floors, nor did he want to work with the equipment he had been forced to use during this operation. Rather than discuss this situation with his supervisor, however, he had brought the problem to his doctor. By securing and reviewing the job analysis, the doctor and her patient were able to save his job and eliminate future problems.

REFERENCES

Akabas SH: Commentary: a rose by another name may smell sweeter. In Remenyi AG, Swerissen H, Thomas SA, contributing editors: *New developments in worker rehabilitation: the workcare model in Australia,* New York, 1987, World Rehabilitation Fund.

The American coal miner: a report on community and living conditions in the coalfields, Washington, DC, 1980, The President's Commission on Coal.

Bitter JA: *Introduction to rehabilitation,* St. Louis, 1979, Mosby-Year Book.

Corn J: Protective legislation for coal miners, 1870-1900: response to safety and health hazards. In Rosner D, Markowitz G, editors: *Dying for work: workers' safety and health in 20th century America,* Bloomington, In, 1989, Indiana University Press.

Demore-Taber M, Cohen-Siskind BM: The role of the vocational rehabilitation counselor. In Sheer SJ, editor: *Multidisciplinary perspective in vocational assessment of impaired workers,* Rockville, Md, 1990, Aspen Publishers.

Deneen LJ, Hessellund TA: *Counseling the able disabled: rehabilitation consulting in disability compensation systems,* San Francisco, 1986, Rehab Publications.

Freireich D: A call for case study and serious consideration. In Remenyi AG, Swerissen H, Thomas SA, contributing editors: *New developments in worker rehabilitation: the work-*

care model in Australia, New York, 1987, World Rehabilitation Fund.

Hay DI: Socioeconomic status and health status: a study of males in the Canada health survey. *Social Science and Medicine* Vol 27(12): 1317-1325, 1988.

Jarvikoski A, Lahelma E: *Early rehabilitation at the work place,* New York, 1980, World Rehabilitation Fund.

Kitagawa EM, Hauser PM: *Differential mortality in the United States: a study in socioeconomic epidemiology.* Cambridge, 1973, Harvard University Press.

Levitan S, Taggart R: Rehabilitation, employment, and the disabled. In Rubin J, LaPorte V, editors: *Alternatives in rehabilitating the handicapped,* New York, 1982, Human Sciences Press.

Lilienfeld DE, Lilienfeld AM: The French influence on the development of epidemiology. In Lilienfeld AM, editor: *The times, places, and persons: aspects of the history of epidemiology,* Baltimore, 1980, The John Hopkins University Press.

Matkin RE: The state of private sector rehabilitation. In Taylor LJ, Golter M, Golter G, Backer TE, editors: *Handbook of private sector rehabilitation,* New York, 1985, Springer Publishing Company.

McGowan JF, Porter TL: *An introduction to the vocational rehabilitation process,* Washington, 1967, US Department of Health, Education, and Welfare.

Nagi SZ: *Disability and rehabilitation: legal, clinical, and self-concepts and measurement,* Columbus, 1970, Ohio State University Press.

Nagi SZ: Early rehabilitation and the role of industry. In Jarvikoski A, Lehelma E, editors: *Early rehabilitation at the work place,* New York, 1980, World Rehabilitation Fund.

Robertson L: Behavioral research and strategies in public health. *Social Science and Medicine* Vol 9: 165-170. 1975.

Rothstein MA: Legal issues related to vocational capacity. In Scheer SJ, editor: *Multidisciplinary perspective in vocational assessment of impaired workers,* Rockville, Md, 1990, Aspen Publishers.

Rubin SE, Roessler RT: *Foundations of the vocational rehabilitation process,* Baltimore, 1978, University Park Press.

Rusk HA: *Rehabilitation medicine,* St. Louis, 1971, Mosby-Year Book.

Scheer SJ: Commonalities of measuring capacity to work. In Scheer SJ, editor: *Multi-disciplinary perspectives in vocational assessment of impaired workers,* Rockville, Md, 1990 Aspen Publishers.

Thomas SW, Vocational assessment of multiple and severe physical impairments. In Scheer SJ, editor: *Multidisciplinary perspectives in vocational assessment of impaired workers,* Rockville, Md, 1990, Aspen Publishers.

US Department of Health and Human Services: Setting the national agenda for injury control in the 1990s. Papers from the Third National Injury Control Conference, 1992, Centers for Disease Control.

Weeks JL: Occupational health and safety regulation in the coal mining industry: public health at the workplace. *Annual Review of Public Health* Vol 12: 195-207, 1991.

Weeks JL, Levy BS, Wagner GR: *Preventing occupational disease and injury,* Washington, DC, 1990, American Public Health Association.

Wickstrom RJ: Functional capacity evaluation. In Scheer SJ, editor: *Multidisciplinary perspectives in vocational assessment of impaired workers,* Rockville, Md, 1990, Aspen Publishers.

Winkleby MA, Jatulis DE, Frank E, Fortmann SP: Socioeconomic status and health: how education, income, and occupation contribute to risk factors for cardiovascular disease. *American Journal of Public Health* Vol 8(6): 816-820, June 1992.

The Workers' Compensation Laws of California, New York, 1993, Matthew Bender and Co., Inc.

37 Drug Testing and Occupational Injuries

Drug testing is being marketed as the prevention solution to rising workers' compensation costs from industrial accidents. Occupational health clinics in many areas are besieged by employers requesting 24-hour drug testing services for preemployment, random, and postinjury tests (forensic drug tests).

There is no question that substance abuse is a cause of industrial accidents, and appropriate drug testing with scrupulous attention to the points discussed below is a much-needed service to industry. Because of the legal ramifications and exposure as well as major ethical issues, however, program involvement with forensic drug testing needs to be carefully thought out and well planned.

Moreover, occupational health clinicians must remind employers that drug testing is not a panacea, and will not, in isolation, solve work injury and illness problems. The full range of safety services is needed for an effective prevention program. A workplace can be drug-free and yet at high risk for serious accidents if appropriate engineering and administrative control of hazards are not in place, equipment is poorly maintained, the plant facility is cluttered and slippery, and staff are not trained or provided with appropriate safety and personal protective equipment.

Before a physician becomes involved in forensic urine drug testing for local employers, she should review the company's written policy concerning drug use and testing procedures. The guidelines developed by the American College of Occupational and Environmental Medicine (ACOEM) regarding workplace drug screening are helpful in reviewing such policies. Essential components of an effective workplace drug testing program include clear communication of the policy, rationale for drug testing, and impartial application of the policy. Affected employees must be informed in advance about drug testing and the consequences of refusing to participate. Although Department of Transportation (DOT) regulations do not require written consent for drug screening, such consent should be obtained and should include consent for communicating the test results to the employer. The ACOEM guidelines also in-

clude recommendations regarding the training and qualifications of the medical review officer that are more extensive than those required by federal regulations.[3]

Physician involvement can include collection of specimens, reviewing laboratory results as medical review officers, and providing factual information in legal depositions and courtroom testimony. The term "medical review officer" (MRO) comes from federal regulations describing physicians who review forensic urine drug test results. The DOT regulations describe an MRO as "a licensed physician . . . who has knowledge of substance abuse disorders and has appropriate medical training to interpret and evaluate an individual's positive test result together with his or her medical history and any other relevant biomedical information." Although no regulatory or professional requirement exists for certification or training of physicians as MROs, voluntary accreditation programs are in place. Given the various technical issues and legal issues, formal accreditation requirements are probably a matter of time.

SPECIMEN COLLECTION

Physicians involved in forensic substance abuse testing need to understand how it differs from diagnostic testing. Forensic urine drug testing is much more a legal test than a medical test. The weakest link in the entire forensic drug testing process is the documentation known as the chain of custody or custody and control form, which must be accurately completed for every test. Documentation and the paperwork accompanying the specimen are equally important to the final test result. Any positive test result should be handled as though it will result in a legal challenge. Unless all paperwork is completed as required, a test result should be declared negative if the entire chain of custody and documentation has not been adequately completed.

Clinics that are considering providing collection services for an employer as part of their drug-free workplace program need to have standard operating procedures related to such collections. The Department of Transportation's specimen collection workbook contains the key procedures for collection. In the collection process, it is critically important that the person responsible for completing the paperwork and giving directions to the client have this as a sole assignment. The collection site person should be uninterrupted, maintain direct observation of the client outside the restroom, and be able to concentrate during the entire process to correctly and accurately complete all the necessary paperwork. In general, the provision of a specimen can be permitted in private unless certain specific conditions require direct observation. Such circumstances are clearly defined in federal regulations. If the testing is not done under the guidelines of a federal regulatory agency, the employer's written policy should clearly delineate the situations under which direct observation is required.

The staff member responsible for collection is critically important in documenting the validity of a specimen. Having strict guidelines for an acceptable specimen will go a long way to preventing alteration or specimen tampering and/or substitution. The DOT guidelines are highly specific about how the specimen is to be evaluated and handled at the time of collection. At present, the DOT guidelines allow the urine temperature to range between 90.5° to 99.8° F, unless the client providing the specimen has a fever. Under Nuclear Regulatory Commission (NRC) regulations or for nonregulated testing, temperature guidelines may be much stricter and a temperature range of 96° to 99.8° F, or if febrile, within 1° F of body temperature will go a long way to preventing urine substitution or tampering.

At the time of collection, specific gravity testing and pH testing are also effective maneuvers to ensure a valid specimen. These latter two procedures are at present prohibited by DOT guidelines. However, again for the NRC or nonregulatory testing, having a specific gravity requirement of 1.005 up to 1.030 will identify those persons who overhydrate to pass a urine drug test. pH guidelines between 5.0 and 8.0 will also help detect adulteration such as the addition of drain cleaner or bleach to the urine specimen.

Split specimens are allowed under federal regulations and have often been performed as an accommodation to labor relations concerns regarding accuracy of the drug-testing process. If appropriately done, the split specimens are useful in providing additional assurances that the testing process is valid. A complete set of paperwork is required for the split specimen. Also, the laboratory needs to be told when handling a split specimen that it should go directly to confirmation testing regardless of the results of any screening test performed. Some substances (especially mari-

juana) often degrade over time and on a split specimen may screen negative several days after the initial specimen is processed. Split specimens should always be processed as a qualitative test for the presence of substance only. Quantitation of results should only be done on the initial specimen.

MEDICAL REVIEW OFFICER

The second important function that physicians may fill in forensic urine drug testing is that of a medical review officer. Federal regulations require that all urine test results be received from the laboratory by a medical review officer who reviews the results and determines whether there is any legitimate reason for the test to be positive for drugs. The MRO's responsibilities defined by the Department of Health and Human Services and DOT regulations include the following:

1. Receive negative and confirmed positive test results from the laboratory.
2. Receive a certified copy of the original chain of custody (or custody and control) form.
3. Reject results of specimens that are not obtained or processed in accordance with the employer's policy and procedures.
4. Review and interpret positive test results.
   A. Give the client an opportunity to discuss his or her test results.
   B. Review the client's medical history or any other relevant biomedical factors.
   C. Request, if appropriate, a quantitative description of test results.
   D. Authorize, if indicated, reanalysis of the original sample.
   E. Consult with laboratory officials or other experts as needed.
   F. Determine whether there is a legitimate medical explanation for the positive test result. If not, then the result is verified positive.
   G. Determine that opiate positive results are verified as positive only if there is other clinical evidence of illegal opiate use or if gas chronography mass spectrometry analysis shows the heroin metabolite 6-monoacetylmorphine.
5. Report persons with verified positive test results through the employer's employee assistance program (EAP) and to the management official empowered to take administrative action. A detailed explanation of these requirements can be found in the *Medical Review Officer Guide* published by the U.S. Department of Transportation, October 1990.

LABORATORY TESTING

The testing process includes an initial or screening test followed by a confirmatory test for all positive specimens. The initial test requires an amino acid process that has been standardized and meets the requirements of the Food and Drug Administration (FDA) for commercial distribution. If the specimen is tested negative, no further tests are done. The confirmatory test is the analytical procedure that identifies the specific drug or metabolite independent of the initial test result. It uses a different technique or chemical principal from that in the initial test. For a regulated drug test, this confirmatory test is a gas chromatography/mass spectrometry (GC/MS) process. GC/MS has become the gold standard in forensic urine drug testing and should always be the procedure of choice for confirmatory testing.

The administrative cut-off levels are used to divide samples into negative and positive specimens. The cut-off level is a relative, arbitrary point on a continuum of possible analytic concentrations. It is generally set at such a point that passive inhalation of illegal substances will not trigger a positive test result. The initial cut-off levels for the five drugs primarily tested in regulated situations are as follows: marijuana metabolites, 100 nanograms per milliliter (ng/ml); cocaine metabolites, 300 ng/ml; opiate metabolites, 300 ng/ml; PCP, 25 ng/ml; amphetamines, 1,000 ng/ml.

For the confirmation testing done by GC/MS, cut-off levels are: marijuana, 15 ng/ml; cocaine, 150 ng/ml; morphine, 300 ng/ml; codeine, 300 ng/ml; PCP, 25 ng/ml. In the case of marijuana and cocaine the marked difference in cut-off levels between the initial test and the confirmatory test is due to the fact that the confirmatory test looks at one principal metabolite only. The initial screening test looks at the entire class of marijuana and cocaine metabolites. Therefore, a test result that screens positive for marijuana at a screening level of 100 ng/ml and then goes to GC/MS and is quantitated at 45 ng/ml is indeed a positive test, despite being lower than the initial screening cut-off level. In the case of marijuana, for example, more than 60 different metabolites are formed after marijuana is ingested. The initial aminoassay for marijuana looks at an entire class of metabolites, whereas the GC/MS screening process searches for one metabolite only, delta-9 tetrahydrocannabinol (delta-9-THC). This is an often confusing point for clients receiving their test results from the MRO physician.

Interpretation of negative test results is not as simple as would first appear. A negative test result may mean that there has been no drug use by this client. It may mean that there has been no recent drug use by this client. Negative test results may also occur as the result of urine dilution (in vivo or in vitro) or adulteration. Finally, the negative test result may occur with a drug being present but below administrative cut-off levels.

A positive test result is subject to significant limitations. Physicians should understand that a positive test result indicates use only. The test result, even when quantitated with GC/MS, does not correlate to impairment. It also cannot be used to indicate route of administration of the substance. Only in rare circumstances can an estimation of time of use or amount used be gathered from quantitation of a positive test result.

SPECIFIC SUBSTANCES
Marijuana

Marijuana is extensively metabolized to more than 60 different metabolites in the human body. As noted earlier, the initial aminoassay use of the screening test detects the class of a particular administrative cut-off level. The confirmatory test process with GC/MS specifically looks for one metabolite, the delta-9 THC. The time frame for detecting marijuana use depends greatly on the cut-off levels of the aminoassay and the type of user. Under DOT regulations the current aminoassay cut-off level is 100 ng/ml. For NRC testing the cut-off level is recommended at 100 ng/ml, but may be less if the licensee is able to support a different level. Of course, for nonregulated testing other cut-off levels of the aminoassay are used, most commonly 50 ng/ml. Some, however, use 20 ng/ml. It is expected that new Department of Transportation regulations will lower the initial cut-off level to 50 ng/ml.

The type of use is also critical in determining how long marijuana may be detected. A one-time or once-a-month user may have detectable levels 3 to 5 days after use, whereas a daily user could possibly be detected up to 30 days after last use. Route of administration as noted previously cannot be determined by a positive test result. For marijuana, the most common route of administration is smoking. Oral use, however, will also be detected by the test result.

Two somewhat controversial areas in marijuana testing include passive inhalation and unknowing ingestion. Sufficient testing under external conditions rules out passive inhalation when using a cut-off level for the initial test of 50 or 100 ng/ml. It is simply not possible to have passive inhalation account for a positive test with those cut-off levels. Regarding unknowing ingestion it is not infrequent that a client will make the claim that he was at a party and consumed brownies, cookies, or some other substance that contained marijuana without his knowledge. Although this scenario is possible, it is not particularly probable. Many medical review officers, in order to remain objective and consistent in interpretation of marijuana test results, disregard this explanation entirely or offer to consider that explanation seriously if the client files a formal police report against the person or persons who supposedly spiked the food with marijuana.

Another issue regarding marijuana testing for reanalysis of an original specimen or testing the split portion of a specimen is the degradation that occurs after collection. If a specimen initially quantitative for marijuana is retested or a split specimen is tested, the second analysis should be for qualitative identification of substance only. It should not be quantitative. Rare therapeutic uses of synthetic marijuana include experimental use for glaucoma, use as an antiemetic, and use in cancer chemotherapy. Most certified laboratories are unable to differentiate between synthetic THC given for therapeutic purposes and the illegal natural version of THC. Roger Fulls, MD, of Northwest Toxicology in Salt Lake City, Utah, has developed a protocol to differentiate between synthetic and natural THC. Marijuana test results should routinely be quantified, particularly when an individual would be required to go through a rehabilitation program before being allowed to return to work. Although marijuana may persist in a person's body for a significant period of time, it would not be uncommon for a postsuspension test to remain positive after initial test failure. Evidence of a decreasing level over time should therefore be considered a past test. When following an individual closely, a test result should be considered a positive or failed test result any time the quantitation increases by 50%.

Opiates

Opiates have caused the bulk of controversial issues in substance abuse tests because most test results are due to the use of illegally prescribed substance. Heroin is administered through injection, smoking, and via oral and rectal routes. However, ingestion of poppy seeds will also give a positive test for opiates. The poppy seed has generated many articles in technical literature regarding quantitation levels at which perhaps a test could be interpreted to mean abuse and/or addiction versus only ingestion. Some of these studies, however, have shown that high levels, even as high as 10,000 ng/ml, of morphine can be generated by healthy young males ingesting large quantities of poppy seed pastries. Therefore, use of GC/ML/GC/MS quantitation results for opiates to

make a determination as to a legitimate ingestion versus opiate abuse is not recommended. The screening test looks for metabolites of morphine and codeine which can be found for days after use. 6-monoacetyl-morphine (6-MAM) is the major metabolite from heroin and if detected is the evidence for use of heroin. No other alternate explanation exists. However, it is highly unlikely that 6-MAM will be detected as a result of its extraordinarily short half-life. The aminoassay screening test will also pick up some synthetic narcotics but would then be read as negative with a GC/MS test that is looking only for codeine or morphine.

Perhaps the single most controversial issue for physicians acting as medical review officers regards familiar use of opiates. As a group, MROs appear to be about equally divided with regard to interpretation of positive results when a client admits to use of a family member's opiate prescription medication. Some would report the test result as positive to an employer with the comment that it was a family member's prescription that was used, and allow the employer to make a determination of whether that constitutes appropriate or inappropriate use of medication. Other MROs would evaluate the clinical situation in which medication was used and, if the situation was clinically appropriate, the MRO would report to the employer a negative test result. If use of the family member's medication was clinically inappropriate or there was abuse of the medication, the test result would be reported to the employer as positive.

Cocaine

Cocaine is detected by aminoassay as a class of metabolites and then confirmed with GC/MS screening for a single metabolite. Cocaine is administered by smoking, injection, and snorting. In general, oral ingestion is not used because it does not provide the effect that the substance abuser is looking for. There are indeed therapeutic uses for cocaine, primarily by ear, nose, and throat (ENT) specialists who apply it when working in the nasal area. A few eye drops also contain cocaine. Many substance abusers believe that novocaine or any word with "caine" in it will test positive for cocaine. This is, of course, not correct. The GC/MS is specific for the cocaine molecule itself and no other medications or cross contaminates interfere with the assay for cocaine.

As with marijuana, some of the controversies in cocaine include passive inhalation and unknowing ingestion. Again, administrative cut-off levels are set so that passive inhalation is not an issue. Unknowing ingestion may occur, and some physicians acting as MROs have used as a standard that this would not change their call of a positive test or they would allow the client tested to formally file a police report against the person or persons thought to have provided cocaine in this manner. A much more rare situation does occur, however, with tea made from the cocoa leaf, which is forbidden to be sold commercially in the United States. It is not impossible that a person could unknowingly consume tea made from cocoa leaves brought in from another country. As with marijuana, cocaine will degrade post collection. Therefore, any retesting or testing of split specimens should be for qualitative presence, not quantitative.

Amphetamines

The aminoassay test is used to screen methamphetamine and its metabolite amphetamine as well as other hydroxylated metabolites. Route of administration includes injecting, snorting, smoking, and taking orally. Amphetamines are rarely used therapeutically in disorders that include narcolepsy, attention deficit disorder, and obesity. In all cases, a legitimate prescription would be identified.

A controversial aspect of amphetamine testing has to do with over-the-counter medications that cause reaction with the aminoassay. Methamphetamine, amphetamine, and D and L isomers exist. Prescription amphetamines and illegal amphetamines are nearly 100% the D isomer. Over-the-counter amphetamines, particularly the Vicks inhaler that contains desoxyephedrine, a synonym for methamphetamine, is 100% the L isomer. When methamphetamine and/or amphetamines have been confirmed by GC/MS testing, the laboratory should routinely be asked to differentiate between the presence of D and L isomer. Only if the specimen is 100% L isomer should an explanation of Vicks inhaler use be accepted. Amphetamine testing emphasizes the importance of always obtaining sophisticated confirmatory testing before declaring a specimen positive or negative. In the realm of unregulated testing, some companies would ask the physician to make the determination based on a screening test only. This would never be acceptable in any legitimate forensic urine testing program. In the case of amphetamines, numerous over-the-counter medications would indeed trigger a positive screen test based on aminoassay alone. Today's GC/MS testing is reliable and valid in differentiating between over-the-counter medications that may cause an aminoassay cross-reaction versus prescription or illegal methamphetamine.

Phencyclidine (PCP)

There is no legitimate use for PCP, which is ingested via smoking. The local physician's knowledge of substance abuse will be helpful in knowing the expectant frequency of a positive phencyclidine test result. There are no significant cross-reactivity issues with phencyclidine. The experience in testing that most laboratories have is during the blind sampling program or proficiency program, which drug testing labs are required to go through to be certified.

Other substances

Testing for drugs other than marijuana, cocaine, opiates, amphetamines, and phencyclidine is forbidden under DOT regulations but permitted under NRC regulations and, of course, nonregulated drug testing programs. Most commonly these extended panels for urine testing include barbiturates, benzodiazepine, provoxidines, and methadone. Some employers are concerned about these classes of drugs particularly in regard to employees with safety-sensitive occupations.

FORENSIC ALCOHOL TESTING

At the present time, forensic alcohol testing in the employment setting is performed under NRC regulations. The DOT has post regulations that would require alcohol testing. It is expected that the screening for alcohol will be in the form of breath testing with confirmation done by evidentiary grade breath test devices or a blood alcohol test. In general, blood specimens are preferred over breath and urine specimens for alcohol testing because of technical and legal reasons. Most state laws define "legal intoxication" in terms of blood alcohol concentration (BAC). Although blood alcohol concentrations can be correlated with impairment, breath alcohol concentration cannot. It is important to understand that the evidential grade breath testing devices generally use a conversion ratio of 2,100:1 blood/breath alcohol ratio. The mean value of the blood/breath alcohol ratio is approximately 2,300:1 per populations of healthy men in the post-absorptive state of alcohol distribution. The actual ratio, however, varies substantially, from as low as 1,155:1 to as high as 3,500:1. Using the ratio of 2,300:1, a reported BAC of 0.04 could actually range from 0.02 to 0.06. Evidentiary grade blood testing devices report the BAC to two significant digits, the third digit simply being dropped. Therefore, there may be little difference between a breath test level of 0.04 and 0.05 if the digits were also reported as 0.048 and 0.052, respectively. For these reasons, doing backward extrapolation of a blood alcohol concentration should be based on blood test results only. The rate of metabolism of alcohol ranges from 0.015% per hour to 0.02% per hour. Using the slower rate of 0.015% is therefore appropriate for making conservative predictions.

Urine alcohol test results, though obtained readily in the laboratory by gas chromatography are difficult for the MRO to interpret. The concentration of alcohol in urine is on average 1.3 times greater than blood concentration in the post-absorptive phase. The actual distribution ratio ranges from 1.16 to 1.57. Urine can be a reliable estimate of blood alcohol concentration only in the post-absorptive phase and only if the subject completely empties his bladder so that the first specimen may be discarded and another specimen can be examined about 30 minutes later.

For those physicians wishing a comprehensive review of the technical issues of forensic drug testing, a good review has been compiled by the NRC in the form of what are called nureg/CR-5227 and nureg/CR-5227 supplement 1, 1988. These contain excellent reviews of the technical issues in forensic drug testing including alcohol testing. Another excellent reference regarding breath alcohol analysis has been authored by Kurt Dubowski and published by the Department of Health and Human Services in 1991.

COURT TESTIMONY

The physician may have a less common but important role in forensic substance abuse testing: legal deposition and courtroom testimony. As noted earlier, physicians should assume that all failed drug tests will be challenged legally. It is therefore important that all confirmation testing be done GC/MS (or GC in the case of alcohol only). For this reason, the physician should never hesitate to contact the laboratory toxicologist directly and authorize any additional testing such as D and L isomers of amphetamines, the 6-MAM test, and so forth.

To reduce a physician's professional legal liability, written consent for performing tests and releasing results to an employer should be obtained from employees and applicants before any test is administered. It is also recommended that the employer agree in writing to indemnify the physician for any expenses incurred as a result of the testing program, such as attorney fees or damage awards.

If the physician acting as an MRO has appropriately documented standard operating procedures, reviewed the chain of custody (or custody and control) form, and documented the interview with the client, little is to be feared about a legal proceeding. In this case, the physician would be participating as a technical expert only and is not required to represent the employer about the testing program, or in particular, the legality of such a testing program. Documentation of all aspects of the testing process, including collection, facility checklist, chain of custody documentation, and interview with the client should be maintained in a record separate from a client's medical file. Any positive test result must be maintained at least 5 years, although most attorneys would recommend maintaining positive test results indefinitely. Records of negative tests need be maintained only for 1 year. In any deposition or legal proceedings, it should be remembered that a positive test result indicates presence of the substance only. It does not state how the substance came to be present and does not signify impairment except in the case of alcohol. By clearly understanding the limitations of forensic testing and communicating those limitations to client employers, a physician can minimize legal liability.

SUMMARY

Forensic urine drug testing can be a useful service to employees. It is important to understand the need for strict documentation and record keeping. It is also necessary to understand that a drug test is not a medical examination and does not constitute a doctor/patient relationship. By clearly understanding the limits of forensic drug testing a physician may properly advise an employer on its appropriate uses. Properly performed and documented, forensic drug testing appears to have little legal or malpractice liability for the individual physician. Primary care/occupational medicine physicians with an understanding of substance abuse and the broad array of clinical factors that may influence the interpretation of a test result, can be highly effective as medical review officers, and provide important service to employers seeking to reduce injury rates.

Appendix A

Safety/Industrial Hygiene Resources

American Board of Industrial Hygiene
4600 West Saginaw, Suite 101
Lansing, MI 48917
(517)321-2638

American Conference of Governmental Industrial
 Hygienists
6500 Glenway Ave, Bldg D-7
Cincinnati, OH 45211-4438

American Industrial Hygiene Association
2700 Prosperity Ave, Suite 250
Fairfax, VA 22031
(703)849-8888

American Society of Safety Engineers
1800 East Oakton St
Des Plaines, IL 60018-2187
(708)692-4121

Board of Certified Safety Professionals
208 Burwash Ave
Savoy, IL 61874-9510
(217)359-9263

Health Physics Society
8000 West Park Dr, Suite 130
McLean, VA 22102
(703)790-1745

Society of Toxicology
1101 14th St, NW, Suite 1100
Washington, DC 20005-5601
(202)371-1393

U.S. Department of Labor

**Regional Offices for the Occupational Safety &
Health Administration (OSHA)**

States marked with asterisk operate their own federally
 approved OSHA programs.

Region I (CT,* MA, ME, NH,VT*)
133 Portland St, 1st Floor
Boston, MA 02114
(617)565-7164

Region II (NJ, NY,* PR,* VI*)
201 Varick St, Rm 670
New York, NY 10014
(212)337-2378

Region III (DC, DE, MD,* PA, VA,* WV)
Gateway Bldg, Suite 2100
3535 Market St
Philadephia, PA 19104
(215)596-1201

Region IV (AL, FL, GA, KY,* MS, NC,* SC,* TN*)
1375 Peachtree St, NE, Suite 587
Atlanta, GA 30367
(404)347-3573

Region V (IL, IN,* MI,* MN,* OH, WI)
230 South Dearborn St, Rm 3244
Chicago, IL 60604
(312)352-2220

Region VI (AR, LA, NM,* OK, TX)
525 Griffin St, Rm 602
Dallas, TX 75202
(214)767-4731

Region VII (IA,* KS, MO, NE)
911 Walnut St, Rm 406
Kansas City, MO 64106
(816)426-5861

RegionVIII (CO, MT, ND, SD, UT,* WY*)
Federal Bldg, Rm 1576
1961 Stout St
Denver, CO 80294
(303)844-3061

Region IX (Am. Samoa, AZ,* CA,* Guam, HI,* NV,*
Trust Territories of Pacific)
71 Stevenson St, 4th Floor
San Francisco, CA 94105
(415)744-6670

Region V (AK,* ID, OR,* WA*)
1111 Third Ave, Suite 715
Seattle, WA 98101-3212
(206)553-5930

USEFUL TELEPHONE NUMBERS

Equal Employment Opportunity Commission – Publications Office	(800)669-3362
American Assoc. of Occupational Health Nurses	(404)262-1162
American College of Environmental/Occupational Medicine	(708)228-6850
American Public Health Association	(202)789-5667
Bureau of Labor Statistics	(202)606-7828
C.D.C. Center for Disease Control and Prevention	(404)639-3311
Environmental Protection Agency	(202)260-2090
National Assoc. of Occupational Health Professionals	(800)666-7926
National Safety Council	(800)621-7619
NIOSH National Institute for Occupational Safety and Health	(513)533-8236
O.S.H.A. Occupational Safety and Health Administration	(202)219-8148
Workers' Comp Research Institute	(617)494-1240

Appendix B

Alabama

Workmen's Compensation Division, Department of Industrial Relations, Industrial Relations Building, Montgomery, AL 36131. (205)242-2868.

Alaska

Workers' Compensation Division, Dept. of Labor, P.O. Box 25512, Juneau, AK 99802. (907)465-2790.

Arizona

Industrial Commission, 800 West Washington, P.O. Box 19070, Phoenix, AZ 85007. (602)542-4661.

Arkansas

Workers' Compensation Commission, 625 Marshal St., Justice Building, State Capitol Grounds, Little Rock, AR 72201. (501)682-3930.

California

Division of Workers' Compensation, P.O. Box 420603, San Francisco, CA 94102. (415)703-3731.

Colorado

Workers' Compensation Section, Division of Labor, 1120 Lincoln, #1401, Denver, CO 80203. (303)764-2929.

Connecticut

Workers' Compensation Commission, 1890 Dixwell Ave., Hamden, CT 06514. (203)789-7783.

Delaware

Industrial Accident Board, State Office Building, 6th Floor, 820 North French St., Wilmington, DE 19801. (302)577-2884.

District of Columbia

Dept. of Employment Services, Office of Workers' Compensation, P.O. Box 56098, Washington, DC 20011. (202)576-6265.

Florida

Division of Workers' Compensation, Dept. of Labor and Employment Security, 2728 Centerview Dr., Ste. 301, Forest Bldg., Tallahassee, FL 32399-0680. (904)488-2514.

Georgia

Board of Workers' Compensation, South Tower, Ste. 1000, One CNN Ctr., Atlanta, GA 30303-2788. (404)656-3875.

Guam

Workers' Compensation Commission, Dept. of Labor, Govt. of Guam, P.O. Box 9970, Tamuning, GU 96911. 647-4222.

Hawaii

Disability Compensation Commission, Dept. of Labor & Industrial Relations, 830 Punchbowl St., Rm. 209, Honolulu, HI 96813. (808)586-9200.

Idaho

Industrial Commission, 317 Main St., Boise, ID 83720. (208)334-6000.

Illinois

Industrial Commission, 100 W. Randolph St., Ste. 8-200, Chicago, IL 60601. (312)814-6500.

Indiana

Workers' Compensation Board, 402 W. Washington St., Rm. W196, Indianapolis, IN 46204. (317)232-3808.

Iowa

Div. of Industrial Services, Dept. of Employment Services, 1000 E. Grand Ave., Des Moines, IA 50319. (515)281-5934.

Kansas

Division of Workers' Compensation, 800 SW Jackson, Ste. 600, Topeka, KS 66612-1227. (913)296-3441.

Kentucky

Dept. of Workers' Compensation, Perimeter Park Width, 1270 Louisville, Bldg. C, Frankfort, KY 40601. (502)564-5550.

Louisiana

Dept. of Labor, Office of Workers' Compensation Administration, P.O. Box 94040, Baton Rouge, LA 70804-9040. (504)342-7555.

DIRECTORY OF WORKERS' COMPENSATION ADMINISTRATORS   *(Continued)*

Maine

Workers' Compensation Board, State House Station 27, Deering Bldg., Augusta, ME 04333. (207)289-3751.

Maryland

Workers' Compensation Commission, 6 N. Liberty, Baltimore, MD 21201. (410)333-4700.

Massachusetts

Dept. of Industrial Accidents, 600 Washington St., 7th Flr., Boston, MA 02111. (617)727-4300.

Michigan

Bureau of Workers' Disability Comp., Dept. of Labor, P.O. Box 30016, Lansing, MI 48909. (517)373-3480.

Minnesota

Workers' Compensation Division, Dept. of Labor & Industry, 443 Lafayette Rd., St. Paul, MN 55155. (612)296-6107.

Mississippi

Workers' Compensation Commission, 1428 Lakeland Drive, P.O. Box 5300, Jackson, MS 39296-5300. (601)987-4200.

Missouri

Division of Workers' Compensation, Dept. of Labor & Industrial Relations, P.O. Box 58, Jefferson City, MO 65102. (314)751-4231.

Montana

State Compensation Mutual Insurance Fund, P.O. Box 4759, Helena, MT 59604. (406)444-6518.

Nebraska

Workers' Compensation Court, State House, 13th Flr., Lincoln, NE 68509. (402)471-2568.

Nevada

State Industrial Insurance System, 515 East Musser St., Carson City, NV 89714. (702)687-5220.

New Hampshire

Dept. of Labor, 95 Pleasant St., Concord, NH 03301. (603)271-3171.

New Jersey

Division of Workers' Compensation, Dept. of Labor, Call Number 381, Trenton, NJ 08625. (609)292-2414.

New Mexico

Workers' Compensation Division, Dept. of Labor, 481 Broadway NE, Albuquerque, NM 87103. (505)841-8600.

New York

Workers' Compensation Board, 180 Livingston St., Brooklyn, NY 11248. (718)802-6600.

North Carolina

Industrial Commission, Dobbs Bldg., 430 North Salisbury St., Raleigh, NC 27611. (919)733-4820.

North Dakota

Workers' Compensation Bureau, Russell Bldg., Highway 83 North, 4007 North State St., Bismarck, ND 58501. (701)224-3800.

Ohio

Bureau of Workers' Compensation, 30 West Spring St., Columbus, OH 43266-0581. (614)466-2950.

Oklahoma

Oklahoma Workers' Compensation Court, 1915 North Stiles, Oklahoma City, OK 73105. (405)557-7600.

Oregon

Dept. of Insurance and Finance, 21 Labor and Industries Bldg., Salem, OR 97310. (503)378-4100.

Pennsylvania

Bureau of Workers' Compensation, Dept. of Labor and Industry, 1171 South Cameron St., Rm. #103, Harrisburg, PA 17104. (717)783-5421.

Puerto Rico

Industrial Commissioner's Office, G.P.O. Box 4466, San Juan, PR 00936. (809)783-2028.

Rhode Island

Dept. of Workers' Compensation, 610 Manton Ave., P.O. Box 3500, Providence, RI 02909. (401)272-0700.

South Carolina

Workers' Compensation Commission, 1612 Marion Street, P.O. Box 1715, Columbia, SC 29202. (803)737-5700.

South Dakota

Division of Labor and Mgmt., Dept. of Labor, Kneip Bldg., Third Flr., 700 Governors Dr., Pierre, SD 57501-2277. (605)773-3681.

Tennessee

Workers' Compensation Division, Dept. of Labor, 501 Union Bldg., Second Flr., Nashville, TN 37243-0661. (615)741-2395.

Texas

Texas Workers' Compensation Commission, 4000 South IH35, Austin, TX 78704. (512)448-7900.

Utah

Industrial Commission, 160 East 300 South, Salt Lake City, UT 84111. (801)530-6800.

Vermont

Dept. of Labor and Industry, National Life Bldg., Drawer 20, Montpelier, VT 05620-3401. (802)828-2286.

DIRECTORY OF WORKERS' COMPENSATION ADMINISTRATORS *(Continued)*

Virgin Islands

Dept. of Labor, 2131 Hospital St., Christiansted, St. Croix, VI 0084-666. (809)773-1994.

Virginia

Workers' Comp. Comm., 1000 DMV Bldg., Richmond, VA 23220. (804)367-8600.

Washington

Dept. of Labor and Industries, P.O. Box 44001, Olympia, WA 98504. (206)956-4213.

West Virginia

Workers' Compensation Commissioner's Office, P.O. Box 3151, Charleston, WV 25332. (304)558-2580.

Wisconsin

Workers' Compensation Div., Dept. of Industry, Labor, and Human Relations, P.O. Box 7901, Rm. 162, 201 East Washington Ave., Madison, WI 53707. (608)266-1340.

Wyoming

Workers' Compensation Div., 122 West 25th St., 2nd Flr., East Wing, Herschier Bldg., Cheyenne, WY 82002. (307)777-7441.

United States

Dept. of Labor, Employment Standards Administration, Washington, DC 20210. (202)219-6191.

Office of Workers' Compensation Programs. (202)219-7503.

Division of Coal Mine Workers' Compensation. (202)219-6692.

Division of Federal Employees' Compensation. (202)219-7552.

Div. of Longshore & Harbor Workers' Compensation. (202)219-8721.

Office of State Liaison and Legislative Analysis. (202)219-4560.

Div. of State Workers' Comp. Programs. (202)219-4560.

Benefits Review Board, Tech World Plaza, 5th Flr., 800 K. St., NW, Washington, DC 2001-8002. (202)633-7500.

Alberta

Workers' Compensation Board, P.O. Box 2415, 9912 107th St., Edmonton, AB T5J 2S5. (403)427-1131.

British Columbia

Workers' Compensation Board, 6951 Westminster Highway, Richmond, BC V7C 1C6. (604)273-2266.

Manitoba

Workers' Comp. Board, 333 Maryland St., Winnipeg, MB R3C 1M2. (204)786-5471.

New Brunswick

Workers' Compensation Board, 1 Portland, Saint John, NB E26 3X9. (506)632-2200.

New Foundland

Workers' Compensation Commission, P.O. Box 9000, Station B, St. John's NF A1A 3B8. (709)778-1000.

Northwest Territories

Workers' Comp. Board, P.O. Box 1390, Northwest Territories, Postal Code X1A 2L9. (403)873-7745.

Nova Scotia

Workers' Compensation Board, 5668 South Street, P.O. Box 1150, Halifax, NS B3J 2Y2. (902)424-8440.

Ontario

Workers' Compensation Board, 2 Bloor St. East, Toronto, ON M4W 3C3. (416)927-9555.

Prince Edward Island

Workers' Compensation Board, 60 Belvedere Ave., P.O. Box 757, Charlottetown, PE C1A 7L7. (902)368-5680.

Quebec

Commission de la Sante et de la Secuite du Travail, 524 Boudages St., Quebec, PQ G1K 7E2. (418)643-5850.

Saskatchewan

Workers' Compensation Board, Suite 200, 1881 Scarth, SK S4P 4L1. (306)787-4370.

Yukon Territory

Workers' Compensation Board, 401 Strickland St., Whitehorse, Yukon, Postal Code Y1A 5N8. (403)667-5645.

Canada

Labour Canada, Federal Workers' Compensation Service, Ottawa, ON K1A OJ2. (613)953-8001.

Merchant Seamen Compensaton Board, Labour Canada, Ottawa, ON K1A OJ2. (613)997-2281.

Appendix C

EYE EXAMINATION TECHNIQUES
1. Visual acuity

Measurement of visual acuity is the first step in any eye examination. The only exception is in the case of a chemical burn when vision should be tested after emergency eye irrigation.

A standard Snellen Eye chart is recommended for determining visual acuity. Record the vision for each eye separately. Record the patient's distance from the chart and the smallest letter size correctly identified. If the patient normally wears distance glasses, they should be worn during the eye test. If the distance glasses are broken or lost, use a multiple pinhole aperture. If a Snellen chart is not available, use a near vision card, newspaper, or magazine and record the smallest-sized word and the distance at which the patient can read it accurately. Patients over 40 may require their reading glasses for such near vision acuity measurements.

In many cases of serious injury, the patient is unable to read even the largest letter on an eye chart. If this is the case, record the distance at which he or she can count fingers with the affected eye. If the patient cannot count fingers, determine the distance at which hand movement can be detected. If the patient is unable to detect hand movement, determine whether he or she can perceive light. Accurate differentiation between vision capable of light perception, hand motion, and counting fingers can have great diagnostic and therapeutic implications.

2. External examination (lids and orbit)

Examine the lids to determine whether they open and close completely. Ensure the integrity of the lid margins and note any swelling or change in color. In cases of trauma, examine the orbit for subcutaneous emphysema, defects in the orbital rim, localized areas of anesthesia, and exophthal-

mos or enophthalmos. Orbital x-rays may be required.

Foreign bodies on the surface of the eye may be hidden under the inner surface of the upper lid or high up in the cul-de-sac formed by the reflection of upper lid and globe conjunctiva. In order to check for such foreign bodies, examiners must be able to perform single and double eversions of the upper eyelids.

1. Single eversion of the upper eyelids to expose undersurface of the upper lid is performed as follows:
   a. Instill topical anesthetic and tell patient to look down.
   b. Place the handle of a cotton swab just below the orbital rim.
   c. Grasp the eyelashes with the other hand and pull straight out from the globe.
   d. Pull the lashes up toward the forehead and flip the eyelid over using the applicator stick as a fulcrum.
   e. Hold the eyelashes against the orbital rim and remove the applicator.
2. Double eversion of the upper eyelids to expose the upper cul-de-sac is performed as follows:
   a. Ask the patient to lie down.
   b. Instill topical anesthetic.
   c. Place a lid retractor on the lid above the tarsal plate, grasp the eyelashes, and evert the lid over the retractor.
   d. Tilt the retractor back toward the forehead and hold the lid outward to expose the upper cul-de-sac.

3. Pupils

The pupils should be black, round, equal in size, and should react to light. Any deviation from these norms may indicate a serious problem. In any case of trauma or decreased vision, check the eye for

545

afferent pupillary defect (Marcus-Gunn pupil). To perform this test, shift a light back and forth from pupil to pupil, and wait for several seconds at each eye to watch for dilation. A normal pupil will constrict in response to illumination, but a lesion of the optic nerve (or certain retinal problems) will cause the pupil to dilate when the light is transferred to its side from the previously illuminated normal eye. A positive afferent defect confirms the presence of an organic defect, and identifies the lesion with the optic nerve or retina.

4. Motility examination

Check each eye for fullness of excursion and nystagmus in four positions of gaze—up, down, right, and left. Extraocular movements should be symmetrical between the two eyes.

5. Anterior segment of the globe

Inspect the sclera/conjunctiva or white of the eye for color change, swelling (chemosis), discharge, foreign bodies, or lacerations. Desmarres lid retractors or folded paper clips may be used to retract the lids for adequate exposure.

The cornea is the clear window of the eye. It should appear lustrous and compact and should demonstrate a sharp light reflex when inspected with a hand-held flashlight.

The anterior chamber is the space between the cornea and the lens/iris plane. The depth of the anterior chamber should be symmetrical between the two eyes and the space should be free of blood (hyphema) or pus (hypopyon). The lens should appear optically clear to flashlight inspection.

6. Ophthalmoscopy

Use the direct ophthalmoscope to examine the optic nerve, blood vessels, and retina of each eye. If the ocular media are clear, the examiner will observe a brilliant red reflex through the ophthalmoscope when the light fills the pupil. Use the direct ophthalmoscope with appropriate focusing to assess optic nerve color and elevation. Follow the vessel arcades in each direction to look for retinal hemorrhages or exudates. View the macular region last by having the patient look directly at the examination light.

7. Intraocular pressure (IOP)

Measurement of intraocular pressure is part of a routine ophthalmologic examination. It is particularly important in the emergency center in cases of suspected angle closure glaucoma, sudden visual loss, and iritis. Compare the pressure of the two eyes by using digital pressure on the globe through closed lids or by Schiøtz tonometry. Schiøtz tonometry is accurate and reasonably easy to perform.

1. First check the tonometry on the metal foot plate in the case; the instrument should read "O" units on the scale.
2. Ask the patient to lie down.
3. Use the tonometer weight of 5.5 grams.
4. Instill one drop of topical anesthetic in each eye.
5. Ask the patient to stare at the ceiling or at his or her thumb held about two feet in front of the nose.
6. Gently retract the lids against the orbital rims, being sure to avoid pressure on the globe.
7. Holding the tonometer as vertical as possible, gently place it on the central cornea.
8. Observe and record the position of the pointer on the scale.
9. If the pointer reads 3 scale units or less, the intraocular pressure is elevated.
10. Use the card in the tonometer case to convert scale units to millimeters of mercury (mm Hg).
11. Follow the manufacturer's recommended procedure for sterilizing the tonometer. If the tonometer is not cleaned between patients and sterilized at the appropriate intervals, erroneous readings may result and infection can be transmitted from patient to patient.

Do not attempt Schiøtz tonometry or digital evaluation of intraocular pressure if a ruptured globe is suspected. Also avoid Schiøtz tonometry in cases of active conjunctival or corneal infection.

8. Visual field

In cases of altered vision or head trauma, it is also important to test the patient's peripheral vision. The confrontation method, described below, is useful for such documentation.

1. Carefully occlude the fellow eye of the patient in order to test one eye at a time.
2. Sit opposite the patient.
3. Instruct patient to fix, using the eye to be tested, on the examiner's open eye directly opposite.
4. Hold fingers of each hand in the nasal and temporal fields simultaneously and instruct patient to count the fingers of each hand while looking straight ahead.
5. Test all four quadrants for each eye.

Table C-1 The "red eye": differential diagnosis

	Conjunctivitis	Iritis	Keratitis (corneal inflammation or foreign body)	Acute glaucoma*
Vision	Normal or intermittent blurring that clears on blinking	Slightly blurred	Slightly blurred	Marked blurring
Discharge	Usually significant with crusting of lashes	None	None to mild	None
Pain	None or minor and superficial	Moderately severe; aching and photophobia	Sharp, severe foreign body sensation	Very severe; frequently nausea and vomiting
Pupil size	Normal	Constricted	Normal or constricted	Dilated
Conjunctival injection	Diffuse	Circumcorneal	Circumcorneal	Diffuse with prominent circumcorneal injection
Pupillary response to light	Normal	Minimal further constriction	Normal	Minimal or no reaction of dilated pupil
Intraocular pressure	Normal. Caution: do not measure if discharge is present.	Normal to low	Normal. Caution: do not measure.	Elevated
Appearance of cornea	Clear	Clear or slightly hazy	Opacification present; altered light reflex; positive fluorescein staining	Hazy; altered light reflex
Anterior chamber depth	Normal	Normal	Normal	Shallow

* **Special note on acute glaucoma:** It is highly desirable for an ophthalmologist to examine the patient during an acute attack to confirm the diagnosis.

Appendix D

EXAMINATION OF PROSPECTIVE DIVERS

MEDICAL STANDARDS
AND RECOMMENDATIONS
Introduction

The following recommendations are set forth by the Association of Diving Contractors Safety, Medical and Education Committee. They are intended to be used with the ADC medical history/ physical examination forms. They deal with specific aspects of the subjects's physical fitness to dive by item number. These standards are offered as, in most cases, the minimum requirements and the use of these standards is intended to be tempered with the good judgement of the examining physician. The examining physician in doubt about the medical fitness of the subject should seek further opinion/consultation and recommendations of an appropriate specialist in that field. Particular attention must be paid to medical and diving history. In general, a high standard of physical and mental health is required for diving. Consequently, in addition to excluding major disqualifying medical conditions, examining physicians should identify and give careful consideration to minor, chronic, recurring, or temporary mental or physical illnesses that may distract the diver and cause him to ignore factors concerned with his own or others' safety.

The spectrum of commerical diving includes industrial tasks performed from just below the surface to deep saturation diving. Job descriptions and job-limiting disabilities may vary widely. The standards, in general, apply to all divers. Some consideration must be given to the subject's medical history, work history, age, and so forth.

There is no minimum or maximum age limit, providing all the medical standards can be met. Serious consideration must be given to the need for all divers to have adequate reserves of pulmonary and cardiovascular fitness for use in an emergency. The lack of these reserves may possibly lead to the termination of a professional diving career. The examining physician should exercise the appropriate professional judgment to determine whether, in particular circumstances, additional testing may be warranted. Disqualification for the inability to meet any of these standards must be done on a case by case basis related only to the specific job functions of the position being applied for, and assuming reasonable accommodations can not be made (see box).

On application of the company to ADC, and concurrence by the examining physician, in partic-

---

DISQUALIFYING CONDITIONS

A person with any of the following conditions as determined by a physician's examination should be disqualified from engaging in diving or hyperbaric activities:

- History of seizure disorder other than early childhood febrile convulsions
- Cystic or cavitary disease of the lungs, significant obstructive or restrictive lung disease, or recurrent pneumothorax
- Chronic inability to equalize sinus and middle ear pressure
- Significant central or peripheral nervous system disease or impairment
- Significant cardiac abnormalities
- Chronic alcoholism, drug abuse, or history of psychosis
- Significant hemoglobinopathies
- Significant malignancies
- Grossly impaired hearing
- Significant osteonecrosis
- Chronic conditions requiring continuous control by medication
- Pregnancy

From Medical Examination of Prospective Diver, *Consensus Standards for Commercial Diving Operations,* 4th ed, Houston, TX, 1992, Association of Diving Contractors.

549

ular medical circumstances, a permitted variance may be granted to be in effect until the diver's next periodic diving physical. At this time the permitted variance is to be subject to the examining physician's review and comment. Examining physicians must have a list of the essential job functions (job description) to review with each commerical diving physical examination. The examining physician is encouraged to make any recommendations for reasonable accommodations necessary for a person to meet these standards.

The numbered items within these standards refer to boxes on the ADC medical history/physical examination form. These forms are available from the offices of the ADC and should be used by all examining physicians conducting ADC diving physical examinations.

If any further clarification of this recommended standard is desired, please contact the ADC Safety Medical and Education Committee.

ADC physical examination standards

The following headings refer to and explain the numbered boxes on the ADC physical examination form, pages 3 and 4. Patient history is recorded on pages 1 and 2 of the form set. Use of these forms ensures quality and consistency throughout the commercial diving industry. They may be obtained from the office of the ADC. Medical tests for diving are listed in Table 1.

1. Name
   Record
2. Social Security Number
   Record
3. Height
   No set limits.
4. Weight
   The weight standards listed below should apply. If a diver exceeds these standards and the cognizant physician feels the increase is due to muscular build and physical fitness, a variance is appropriate. Furthermore, individuals who fall within these weight standards but who present an excess of fatty tissue should be disqualified.

Height in. (cm)	Max. weight lbs. (kg)	Height in. (cm)	Max. weight lbs. (kg)
64 (162.56)	164 (73.80)	72 (182.88)	205 (92.25)
65 (165.10)	169 (76.05)	73 (185.42)	211 (94.95)
66 (167.64)	174 (78.30)	74 (187.96)	218 (98.10)
67 (170.18)	179 (80.55)	75 (190.50)	224 (100.80)
68 (172.72)	184 (82.80)	76 (193.04)	230 (103.50)
69 (175.26)	189 (85.05)	77 (195.58)	236 (106.20)
70 (177.80)	194 (87.30)	78 (198.12)	242 (108.90)
71 (180.34)	199 (89.55)		

5. Temperature
   The diver should be free of any infection/disease that would cause an abnormal temperature.
6. Blood Pressure
   Ideally the resting blood pressure should not exceed 140/90 mm Hg. In cases of apparent hypertension, repeated blood pressure determinations should be made before a final decision.
7. Pulse/Rhythm
   Persistent tachycardia, marked arrhythmia except of the sinus type or other significant disturbances of the heart or vascular system should be disqualifying.
8. Hygiene
   Should be good.
9. Nutrition
   Should be good.
10. Build
   Record
11. Distant Vision
   Should have vision in both eyes, corrected to 20/40, O.U.
12. Near Vision
   Uncorrected—J16
13. Color Vision
   Record
14. Field of Vision
   Should be normal with any discrepancies documented.
15. Contact Lenses
   Record if used.
16. Head, Face, and Scalp
   The causes for rejection may be:
   a) Deformities of the skull in the nature of depressions, exostosis, etc. of a degree that would prevent the individual from wearing required equipment.
   b) Deformities of the skull of any degree, associated with evidence of disease of the brain, spinal cord or peripheral nerves.
   c) Loss or congenital absence of the bony substance of the skull.
17. Neck
   The causes for rejection may be:
   a) Cervical ribs if symptomatic.
   b) Congenital cysts of branchial cleft origin or those developing from the remnants of the thyroglossal duct, with or without fistulous tracts.
   c) Fistula, chronic draining, of any type.
   d) Spastic contraction of the muscles of the neck, persistent and chronic.

18. **Eyes**

Active pathology or previous eye surgery may be cause for restriction or rejection.

19. **Fundus**

No pathology.

20 **through 24. Ears, Nose, Throat and Eustachian Tube**

The following conditions are disqualifying: acute disease, chronic serious otitis or otitis media, perforation of the tympanic membrane (23), any significant nasal or pharyngeal respiratory obstruction, chronic sinusitis if not readily controlled, speech impediments from organic defects, or inability to equalize pressure because of any cause.

25. **Mouth**

a) Candidates should have a high degreee of dental fitness; any abnormalities of dentition or malformation of the mandible likely to impair the diver's ability to securely and easily retain any standard diving equipment mouthpiece should disqualify.

b) Removable dentures should not be worn while diving.

c) Record the date of most recent dental x-ray films. Record dentist's name and address to enable x-ray film location if needed for post-mortem identification.

26. **Lungs and Chest (including breasts)**

Pulmonary: congenital and acquired defects that may restrict pulmonary function, cause air entrapment or affect the ventilation-perfusion balance shall be disqualifying for both initial training and continuation. In general, chronic obstructive or restrictive pulmonary disease of any type shall be disqualifying.

27. **Heart (thrust, size, rhythm, sounds)**

Cardiovascular system: There should be no evidence of heart disease. Any arrhythmias must be fully investigated.

28. **Pulse**

Record

29. **Vascular System**

Cardiovascular system: The cardiovascular system shall be without significant abnormality in all respects as determined by physical examination and tests as may be indicated. Persistent tachycardia and arrhythmia except of sinus type, evidence of arteriosclerosis (an ophthalmoscopic examination of the retinal vessels shall be included in the examination), severe varicose veins, and marked symptomatic hemorrhoids, may be disqualifying.

30. **Abdomen and Viscera**

a) Peptic ulceration should be a cause for rejection unless healed and the candidate has been asymptomatic for at least 3 months without supportive medication.

b) Any other chronic gastrointestinal disease (e.g. ulcerative colitis, cholelithiasis) should be cause for rejection.

31. **Hernia**

Any significant abdominal herniation should be a cause for rejection until satisfactory repair has taken place.

32. **Endocrine System**

Any endocrine disorder requiring daily or intermittent medications for control is disqualifying. Diabetes mellitus, controlled by insulin, oral hypoglycemic agent, or diet, is disqualifying.

33. **G.U. System (genital-urinary) system:**

a) Venereal disease will disbar until adequately treated.

b) Evidence or history of nephrolithias is must be fully investigated and treated.

c) Evidence or history of urinary dysfunction or retention must be fully investigated and treated.

34. **Upper Extremities (strength, range of motion)**

Any impairment of musculoskeletal function that would interfere with the individual's performance as a diver should be carefully assessed against the general requirements.

35. **Lower Extremities (except feet)**

Any impairment of musculoskeletal function that would interfere with the individual's performance as a diver should be carefully assessed against the general requirements.

36. **Feet**

Any impairment of musculoskeletal function that would interfere with the individual's performance as a diver should be carefully assessed against the general requirements.

37. **Spine**

Any impairment of musculoskeletal function or skeletal structure that would interfere with the individual's performance as a diver should be carefully assessed against the general requirements.

38. Skin-Lymphatics

There should be no active, acute, or chronic disease of the skin or lymphatic system.

39. Anus and Rectum

Any conditions that interfere with normal function (such as stricture, prolapse, severe hemorrhoids) may be disqualifying.

40. Sphincter Tone

Note and record.

41. Pelvic Exam

Must be within normal limits. Pregnancy at any stage may be disqualifying. Any menstrual disorder manifested by abnormal or prolonged bleeding, as well as excessive pain, may be disqualifying.

42. Neurologic Exam

A full examination of the central and peripheral nervous system should show normal function, but localized minor abnormalities, such as patches of anesthesia, are allowable provided generalized nervous system disease can be excluded. Any history of seizure (apart from childhood febrile convulsions), intracranial surgery, loss of consciousness, or severe head injury involving more than momentary unconsciousness or concussion should be cause for rejection. If the severity of head injury is in doubt, special consultation and studies should be considered.

43. Cranial Nerves

Examine and record.

44. Reflexes

Should be normal and free from pathology. Document any abnormality.

45. Cerebral Function

Test and record.

46. Power and Tone of Muscles

Examine and record.

47. Proprioception—Stereognosis

Examine and record.

48. Romberg

Do and record.

49. Unterberger

Optional. (If done, record.)

50. Nystagmus

Do and record.

51. Sensations

Test and record.

52. Miscellaneous Remarks and Dermatome Diagram

Record findings and comments.

53. Urinalysis

Includes color, pH, specific gr., glucose, albumin, micro. All results should be within normal limits.

54. Blood Tests

a) Hematology: Any significant anemia or history of hemolytic disease must be evaluated. When caused by a variant hemoglobin state, it shall be disqualifying.

b) Serology test done. If positive, cause for rejection until properly treated and cleared.

c) All applicants for diving duty should have a sickle cell and acquired immunodeficiency syndrome (AIDS) test done and recorded.

55. Pulmonary Function

Pulmonary function tests:

a) All divers must have periodic pulmonary function tests to establish forced expiratory volume at one (1) second (FEV1) and forced vital capacity (FVC) recording best of three measurements.

b) A FEV1/FVC × 100 ratio of less than 75% requires additional specialized pulmonary function tests to determine suitability.

56. X-ray films

a) 14 × 17 chest: no pathology, within normal limits

b) Lumbar sacral spine

c) Long bones: any lesions, especially juxtaarticular, should be evaluated to determine patient's fitness to dive.

57. Electrocardiogram

ECG examinations: all divers should have a resting standard 12 lead electrocardiogram (ECG) at initial examination and annually after age 35.

58. Audiogram Pure Tone

A hearing loss in either ear of 35 dB or more at frequencies up to 3000 Hz and 50 dB or more at frequencies above 3000 Hz to a minimum of 6000 Hz is an indication for referral of the candidate to a specialist for further opinion, unless the examining doctor is convinced that such hearing loss is unlikely to be significantly increased by continuous diving activities. Doubts about function of labyrinths require specialized examination.

59. SMA-12

Optional, if done, record.

60. Drug Screen

Do and record.

Table D-1 Medical tests for diving

Test	Initial	Periodic	Comments
History and physical	X	X	Include predisposition to unconsciousness, vomiting, cardiac arrest, impairment of oxygen transport, serious blood loss, or anything which in the opinion of the examining physician will interfere with effective underwater work
Chest x-ray film	X	X	PA (Projection: $14'' \times 17''$ minimum)
Bone and joint x-ray survey	X		Required initially and as medically indicated
EKG: standard (12 L)	X		Required initially to establish baseline, annually after age 35, and as medically indicated
EKG: stress			Required only as medically indicated
Pulmonary function	X	X	Do
Audiogram	X	X	Threshold audiogram by pure tone audiometry; bone conduction audiogram as medically indicated
EEG			Required only as medically indicated
Visual acuity	X		Required initially and as medically indicated
Color blindness	X		Required initially
Hematocrit, hemoglobin, white blood count	X	X	
Routine urinalysis	X	X	

Psychiatric

The special nature of diving duties requires a careful appraisal of the individual's emotional and temperamental fitness. Personality disorders, psychosis, immaturity, instability, and asocial traits shall be disqualifying. Severe stammering or stuttering shall disqualify. Any past or present evidence of psychiatric illness shall be cause for rejection unless the examining doctor can be confident that it is of a minor nature and unlikely to recur. Particular attention should be paid to any past or present evidence of alcohol or drug abuse. Any abnormalities should be noted in block 52 of the physical examination form.

Temperament

The special nature of diving duties requires a careful appraisal of the candidate's emotional, temperamental, and intellectual fitness. Past or recurrent symptoms of neuropsychiatric disorder or organic disease of the nervous system shall be disqualifying. No individual with a history of any form of epilepsy, head injury with sequelae, or personality disorder shall be accepted. Neurotic trends, emotional immaturity or instability, and asocial traits, if of sufficient degree to militate against satisfactory adjustment, shall be disqualifying. Stammering or other speech impediment which might become manifest under excitement is disqualifying. Intelligence must be at least normal. Any abnormalities should be noted in block 52 of the physical examination form.

Index

Page numbers in italics indicate illustrations; *t* indicates tables.